Current Management of the Menopause

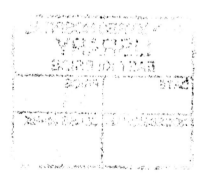

Current Management of the Menopause

Edited by

CHRISTIAN LAURITZEN AND JOHN STUDD

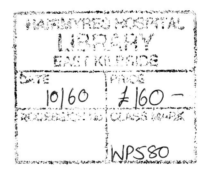
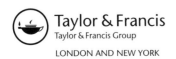

Taylor & Francis
Taylor & Francis Group

LONDON AND NEW YORK

© 2005 Taylor & Francis, an imprint of the Taylor & Francis Group

First published in the United Kingdom in 2005
by Taylor & Francis, an imprint of the Taylor & Francis Group, 2 Park Square,
Milton Park, Abingdon, Oxon OX14 4RN

Tel.: +44 (0) 20 7017 6000
Fax.: +44 (0) 20 7017 6699
E-mail: info.medicine@tandf.co.uk
Website: http://www.tandf.co.uk/medicine

Although every effort has been made to ensure that all owners of copyright material
have been acknowledged in this publication, we would be glad to acknowledge in
subsequent reprints or editions any omissions brought to our attention.

Although every effort has been made to ensure that drug doses and other
information are presented accurately in this publication, the ultimate
responsibility rests with the prescribing physician. Neither the publishers nor the
authors can be held responsible for errors or for any consequences arising from the
use of information contained herein. For detailed prescribing information or
instructions on the use of any procedure discussed herein, please consult the
prescribing information or instructional material issued by the manufacturer.

A CIP record for this book is available from the British Library

Library of Congress Cataloging-in-Publication Data
Data available on application

ISBN 1-84184-232-X

Distributed in North and South America by
Taylor & Frances
2000 NW Corporate Blvd
Boca Raton, FL 33431, USA

Within Continental USA
Tel: 800 272 7737; Fax: 800 374 3401
Outside Continental USA
Tel: 561 994 0555; Fax: 561 361 6018
E-mail: orders@crcpress.com

Distributed in the rest of the world by
Thomson Publishing Services
Cheriton House
North Way
Andover, Hampshire SP10 5BE, UK
Tel.: +44 (0)1264 332424
E-mail: salesorder.tandf@thomsonpublishingservices.co.uk

Composition by Wearset Ltd, Boldon, Tyne & Wear, Great Britain

Printed and bound in Spain by Grafos SA

Contents

Contributors vii

Foreword *Egon Diczfalusy* xi

Preface *C Lauritzen and J Studd* xiii

After the Women's Health Initative and Million Women Study *J Studd and C Lauritzen* xv

Section 1: The Third Part of Life

1. Basic facts and definitions *C Lauritzen* 3

2. Social structure and social medicine *A Rieder* 9

3. Menopausal changes of ovaries and hypothalamic–pituitary and cerebral function
    AR Genazzani, F Bernardi, N Pluchino, C Ceccarelli and M Luisi 19

4. Premenopausal cycle anomalies *M Neves-e-Castro* 31

5. History of estrogen–progestogen replacement therapy *H Rozenbaum* 35

Section 2: The Patient's Perspective

6. The awareness of the menopausal woman concerning the menopausal transition
    S Palacios 43

7. The considerations, hopes and fears of the menopausal woman *G Zelinsky* 51

Section 3: Hormone Therapy and Replacement

8. The climacteric syndrome *GA Hauser* 57

9. Practice of hormone substitution *C Lauritzen* 79

10. Mechanisms of action of sex steroid hormones and their analogs
    C Ibanez and EE Baulieu 93

11. Estrogens, progestogens and the endometrium *DW Sturdee* 105

12. Estrogen deprivation and hormone replacement therapy: effects on glucose and insulin
    metabolism and the metabolic syndrome *IF Godsland* 117

13. Possible side-effects of sexual hormones *G Creatsas* 131

Section 4: Role of Hormones in Preventive Gynecology

14. Osteoporosis *NH Bjarnason and C Christiansen* 139

15. Hormone replacement therapy and atherosclerotic vascular disease
    E Windler and B-Chr Zyriax 151

16. Direct vascular actions of estrogens *AO Mueck and H Seeger* 159

17. Neurotropic and psychotropic action of estrogens: implications for Alzheimer's disease
    P Schönknecht, J Pantel, J Schröder and K Beyreuther 173

18.   Sexuality in postmenopause and senium   *A Graziottin* 185

19.   Estrogens and urogenital atrophy   *D Robinson and L Cardozo* 205

20.   Estrogens in the treatment of premenstrual, postnatal and perimenopausal depression
      J Studd 219

21.   Anti-aging and esthetic endocrinology   *CJ Gruber and JC Huber* 229

22.   Skin and connective tissue   *MP Brincat, Y Muscat Baron and R Galea* 243

23.   Lifestyle counseling   *AS Wolf* 251

24.   Phytoestrogens   *H Adlercreutz* 271

25.   Possible risks of hormone replacement therapy (HRT): venous thromboembolism (VTE)
      I Greer 285

26.   Gallbladder, liver, pancreas   *H Kuhl* 293

27.   Carcinogenesis and the role of hormones: promotion and prevention
      HPG Schneider 303

28.   Strategies for the prevention of breast and gynecologic cancer   *C Lauritzen* 317

29.   Benefits, risks and costs of estrogen and hormone replacement therapies
      C Lauritzen 351

Section 5: Miscellaneous

30.   Information sheet for climacteric women   *C Lauritzen* 391

31.   The aging male   *B Lunenfeld* 399

32.   Future developments   *C Lauritzen* 421

Index 435

Contributors

H Adlercreutz
Folkhaelsan Research Center
University of Helsinki
FIN-00014
Finland

EE Baulieu
ISERM-U488
College de France
11 Place Marcelin-Berthelot
75005 Paris
France

F Bernardi
Department of Obstetrics and Gynaecology
University of Pisa
Via Roma 35
56100 Pisa
Italy

K Beyreuther
Center for Molecular Biology
University of Heidelberg
Im Neuenheimer Feld 280
69120 Heidelberg
Germany

NH Bjarnason
Gentofte University Hospital
Department of Clinical Biochemistry
Nils Anderson Vej 65
2900 Hellerup
Denmark

MP Brincat
Department of Obstetrics and Gynaecology
St Luke's Hospital Medical School
Msida MSD 06
G'Mangia
Malta

L Cardozo
Department of Obstetrics and Gynaecology
Kings College Hospital
Denmark Hill
London SE5 9RS
UK

C Ceccarelli
Department of Obstetrics and Gynaecology
University of Pisa
Via Roma 35
56100 Pisa
Italy

C Christiansen
Center of Clinical and Basic Research
Ballerup Byvej 222
Denmark

G Creatsas
Professor of Obstetrics and Gynaecology &
Dean
Department of Obstetrics and Gynaecology
Aretaieion Hospital
University of Athens Medical School
10671 Athens
Greece

E Diczfalusy
Roenningevaegen 21
SE-144 61 Roenninge
Sweden

R Galea
Consultant Obstetrician and Gynaecologist
St Luke's Hospital Medical School
Msida MSD 06
G'Mangia
Malta

AR Genazzani
Department of Obstetrics and Gynaecology
University of Pisa
Via Roma 35
56100 Pisa
Italy

IF Godsland
Reader in Human Metabolism
Endocrinology and Metabolic Medicine
St Mary's Hospital
Mint Wing 2nd Floor
Praed Street
London W2 1NY
UK

A Graziottin
Chief of Medical Sexology and Gynaecology
Center
Casa de Policlinico
Via San Secondo 19#
10128 Turin
Italy

I Greer
Department of Obstetrics and Gynaecology
Glasgow Royal Infirmary
Queen Elizabeth Building
10 Alexandra Parade
Glasgow G31 2ER
UK

CJ Gruber
Universitatsklinik fur Frauenheilkunde
Klin. Abt. Gynaekol. Endokrinologie
Waehringer Guertel 18–20
A-1090 Wien
Austria

GA Hauser
Specialist for Gynaecology
Former Director of the Gynaecology and
Obstetric Clinic
Kanton-Spital
Now: Faculty of Gynaecology
6004 Luzern
Switzerland

JC Huber
Universitatsklinik fur Frauenheilkunde
Klin. Abt. Gynaekol. Endokrinologie
Waehringer Guertel 18–20
A-1090 Wien
Austria

C Ibanez
INSERM U-488
80 Rue du General Leclerc
94276 Le Kremlin-Bicètre Cedex
France

H Kuhl
Professor of Experimental Endocrinology
Head of the Endocrinology Laboratory
Division of Gynaecology and Obstetrics
JW Goethe-University Frankfurt am Main
Theodor-Stern-Kai 7
D-60590 Frankfurt am Main
Germany

C Lauritzen
Professor Emeritus
Former Director of the Department of
Gynaecology and Obstetrics
University of Ulm
Now: Director of the Christian Lauritzen
Research Institute
Honorary President of the German Menopause
Society
Honorary Member of the International, Swiss
and Austrian Menopause Societies
Private address: Alpenstrasse 49, 89075 Ulm
Germany

M Luisi
Department of Obstetrics and Gynaecology
University of Pisa
Via Roma 35
56100 Pisa
Italy

B Lunenfeld
Professor Emeritus of Endocrinology at Faculty
of Life Sciences
Bar Ilan University
Treasurer of the International Society of
Gynaecological Endocrinology
President of the International Society for Study
of the Aging Male ISSAM
Member of the Israel Government National
Council for Obstetrics, Genetics and
Neonatology

AO Mueck
Head of Endocrinology and Menopause
University Hospital for Women
Calwerstrasse 7
72076 Tuebingen
Germany

Y Muscat Baron
Senior Registrar
Department of Obstetrics and Gynaecology
St Luke's Hospital Medical School
Msida MSD 06
G'Mangia
Malta

M Neves-e-Castro
Honorary President of the Portuguese
Menopause Society
Founder, Honorary Member and Past Vice
President of the European Menopause and
Andropause Society EMAS
Head of Clinica de Feminalogia Holistica
Av. Antonio Augusto Aguilar 24–2 DTo
Lisbon
Portugal

S Palacios
Instituto Palacios
Salud y Medicina de la Mujer
Calle Antonio Acuna 9
28009 Madrid
Spain

J Pantel
Ruprecht Karls University Heidelberg
Department of Psychiatry
Voss-Str.4
69115 Heidelberg
Germany

N Pluchino
Department of Obstetrics and Gynaecology
University of Pisa
Via Roma 35
56100 Pisa
Italy

A Rieder
Full Professor of Social Medicine
Health Pathologist
Vice Chair, Institute of Social Medicine
Medical University of Vienna
Rooseveltplatz 3
1090 Vienna
Austria

D Robinson
Department of Obstetrics and Gynaecology
Kings College Hospital
Denmark Hill
London SE5 9RS
UK

H Rozenbaum
President of the French Menopause Society
(AFEM)
and the Federation of European Menopause
Society
15 Rue Daru
75008 Paris
France

HPG Schneider
President of the International Menopause
Society
Former Director Universitats Frauenklinik
Albert Schweitzer Strasse 33
48149 Munster
Germany

P Schönknecht
Ruprecht Karls University Heidelberg
Department of Psychiatry
Voss-Str.4
69115 Heidelberg
Germany

J Schröder
Ruprecht Karls University Heidelberg
Department of Psychiatry
Voss-Str.4
69115 Heidelberg
Germany

H Seeger
Head of Endocrinology and Menopause
Laboratory
University Hospital for Women
Calwerstrasse 7
72076 Tuebingen
Germany

J Studd
Professor, University of London
Chief of Fertility and Gynaecological
Endocrinology Centre
The Lister Hospital
Chelsea Bridge Road
London SW1 8RH
UK

DW Sturdee
Consultant Obstetrician and Gynaecologist
Birmingham Hartlands and Solihull
Solihull Hospital
Wome
Lode Lane
West Midlands B91 2JL
UK

E Windler
Professor of Medicine
University of Hamburg-Eppendorf
Martinistrasse 52
20245 Hamburg
Germany

AS Wolf
Praxis Klinik
Frauenstrasse 51
89073 Ulm
Germany

G Zelinsky
Schloss Haltenbergstetten 5
Pinzessinnenhaus
97996 Niederstetten
Germany

BC Zyriax
University of Hamburg-Eppendorf
Martinistrasse 52
20245 Hamburg
Germany

Foreword

Had I been present at the creation
I would have given some useful hints
For the better ordering of the Universe.

Alphonso X, the Learned (1252–1284)
King of Spain

It is an honour and a privilege to write a foreword to such an important book as this one, but
it is also a rather difficult task, particularly if
one wishes to resist the temptation of the
autumnal mind to draw rapid conclusions
about the human condition in a fundamentally
uncertain world, where the present is just as
uncertain as the future.

When the former Secretary of State of the
USA, Dean Acheson, described his years at the
Head of the State Department, his book was
entitled *Present at the Creation* (1969) in reference to the above epigraph. In a much more
modest way, I was also present at the creation
of the great revolutions of our time in contraception, reproductive health and gender equity
which have changed the world around us and
our perception of it. I have also witnessed the
biggest of all demographic revolutions in history and could sense the increasing impact of
rapidly changing population structures on our
social, economical, health and even political
infrastructures.

Just 1000 years ago the global population
was around 280 million people; today it exceeds
6 billion and the United Nations projects that it
may reach 9.3 billion people by the middle of
this century. Virtually all of this growth will
take place in the less developed regions and the
number of people living in the more developed
regions is projected to remain unchanged.

The most important demographic change
will take place in the population structure of
the world, with a rapidly declining number of
children and an even more rapidly increasing
proportion of elderly people. Between 1950 and
2050 the proportion of the world's children
(people aged 14 or less) is projected to decline
from 34.3% to 21.0% and that of its elderly population (people aged 60 and over) to increase
from 8.2% to 21.1%. During the same period,
the proportion of children in Europe is projected to decline from 26.2% to 14% and the
elderly population to increase from 13.2% to
46.6%.

The United Nations estimate that today some
335 million elderly women live on our Earth
and project that by year 2050 their number will
exceed one billion. Of course, projections are
always uncertain; however, some of them – like
this one – are less uncertain than others, simply
because those one billion women are already
among us as teenagers or young women.
Hence, the overwhelming challenge facing the
next generations will be to find imaginative

new approaches to the delivery of quality health care which will be affordable in such a brave new world.

If King Alphonso X had lived in the 20th century, perhaps he could have advised us that – in logical terms – a *contraceptive revolution* can hardly exist as a separate idea, without placing it into its wider context of *reproductive health* and that a *revolution in reproductive health* cannot materialize without making major progress in the achievement of gender equity. Our generation has to learn this in a difficult, sequential manner, 'discovering' each of these ideas as separate concepts. Who knows, perhaps Alphonso X could also have predicted for us that true gender equity may not materialize without also achieving health equity.

In Shakespeare's *Measure for Measure* (Act III, Sc. 1, 1.2) Claudio exclaims, 'The miserable have no other medicine but only hope', and since the dawn of civilization this dictum has applied to the living conditions of the overwhelming majority of human beings. However, there is a change in the air: our generation seems to be the first in history that has dared to think it possible to create a new world on this planet in which medical care may be provided to every human being. For the time being, health equity is still a dream, but a very important one. In fact, dreams are more important than we may think since, as Yates stated, 'in dreams begins responsibility'.

Worldwide life expectancy for women more than doubled over the past two centuries from about 25 to 68 years and it is projected to reach 79 years by the year 2050. However, menopause will still occur at 50 years of age, or so. Hence, when reaching the menopause in the next few decades, one billion women will depend to a considerable extent on the preventive measures, management and advice provided to them by the medical community in general and by the gynaecologists of this world in particular. To enable them to properly do so, access to reliable, up-to-date scientific information will be of paramount importance. Therefore the value of a textbook such as this one cannot be overestimated.

A final reflection: the United Nations project that by the year 2050, women aged 60 and over will constitute 40% of the female population of Europe and 23% of that of the entire world. Hence, it is rather easy to see that the present book will be a most valuable source of information not only to gynaecologists and other members of the medical community, but virtually to everyone involved in the provision of health care to women in general and elderly women in particular.

Egon Diczfalusy MD PhD DSc(Hon) Drhc(mult)
FRCOG FACOG(Hon)
Professor Emeritus
Karolinska Institute
Stockholm, Sweden

Preface

At a time when doubts and criticisms concerning the real benefit and the justification of peri-to-postmenopausal estrogen–progestogen substitution, especially of long-term primary prevention, is widely questioned in the name of evidence-based medicine, it is pertinent to summarize the established facts in a critical authoritative monograph. Such a summary should formulate the experiences of competent critical experts on a correct, successful and low-risk management of menopausal women. These experiences are often in contrast to experimental, largely artificial, interventional studies, which are far from practice. An answer must be given and a firm stance must be taken concerning the undoubtable value and benefits of estrogen and hormone replacement therapies (ERT and HRT, respectively) against current disinformation. In this regard, the postmenopausal women affected must be heard.

Not all observational and epidemiological trials, and not all results of account reports dealing with treatment results, are invalid in the light of evidence testing. Some of them have, because of their proximity to practice, their careful design, conscientious performance and perfect plausibility, a strong degree of credibility and must be ranked high in the score of evidence. Many good data and identical positive results of a great number of critical scientists must not be rated low.

We do not intend to regress behind the welcome progress marked by the establishing of evidence-based medicine. However, the danger exists that controlled trials are now widely accepted without the necessary criticism. There is a tendency, originating from poorly planned and conducted randomized controlled trials, which are very construed and unrealistic, that physicians, statisticians, internists, commissions, governmental authorities and health insurance companies draw consequences and conclusions concerning ERT and HRT which are premature and inappropriate. Such examples can regrettably already be given such as following publication of the Heart and Estrogen/progestin Replacement Study (HERS) and the Women's Health Initiative (WHI) study.

The results of these studies were, against all scientific rules (and against the authors' and commenting scientists' wishes) by some self-appointed experts and the lay press, unduly generalized and considered to be valid for all estrogen and progestogens, all doses and all forms of application, whether arranged sequentially or combined, given orally or by the different parenteral ways. This is against the basic rules of science, with the gravest of faults made when results are interpreted to reach conclusions which are not supported by the data.

Experience teaches that the latest published results are not always the final truth.

The ad hoc comments of recognized experts and commissions have stated that the WHI study was faulty in design and management, used a badly suited combined preparation, and that the value of ERT/HRT for treatment of climacteric complaints as well as for some aims of primary prevention is valuable and unchanged. Treatment according to the established rules will, as demonstrated in innumerable account reports and epidemiological studies, not cause substantial side-effects.

Substitution with estrogens and progestogens during menopause will probably become of even greater importance in the future. Biochemical innovations and the development of selective estrogen receptor modulators (SERMs), designer hormones, phytoestrogens and new methods of application will open a wide promising field of new possibilities of individualized treatment and of substitution without unwanted side-effects. The prospective risk assessment will probably be improved by genetic tools, which will influence indications, contraindications and the mode of medication.

This monograph is intended to bring together the contemporary knowledge on the management of the menopause. It aims to give the scientist state-of-the-art information to guide where to go with his/her research. For the gynecologist and the practitioner a guide for his/her practice and for the counseling of menopausal patients when they consider ERT/HRT is given.

The science of estrogens, menopause and its management owes research from the United States a lot of data and knowledge. However, many wrong points were also followed from those results. Many problems and questions are posed differently in Europe. Therefore, this book intends to describe mainly European facts, views, possibilities of menopausal management, problems, conclusions and solutions.

It is a hard task to bring together so many known scientists who are swamped with work, and to make them deliver their contributions. The editors have to thank all authors for their cooperation and for sharing their knowledge and expertise with the readers of this publication.

Our publishers, Martin Dunitz, have been very patient, understanding and professional in their assistance. We sincerely thank Robert Peden, Commissioning Editor, and Maire Harris, Development Editor, for their valuable help in all stages of collecting and editing our book.

One of the most important and still unsolved problems is the missing conversion of scientific facts and knowledge into daily work. We hope that this monograph will provide the interested reader with the desired information on all aspects of the menopause and will give him/her a solid standpoint to find his/her individual attitude. May the book help to attain orientation in the sometimes overwhelming amount of information, and to acquire the knowledge which the therapist has to transfer into his/her medical practice for the benefit of his/her patients.

C Lauritzen
J Studd

After the Women's Health Initiative and Million Women Study

John Studd and Christian Lauritzen

Introduction • Recent adverse publicity • HERS study • Women's Health Initiative study • NAMS response • Breast cancer • The Million Women Study • Current advice for hormonal replacement therapy prescribing • References

INTRODUCTION

Until recently, hormone replacement therapy (HRT) was quite straightforward. Estrogen prevented climacteric symptoms, in particular, flushes, sweats, vaginal dryness, depression, loss of energy and loss of libido, and cyclical or continuous progestogen, although possibly producing premenstrual syndrome (PMS)-type side effects in women who were progestogen-intolerant, protected the endometrium. There were also long-term benefits such as protection from osteoporosis, reduction in colon cancer and both primary and secondary prevention of heart attacks. It is possible that part of this 50% reduction of coronary artery disease was due to selection of patients – with the healthier, non-smoking, normotensive patients receiving HRT – but most laboratory studies in primates and trials in women supported the hypothesis of this protective role.

There was a possible slight increase in breast cancer but as virtually all studies showed an increased survival in these women, it was easy to believe that this apparent increase was an artefact due to increased surveillance in women receiving HRT or a problem of precise pathological diagnosis in the gray area between ductal carcinoma in situ or invasive cancer.

RECENT ADVERSE PUBLICITY

The Heart and Estrogen/progestin Replacement Study (HERS) study[1] first challenged the optimism that estrogens exerted a protective effect in women with established coronary artery disease and, more recently, articles from the Women's Health Initiative (WHI)[2] study and the Million Women Study (MWS)[3] have caused considerable alarm by reporting that heart attacks, strokes, venous thromboembolism (VTE) and breast cancer are more common in women who are receiving treatment. In December 2003 in the UK, the Committee on Safety of Medicines (CSM), following the lead of the European Menopause and Andropause Society (EMAS), advised that HRT should no longer be the first choice for the prevention and treatment of osteoporosis. We strongly disagree with this opinion as did one of the two gynecologists on the committee, who resigned in protest. The MWS was attended by a hostile and superficial editorial[4] that reads as a political polemic.

Although the WHI and MWS are now recognized to be greatly flawed at many levels, they were both the subject of press conferences before publication with the front pages of the newspapers reporting the bad news before the studies were in any way discussed by the scientific community.[5] The errors in the studies were so manifest that they would have been improved by prior discussion but we are left with the fact that the putative side effects of HRT are now fixed in the public memory regardless of any final scientific revision of the conclusions from these papers. If that were not enough, a subsequent paper from the WHI study indicated that quality of life was not improved with treatment after all.[6] Not surprisingly there has been a 50% reduction of HRT taking in the USA and a significant, but rather less, reduction in Europe.

One can only wonder at the motives of these authors who have paraded their data to the press before their clinical colleagues have exam-ined the evidence. This discourages critical discussion by experts before publication. Although the design and conclusions of these two studies have been roundly criticized by epidemiologists and clinicians, the damage has been done.

The results of the estrogen arm of the WHI study were published after it was disbanded because of an increased incidence of stroke among participants in the higher age group (60–69 years).[7] However, in practice this group was never treated primarily with oral estrogens (Table 1). After 6.8 years, treatment with conjugated estrogens given continuously gave more favourable results than treatment with conjugated estrogens + medroxyprogesterone acetate

Table 1 Relative and absolute risks (hazard ratio, HR) for preventable postmenopausal diseases.* An estrogen monotherapy study, randomized and controlled against placebo: hysterectomized women; mean age at start of treatment 63.8 years (50–79 years); mean duration of treatment 6.8 years; 0.625 mg conjugated estrogens given continuously; n = 5310 estrogen, n = 5429 placebo. The medication was experimental without any clear indication and without any evidence of estrogen deprivation. Patients were older than usual for estrogen treatment and in part not healthy

Disease	Relative risk against placebo (HR); nominal 95% confidence limits	Absolute risk, no. of probands/ 10,000 women/year		Risk ERT[1]	Benefit ERT[1]
		Conjugated estrogens	Placebo		
Breast cancer	0.77 (0.59–1.01)	26	33	–	7
Coronary infarction	0.91 (0.75–1.12)	49	54	–	5
Stroke	1.39 (1.01–1.77)[2]	44	32	12	–
Thromboembolism	1.33 (0.99–1.79)	28	21	7	–
Colorectal cancer	1.08 (0.75–1.55)	17	16	1	–
Osteoporotic fractures	0.70 (0.63–0.79)[3]	139	195	–	56
Sum of events	–	–	–	20	68
Mortality	0.98	–	–	–	–

* Source: WHI Steering Committee. Effects of conjugated equine estrogen in postmenopausal women with hysterectomy. *JAMA* 2004; **291**: 1701–12.
[1] Comparison of risk versus benefit is of course difficult.
[2] Not significant; also mortality of stroke under estrogen was not significantly increased (HR 1.13); embolism following thrombosis was not increased.
[3] Hip fractures HR 0.61 (0.41–0.91); vertebral fractures HR 0.62 (0.42–0.93).

(MPA) given continuously (Table 2). Breast cancer showed a 23% reduction in the hazard rate (HR). Osteoporotic fractures, including hip fractures, were significantly reduced. Stroke was slightly, but not significantly, increased (HR 1.29) but the mortality of stroke was not significantly increased. Thromboembolism was not significantly increased. When the results were stratified for age, the preventative effect of estrogen treatment was clearly confirmed in the 50–59 years age group, which is normally treated with estrogen, for coronary heart disease (CHD), col-

orectal cancer, bone fractures, including hip fractures, and overall mortality (Table 3). The data, moreover, confirmed the suspected adverse effects of the addition of the progestogen MPA administered continuously because of its proliferative effects on the breast epithelium and its thrombogenic effects. Table 4 shows that the population treated in the WHI study was by no means healthy but exhibited multiple clear contraindications and risk factors against treatment with estrogens.

Table 2 Relative and absolute risks (hazard ratio, HR) for preventable postmenopausal diseases.* An estrogen + MPA study, randomized and controlled against placebo: mean age at start of treatment 63.2 years; mean age at end of treatment 69.4 years; mean duration of treatment 5.2 years with correction in 2003; 0.625 mg conjugated estrogens + 2.5 mg MPA given combined and continuously; *n* = 8506 estrogen + MPA, *n* = 8102 placebo

Disease	Relative risk against placebo (HR); nominal 95% confidence limits	Absolute risk, no. of probands/ 10,000 women/year		Risk HRT[1]	Benefit HRT[1]
		Conjugated estrogens + MPA	Placebo		
Breast cancer	1.24 (1.01–1.54)[2]	41	33	8	0
Coronary infarction	1.24 (1.00–1.54)[3]	37	30	7	0
Stroke	1.41 (1.07–1.85)[4]	29	21	8	0
Thromboembolism	2.11 (1.58–2.82)	34	16	18	0
Colon cancer	0.63 (0.43–0.92)[5]	10	16	–	6
Osteoporotic fractures	0.76 (0.69–0.83)	152	199	–	47
Diabetes	0.79	20	15	–	5
Sum of events	–	–	–	41	59
Mortality	–	52	53	–	1

* Source: WHI Steering Committee. Effects of conjugated equine estrogen in postmenopausal women with hysterectomy. *JAMA* 2004; **291:** 1701–12 and Roussow et al. Writing Group for the Women's Health Initiative Investigators. Risks and benefits of estrogen plus progestin in healthy postmenopausal women: principal results from the Women's Health Initiative randomized controlled trial. *JAMA* 2002; **288:** 321–33.
[1] Comparison of risk versus benefit is of course difficult.
[2] The risk to women who had not received estrogen–progestogen prior to beginning the WHI study showed HR 1.09 (0.86–1.39) under HRT; verum against placebo, not significant.
[3] In probands < 10 years since menopause HR (0.5–1.5), not significant.
[4] In probands < 10 years since menopause HR 1.08 (0.57–2.04): no difference in verum/placebo.
[5] Endometrial and ovarian cancer were not increased.

Table 3 Influence of age on the hazard ratio (HR) of preventable postmenopausal diseases with the intervention of conjugated estrogen.* An estrogen monotherapy study, randomized and controlled against placebo: mean duration of treatment 6.8 years; 0.625 mg conjugated estrogens given continuously

Disease	Age (years)			Total HR for all ages
	50–57[1]	60–69	70–79	
Total of probands population (%)	33.4	45.3	27.3	–
Coronary heart disease	0.56	0.92	1.04	0.91
Stroke	1.08	1.65[2]	1.25	1.29
Venous thromboembolism	1.22	1.31	1.44	1.33
Mammary cancer	0.72	0.72	0.94	0.77
Colorectal cancer	0.59	0.88	2.09	1.03
Hip fractures	–	0.33[3]	0.62	0.70[3]
Mortality	0.73	1.01	1.20	1.08

* Source: WHI Steering Committee. Effects of conjugated equine estrogen in postmenopausal women with hysterectomy. *JAMA* 2004; **291**: 1701–12.
[1] Usual age when HRT or ERT is begun.
[2] Significant on the basis of nominal confidence intervals.
[3] All fractures.

HERS STUDY

The anxiety about HRT started with the HERS study,[1] which evaluated the effect of estrogens on women with established coronary artery disease. There had been many clinical papers and studies of lipids and coronary blood flow and physiology which indicated that estrogens had a profound protective effect on the normal coronary arteries and there was also persuasive clinical evidence that this treatment could be used with advantage in women who had had coronary artery disease. Although a primary prevention study (the future WHI study) was being considered, it was also considered that a secondary protection study would give the answer with fewer patients over a shorter period of time.

The HERS study consisted of a randomized placebo-controlled trial of 2763 women (mean age 66.7 years) with established coronary artery disease. They were given either 0.625 mg of conjugated equine estrogen with 2.5 mg of MPA or placebo. The follow-up was for 6.8 years. Although this therapy produced the expected beneficial biochemical effects on lipids, such as lowering the low-density lipoprotein (LDL) by 11% and increasing high-density lipoprotein (HDL) by 10%, there was an increased rate of venous thromboembolic events and no change in the overall rate of CHD events, either nonfatal myocardial infarction or CHD death in either group. There was, in fact, a small increase in heart attacks in the first year but this had ceased and there was even a nonsignificant decrease by the end of the fourth year. The concept of estrogens producing 'early harm', even if they might ultimately produce benefit, was born, although some of the side effects were probably due to MPA.

The study was discontinued prematurely and hence an important opportunity was missed. The conclusion from this study was that HRT in this form was not recommended

Table 4 Data for manifold pre-existing diseases, anomalies and medicaments of probands of the WHI study.* An estrogen monotherapy study, randomized and controlled against placebo: mean duration of treatment 6.8 years; 0.625 mg conjugated estrogens given continuously; n = 5310 estrogen, n = 5429 placebo. A high percentage of probands exhibited contraindications to estrogen medication and relevant risk factors were present, as evidenced by the use of specific medicaments. Probands were mostly too old for oral estrogen administration and no indication for replacement was existent in the majority of cases. No proof of estrogen deficiency was performed. Therefore the study was not one of replacement but of experimental medication, embedded in a worst-case scenario

Anamnestic data	No. of probands	Probands (%)
Hypertension	2308	48
Cholesterol increase	694	14.5
Medication of statins	394	7.4
Medication of acetyl salicyclic acid	1030	19.4
History of myocardial infarction	165	3.1[1]
Angina pectoris	308	5.8[1]
History of stroke	76	1.4[1]
Bypass operation (angioplasty)	120	2.3[1]
History of thromboembolism	87	1.6[1]
Diabetes mellitus	410	7.7
Smokers	2529	47.6[2]
Overweight (BMI > 30)	2376	45.0[2]
ERT before study	2540	47.8
Nulliparae	489	9.3[2]
First child after 30 years of age	210	4.9[2]
Breast cancer in family	839	18.0[2]

* Source: WHI Steering Committee. Effects of conjugated equine estrogen in postmenopausal women with hysterectomy. *JAMA* 2004; **291:** 1701–12.
[1] Estrogens absolutely or relatively contraindicated.
[2] Risk cases: at least individualization of treatment indicated.

for the secondary prevention of CHD. There now seems to be much agreement on this point.

WOMEN'S HEALTH INITIATIVE STUDY

The WHI study, which so adversely affected patients' confidence, was a large trial using the wrong hormone combination on the wrong patients and bears no relationship to the treatment that is given to patients of the appropriate age with the appropriate symptoms.

A total of 16,809 women aged 50–79 years (mean 63 years; 21% between 70 and 79 years) were recruited from 40 centers in the USA and randomized to active HRT and placebo. Prior cardiovascular disease was present in 7.7%, and 1.1% (HRT group) and 1.5% (placebo group) had had a previous coronary artery bypass operation. Thirty-six per cent were hypertensive and 7% were taking statins at commencement of the study. They were asymptomatic but a further report from this group informs us that

10% had vasomotor symptoms. Many were overweight.

The treatment consisted of continuous combined estrogen and progestogen therapy (CCEP) in the form of conjugated equine estrogen 0.625 mg daily and MPA 2.5 mg daily, or for hysterectomized women conjugated equine estrogen (Premarin) 0.625 mg daily. In spite of this 42% of the treatment group dropped out compared with 38% of the placebo group. Thus this is one of the rare studies when the dropout is more in the treatment group than the placebo group. The CCEP arm was discontinued after 5.2 years because of an excess of complications but the E-only study continued. We do not know the change in the percentage of women on statin therapy when the study was discontinued. It is very likely that these high-risk American patients chose to take statins when, in this barely blinded study, they soon realized that they were on placebo.

The results of CCEP therapy in this population make depressing reading. There was an increase in coronary artery disease, with a risk ratio (RR) of 1.29 (confidence interval (CI) 1.02–1.63). Stroke was increased (RR 1.41; CI 0.7–1.85). There was double the incidence of VTE with an RR of 2.11 (CI 1.58–2.82) and an increase in breast cancer (RR 1.26; CI 1.0–1.94).

In spite of this negative information the WHI was the first randomized study that showed a decrease in hip fracture of 34% (CI 0.45–0.98) and a similar decrease in vertebral fracture (CI 0.44–0.98). There was also a demonstrable decrease in colon cancer of 37% (CI 0.43–0.92). No doubt this improvement was seen because the age group in this study was appropriate for prevention of osteoporotic fractures and occurrence of colon cancer regardless of the type of estrogen and progestogen preparation used.

The increase in coronary heart disease and VTE began in year 1 and the increase in stroke appeared in year 2, supporting the view of early harm. The increase in breast cancer was only apparent after 4 years.

There is a great difference between the reassuring observational studies compared with the interventional (randomized controlled trials) studies in HRT users. There are now more than 30 observational case-control studies showing protection. The most important of these is the Nurses' Health Study[8] of 70,533 postmenopausal women followed up from 1976 to 1996 with 1258 major coronary events.[9] The risk ratio in current users of HRT was reduced to 0.61 (CI 0.52–0.71). Regardless of the other recent large studies showing no change or a decrease in breast cancer[10] or cardiac deaths,[11] the large greatly flawed WHI study has been used unwisely to erase all of the clinical, laboratory and animal studies supporting the use of HRT in the primary prevention of CHD. These publications of inappropriate optimistic therapy seemed to impress the North American Menopause Society (NAMS) and other American medical bodies.

NAMS RESPONSE

The NAMS Advisory Panel report (dated 3 October 2002) on the HERS and WHI studies made the following recommendations:

- treatment of menopausal and vasomotor symptoms and pelvic atrophy remain the major indications for HRT;
- progestogens are to be used in women with a uterus. HRT is not suited for primary or secondary prevention of coronary vascular disease;
- physicians should try alternatives to HRT for osteoporosis;
- use for the shortest duration;
- lower than standard dosage should be considered; and
- alternative medications should be tried.

Two weeks later at a meeting (dated 23/24 October 2002) with NAMS/ACOG and AHA (American College of Obstetricians and Gynecologists and American Heart Association) the panel confirmed that:

- HRT is not to be used for prevention of coronary vascular disease;
- it had no place for the prevention of chronic conditions;

- HRT is indicated for treatment of vasomotor symptoms 'if severe enough';
- 'lowest possible dose should be used for as short as possible'.

They continue that:

- estrogen/progestogen HRT is not the first choice for prevention or treatment of osteoporosis but can be used if other treatments are not tolerated and if there are vasomotor symptoms.

This meeting concluded that:

- the conjugated estrogen/MPA formulation in WHI cannot be extrapolated to other estrogen/progestogen HRTs but the safety of other formations cannot be assumed until proved.

There recommendations continue to produce outrage from experienced workers in the field of menopause. The advice concerning cardiovascular disease, particularly primary prevention, was too negative.

In years 2, 3, 4 and 6 of the WHI there was no significant increase in CHD. There was, as in the HERS study of secondary protection, a slight increase in the first year. The number of CHD events in years 2–6 was relatively the same, although there was a trend towards reduction (Table 5). The statistically significant risk ratio in year 5 is because of an unexplained large fall in the number of placebo cases. It was this as much as the data on breast cancer that triggered the alarm bells to stop the study. There was in fact no increase in incidence of CHD in the treatment group in spite of the high cardiovascular risk of this group.

As these older, 60- and 70-year-old, hypertensive women are not the patients who would normally commence treatment with HRT, we must ask what the information specifically about the younger patients is. Naftolin[12] has deduced the following: this study had 287 patients aged 50–54 years, and since the age-corrected number of expected events found in the Nurses' Health Study is 0.7 events per 275 women per 5 years, it would require greater than 4000 women in each arm to show a statistically significant difference between the groups. So with a 42% dropout rate the number of women needed per group becomes 9000. Thus the WHI randomized controlled trial is ten-fold underpowered to test the cardioprotective effect of HRT in women entering the menopause. Although the authors claim to show the same increase in risk at each decile of age, there is clearly inadequate or virtually no

Table 5 Inspection of the year by year analysis of incidence of coronary heart disease (CHD) in the treatment and placebo groups of the Women's Health Initiative (WHI) study

	No. of CHD events		Hazard rate (risk ratio)
	Treatment	Placebo	
Year 1	43	23	1.78[1]
Year 2	36	30	1.15
Year 3	20	18	1.06
Year 4	25	24	0.99
Year 5	23	09	2.38[1]
Year 6	17	18	0.78

* Source: WHI Steering Committee. Effects of conjugated equine estrogen in postmenopausal women with hysterectomy. *JAMA* 2004; **291:** 1701–12.
[1] Significant.

information about the 45–55-year-old typical menopausal patients whom we treat.

As the misguided advice based on the WHI study is pervasive in that recent guidelines from the Royal College of Physicians of Edinburgh[13] begin by stating that 'the administration of oestrogens may produce heart attacks', it is worth pointing out again that the cardioprotective effect of starting hormone treatment at the time of the menopause cannot be ruled out by the WHI study. Similarly, the cardiovascular consequences of stopping hormone therapy that began at the time of the menopause cannot be evaluated by these data.

This study is of the wrong population, the wrong drug, and clearly came to the wrong conclusions concerning the early symptomatic woman as it used treatment that is rarely used in Europe in women whom we do not treat. It will take time to erase the unjustified conclusions from the WHI study but many smaller studies including the WISP study of Stevenson using the correct hormone – estradiol – in well supervised patients of the correct age for the appropriate pathology or symptoms are likely to produce a message, one way or another, which we can believe.

BREAST CANCER

The data on the extra risk of breast cancer are mixed and confused with almost as many publications reporting a decrease as those reporting an increase. However the conclusion from Beral's[11] meta-analysis which reports a duration-dependent increase in incidence seems now to be increasingly accepted. It has been reported that after 5, 10 and 15 years of HRT use there are 2, 6 and 12 extra diagnosed cases/1000 HRT users, respectively.

The majority of papers looking at mortality from breast cancer in women taking HRT have found this to be greatly reduced by as much as 30%. An exception is Chlebowski et al[14] from the WHI group reporting a higher mortality in these tumours, which were more commonly metastatic at the time of diagnosis. These authors are alone in this finding.

THE MILLION WOMEN STUDY (MWS)

The MWS did not meet any requirements of the principles of evidence-based medicine but stands as a very influential study of a large group of patients. 1,084,110 women in the UK, aged 50–64 years attending for mammography were evaluated using questionnaires. There were 9364 cases of invasive breast cancer at 2.6 years of follow-up but only 7140 were analysed. These exclusions are important as they have biased the conclusions by turning the control group into low risk while the active group remained the same.

There were 637 breast cancer deaths at 4.1 years of follow-up of current users. This gave an overall relative risk (RR) of 1.66 with a 1.22 risk ratio of death from breast cancer. The results were shown to be worse in the estrogen plus progestogen group (RR 2.0; CI 1.88–2.12). Estradiol-only group had an RR of 1.30 (CI 1.21–1.40). Being a large study, it was able to evaluate different estrogens and different routes of administration. There was no significant difference between estrogens taken by the oral route, as a patch or an implant. The tibolone group also showed an increase of breast cancer (RR 1.44; CI 1.25–1.68).

The breast cancers were diagnosed on average 1.2 years after recruitment with the mean time of death from diagnosis of only 1.7 years. These are extraordinary results as it takes 5–8 or more years for a few malignant cells to become a 1-cm tumour. Many of these must have been interval tumours not related to estrogen therapy. Although such tumours have a poor prognosis, the short survival of 1.7 years from diagnosis in this study is hard to explain being less than the 3-year survival of women diagnosed with metastatic breast cancer. Can these MWS data really be correct? The study should have excluded all cancers, mostly interval cancers, found in the first and perhaps even the second year of taking estrogen, as our knowledge of the biology of breast cancer makes the therapeutic association unlikely. Any real excess of cancer would have shown up after 5 or more years if there was a causal link.

In current users of each type of HRT the risk of breast cancer increased with increasing total duration of use. The authors estimate that 10 years' use of HRT results in 5 additional diagnosed breast cancers per 1000 users of estrogen-only preparations and 19 additional cancers per 1000 users of estrogen and progestogen combinations. Furthermore, the authors extrapolate the data by claiming that HRT used by women aged 50–64 years in the UK within the past decade has resulted in an estimated 20,000 extra breast cancers. This claim is not supported by the UK cancer statistics according to which breast cancer numbers have reached a plateau since 1993.

Another oddity is the finding of no increase in breast cancer incidence (1.01) or breast cancer deaths (RR 1.05) in past users. If estrogens really were carcinogenic this is different from other promoters of malignancy such as tobacco, asbestos or even nulliparity or a late menopause where the excess risk does not reach zero 5 years after the exposure. But the cancers which were excluded made a difference in the direction of risk. Forty-eight per cent of the fatal cases (485 out 1002) were excluded, creating an imbalance which cannot be calculated from the information given. The authors excluded 60,606 50–52-year-old HRT users with low mortality (18 deaths) because they considered that the menopausal status would be confused by treatment.

There are many critiques of this study[16–18] but in our view the following points need to be addressed.

- Is the percentage of women taking HRT in the UK correct?

Fifty per cent of the women recruited for MWS were ever-users and 33% were current users. These very high percentages contradict publications concerning the frequency of HRT use in the UK. This is an atypical population as at least two-thirds of estrogen replacement therapy (ERT)/HRT users stop hormonal intake within 1 year, and according to the study of European countries including the UK only 10% of all women use ERT long term. Unfortunately, after the initial questionnaire study and categorization it was not possible for the authors of the MWS to get information about continuation of HRT or changes in treatment as there was no follow-up questionnaire. This inadequacy is not

corrected by the large numbers involved in the study since, as claimed by Beral and colleagues,[11] it will reinforce the errors rather than cancelling them out.

Not only are the results of the MWS based on one-time data collection by questionnaire with no follow-up but also not all centres have reported back. No clinical statements concerning the conditions of treatment can be made on the basis of these data as indications for treatment, dosage, route, consideration of contraindications and compliance are not recognizable from the paper. This is an important point since the rate of side effects is directly related to the quality of treatment such as individualization, choice of preparation and dose according to the symptoms or pathology to be treated.

- Are women attending for mammography in some way selective regarding risk and anxiety?

It is likely that a high-grade selection has occurred in that women registered voluntarily for screening on long-term HRT. These may be risk cases with a fear of ongoing breast cancer risk. Also women taking ERT are more willing to register for safety screening.

- Why is the excess of breast cancers during the first year of HRT not excluded since it is a biological impossibility for such tumour, if caused by estrogen, to be apparent as an invasive tumour within the first year?
- If estrogens were carcinogenic why are recent past-users clear of risk? This sudden return to normality does not occur with other carcinogens.
- The pathology was not checked by a second independent pathologist. This has been the fault of almost all of the previous reports that showed an excess of breast cancer with a better prognosis in women taking HRT.

A Swedish study[18] re-evaluated the histology of endometrial cancer associated with estrogen use and downgraded more than 33% to a lesser diagnosis of atypical or adenomatous hyperplasia. This should be done with the MWS data which show an increase in the first 2 years and no excess on stopping HRT as this sounds more like ductal carcinoma in situ stimulated with estrogens than invasive cancer. This diagnostic grey area occurs in about 4% of cases and should be excluded.

- The increased risk from tibolone is surprising. There is a belief that tibolone, acting like a selective estrogen receptor modulator (SERM), may have a protective effect upon the breast – a view supported by considerable laboratory and clinical work. It has therefore been commonplace to prescribe tibolone for higher-risk women with a family history, or in the presence, of benign breast disease. There must have been a degree of selective prescribing.

The table referring to ethinylestradiol, at 10 times the correct dose (even if this estrogen was ever used in HRT) is clearly a mistake missed by the authors, the reviewers and the editors. It would have been picked up if there had been the most rudimentary clinical input into the study which would also have revealed the more eccentric claims and conclusions of the study. There are also at least 15 other errors of data presentation in the text and tables including multiple discrepant estimates given in the abstract, the text and the figures together with incorrect arithmetic in both text and tables. As things stand we have an influential and hastily written paper of such carelessness that it brings into question the validity of the statistics and any of the conclusions made.

CURRENT ADVICE FOR HORMONAL REPLACEMENT THERAPY PRESCRIBING

1. Estrogen treatment should be used for the treatment of specific symptoms and low bone density.
2. Although estrogen appears to have no place for the secondary prevention of cardiovascular disease, we believe it is still indicated in the early menopausal woman for protection against CHD, stroke and Alzheimer's disease. There is a window of opportunity in 45–60-year-old symptomatic women who may show long-term cardiovascular and neurological benefits from early estrogen therapy.
3. Estrogens commenced in older 60–79-year-old women may do 'early harm' before any benefit is achieved.
4. The dose and route will depend upon the symptoms and the age of the patient. Perimenopausal and post-menopausal patients with vasomotor symptoms should be given either oral or transdermal estradiol with cyclical progestogen for endometrial protection.
5. The usual duration of progestogen is 14 days but if the extra risk to the breasts from progestogen is confirmed it would be sensible to reduce the duration to 7–10 days. A shortened course is useful in women with progestogen intolerance.
6. Patients may wish to avoid bleeding by using low dose estrogen and progestogen or have a Mirena IUS (Mirena intrauterine system) inserted or take tibolone.
7. Patients with hormone-responsive mood disorders should have a higher dose of transdermal estrogens either by patch, gel or implant. As these patients are often progestogen-intolerant, short cycles of progestogen are permissible rather than the orthodox 14-day cycles.
8. If loss of libido and loss of energy remain a problem, the addition of testosterone should be considered.
9. The lowest effective dose should be used remembering that the dose for the elimination of vasomotor symptoms will be less than the dose required for mood disorders or low bone density.
10. The indication and the need for HRT should be reviewed each year with discussion of the current views on risk.
11. A 5-year duration has been recommended but in reality women remain on HRT if they are feeling well with relief of symptoms. It is difficult to persuade these women to stop even after 10 or more years. Long-term ERT or HRT is possible if symptoms persist and no side effects have occurred.
12. A mammogram should be done each year and breast examination every 6 months.[19]

REFERENCES

1. Hulley S, Grady D, Bush T et al. Randomized trial of estrogen plus progestin for secondary prevention of coronary heart disease in post-menopausal women. *JAMA* 1998; **280:** 605–13.
2. Writing Group for Women's Health Initiative Investigators. Risks and benefits of estrogen plus progestin in healthy postmenopausal women; principal results from the Women's Health Initiative randomized controlled trial. *JAMA* 2002; **288:** 321–33.
3. Beral V. Million Women Study Collaborators. Breast cancer and hormone-replacement therapy in the Million Women Study. *Lancet* 2003; **362:** 419–27.
4. Lagro-Jannsen T, Rosser WW, van Weel C. Breast cancer and hormone-replacement therapy; up to general practice to pick up the pieces. *Lancet* 2003; **362:** 414–15.
5. Studd J. 'Up to general practice to pick up the pieces' – what pieces? – a response to WHI and MWS. *Maturitas* 2003; **46:** 95–7.
6. Hays J, Ockene JK, Brunner RL et al, Women's Health Initiative Investigators. Effects of estrogen plus progestin on health-related quality of life. *N Engl J Med* 2003; **348:** 1839–56.
7. Anderson GL, Hutchinson F, Limacher M et al for the WHI Steering Committee. Effects of conjugated equine estrogen in postmenopausal women with hysterectomy. *JAMA* 2004; **291:** 1701–12.
8. Stampfer MJ, Colditz GA Willett WC et al. Post menopausal estrogen therapy and cardio-vascular disease; ten year follow-up from the Nurses' Health Study. *N Engl J Med* 1991; **325:** 756–62.
9. De Lignieres B, de Vathaire F, Fournier S et al. Combined hormone replacement therapy and risk of breast cancer in a French cohort study of 3175 women. *Climacteric* 2002; **5:** 332–40.
10. Sourander L, Rajala T, Raiha I, Makinen J, Erkkola R, Helenius H. Cardiovascular and cancer morbidity and mortality and sudden cardiac deaths in postmenopausal women on estrogen replacement therapy (ERT). *Lancet* 1998; **352:** 1965–9.
11. Collaborative Group on Hormonal Factors in Breast Cancer. Breast cancer and hormone replacement therapy; collaborative reanalysis of data from 51 epidemiological studies of 52,705 women with breast cancer. *Lancet* 1997; **350:** 1047–59.
12. Naftolin F, Taylor HS, Karas R. Early initiation of hormone therapy and clinical protection: the Women's Health Initiative (WHI) could not have detected cardioprotective effects off starting hormone therapy during the menopausal transition. *Fertil Steril* 2004; **81:** 1498–1501.
13. Royal College of Physicians of Edinburgh. Concensus Conference, RCP, Edinburgh, 2003.
14. Chlebowski RT, Hendrix SL, Langer RD et al, WHI investigators. Influence of estrogen plus progestin on breast cancer and mammography in healthy postmenopausal women: the Women's Health Initiative randomised trial. *JAMA* 2003; **289:** 3243–53.
15. Speroff L. The Million Women Study and breast cancer. *Maturitas* 2003; **46:** 1–6.
16. Genazzani AR, Gambacciani M. The sound of an international anti-HRT herald. *Maturitas* 2003; **46:** 105–6.
17. Sturdee DW, MacLennan AH. Is combined estrogen/progestogen hormone therapy worth the risk? *Climacteric* 2003; **6:** 177–9.
18. Persson I, Adami HO, Lindgren A, Norlinder H, Pettersson B, Silver S. Reliability of endometrial cancer diagnoses in a Swedish Cancer Registry – with special reference to classification bias related to exogenous estrogens. *Acta Pathol Microbiol Immunol Scand* 1986; **94:** 187–94.
19. Naftolin F, Schneider HPG, Sturdee DW et al. Guidelines for hormone treatment of women in the menopausal transition and beyond. Revised Position Statement of the International Menopause Society. *Climacteric* 2004; **7:** 333–7.

Section 1

The Third Part of Life

Chapter 1   Basic facts and definitions

Chapter 2   Social structure and social medicine

Chapter 3   Menopausal changes of ovaries and hypothalamic–pituitary and cerebral function

Chapter 4   Premenopausal cycle anomalies

Chapter 5   History of estrogen–progestogen replacement therapy

1

Basic facts and definitions

C Lauritzen

Basic biological facts • Justification for estrogen–progestogen substitution • Definitions • ERT • HRT • New definitions and abbreviations

BASIC BIOLOGICAL FACTS

The ovaries are endocrine glands exhibiting exocrine (eggs) and endocrine functions. Their hormones (estradiol, androstendione, testosterone, progesterone and inhibin) are not necessary for maintaining life as are those of the adrenal, pancreas and thyroid glands. Ovarian function is to create life, safeguarding the procreation of humankind. To prepare a woman for this most important task, the ovarian hormones stimulate growth, differentiation and functions of the reproductive organs through puberty to maturity. Moreover, all vital important organs and physiological functions are positively influenced by estrogens, as pregnancy exerts a high demand on the whole organism.

To incite male–female sexual relations, leading to procreation, sexual hormones instigate sexual desire and development, and secondary sexual characteristics, e.g. breast development. To secure the safety of the the embryo/fetus and to satisfy the high demand of pregnancy, the ovarian hormones exert profound effects on cell mitosis, organ growth and function, general metabolism, cardiovascular and brain function, on lipids and proteins, on the function of the heart and, via a stimulation of nitroxid (NO) production, on the maintenance and improvement of arterial endothelial function.

JUSTIFICATION FOR ESTROGEN–PROGESTOGEN SUBSTITUTION

While the male gonads may exhibit their exocrine and endocrine functions up to a high age, the ovaries are the only endocrine glands (except the thymus and placenta) that cease to function before the end of life. Follicles, eggs and endocrine substrates are exhausted after about 50 years of age. The coming to an end of ovulation and ovarian endocrine function in the aging female is meaningful from an evolutionary standpoint, as it prevents mothers having difficult or complicated pregnancies and endangering their children, and because it prevents children having mothers too old to rear them. Accordingly, the lifespan of women was 50 years or less in earlier centuries.

However, improvements in living conditions and progress in medical science have led to an increased life expectancy for women in affluent societies of about 30 years after menopause. As ovarian function ceases at about 50 years of age, the woman has to live the last 30 years of her life without the benefits exerted by ovarian hormones. Indeed, the majority of postmenopausal women suffer a syndrome of estrogen withdrawal and deficiency symptoms, called climacteric complaints, which are characterized by frustrated attempts of the endocrine system to restore the endocrine balance by increasing the output of gonadotrophin-releasing hormone

(GnRH) and gonadotrophins. However, the burnt-out ovaries cannot react; estrogen levels remain low, and follicular hormone production, ovulation and luteinization cannot be resumed.

The loss of ovarian hormones has consequences limited not only to classic target organs but also to the performance of the whole organism. In most cases, withdrawal of ovarian hormones leads to many complaints such as hot flushes, sweating, sleeplessness, arthralgia and depressive moods, indicating an imbalance in the autonomous nervous system, which usually diminishes the quality of life and may reduce the capacity to work and for creativity.

Some years after menopause atrophic changes of the skin, mucous membranes and the urogenital system will frequently result in disadvantageous consequences for sexuality and social behavior (e.g. aging of the skin, atropy of mucous membranes and conjunctivae, pruritus, dry vagina, dys- and stranguria, urinary frequency, incontinence). Years later a steep increase in diseases will occur due to chronic estrogen deficiency, such as osteoporosis, cardiovascular events and worsening of cognitive functions. The incidence of many other diseases also increases due to estrogen deficiency.

If estrogen deficiency indeed plays a role in these events, logically some may be prevented by lifestyle counseling and a competent individual estrogen–progesterone or androgen substitution.

This is the philosophy of physicians and scientists dealing with the problems of the menopause. Innumerable menopausal women have experienced the valuable help of peri-postmenopausal estrogen substitution, as witnessed by many physicians. Estrogen–progestogen–androgen treatment and substitution have some side-effects, but safety is secured by a proper indication, consideration of contraindications and risks, careful supervision and additional treatment if necessary.

By prudent selection of hormones, doses and application forms, i.e. an individually tailored treatment, along with regular adaptation to meet needs, side-effects may be minimized. If so performed, the benefits of estrogen and hormone replacement therapies (ERT and HRT, respectively) greatly outweigh the few possible side-effects and associated risks.

Thus, HRT during the third phase of life is a method of preventing unnecessary complaints, diseases and suffering, and can be seen as an attempt to create equality between the sexes in so far as is possible by administration of hormones and additional lifestyle counseling.

The decision to use estrogen or not during postmenopause is a very important one for a woman, with implications for her health in later life. Therefore, it is to be hoped that all women will find a competent therapist.

DEFINITIONS

The definitions given here and used in this monograph follow the formulations of the World Health Organization (WHO) and the International Menopause Society (IMS).

Menopause

WHO: 'The term menopause is defined as the permanent cessation of menstruation resulting from the loss of ovarian follicular activity. Natural menopause is recognized to have occurred after 12 consecutive months of amenorrhea, for which there is no other obvious pathological or physiological cause. Menopause occurs with the final normal period, which is known with certainty only in retrospect a year or more after the event. An adequate marker for the event does not exist.'

Menopause is the last menstruation governed by ovarian function – bleeding caused by nonhormonal endometrial pathology (e.g. polyps, myomata) are excluded. Existing amenorrhea, climacteric age, exclusion of pregnancy, of intake of medications causing amenorrhea, of endocrine pathology or consuming diseases, repeated determinations of estradiol (< 30 pg/ml) and of follicle-stimulating hormone (FSH) in plasma (> 40 IE/l), measurement of ovarian volume, exclusion of ovulatory follicles and measurement of endometrial thickness (< 5 mm) may help establish a definite diagnosis of menopause.

Perimenopause

WHO: 'The term perimenopause should include the period immediately prior to the menopause (when the endocrinological, biological and clinical features of approaching menopause commence) and the first year after menopause.'

Menopausal transition

WHO: 'The term menopausal transition should be reserved for that period of time before the final menstrual period when variability of the menstrual cycle is usually increased.'

Climacteric

IMS: 'This phase in the aging of women marks the transition from the reproductive phase to the non reproductive state. This phase incorporates the perimenopause by extending for a longer variable period before and after the menopause.'

Climacteric syndrome

IMS: 'The climacteric is sometimes, but not necessarily always, associated with symptomatology. When this occurs, it may be terminated the "climacteric syndrome".'

The climacteric syndrome is caused mainly by estradiol deficiency. The main climacteric symptoms, e.g. hot flushes and sweating, are typical for the perimenopause but admittedly are not specific. Differential diagnostic considerations must include mainly vegetative dytonia and dysthyreosis.

Premenopause

WHO: 'The term premenopause is often used ambiguously to refer to the one or two years immediately before the menopause or to refer to the whole of the reproductive period prior to the menopause. The WHO group recommended that the term be used consistently in the latter sense to compass the entire reproductive period up to the final menstrual period.'

The definition of premenopause as the beginning of the climacteric transition, which starts a few (2–5) years before menopause, is preferred by the editors.

Postmenopause

WHO: 'The term postmenopause is defined as dating from the final menstrual period, regardless whether the menopause was induced or spontaneous.'

The postmenopause lasts about 10–15 years and is followed by the senium from about 65 years of age to the end of life. This age limit of 65 years is marked by the cessation of employment and the successive occurrence of the maximum rate of cardiovascular, orthopedic and oncologic diseases. At 65 years of age estrogen substitution may be accompanied by higher vascular and oncologic risks.

Premature menopause

WHO: 'Ideally, premature menopause should be defined as menopause that occurs at an age more than two standard deviations below the mean estimated for the reference population. In practice, in the absence of reliable estimates of the distribution of age at natural menopause in developing countries, the age of 40 years is frequently used as an arbitrary cut-off, below which menopause is said to be premature.'

In Western countries the menopause presently occurs at about 52±4 years of age. Premature menopause is usually defined as occurring before the age of 40, but estrogen–progesterone substitution should be prescribed only from a menopausal age of 45. Causes of premature menopause are: (1) primary diminution of germ cells; (2) increased atresia of follicles and eggs, caused by chromosomal anomalies; (3) autoimmune diseases and enzyme defects; (4) postnatal damage of germ cells by ionizing radiation or cytotoxic medications. *Late menopause* would then be defined as occuring after 56 years of age.

Induced menopause

The term induced menopause is defined by the WHO as the cessation of menstruation, which follows either surgical removal of both ovaries (with and without hysterectomy) or iatrogenic ablation of ovarian function (e.g. by radiation or chemotherapy).

Estrogen replacement therapy (ERT)

ERT refers to substitution of missing estrogen if symptoms of estrogen deprivation are present. Estrogen monotherapy is restricted to women who have had a hysterectomy.

Hormone replacement therapy (HRT)

This is the substitution of both estrogen and progesterone or of a progestogen, if a uterus is present, to secure a stable cycle with normal uterine bleedings and to prevent hyperplasia of the endometrium and endometrial cancer that may be caused by a long-term estrogen monotherapy. The replacement is not always a therapy but may have a preventative aim.

Sequential treatment

Medication of an estrogen followed by medication of progesterone or a progestogen for at least 10 days, but ideally 14 days. This arrangement secures regular uterine bleedings during the perimenopause through a normal endometrial histology and prevents endometrial hyperplasia and endometrial cancer caused by estrogen monotherapy.

Combined treatment

Daily medication of an estrogen combined with progesterone or a progestogen. This arrangement leads, in the majority of cases, to attainment or the maintainance of a desired postmenopausal uterine amenorrhea. Usually, combination therapy is given continuously without interruption.

Combined continuous estrogen–progestogen treatment seems to be optimal in diminishing endometrial and ovarian cancer risk and osteoporosis (norethisterone derivates). It is however questionable whether the combined continuous estrogen–progestogen treatment is optimal for the prevention of cardiovascular diseases and for the incidence of breast cancer. The choice of the progestogen may play a role in determining benefits and risks. The use of genuine progesterone is recommended.

Androgen replacement therapy (ART)

Androgen replacement may be indicated (together with estrogens) in cases of early bilateral oophorectomy (with a 50% reduction of testosterone production) and in cases of low androgen levels, which are symptomatic, for example, of chronic fatigue syndrome. A pharmacological indication may be given in cases of loss of drive and of the capabiltity to make decisions, in apathic melancholia, loss of libido and anorgasmia.

Natural estrogens

Natural estrogens are obtained from natural sources, e.g. human beings, equides (horses) and plants. Most sexual hormones are at present produced from plant sources using chemical methods for final preparation of estradiol, estriol, progesterone or androgens.

The definition of natural estrogens is historical. At the beginning of hormone therapy, extracts of animal ovaries and estradiol were orally ineffective. Thereafter the orally highly effective ethinylestradiol and stilbestrol were introduced. In 1942 conjugated estrogens, extracted from the urine of pregnant mares, were developed and were the first and only effective oral estrogens from a natural source, in contrast to synthetic estrogens that are excusively laboratory products.

Conjugated estrogens

These are formed from estrogen extract from the urine of pregnant mares conjugated with natrium sulfate. Conjugation is normally a metabolic process, making the hormones more water soluble and ready for excretion.

Conjugated estrogens, a mix of several estrogens, contain mainly estrone sulfate (about 50%) and equilin sulfate (about 25%), 17α-dehydroequilenin sulfate (15%), equilenin sulfate (3%), 17α- and 17β-dihydroequilenin sulfate (5%), 17α-estradiolsulfate (2%) and 17β-estradiol sulfate (3%). Recently, delta (8,9)-dehydroestrone sulfate (DHES) was identified (4.4%). This compound comprises approximately 34% of the combined concentration of metabolites of the ingredients estrone sulfate and equilin sulfate or 26% of the metabolites from three estrogens. Several additional estrogenic substances, exhibiting mostly weak estrogenic activity, are still unidentified.

The belief that all estrogenic substances act similarly in the body, which was held for some time, is not true. The pharmacologic activity of such a complex of compounds cannot be described in terms of its total estrogenic potency, which may in addition vary in different batches. Pharmacokinetics, tissue metabolism and tissue-specific reception is different for each compound.

The preparation from the urine of pregnant mares contains estrogens that do not occur in the human body. Since 1942, conjugated estrogens are the most frequently used estrogens in the United States. Most of the physiopathological knowledge and epidemiological evidence available has been produced by investigating the effects of conjugated estrogens.

Since oral and parenteral estradiol are available and therapeutically effective, this genuine human female hormone will in time replace the conjugated estrogens.

Esterified estrogens

Conjugated estrogens marketed by some companies, not produced from the urine of pregnant mares but prepared by synthesis from precursor substances, must not be called conjugated estrogens according to jurisdiction. Such preparations contain estrone sulfate and equilin sulfate in defined amounts.

Artificial estrogens

Artificial estrogens produced in vitro, which do not naturally occur in the human body or in nature, are not to be confused with synthetic estrogens, as most estrogens used (e.g. estradiol) are made by partial synthesis from precursor steroids or plant steroids. Examples of artificial estrogens are ethinylestradiol and stilbestrol.

Synthethic estrogens

All synthetic estrogens in use are prepared by synthetic manipulations. Most estrogens used for treatment or substitution are synthesized in big industrial processes.

Estradiol

Estradiol is available as a micronized compound and as estradiol valerate. After oral administration most of the estradiol is converted to estrone in the body. Transdermal, rectal, vaginal, buccal and nasal estradiol is resorbed mostly unchanged. Protracted injectable estradiols are esterified with fatty acids of different chain lengths, such as benzoate, propionate and valerate. The chain length mostly corresponds to the duration of effect. Also available are estrone sulfate and estriol.

Pulsed estrogen therapy

Intranasal administration of estradiol avoids the first-pass effect and leads to a very rapid increase of its plasma levels, resulting, by intermittent exposure in a pulse-like application, in an estrogen profile that is different from the sustained estrogen profile observed after oral, transdermal or other parenteral administration.

Long-term treatment and substitution

Treatment or substitution given over a period of more than 5 years.

Progesterone

The genuine human ovarian steroid hormone secreted by the corpus luteum, produced from granulosa cells or by partial pharmacological synthesis.

Progestins

Summarizing expression for artificial hormones exerting similar but by no means identical effects to progesterone.

Progestogens

Like progestins, artificial compounds exerting similar but not identical effects to genuine progesterone.

Selective estrogen receptor modulators (SERM)

SERM exert only partial effects of estradiol by modulating the estrogen receptor proteins, e.g. beneficial effects on organ perfusion, bone and lipids, but no stimulation on endometrium and breast epithelium.

Selective progestogen receptor modulators (SPRM)

By modulating the proteins of the progesterone receptors, SPRM exert only the desired partial effects of progesterone.

Selective androgen receptor modulators (SARM)

By modulating the androgen receptor, SARM may exert desired partial effects of testosterone.

Primary prevention

Prevention of diseases before they become organic and clinically symptomatic. Primary prevention for most diseases must begin in youth or at maturity, or at the latest at the time of menopause.

Secondary prevention

Prevention of organic changes and disease events when an organic pathology is already present and when disease events have already occurred. Secondary prevention is, in most cases, truly a treatment of the existing disease.

NEW DEFINITIONS AND ABBREVIATIONS

In March 2003, in *Climacteric* (the journal of the IMS), a new nomenclature for hormonal treatment was proposed. These new definitions and abbreviations – Box 1.1 – will now be used in all papers of *Climacteric* and other publications of the IMS.

Box 1.1 Proposals of the IMS, March 2003	
CCEPT	Combined continuous estrogen–progestogen therapy
CSEPT	Combined sequential estrogen–progestogen therapy
EAT	Estrogen–androgen therapy
EPT	Estrogen–progestogen therapy
ET	Estrogen therapy

2

Social structure and social medicine

A Rieder

The demographic challenge • **Life expectancy and healthy life expectancy** • **Self-perceived health**
• **Employment and health** • **Income of elderly women** • **Sociobehavioral changes** • **Caring for others**
• **Mortality and morbidity** • **Cardiovascular diseases (CVD) in women** • **Cancer** • **Diabetes**
• **Lifestyle facts and risks** • **Socioeconomic inequalities in mortality among women and men**
• **Importance of prevention** • **References**

THE DEMOGRAPHIC CHALLENGE

The population of the European Union (EU) is
characterized by growing life expectancy,
decreasing fertility rates, growth of the population over 65 years of age and an even faster
increase of the very old, i.e. people above the
age of 80.

Growing life expectancy is resulting in a
larger proportion of females in the older population. Women – totalling 191 million – constitute 51.2% of the population in the EU. This
percentage is very stable across the member
states, varying from 50.4% in Ireland to 51.8%
in Portugal. In the older population the ratio of
women to men varies across the different countries in the EU. For instance, in Greece there are
only 120 women to 100 men in this age group
whereas in Germany there are almost 160
women to 100 men over the age of 60.[1,2]

The process of fertility decline started in the
1960s, first in the Nordic member states and a
decade later in the southern member states.
Today the lowest fertility rates can be found in
the Mediterranean member states, with the
minimum falling below 1.2 children/woman in
Spain and Italy. This means that the southern

member states are aging more quickly than the
northern ones.[3]

The large differences between male and
female life expectancy and the lingering effects
of the Second World War have resulted in
elderly female:male ratios that remain as high
as 2:1 in Russia and other parts of the former
Soviet Union. Among the old (80 years of age
and over), the proportion of females often
exceeds 70% (e.g. in Belgium and Germany,
and the Ukraine) and has reached 80% in
Russia. It can be said that the social, economic
and health problems of elderly people are to a
large extent the problems of elderly women.[4]

LIFE EXPECTANCY AND HEALTHY LIFE EXPECTANCY

In Europe over the past 50 years, life expectancy
of men and women has risen steadily. In 1998,
the life expectancy of women in the EU-15 was
80.8 years while that for men was 74.5 years
(Tables 2.1 and 2.2). Eurostat (Statistical Office
of the European Communities) estimates that
the life expectancy of men and women will
reach 83 and 87 years, respectively, by 2050. The

Table 2.1 Life expectancy and life expectancy without disability in Europe*

	EU-15	B	DK	D	EL	E	F	IRL	I	L	NL	A	P	FIN	S	UK
Life expectancy, 1998																
Males	74.5	74.1	73.6	74.1	75.5	74.4	74.6	73.4	74.9	74.1	75.1	74.6	71.7	73.5	76.7	74.6
Females	80.8	80.6	78.5	80.4	80.8	81.7	82.2	78.6	81.3	79.8	80.5	80.8	78.8	80.8	81.8	79.6
Life expectancy without any disability, 1994																
Males	60	60	61	57	63	62	60	61	60	59	59	–	55	–	–	59
Females	62	61	61	60	65	64	65	64	61	61	59	–	57	–	–	61

*Source: Eurostat, Demographic Statistics and European Community Household Panel, 2000.

Table 2.2 Life expectancy of men and women at age 65 in Europe, 1998*

	EU-15	B	DK	D	EL	E	F	IRL	I	L	NL	A	P	FIN	S	UK
Males	–	16.6	14.7	15.3	16.2	16.3	–	–	–	–	14.7	15.6	14.4	14.9	16.3	–
Females	–	19.8	17.9	19.0	18.7	20.3	–	–	–	–	18.8	19.3	17.9	19.1	20.0	–

	CH	USA	EST	PL	SLO	CZ	H
Males	16.7	16.0	12.4	–	13.9	13.5	12.3
Females	20.6	19.1	16.6	–	18.1	17.1	16.1

*Source: OECD Health Data, 2000, WHO Health for all Data Base, 2000.

greatest gender difference in life expectancy at the time of birth was found in France (8 years longer in baby girls). The smallest difference was found in the UK (5 years).

The southern member states have made great strides to close the gap with the north. Since 1960, the life expectancy of men and women in Portugal has improved by 10.5 and 12 years, respectively, compared with an average of 3.2 and 4.1 years, respectively, in Denmark.[3]

Healthy life expectancies at birth are higher for females than males in most regions of the world and the difference between the sexes generally increases as average life expectancy increases. In the twenty-first century most dependants will be older people due to greater longevity, particularly women.[3]

Health expectancies are a group of health indicators combining data on mortality and disability/morbidity. Women in the EU can expect to live to 62 years of age without any disability and 74 years of age without any severe disability. The corresponding figures for men are 60–69 years (Table 2.1).[3]

To describe population health the World Health Organization (WHO) calculated the disability adjusted life expectancy (DALE) for 191 countries, which measures the equivalent number of years of life expected to be lived in full health, i.e. healthy life expectancy. Global healthy life expectancy at birth was 56.8 years, 7.7 years lower than total life expectancy at birth. Healthy life expectancy at the global level was 57.8 years for women, 2.0 years higher than that for men at 55.8 years. DALE at birth in 1999 ranged from a low of 37 years for African men to a high of almost 70 years for women in the low mortality countries of mainly Western Europe.[5]

SELF-PERCEIVED HEALTH

Almost one in four elderly people describe their health as bad. In all age groups more women than men perceive their health as (very) bad. Among 65 year olds about 26% of women perceive their health as bad or very bad compared to 20% of men (Fig. 2.1).[3] All the southern member states reported lower levels of perceived

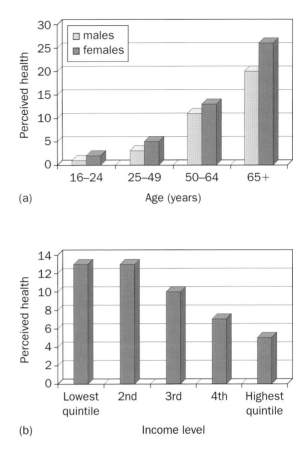

(a)

(b)

Fig. 2.1 Proportion of population whose perceived health is bad or very bad, (a) by age and sex, (b) EU-15, 1995. (Source: Eurostat, European Community Household Panel, 2000.)

health. In total, poorer health is more frequently reported by women. On average 63% of women declare their health as good or very good compared to 70% of men. The highest percentages of good and very good health are found in The Netherlands, Austria, Denmark and Ireland. The lowest percentage and the greatest sex differences are observed in Portugal, followed by Greece, Luxembourg and Italy.[3]

Based on self-reports, the most prevalent chronic disease among the elderly is arthritis followed by high blood pressure for both men and women. Heart disease is next for men and chronic obstructive pulmonary disease for women. The chronic diseases responsible for the most disability in both sexes are arthritis and heart disease, while high blood pressure is more significant in women and chronic obstructive pulmonary disease in men.[6]

EMPLOYMENT AND HEALTH

EU-wide, 68% of the population aged 15–64 are economically active, the rate for males (77.8%) is considerably higher than that for females (58.2%). In the vast majority of member states, women (11.7%) are more likely to be unemployed than men (8.6%). Ireland, Sweden and, in particular, the United Kingdom (UK) (5.5% women and 7.0% men) are the exceptions.

The employment rates of elderly people (55–64 years of age) differ between the countries of the EU, ranging from 22.5% in Belgium to 50.4% in Denmark. Elderly women show lower employment rates than men (EU average 47 versus 29%). With respect to age, the employment rates of women range from 55% among the age group of 50–54 years of age to about 12–14% among the age group of 60–64 years of age.

As with younger workers, females (41%) have a greater tendency than males (8%) to work part time. Females are more affected than males by long-term unemployment (unemployment for > 1 year).[3] Unemployment rates are highest among poorly educated women and men, but in women the unemployment rates are higher than among men at each educational level. In the countries applying for EU membership unemployment rates among men are higher than among women, the biggest gap can be found in the Baltic countries.[3]

Employed women are physically and psychologically healthier than nonemployed women. Paid employment for women is mediated through a higher degree of self-esteem and improved opportunities to exert influence over their own lives by becoming economically less dependent.[7]

Krantz and Östergren[7] report that Swedish women have higher rates of sickness absence and disability pensions than men. The reasons for women above 40 years of age to be sick-listed are manifold, with factors related to paid employment and family situations being dominating causes. Nonemployment, job strain, completed primary education, poor social support, low social anchorage and low social participation were significantly associated with a high level of common symptoms. Among the employed women job strain was significantly associated with a high level of common symptoms.[7]

INCOME OF ELDERLY WOMEN

Throughout the EU poverty is slightly more prevalent among women than among men (EU average of 19 versus 17%). The gender gap is even larger among persons living alone, particularly among the elderly. Older women are poorer than elderly people in general, and older women living alone are the poorest of elderly people.[4] In all member states of the EU men living on their own have a higher median income than women. The group worst off are women aged 65 and over (75% of the national median).

The gross monthly earnings of women were 26% less than the earnings of men in 1995 in the EU. The smallest differences were found in Belgium, Denmark, Luxembourg and Sweden. Although it is not possible to determine whether women are paid less for equal work, it can be concluded that women are generally in lower paid positions. Comparing the inequality structure by age shows that pay differences between men and women increase rapidly with age.[3]

There is more diversity among elderly people in terms of poverty and income distribution than in terms of income sources. Elderly people at low and middle income levels rely heavily on social security, while the more well-to-do elderly in all nations benefit proportionally more from earnings, property income and occupational pensions.

Growing female economic and social participation has been a very significant development. In the last three decades, patterns of education and employment for men and women have become more similar. Women have been experiencing entitlement to more individualized social rights. However, within the family, women still assume most of the caring responsibilities. In the future, these responsibilities are also likely to contribute to increasing the demand for social services.[3]

SOCIOBEHAVIORAL CHANGES

The structure of the family is being transformed in EU member states as changes are occurring in the patterns of marriage, family formation and dissolution. People are marrying less and later. The average age of women when they marry is about 26.5 years (1995) compared to 24.5 years in 1985; for men this figure is 29 years compared to 27 in 1985. Divorce is more frequent and a growing number of one-person households can be observed.

Today, patterns of marital status are very different among elderly men and women. The large majority of men aged 65 and over are married, whereas on average about half of all elderly women are widowed. Comparing European countries, the highest percentages of women (65 years of age and over) living alone are found in Denmark and Sweden (52 versus 23.3% of men and 49.9 versus 25.1% of men, respectively): the lowest percentages are found in Greece (22.8 versus 8.7%, of men), Portugal (23.9 versus 9.4% of men and Ireland (27.7 versus 18.9% of men).[3,4]

CARING FOR OTHERS

Women are twice as likely as men to be caring for sick or disabled persons. But not only the younger age groups are caring for others, 11% of 50–59 year olds, 9% of 60–69 year olds, 7% of 70–79 year olds and 3% of those aged 80 years and above are providing care for sick, disabled or frail adults in Europe. So, the life of most women is characterized by four phases of caring, with the fourth phase being the need for someone who cares for them.[3]

MORTALITY AND MORBIDITY

There has been a consistent decline in mortality rates in all EU member states but not in all age groups. The mortality trend in the 25–35-year-old group in recent years shows slight increases for men and has remained at similar levels for women. This is mainly explained by accidents, suicides and, to a lesser extent, AIDS. Women are at lower risk of dying at all ages.

The current major causes of death are cardiovascular diseases (CVD), cancer and respiratory diseases, but of course causes of death vary significantly with age. CVD and cancer start to be the main causes of death in middle age. Around 50% of deaths in the population of 60 years of age and above are due to CVD. Cancer is the second most common cause of death in Europe after CVD, accounting for half of all deaths of women aged between 45 and 54.[8]

Osteoporosis is one of the main causes of chronic illness and disability. In the EU it is expected that there will be a significant increase in hip fractures of between 0.5 and 3%. Age-specific incidence rates of hip fractures are about 140/10,000 among 80–84-year-old women and about 350/10,000 among those aged 85 and above. In the EU ratio of the female:male is 3.71:1.[9]

Incontinence affects 40% of women above 60 years of age and causes 25% of admissions to nursing homes. Incidence rates of Alzheimer's disease are estimated to be around 28/100,000 in women.[10]

According to the 1996 'Euro-barometer' average, almost one in four women report limitations in their daily activities to some extent (17.3%), or severely (6.3%), because of long-standing illness. This average varies from a high of 30% (in Finland and Portugal) to a low of 15% (in Luxembourg) and increases with age. More than half of all women 75 years of age and older report such activity limitations.[2]

CARDIOVASCULAR DISEASES (CVD) IN WOMEN

CVD is the most common cause of ill health and is the leading cause of death in women, responsible for more deaths each year than all other causes combined. The incidence of myocardial infarction in women, although lower than in men, increases dramatically after the menopause. A number of important cardiovascular risk factors affect both men and women. There is evidence, however, that hormonal status, diabetes, smoking and a family history of premature coronary heart disease (CHD) are more important in women than in men.[11]

In the elderly population women are less likely to die from CVD and cancer compared to men, but slightly more likely to die of cerebrovascular disease. Lifetime risk for stroke is 18% for men and 24% for women. All in all, standard deaths rates in 1996 show that slightly more women than men die from diseases of the circulatory system.[8]

Peeters et al[12] constructed multistate life tables of the Framingham Heart Study cohort to calculate dwelling times with a history of CVD. The lifetime risk of developing CVD for individuals free of CVD at 40 and 60 years of age are slightly higher in women than in men for stroke and congestive heart failure (21 and 19% for women aged 40 and 60, respectively, compared to 16 and 18% for men aged 40 and 60, respectively, for stroke, and 17% for congestive heart failure). Lifetime risk for stroke and congestive failure before the age of 85 is slightly higher in men. Lifetime risk for developing CVD and acute myocardial infarction is always higher in men, for lifetime and before the age of 85. Lifetime risk for CVD before the age of 85 for a 60-year-old woman is 49% and for 60-year-old men is 57%. Any CVD will potentially cause a 50-year-old woman to lose 12 years of life and a 70-year-old woman to lose 6 years of life.

From the Swedish data of the MONICA Study it is known that low socioeconomic status (SES) exerts a stronger adverse influence on cardiovascular risk factors for women than it does for men.[13]

CANCER

Incidence and mortality rates are higher in northern EU countries than in southern EU countries, although incidence rates have increased in all European countries. The age-standardized incidence and mortality rate per 100,000 of population for all the cancer groups is highest for women in Denmark (272.4), and for men in France (300.5). The lowest incidence rates for both sexes were found in Spain, Greece and Portugal. In Europe, the 5-year prevalence rate reported by the International Agency for Research on Cancer (IARC) is 2.1 million for women.

Lung cancer is responsible for 9% of all cancer deaths and represents 5.9% of all new cancer cases in women.

Among the elderly, 20% of all deaths are caused by cancer. Breast cancer is the most common cancer in women. The aging impact in breast cancer is severe because as many as 60% of deaths occur after the age of 65. There is an increasing trend for breast cancer among elderly women in the EU, which is responsible for 19% of all cancer deaths and 28.5% of all new female cancer cases.[8]

Differences in incidence rates between northern and southern EU countries are also found for cancer of the body of the uterus and ovarian cancer. Cancers of the body of the uterus, which are mainly cancers of the endometrium, show the lowest cancer incidence rate in the southernmost countries and resemble the pattern of breast cancer incidence and mortality rates. This is also the case for ovarian cancer, with quite large differences between countries. Incidence rates are twice as high in Denmark compared with Greece, with mortality rates three times higher in Denmark.

About 40% of women in European countries report having had a cervical smear in the past year, the same percentage as having had a breast examination by hand. About 18% of the women reported having had a mammography during the past year. More than 90% of women endorsed (free) mammography screening in the age groups where it has the potential to reduce mortality.[2] The burden of cancer is even more important in populations with long life expectancies.[8]

DIABETES

Today diabetes is a common disease and a major public health problem. Incidence rates are expected to increase as a result of the aging population and because of the increasing prevalence of unhealthy diets, obesity and sedentary lifestyles. The estimated prevalence rates of diabetes mellitus provided by the International Diabetes Institute in 1994 was 3.4% for the total population of the EU (not including Greece). The increase in the numbers of cases for the period 1994–2000 has been projected as 22.5% for the year 2010.[8] A Danish study investigated the age-specific increase of diabetes and impaired glucose tolerance (IGT) among 60-year-old men and women. Between 1974/75 and 1996/97 they found a 21% increase in diabetes among women (6.8% of women were diagnosed with diabetes) and a 16% increase in the prevalence of IGT (prevalence of IGT was 13.1%). The increases were lower among women than men.[14] The increase was fully explained by a concurrent increase in body mass index (BMI).

The Framingham Heart Study has shown that women with diabetes have a 200% increased risk of developing coronary heart disease (the increased risk in men is 70%).[15]

Only 22% of European women have had a diabetes test in the past year, although among the severely overweight (aged 40 and above) the rate is 44%.[2]

LIFESTYLE FACTS AND RISKS

If all premature deaths among women below 65 years of age could be eradicated, life expectancy for women in the EU would increase by almost another 4 years.[2] The Nurses Health Study found that reductions in smoking, improvements in diet and postmenopausal hormone use were the biggest factors accounting for the decline in CHD observed in this population of women.[16] An increase in obesity had the opposite effect.

Cardiovascular risk factors in postmenopausal women – women aged 60 and above – are most commonly hypertension, hypercholesterolemia, diabetes and obesity. In a French study only 39% of postmenopausal women had no CVD risk factors, and only 51% of the perimenopausal women.[17] An Italian study shows the north–south differences within one country. CVD risk factors are more preva-

lent in southern Italy than in the north and in general they are most prevalent in the most poorly educated.[18] In the Munster Heart Study (PROCAM) some results have been more marked in women than in men. Increasing levels of elevated fasting blood glucose levels and BMI increased with age in both sexes, the increase was more marked in women.[19]

Smoking

The single most dangerous health habit among women in the EU is smoking. Twenty-eight per cent of all women in the EU smoke, although the rate varies across the member states. Denmark and Portugal stand out because of their very high (42%) and low (12%) rates of smoking among women, respectively.

As expected, smoking-related cancers and CVD are increasing in women. Mortality from cancer of the respiratory system – predominantly lung cancer – has increased by almost 70% since 1970. Sacker et al[20] investigated social inequality in the health of women in England. They found, consistent with other studies, the strongest independent effect on women's health comes from smoking: social support was the next strongest independent predictor.

Alcohol

There are no data on average alcohol consumption by women in European countries, although it is known that women drink less than men.[8] In the study by Sacker et al[20] alcohol consumption in women was associated with good rather than poor health. They even found that alcohol consumption was positively associated with participation in sport and with social support, both of which were related to better health (comparing women who drink moderately to women who do not drink at all).

Overweight

It is estimated that one out of every five women in the EU is overweight or severely overweight as measured by the BMI, while 15% are underweight.[8] Referring to data of the World

Health Organization–Countrywide Integrated Noncommunicable Disease Intervention (WHO–CINDI) study the lowest percentages of obese women can be found in Denmark (10%), The Netherlands (11%) and Sweden (12%), the highest percentages are found in Spain (24%), Portugal (21%), Italy (21%) and Greece (20%). Being overweight is a significant risk factor for a number of diseases that affect women after the menopause, in particular heart disease, diabetes and cancer. Bergström et al[21] reviewed the epidemiological literature and found that, overall, excess body mass accounts for 5% of all cancers in the EU, 6.4% in women and 3.4% in men, corresponding to 45,000 female cancer cases yearly. For women the proportion varied from 3.9% for Denmark to 8.8% for Spain. The highest proportions were obtained for cancers of the endometrium (39%), kidney (25% in both sexes) and gallbladder (24% in women and 25% in men). The number of new cancer cases attributable to overweight and obesity are 12,870 for breast cancer, 14,230 for endometrial cancer and 10,460 for colon cancer: in total, 44,750 female cancer cases in Europe. Thousands of cancer cases could be avoided by halving the prevalence of overweight and obese people in Europe.[21]

Exercise

There are no gender-specific representative data about exercise in the EU but it is generally accepted that, in particular, elderly women do not exercise sufficiently. Older women show higher rates of ADL (activities of daily living) and IADL (instrumental activities of daily living) disability than men do, which might be one reason why women are more commonly thought to have poorer health-related quality of life (HRQL).[6]

SOCIOECONOMIC INEQUALITIES IN MORTALITY AMONG WOMEN AND MEN

Mackenbach et al[22] investigated socioeconomic inequalities in total and causes of specific mortality by sex in six European countries (Finland, Norway, Italy, the Czech Republic, Hungary

and Estonia) and the USA. They found that in all countries mortality was lowest among women with a high level of education and highest among men with a low level of education. Men with a high level of education always had higher mortality rates than women with a low level of education. The only cause of death for which (relative) inequalities were often larger among women than among men was CVD (with the exception of Hungary and the Czech Republic).

In most countries, poorly educated women had higher mortality rates than highly educated women for most causes of death, including all CVD, ischemic heart disease, cerebrovascular disease, respiratory diseases and gastrointestinal diseases. For neoplasms, mortality was not clearly higher among poorly educated women and in some countries (the Czech Republic and Hungary) it was actually higher among highly educated women. Breast cancer was less common among poorly educated women in all countries. They summarized that socioeconomic inequalities in total mortality tend to be smaller among women than among men. Sex differences in the size of the inequality vary between countries, from almost none in Norway to huge in the Czech Republic. At the level of specific causes of death, relative inequalities in mortality among women are usually smaller than those among men (e.g. neoplasm), but are sometimes larger (e.g. CVD). While differences in cause of death patterns explain a larger part of the sex differences in the size of inequalities in total mortality in the USA and western Europe, this does not apply to the Czech Republic and Hungary, the countries where inequalities among men were larger than elsewhere.[22]

IMPORTANCE OF PREVENTION

Although people in the EU are now living longer, one in five citizens still dies prematurely, often due to preventable diseases. New risks to health, especially communicable diseases, are emerging, there are disturbing inequalities in health status between social classes, and longer life expectancy is itself creating problems such as sharp rises in age-related diseases such as Alzheimer's disease. Studies from the USA, Canada and the EU member states have shown the future needs of both social and health care. The average cost of those aged 65–74 is estimated to be more than twice that for those aged 65 or younger. Regarding Europe, the average population will increase by 3% by 2010, the age-adjusted cost of health will increase by 10%. This increase only takes into account the demographic effect.

In addition, health risks associated with respiratory illnesses, stress and musculoskeletal problems are arising from environmental changes, lifestyle habits and working conditions.[8]

Due to the higher female life expectancy in absolute numbers, women will become the greater concern. Specific action is required to improve the condition of women's health, to provide for their special needs and to create awareness among women about the importance of preventive action, continuing during the aging process. With respect to social programs promoting lifestyle changes, potential health gains are greatest among persons with less wealth.[23] It is well known that health and wealth are strongly correlated and women are at higher risk of poverty, living alone and chronic illness. On the other hand, it is difficult to reach people of low SES effectively with health promotion programs. Efforts have to be made to implement effective gender-specific prevention programs targeting low socioeconomic groups, bearing in mind the aging population and aging as a risk factor, as well as the increasing prevalence of risk factors and diseases, such as overweight, smoking and diabetes.

REFERENCES

1. Rozenberg L, Fellemans C, Kroll M, Vandromme J. The menopause in Europe. *Int J Fertil* 2000; **45:** 182–9.
2. *The state of women's health in the European Community*. Report from the Council, the European Parliament, the Economic and Social Committee of the Regions, European Communities, 1997.
3. *Report on the social situation in the European Union*. The European Commission, Employment and Social Affairs, 2000.
4. Kinsella K, Suzman R, Robine J-M, Myers G. Demography of older populations in developed countries. In: (Evans G, Williams TF, Michel J-P, Beattie L, Eds) *Oxford Textbook of Geriatric Medicine*, 2nd edn. (Oxford University Press: New York, 2000) 7–19.
5. Mathers CD, Sadana R, Salomon JA et al. Healthy life expectancy in 191 countries, 1999. *Lancet* 2001; **357:** 1685–91.
6. Clark DO. Social aspects of ageing. In: (Evans G, Williams TF, Michel J-P, Beattie L, Eds) *Oxford Textbook of Geriatric Medicine*, 2nd edn. (Oxford University Press: New York, 2000) 20–6.
7. Krantz G, Östergren P-O. Common symptoms in middle aged women: their relation to employment status, psychosocial work conditions and social support in a Swedish setting. *J Epidemiol Commun Health* 2000; **54:** 192–9.
8. *Key data on health 2000*. European Commission, Eurostat, European Communities. Luxemburg, 2001.
9. *The European Union report on osteoporosis – action for prevention*. European Communities. Luxemburg, 1998.
10. Kytir J, Schmeiser-Rieder A, Böhmer F et al. Gesund und krank älter werden In: (*Gesundheitministerium für Soziale Sicherheit und Generationen*, Ed) *Bundesministerium für Soziale Sicherheit und Generationen. Ältere Menschen – Neue Perspektiven, Seniorenbericht 2000*. (Zur Lebenssituation älterer Menschen in Österreich: Vienna, 2000.)
11. Douglas P, Poppas A. Determinants and management of cardiovascular risk in women. Wellesley (MA): Up To Date, 2002.
12. Peeters A, Mamun AA, Willekens F, Bonneux L. A cardiovascular life history, a life course analysis of the original Framingham Heart Study cohort. *Eur Heart J* 2002; **23:** 458–66.
13. Menhem K, Dotevall A, Wilhelmsen L, Rosengren A. Social gradients in cardiovascular risk factors and symptoms of Swedish men and women: the Goteborg Monica Study 1995. *J Cardiovasc Risk* 2000; **7:** 359–68.
14. Drivsholm T, Ibsen H, Schroll M et al. Increasing prevalence of diabetes mellitus and impaired glucose tolerance among 60-year-old Danes. *Diabetic Med* 2001; **18:** 126–32.

15. Kannel WB. Lipids, diabetes, and coronary heart disease: insights from the Framingham. *Am Heart J* 1985; **110:** 1100–7.

16. Stampfer MJ, Hu FB, Manson JE et al. Primary prevention of coronary heart disease in women through diet and lifestyle. *N Engl J Med* 2000; **343:** 16.

17. Tremollieres FA, Pouilles JM, Cauneille C, Ribot C. Coronary heart disease risk factors and menopause: a study in 1684 French women. *Atherosclerosis* 1999; **142:** 415–23.

18. Giampaoli S, Panico S, Meli P et al. Cardiovascular risk factors in women in menopause. *Ital Heart J* 2000; **1** (Suppl 9): 1180–7.

19. Schulte H, Cullen P, Assmann G. Obesity, mortality and cardiovascular disease in the Munster Heart Study (PROCAM). *Atherosclerosis* 1999; **144:** 199–209.

20. Sacker A, Bartley M, Firth D, Fitzpatrick R. Dimensions of social inequality in the health of women in England: occupational, material and behavioral pathways. *Soc Sci Med* 2001; **52:** 763–81.

21. Bergström A, Pisani P, Tenet V et al. Overweight as an avoidable cause of cancer in Europe. *Int J Cancer* 2001; **91:** 421–30.

22. Mackenbach J P, Kunst AE, Groenhof F et al. Socioeconomic inequalities in mortality among women and among men: an international study. *Am J Public Health* 1999; **89:** 1800–6.

23. Laditka J, Laditka S. The morbidity compression debate: risks, opportunities, and policy options for women. *J Women Aging* 2000; **12:** 23–38.

3

Menopausal changes of ovaries and hypothalamic–pituitary and cerebral function

AR Genazzani, F Bernardi, N Pluchino, C Ceccarelli and M Luisi

Introduction • Gonadal hormones and neurotrasmitters • Gonadal hormones, neuropeptides and the hypothalamic–pituitary axis • Gonadal hormones and neurosteroids: clinical implications in menopause • References

INTRODUCTION

The brain is one of the specific target tissues for sex steroid hormones. Estrogens, progestins and androgens are able to induce several effects in brain areas of the central nervous system (CNS), through the binding with specific receptors. The action of sex hormones is not limited to the regulation of endocrine functions and mating behavior: the identification of estrogen, progestin and androgen receptors outside the classical CNS regions, such as pituitary and hypothalamus, justifies their role in controling different brain functions. In particular, specific receptors for gonadal steroids have been localized in the amygdala, hippocampus, cortex basal forebrain, cerebellum locus coeruleus midbrain rafe nuclei, glial cells and central gray matter, confirming an involvement of sex hormones in controling wellbeing, cognitive functions and memory processes in physiological as well as in pathological conditions.[1–3]

The mechanism of action of these steroids in the CNS is similar to that observed in the peripheral target organs, producing both genomic and nongenomic effects. In the genomic mechanism, steroids induce relatively long-term actions on neurons by activating specific intracellular estrogen receptors (ERα and ERβ) that modulate gene transcription and protein synthesis. Thus, gonadal steroids modulate the synthesis, release and metabolism of many neuropeptides and neuroactive transmitters, and the expression of their receptors.[4] ERα and ERβ are differently expressed throughout the rat brain and there is anatomical evidence of distinct roles of each subtype. Hybridization histochemical studies have shown that both receptors are present in the rat cortex, pituitary and hypothalamus (ERα mostly in the arcuate and ventromedial nuclei, while ERβ is mostly present in the paraventricular and ventromedial nuclei), while the cerebellum expresses only ERα and the hippocampus expresses particulary ERβ.[5]

Moreover, sex steroids exert very rapid effects in the brain that cannot be attributed to genomic mechanisms.[2] These rapid nongenomic effects of steroids modulate electrical excitability, synaptic functioning and morphological features. Recently the specific cellular and molecular mechanisms underlying the nongenomic actions of estrogen have begun to be elucidated. Estrogen may utilize direct membrane mechanisms, such as activation of ligand-gated ion channels and G-protein-coupled second messenger systems and regulation of neurotransmitter transporters.[6,7] The existence of an estrogen receptor on the plasma membrane has been supported by experimental data since 1980. Original reports of a cell membrane protein that could bind and rapidly respond to 17β-estradiol (17βE2) are supported by the evidence that a putative membrane receptor could effect a variety of signal transduction events. Recent studies have shown that the nongenomic actions of 17βE2 can be mediated through this plasma membrane ER.[8]

The interaction of genomic and nongenomic mechanisms allows for the wide range of sex steroid actions in the regulation of cerebral function.[9] Additionally the genomic and nongenomic actions of estrogen have the potential to interact, producing synergistic effects.

In postmenopause, neurotransmitters, neuropeptides and neurosteroids undergo important changes as a consequence of the failure of gonadal hormone production, bringing on specific symptoms due to CNS derangement (Table 3.1). Hot flushes, sweating, obesity and hyper-

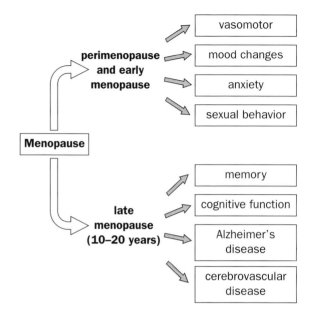

Figure 3.1   Menopause and brain function.

tension are consequences of the neuroendocrine changes in the hypothalamus. Mood changes, anxiety, depression, insomnia, headaches/migraine, alterations of cognitive function are all related to postmenopausal alterations of the limbic system (Fig. 3.1).[10]

This physiological model represents a unique opportunity to investigate the actions of gonadal hormones on their specific receptors in human reproductive organs, cardiovascular system, bone and CNS.[11,12]

GONADAL HORMONES AND NEUROTRANSMITTERS

Sex steroid hormones modulate the noradrenergic and dopaminergic systems at the hypothalamic level, as well as of the extrahypothalamic regions of the brain controling movement and behavior in both animals and humans. Animal studies show an increase of norepinephrine (NE) and dopamine turnover rates induced by estrogens during the proestrus period.[5,13] On the other hand, in castrated female rats an impairment of catecholaminergic neurons has been demonstrated, with an increase in noradrenaline and a decrease in dopamine release.[13]

Table 3.1   Neuropeptide and neurotransmitter levels in postmenopausal women before and after hormone replacement therapy (HRT) administration

	Postmenopause	After HRT
Serotonin	↓	↑
Acetylcholine	↓	↑
Dopamine	↓	↑
Catecholamine	↑	↓
β-Endorphin	↓	↑
Galanine	↓	↑
Neuropeptide Y	↓	↑
Melatonin	↓	?
Neurosteroids	↓	↑

Estrogens administration decreases NE hypothalamic release, while an increase in dopaminergic neuronal activity with a parallel increase in dopamine release in the mediobasal hypothalamus has been shown.[13,14] Regarding the modulation of the different subtypes of adrenergic receptors, in vitro studies suggest that estrogens upregulate α1-adrenergic and downregulate β-adrenergic receptors activity.[15]

Few data are available regarding the effects of progesterone and progestins in experimental or clinical models on the catecholaminergic system: studies in ovariectomized female rats have demonstrated a suppression of the estrogen effects on the pineal gland noradrenergic neurons when progesterone administration was associated.[16] In an animal model, estradiol and progesterone enhance noradrenaline release, leading to increased excitability of ventromedial hypothalamus neuronal activity and to the expression of lordosis behavior.[16] Early studies show that NE turnover and content within the hypothalamus fluctuates in response to gonadal steroid manipulations, indicating that estrogen and progesterone may regulate the activity of NE neurons.[17–19] Indeed, more recent studies in rats have shown that it excites an increase in NE release within the preoptic area on proestrus,[19,20] in the progesteron receptor (PR) expression in NE neurons of the caudal brainstem[21] and in the ability of estrogen to directly upregulate PR gene expression in these neurons.[21] These observations support the hypothesis that the change in gonadal steroids may underlie the ability of estrogen and progesterone to alter NE transmission within the hypothalamus and elsewhere in the brain.[21]

The serotoninergic system is also modulated by the endogenous gonadal hormones. Several findings indicate a gender difference in central serotoninergic pattern: female rats have elevated synthesis, turnover rate and concentration of serotonin in the hypothalamus, cortex, hippocampus, forebrain and raphe compared with values of male rats.[22] Cerebral serotonin concentration and activity are modified during the estrus cycle and in periods characterized by ovarian hormones fluctuations.[23] Estrogens, progesterone or combined treatments in ovariectomized rats positively affect the serotonoinergic system.[24] Estrogens also modify the concentration and availability of serotonin by increasing the degradation rate of monoamino oxidase (MAO), the enzyme that catabolizes serotonin.[25] Experimental data have demonstrated that estrogen displaces tryptophan from its binding sites to plasma albumin; thus more tryptophan is available in the brain to be metabolized into serotonin.[26] Finally, estrogen enhances the transport of serotonin. On the contrary, progesterone is able to increase the MAO concentration in the brain.[27,28]

A positive relationship between circulating levels of estradiol and mood has been demonstrated.[29] A large number of studies concerning the effects of hormone replacement therapy (HRT) on climacteric depression have shown a significant amelioration of mood in depressed postmenopausal women treated with estrogen.[30–32] These positive effects may be related to the direct effect on neural activity, and to the modulation of both adrenergic and serotoninergic tone.

Recently, several lines of evidence have suggested that estrogen may also be important in the protection of the central cholinergic system, which is intimately involved in memory and cognition. Normal aging is associated with a reduction in cholinergic functional markers, such as choline acetyltransferase (ChAT), but a relative preservation of cholinergic cells and terminals.[33]

Studies in experimental animals have suggested that estrogen may influence brain function by effects on the cholinergic system. Receptors for gonadal hormones have been identified in the nuclei of the basal forebrain, the major source of cholinergic innervation to the cerebral cortex, hippocampus and hypothalamus.[34] Estrogen is known to provide trophic support to cholinergic cells and to regulate various markers of cholinergic function, including ChAT and acetylcholine release.[35] Concerning the trophic effect of estrogens on CNS, in addiction to the cholinergic system, it is interesting to note that estrogen and intranuclear estrogen binding sites colocalize and regulate the expression of neurotropins such as nerve growth factor, its receptor tropomyosin-related kinase A (trkA), and brain-derived neurotropic factor.[36] Therefore, estrogens are involved in regulating neuronal survival, regeneration and plasticity.[36]

Alzheimer's disease (AD) is associated with severe reductions in ChAT and diffuse degeneration of cholinergic terminals, which is more prominent in the temporal lobes.[37] Epidemiological data indicate that postmenopausal hormone therapy may reduce the risk or delay the onset of Alzheimer's disease; however, the neurochemical substrates involved in this decreased risk are unknown.[38,39] Therefore these data suggest that estrogen therapy may be beneficial in the prevention of AD but not necessarily in the treatment of established cognitive impairment. Postmenopausal estrogen replacement therapy (ERT) in healthy women is associated with an improvement or reservation of various cognitive functions,[40,41] with a reduction of cognitive decline in memory-impaired postmenopausal women[42] and an improved effectiveness of tacrine, a cholinesterase enzyme inhibitor used in the treatment of AD.[43]

Furthermore, sex steroids influence growth proteins that are associated with axonal elongation and promote synapse formation, particularly in the CA1 region of the hippocampus, an important area for memory processes.[44] Estrogen may also blunt neurotoxic effects of β-amyloid by promoting the breakdown of the amyloid precursor protein.[45]

GONADAL HORMONES, NEUROPEPTIDES AND THE HYPOTHALAMIC–PITUITARY AXIS

At the hypothalamic level, the principal target of sex steroid hormones for the modulation of the reproductive function are the group of neurons producing the pulsatile release of the gonadotropin-releasing hormone (GnRH), localized in the mediobasal hypothalamus and the arcuate nucleus. GnRH release depends upon the complex and the coordinated interrelationships among these peptides, the gonadal steroids and other neurotrasmitter systems, such as the dopaminergic, opiatergic and noradrenergic systems.[46] The interplay of these con-

trol mechanism is governed by feedback mechanisms of peripheral signals; in addition, signals from the higher brain centers could modify GnRH secretion. Regarding the role exerted directly by gonadal hormones on GnRH neuronal activity, estradiol treatment of castrated female rats induces no changes on hypothalamic GnRH, while progesterone treatment induces an increase of the stored decapeptide, suggesting a stimulatory action of progesterone at the hypothalamic level.[46,47] The final effects of the steroid hormones on GnRH synthesis and release occur directly on the gonadotropic neurons, and also indirectly mediated by the influence other neuroendocrine systems and neuroactive trasmitters.[48]

Among those neuropeptides regulated by gonadal steroids, endogenous opioids exert inhibitory or excitatory signals on GnRH hypothalamic neurons. Estrogens directly modulate endogenous opioid activity and directly stimulate the opioid receptor expression. In particular, attention is focused on β-endorphin (β-EP), the most important and biologically active endogenous opioid peptide, which exerts behavioral, analgesic, thermoregulatory and neuroendocrine properties.

Circulating modifications of β-EP levels may be considered markers of neuroendocrine function.[28,29] A decrease in plasma β-EP levels has been detected in postmenopausal women after surgical or spontaneous menopause,[49] and it has been suggested to have a role in the mechanisms of hot flushes and sweating episodes.[50,51] The decrease in plasma β-EP levels has also been related to the pathogenesis of mood, behavior and nociceptive disturbances occurring in this period.[51,52] Indeed, a positive role of HRT on vasomotor and subjective psychobehavioral symptoms may be mediated by acting on the opiatergic pathway.[53] In fact, oral ERT subsequent to spontaneous or surgically induced menopause is followed by a significant increase in circulating β-EP levels.[53]

Concerning the effects of progestins on β-EP, it has been demostrated in ovariectomized female rats that the administration of norethisterone acetate (NETA) or norgestimate increases hypothalamic and circulating β-EP, while medroxyprogesterone acetate or desogestrel do not induce significant changes.[54–56]

The administration of transdermal estradiol, independent of the type of progestin used, induces a significant increase in plasma β-EP levels to premenopausal values.[57] In addition, the lack of response to clonidine (an α_2-presynaptic receptor agonist) and naloxone (an opiate receptor antagonist) in postmenopausal women suggests an impairment of adrenergic and opiatergic receptors in modulating β-EP release. HRT restores basal plasma β-EP levels to those present in fertile women as shown by the response of β-EP to naloxone and clonidine tests.[58]

Moreover, recent studies have described that both raloxifene hydrochloride, a selective estrogen modulator (60 mg/day), and dehydroepiandrosterone (DHEA) administration are able to increase in circulating β-EP and to restore the response of β-EP to clonidine, fluoxetine and naloxone administration, showing that both compounds have an estrogen-like effect on neuroendocrine pathways in postmenopausal women.[59,60]

In addition to β-EP, other neuropeptides such as neuropeptide Y (NPY) and galanin, modulated by gonadal steroids, regulate neuroendocrine functions by the pulsatile release of GnRH and gonadotropins, and regulate nutrient intake by influencing the appetite and satiety center in the hypothalamus.[61] Estrogen is able to stimulate NPY synthesis and release in the hypothalamus. In castrated female rats, gonadal steroid deficiency reduces neurosecretion of NPY-producing neurons.[11] Postmenopausal women show lower NPY plasma levels than young women.[62] Estrogens increase NPY content in the median eminence, and the synthesis of NPY in arcuate nucleus, by inducing NPY gene expression. Indeed, recent findings demonstrate several interactions between NPY and β-EP neurons in the hypothalamus, therefore both estrogens and progestogens may indirectly exert modulatory effects on NPY, thus inducing β-EP release.[63]

Galanin, a 29 amino acid neuropeptide, has been localized in the anterior pituitary gland of rats and humans. Galanin is released in the circulation in pulsatile way and it positively influence luteinzing hormone (LH) secretion. Hypophyseal galanin synthesis is under the control of the sex steroid hormones, particularly the estrogens. Galanin concentration is significatly lower in postmenopausal women than in young women.[64] HRT increases galanin levels but does not restore them to typical concentrations of women of reproductive ages.[65,66] An important action of galanin is to stimulate prolactin release through the inhibition of dopamine hypothalamic release, which inhibits, under basal conditions, lactotrope function. Moreover, significantly increased galanin levels in postmenopausal obese women, coupled with decreased NPY levels, reveal some changes in the neuropeptides regulating eating behavior, which may have an effect on the onset of postmenopausal obesity.[62]

Melatonin is synthesized by the pineal gland, and both synthesis and secretion follow a circadian rhythm, with low rates of production and release during the day and high rates of production and release at night.[67] Several studies show antioxidant property of melatonin.[68] The administration of a physiologic dose of melatonin to female senescence-accelerated mice prevents age-related oxidative DNA damage in the brain.[69] Moreover, melatonin administration in humans synchronizes endogenous rhythms to environmental cycles,[70] favors a propensity to sleep, enhances LH and prolactin (PRL) secretion, and reduces body temperature.[71] In hypertensive individuals, melatonin has been reported to reduce blood pressure[72] and, more recently, in young men and women, to decrease blood pressure and the internal carotid artery pulsatility index (PI).[73,74] Several lines of evidence indicate that aging influences the secretion of and biological responses to melatonin. Aging reduces the circulating levels of the hormone and so reduces the number of melatonin receptors in animals.[75] Since the identification of gonadal steroid receptors in the rat pineal gland, much evidence has suggested that melatonin synthesis may be modulated by the gonadal steroids.[76] However, in humans, the effect of gonadal steroids on pineal secretion of melatonin remains controversial: the effects of estrogen on pineal function varies markedly, depending on the species, the dose of estrogen and the duration of estrogen administration.[77] Moreover, gonadal steroids modulate the number of melatonin receptors in animals, and influence LH and cortisol responses to exogenous melatonin in humans.[78,79]

GONADAL HORMONES AND NEUROSTEROIDS: CLINICAL IMPLICATIONS IN MENOPAUSE

The term *neurosteroids* is applied to those steroids that are formed and accumulate in the nervous system from cholesterol precursors, and, at least in part, do so independently of peripheral steroidogenic glands secretion.[80] Several studies have shown that some psychological functions and symptoms such as depression, anxiety and irritability can be related to the fluctuation of the synthesis and release of neurosteroids, in particular allopregnanolone and DHEA.[81–83] Allopregnanolone is a 3-α, 5-α reduced metabolite of progesterone:[84] the major sources of production are the gonads and adrenal cortex, more so than the CNS.[85] Allopregnanolone acts as an agonist on gamma-aminobutyric acid A (GABA$_A$) receptor, modulating stress, mood and behavior.[86,87] Ovariectomy determines an increased adrenal allopregnanolone content and a reduction of allopregnanolone levels in brain and serum: this event could be explained by the effects of estrogens on the enzymes involved in the synthesis of allopregnanolone.[88–90] On the other hand, 17β-estradiol administration induces a rise in allopregnanolone in the rat hypothalamus, hippocampus, pituitary and serum, and a reduction in its adrenal content.[88] In postmenopausal women, plasma levels of allopregnanolone are similar to follicular phase levels of fertile women.[91] In addition, recent data seem to confirm that the effects of allopregnanolone on GABA$_A$ receptors are influenced by ovarian hormones:[92] estrogen and progesterone may regulate GABAergic responses, and the synthesis and turnover of GABA$_A$ receptors through a long-term genomic action.[93] The present

authors' recent (unpublished) data demonstrate that HRT is able to modify neurosteroid levels in postmenopausal women, leading to an increase in allopregnanolone levels and a decrease in DHEA levels.

The modulation exerted by HRT on allopregnanolone levels might be related to the anxiolitic and sedative effects of HRT in menopause women. On the other hand, it is difficult to explain the role of decreased DHEA levels in response to HRT.

DHEA and its sulfate ester (DHEAS) are the major circulating products of the adrenal glands, the principal source of these steroids. About 20% of DHEA is also produced by ovarian thecal cells under the control of LH and by the CNS, as indicated by the data obtained from ovariectomized and adrenalectomized rats.[94–96] DHEA levels decrease in the third decade of life, independent of the menopausal transition, reaching 20% of the maximum plasma concentration after 70 years of age.[97] Studies performed in postmenopausal women suggest that the reduction of adrenal 17,20-desmolase activity may provoke the decline in DHEA synthesis and secretion.[98] Experimental data suggest that DHEA exerts its effects on the CNS through antagonist action on GABA$_A$ receptors in a dose-dependent manner, with a consequent increase in neuronal excitability.[99] In this way, DHEA is able to improve physical and psychological wellbeing and memory performances in the elderly.[100] In fact, DHEA treatment induces, in animals, memory-enhancing effects: an in vitro study suggested a neurotrophic effect on neurons and glial cells.[101] On the other hand, DHEA administration in rats is able to increase both allopregnanolone and DHEA circulating levels (unpublished data). Some studies have focused on replacement therapy with DHEA in postmenopausal women, demonstrating improvements in sexual and mood disorders, neuroendocrine dysfunction, and metabolic and bone mass effects.[102–105] In addition, DHEA 50 and 25 mg/day promote a sense of wellbeing, and induce endocrinological changes including not only the increase of Δ5- and Δ4-androgens but also a boost in estrogen levels.[106] These endocrinological modifications appear to be in

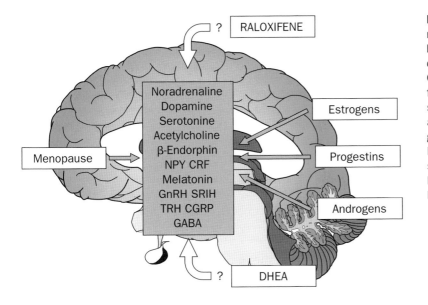

Noradrenaline
Dopamine
Serotonine
Acetylcholine
β-Endorphin
NPY CRF
Melatonin
GnRH SRIH
TRH CGRP
GABA

RALOXIFENE

Menopause

Estrogens

Progestins

Androgens

DHEA

Figure 3.2 Neuropeptides and neurotransmitters are modulated by sex hormones. (CGRP, calcitonin gene-related peptide; CRF, corticotrophin-releasing factor; DHEA, dehydroepiondrosterone; GABA, gamma-aminobutyric acid; GnRH, gonadotropin-releasing hormone; NPY, neuropeptide Y; SRIH, somatoprophin release-inhibiting hormone; TRH, TSH-releasing hormone.

a supraphysiological range at a dose of DHEA 50 mg/day, while at DHEA 25 mg/day they enter a physiological range (unpublished data).[106]

Moreover, recent studies have described that raloxifene hydrochloride administration 60 mg/day is able to increase in plasma allopregnanolone levels. Although the fluoxetine test before therapy failed to show an increase in the release of allopregnanolone, the same test after 6 months of raloxifene administration was characterized by a significant release of allopregnanolone.[59]

In conclusion, mood changes, sweating, anxiety, depression, insomnia and alterations of cognitive functions are some possible clinical consequences of the reduced regulatory effects exerted by gonadal and adrenal hormones on neurotransmitters and neuropeptides in postmenopausal women (Fig. 3.2).[107–109] Certainly, the evidence that gonadal steroids modulate neurosteroids levels open new possibilities in the study of neuroendocrinological menopause-related changes.

REFERENCES

1. Genazzani AR, Petraglia F, Purdy RH, eds. *The Brain: Source and Target for Sex Steroid Hormones.* (Parthenon Publishing, Carnforth UK, 1996.)

2. Speroff L, Glass RH, Kase NH. (eds) *Clinical Gynecological, Endocrinology and Infertility,* 5th edn. (Baltimore, MD: Williams & Wilkins, 1995.)

3. Sherwin BB. Estrogen effects on cognition in menopausal women. *Neurology* 1997; **48:** 21–6.

4. Alonso-Soleis R, Abreu P, Leopez-Coviella I et al. Gonadal steroid modulation of neuroendocrine transduction: a transynaptic view. *Cell Molec Neurobiol* 1996; **3:** 357–82.

5. Couse JF, Lindzey J, Grandien K et al. Tissue distribution and quantitative analysis of estrogen receptor-alpha (ERalpha) and estrogen receptor-beta (ERbeta) messenger ribonucleic acid in the wild-type and ERalpha-knockout mouse. *Endocrinology* 1997; **138:** 4613–21.

6. Wong M, Thompson TL, Moss RL. Non-genomic actions of estrogen in the brain: physiological significance and cellular mechanisms. *Crit Rev Neurobiol* 1996; **10:** 189–203.

7. Kelly MJ, Lagrange AH, Wagner EJ, Ronnekleiv OK. Rapid effects of estrogen to modulate G protein-coupled receptors via activation of protein kinase A and protein kinase C pathways. *Steroids* 1999; **64:** 64–75.

8. Levin ER. Cellular functions of the plasma membrane estrogen receptor. *Trends Endocr Metab* 1999; **10:** 374–7.

9. Fuxe K, Gustafsson JA, Wetterberg L. *Steroid Hormone Regulation of the Brain.* (Pergamon, Oxford, 1981) 27–56.

10. Panay N, Sands RH, Studd JWW. Estrogen and

behaviour. In: (Genazzani AR, Petraglia F, Purdy RH, eds) *The Brain: Source and Target for Sex Steroid Hormones*. (Parthenon Publishing: Carnforth UK, 1996) 257–76.

11. Karla SP. Gonadal steroid hormones promote interactive communication. In: (Genazzani AR, Petraglia F, Purdy RH, eds) *The Brain: Source and Target for Sex Steroid Hormones*. (Parthenon Publishing: Carnforth, UK, 1996), 257–76.

12. Matsumoto A. Synaptogenic action of sex steroids in developing and adult neuroendocrine brain. *Psychoneuroendocrinology* 1991; **16**: 25–40.

13. Etgen AM, Karkanias GB. Estrogen regulation of noradrenergic signaling in the hypothalamus. *Psychoneuroendocrinology* 1994; **19**: 603–10.

14. Ansonoff MA, Etgen AM. Evidence that oestradiol attenuates beta-adrenoceptor function in the hypothalamus of female rats by altering receptor phosphorylation and sequestration. *J Neuroendocr* 2000; **12**: 1060–6.

15. Herbison AE, Simonian SX, Thanky NR, Bicknell RJ. Oestrogen modulation of noradrenaline neurotransmission. *Novartis Found Symp* 2000; **230**: 74–85.

16. Herbison AE. Multimodal influence of estrogen upon gonadotropin-releasing hormone neurons. *Endocr Rev* 1998; **19**: 302–30.

17. Honma K, Wuttke W. Norepinephrine and dopamine turnover rates in the medial preoptic area and the mediobasal hypothalamus of the rat brain after various endocrinological manipulations. *Endocrinology* 1980; **106**: 1848–53.

18. Demling J, Fuchs E, Baumert W, Wuttke W. Preoptic catecholamine, GABA, and glutamate release in ovariectomized and ovariectomized estrogen-primed rats utilizing a push–pull cannula technique. *Neuroendocrinology* 1985; **41**: 212–18.

19. Wise PM, Rance N, Barraclough CA. Effects of estradiol and progesterone on catecholamine turnover rates in discrete hypothalamic regions in ovariectomized rats. *Endocrinology* 1981; **108**: 2186–93.

20. Mohankumar PS, Thyagarajan S, Quadri SK. Correlations of catecholamine release in the medial preoptic area with proestrous surges of luteinizing hormone and prolactin: effects of aging. *Endocrinology* 1994; **135**: 119–26.

21. Haywood SA, Simonian SX, van der Beek EM et al. Fluctuating estrogen and progesterone receptor expression in brainstem norepinephrine neurons through the rat estrous cycle. *Endocrinology* 1999; **140**: 3255–63.

22. Dickinson SL, Curzon G. 5-Hydroxytryptamine-mediated behavior in male and female rats. *Neuropharmacology* 1986; **25**: 771–6.

23. Biegon A, Bercovitz H, Samuel D. Serotonin receptor concentration during the estrous cycle of the rat. *Brain Res* 1980; **187**: 221–5.

24. Mendelson SD, McKittrick CR, McEwen BS. Autoradiographic analyses of the effects of estradiol benzoate on (³H)-paroxetine binding into the cerebral cortex and dorsal hippocampus of gonadectomized male and female rats. *Brain Res* 1993; **601**: 299–301.

25. Luine VN, McEwen BS. Effect of estradiol on turnover of Type A monoamine oxidase in the brain. *J Neurochem* 1977; **28**: 1221–7.

26. Bethea CL, Lu NZ, Gundlah C, Streicher JM. Diverse actions of ovarian steroids in the serotonin neural system. *Front Neuroendocr* 2002; **23**: 41–100.

27. Sherwin BB. Progestogens used in menopause. Side-effects, mood and quality of life. *J Reprod Med* 1999; **44**: 227–32.

28. Luine VN, Rhodes JC. Gonadal hormone regulation of MAO and other enzymes in hypothalamic areas. *Neuroendocrinology* 1983; **36**: 235–41.

29. Studd JWW, Smith RNJ. Estrogen and depression in women. *Menopause* 1994; **1**: 33–7.

30. Best N, Rees M, Barlow D et al. Effect of estradiol implants on noradrenergic function and mood in menopausal patients. *Psychoneurendocrinology* 1992; **17**: 87–93.

31. Montgomery JC, Appleby L, Brincat M et al. Effect of oestrogen and testosterone implants on psychological disorders in the climacteric. *Lancet* 1987; **1**: 297–9.

32. Limouzin-Lamothe MA, Mairon N, Joyce CR, Le Gal M. Quality of life after the menopause: influence of hormonal replacement therapy. *Am J Obstet Gynecol* 1994; **170**: 618–24.

33. Decker MW. The effects of aging on hippocampal and cortical projections of the forebrain cholinergic system. *Brain Res Rev* 1987; **12**: 423–35.

34. Toran-Allerand CD. The estrogen/neurotrophin connection during neural development: is co-localization of estrogen receptors with the neurotrophins and their receptors biologically relevant? *Dev Neurosci* 1996; **18**: 36–48.

35. McMillan PJ, Singer CA, Dorsa DM. The effects of ovariectomy andestrogen replacement on trkA and choline acetyltransferase mRNA expression in the basal forebrain of the adult

female Sprague–Dawley rat. *J Neurosci* 1996; **16:** 1860–5.

36. Luine V, Park D, Joh T et al. Immunochemical demonstration of increased choline acetyltransferase concentration in rat preoptic area after estradiol administration. *Brain Res* 1980; **191:** 273–7.

37. Kuhl DE, Koeppe RA, Minoshima S et al. In vivo mapping of cerebral cetylcholinesterase activity in aging and Alzheimer's disease. *Neurology* 1999; **52:** 691–9.

38. Baldereschi M, DiCarlo A, Lepore V. Estrogen replacement therapy and Alzheimer's disease in the Italian Longitudinal Study on Aging. *Neurology* 1998; **50:** 996–1002.

39. Birge SJ. The role of estrogen in the treatment of Alzheimer's disease. *Neurology* 1997; **48:** S36–S41.

40. Kampen DL, Sherwin BB. Estrogen use and verbal memory in healthy postmenopausal women. *Obstet Gynecol* 1994; **83:** 979–83.

41. Kimura D. Estrogen replacement therapy may protect against intellectual decline in postmenopausal women. *Horm Behav* 1995; **39:** 312–21.

42. Costa MM, Reus VI, Wolkowitz OM et al. Estrogen replacement therapy and cognitive decline in memory-impaired post-menopausal women. *Biol Psychiatry* 1999; **46:** 182–8.

43. Schneider LS, Farlow M. Combined tacrine and estrogen replacement therapy in patients with Alzheimer's disease. *Ann NY Acad Sci* 1997; **826:** 317–22.

44. McEwen BS, Alves SE, Bulloch K, Weiland NG. Ovarian steroids and the brain: implications for cognition and aging. *Neurology* 1997; **48:** 8–15.

45. Greenfield JP, Leung LW, Cai D et al. Estrogen lowers Alzheimer beta-amyloid generation by stimulating trans-Golgi network vesicle biogenesis. *J Biol Chem* 2002; **5:** 12,128–36.

47. Zanisi M, Messi E. Sex steroid and the control of LHRH secretion. *J Steroid Biochem Molec Biol* 1991; **40:** 155–63.

48. Zanisi M, Galbiati M, Messi E. The multiple inputs to the LHRH neurons. In: (Genazzani AR, Petraglia F, Nappi G, Montemagno U, eds) *Neuroendocrinology of Female Reproductive Function.* (Parthenon Publishing Group: Pearl River (NY), 1993) 33–41.

49. Genazzani AR, Petraglia F, Facchinetti F et al. Steroid replacement increase beta-endorphin and beta-lipotropin plasma levels in postmenopausal women. *Gynecol Obstet Invest* 1988; **26:** 153–9.

50. Aleem FA, McIntosh T. Menopausal syndrome: plasma levels of β-endorphin in postmenopausal women using a specific radioimmunoassay. *Maturitas* 1985; **13:** 76–84.

51. Genazzani AR, Petraglia F, Facchinetti F et al. Increase of proopiomelanocortin-related peptides during subjective menopausal flushes. *Am J Obstet Gynecol* 1984; **149:** 775–9.

52. Lightman SL, Jacobs HS, Maguire AK, et al. Climacteric flushing: clinical and endocrine response to infusion of naloxone. *Br J Obstet Gynecol* 1981; **88:** 919–24.

53. Adler MW. Minireview: opioid peptides. *Life Sci* 1980; **261:** 496–510.

54. Donouhe TL, Dorse DM. The opiomelanotropinergic neuronal and endocrine system. *Peptides* 1982; **3:** 383–95.

55. Genazzani AR, Petraglia F, Cleva M. et al. Norgestimate increases pituitary and hypothalamic concentrations of immunoreactive beta-endorphin. *Contraception* 1989; **5:** 605–13.

56. Genazzani AR, Petraglia F, Mercuri N et al. Effect of steroid hormones and antihormones on hypothalamic beta-endorphin concentrations in intact and castrated female rats. *J Endocr Invest* 1990; **13:** 91–6.

57. Stomati M, Bersi C, Rubino S et al. Neuroendocrine effects of different estradiol–progestin regimens in postmenopausal women. *Maturitas* 1997; **28:** 127–35.

58. Petraglia F, Comitini G, Genazzani AR et al. β-Endorphin in human reproduction. In: (Herz A, ed) *Opiods II.* (Springer-Verlag: Berlin, 1993) 763–80.

59. Florio P, Quirici B, Casarosa E et al. Neuroendocrine effects of raloxifene hydrochloride in postmenopausal women. *Gynecol Endocr* 2001; **15:** 359–66.

60. Stomati M, Monteleone P, Casarosa E et al. Six-month oral dehydroepiandrosterone supplementation in early and late postmenopause. *Gynecol Endocr* 2000; **14:** 342–63.

61. Zarjevski N, Cusin I, Vettor R et al. Intracerebroventricular administration of neuropeptide Y to normal rats has divergent effects on glucose utilization by adipose tissue and skeletal muscle. *Diabetes* 1994; **43:** 764–9.

62. Milewicz A, Bidzinska B, Mikulski E et al. Influence of obesity and menopausal status on serum leptin, cholecystokinin, galanin and neuropeptide Y levels. *Gynecol Endocr* 2000; **14:** 196–203.

63. Milewicz A, Mikulski E, Bidzinska B. Plasma

insulin, cholecystokinin, galanin, neuropeptide Y and leptin levels in obese women with and without type 2 diabetes mellitus. *Int J Obes Relat Metab Disord* 2000; **24**: 152–3.

64. Baranowska B, Radzikowska M, Wasilewska-Dziubinska E et al. Relationship among leptin, neuropeptide Y, and galanin in young women and in postmenopausal women. *Menopause* 2000; **7**: 149–55.

65. Kaplan LM, Gabriel SM, Koenig JL et al. Galanin is an estrogen inducible secretory product of the rat anterior pituitary. *Proc Natl Acad Sci USA* 1988; **85**: 7408–12.

66. Meczekalski B, Slopien R, Warenik-Szymankiewicz A. Estimation of hormone replacement therapy influence on serum galanin level in postmenopausal women. *Climacteric* 2001; **4**: 215–18.

67. Reiter RJ. Pineal melatonin: cell biology of its synthesis and of its physiological interactions. *Endocr Rev* 1991; **12**: 151–80.

68. Reiter RJ. Oxidative damage in the central nervous system: protection by melatonin. *Prog Neurobiol* 1998; **56**: 359–84.

69. Morioka N, Okatani Y, Wakatsuki A. Melatonin protects against age-related DNA damage in the brains of female senescence-accelerated mice. *J Pineal Res* 1999; **27**: 202–9.

70. Lewy AJ, Sack RL. Exogenous melatonin's phase-shifting effects on the endogenous melatonin profile in sighted humans: a brief review and critique of the literature. *J Biol Rhythms* 1997; **12**: 588–94.

71. Zhdanova IV, Wurtman RJ, Efficacy of melatonin as a sleep-promoting agent. *J Biol Rhythms* 1997; **12**: 644–50.

72. Cagnacci A. Melatonin in relation to physiology in adult humans. *J Pineal Res* 1996; **21**: 200–13.

73. Birau N, Peterssen U, Meyer C, Gottschalk J. Hypotensive effect of melatonin in essential hypertension. *IRSC Med Sci* 1981; **9**: 906.

74. Cagnacci A, Arangino S, Angiolucci M et al. Influences of melatonin administration on the circulation of women. *Am J Physiol* 1998; **274**: 335–8.

75. Cagnacci A, Arangino S. Effect of exogenous melatonin on vascular reactivity and nitric oxide in postmenopausal women: role of hormone replacement therapy. *Clin Endocr* 2001; **54**: 261–6.

76. Viswanathan M, Laitinen JT, Saavedra JM. Differential expression of melatonin receptors in spontaneously hypertensive rats. *Neuroendocrinology* 1992; **56**: 864–70.

77. Arent J, Laud C, Symons AM, Pryde SJ. Plasma melatonin in ewes after ovariectomy. *J Reprod Fertil* 1983; **68**: 213–18.

78. Okatani Y, Morioka N, Wakatsuki A. Changes in nocturnal melatonin secretion in perimenopausal women: correlation with endogenous estrogen concentrations. *J Pineal Res* 2000; **28**: 111–18.

79. Cagnacci A, Soldani R, Yen SSC. Melatonin enhances cortisol levels in aged women: reversible by estrogens. *J Pineal Res* 1997; **22**: 81–5.

80. Akwa Y, Baulieu EE. Neurosteroids: behavioral aspects and physiological implications. *J Soc Biol* 1999; **193**: 293–8.

81. Mellon SH. Neurosteroids: action and clinical relevance. *J Clin Endocr Metab* 1994; **78**: 1003–8.

82. Majewska MD. Neurosteroids: endogenous bimodal modulators of the GABA A receptors. Mechanism of action and physiological significance. *Prog Neurobiol* 1992; **38**: 379–95.

83. Wolf OT, Neumann O, Helhammer DH et al. Effects of a two-week physiological dehydroepiandrosterone substitution on cognitive performance and well-being in healthy elderly women and men. *J Clin Endocr Metab* 1997; **82**: 2363–7.

84. Monteleone P, Luisi S, Tonetti A et al. Allopregnanolone concentrations and premenstrual syndrome. *Eur J Endocr* 2000; **142**: 269–73.

85. Palumbo MA, Salvestroni C, Gallo R et al. Allopregnanolone concentrations in hippocampus of prepubertal rats and female rats throughout estrous cycle. *J Endocr Invest* 1995; **18**: 853–6.

86. Schumacher M, Coirini H, McEwen BS. Regulation of high affinity GABA$_A$ receptors in the dorsal hippocampus by estradiol and progesteron. *Brain Res* 1989; **487**: 178–84.

87. Serra M, Pisu MG, Littera M et al. Social isolation-induced decreases in both the abundance of neuroactive steroids and GABA(A) receptor function in rat brain. *J Neurochem* 2000; **75**: 732–40.

88. Genazzani AR, Bernardi F, Stomati M, et al. Effects of estradiol and raloxifene analog on brain, adrenal and serum allopregnanolone content in fertile and ovariectomized female rats. *Neuroendocrinology* 2000; **72**: 162–70.

89. Lephart ED, Simpson ER, Trzeciak WH et al. Rat adrenal 5-alpha-reductase mRNA content and enzyme activity are sex hormone dependent. *J Molec Endocr* 1991; **6**: 163–70.

90. Laconi MR, Casteller G, Gargiulo PA et al. The anxiolytic effect of allopregnanolone is associated with gonadal hormonal status in female rats. *Eur J Pharmacol* 2001; **417:** 111–16.

91. Genazzani AR, Petraglia F, Bernardi F et al. Circulating levels of allopregnanolone in humans: gender, age and endocrine influences. *J Clin Endocr Metab* 1998; **83:** 2099–103.

92. Wilson MA. Influences of gender, gonadectomy and estrous cycle on GABA/BZ receptors and benzodiazepine responses in rats. *Brain Res Bull* 1992; **29:** 165–72.

93. Schumacher M, Coirini H, Robert F et al. Genomic and membrane actions of progesterone: implications for reproductive physiology and behavior. *Behav Brain Res* 1999; **105:** 37–52.

94. Yamaji T, Ibayashi H. Serum deydroepiandrosterone sulphate in normal and pathological conditions. *J Clin Endocr Metab* 1969; **29:** 273–8.

95. Parker LN, Odell WD. Control of adrenal androgen secretion. *Endocr Rev* 1980; **4:** 392–410.

96. Corpechot C, Robert P, Axelson M et al. Characterization and measurement of dehydroepiandrosterone sulfate in the rat brain. *Proc Natl Acad Sci USA* 1981; **78:** 4704–7.

97. Davis SR, Burger HG. Androgens and the postmenopausal woman. *Clin Rev J Clin Endocr Metab* 1996; **81:** 2759–63.

98. Utian WH. The true clinical features of postmenopausal oophorectomy and their response to estrogen replacement therapy. *S Afr Med J* 1972; **46:** 732–7.

99. Majewska MD, Demirgoren S, Spivak CE et al. The neurosteroid DHEA is an allosteric antagonist of the GABA A receptor. *Brain Res* 1990; **526:** 143–6.

100. Baulieu EE. Dehydroepiandrosterone: a fountain of youth? *J Clin Endocr Metab* 1996; **81:** 3147–51.

101. Thijssen JH, Nieuwenhuyse H. *DHEA: A Comprehensive Review* (Parthenon Publishing, Carnforth, UK, 1999.)

102. Rubino S, Stomati M, Bersi C et al. Neuroendocrine effect of a short-term treatment with DHEA in postmenopausal women. *Maturitas* 1998; **28:** 251–7.

103. Taelman P, Kayman JM, Janssens X et al. Persistence of increased bone-resumption and possible role of dehydroepiandrosterone as a bone metabolism determinant in osteoporotic women in late menopause. *Maturitas* 1989; **11:** 65–73.

104. Nordin BEC, Robertson A, Seamark RF. The relation between calcium absorption, serum DHEA and vertebral mineral density in postmenopausal women. *J Clin Endocr Metab* 1985; **60:** 651–7.

105. Wolkowitz OM, Reus VI, Roberts E et al. Dehydroepiandrosterone (DHEA) treatment of depression. *Biol Psychiatry* 1997; **41:** 311–18.

107. Genazzani AR, Petraglia F, Purdy RH (eds) *The Brain: Source and Target for Sex Steroid Hormones.* (Parthenon Publishing: Carnforth, UK, 1996.)

108. Ginzburg J, Hardiman P. Adrenergic agonist for menopausal complaints. In: (Genazzani AR, Montemagno U, Nappi C et al (eds) *The Brain and Female Reproductive Function.* (Parthenon Publishing: Carnforth UK, 1987) 623–5.

109. Melis G, Cagnacci A, Gambacciani M. Restoration of luteinizing hormone response to naloxone in postmenopausal women by chronic administration of the antidopaminergic drug veralipride. *J Clin Endocr Metab* 1988; **66:** 964–9.

4

Premenopausal cycle anomalies

M Neves-e-Castro

Introduction • **Symptoms** • **Clinical examination** • **Complementary examinations**
• **Contraception** • **Treatment** • **References**

INTRODUCTION

The important problems of premenopausal cycle anomalies can be discussed very pragmatically from a clinical perspective or they may be the basis for long speculative analysis of their etiopathogenesis. The purpose of this chapter is to emphasize the former, based, whenever possible, on information derived from the latter.

SYMPTOMS

Reported symptoms vary from longer to shorter, regular or irregular menstrual cycles, with scanty or heavy flows, or spotting or breakthrough bleeding, with or without dysmenorrhea. Between menstruation mucous vaginal discharges are also common, which may cause itching (in the absence of infections).

Many women suffer from vasomotor symptoms, e.g. hot flushes and night sweats, that are a cause of a compromised quality of life. Premenstrual tension (PMT) may also be exacerbated. Sensations of bloating and fluid retention are not uncommon. Other symptoms, e.g. emotional disturbances like changes in humor, irritability to depression, insomnia and/or decreased libido, also have unpleasant repercussions on the woman's quality of life. Last, but not least, the appearance of wrinkles and gray hair are triggers of major concerns about the beginning of aging, and decreased feminity, and attractiveness to a male partner.

Most of these symptoms are not necessarily related to the lack of estrogens that characterize the early and late postmenopausal period. On the contrary, what most studies have shown is that in the premenopausal years there is either a relative hyperestrogenism (due to luteal insufficiency) or an absolute hyperestrogenism (caused by persistent follicles that later undergo atresia without ovulating).

Estrogen plasma levels are very erratic: when they are high they may cause PMT, mastodynia or fluid retention, when they suddenly drop to lower levels (without reaching a hypoestrogenic state) this is perceived by the hypothalamus, which responds with vasomotor symptoms and sweating. This endocrine disturbance was termed the *perimenopausal endogenous ovarian hyperstimulative syndrome* by Prior.[1] The trigger seems to be a decrease in inhibin during the luteal phase of the menstrual cycle, as a result of which there is a sharp increase in follicle stimulating hormone (FSH) that hyperstimulates the ovarian follicles. Although many of the follicles may not grow very much, their granulose cells contribute to an overall increase in ovarian estrogen secretion, as mentioned above.

CLINICAL EXAMINATION

In practical terms one should consider a menstrual cycle disturbance as being characteristic of the premenopausal syndrome when it occurs after 45 years of age in a woman who previously had regular cycles. There are many possible causes of menstrual cycle disturbances other than those related to the premenopause that are basically related to ovarian aging.

It is well known that undernutrition or excessive weight, which may cause profound changes in the body mass index (BMI) and in the percentage of fat content, are frequent causes of ovarian dysfunction that are determinants of menstrual cycle irregularities. Therefore, the measurement of BMI and fat is essential.

The distribution of body hair is very important too, because it may be a sign of hyperandrogenism from an adrenal or ovarian origin (both tumoral or dysfunctional). This may often be associated with an oily skin, acne and male implantation of hair (front, hypogastrium, breast), i.e. from hypertrichosis to hirsutism.

A very dry skin, facial and pretibial edema may be signs of hypothyroidism, frequently present in the perimenopause. On the contrary, mild exophthalmoses, hot flushes and profuse sweating, or tachycardia, may be associated with hyperthyroidism. The pelvic examination is very informative to discard adnexal masses or uterine fibroids as causes of cycle irregularities. In their absence, inspection of the cervix will quickly negate a hypoestrogenic state when one sees an opened external os with flowing clear elastic mucus, a sign that indicates that a progestogen challenge test, if there was a delay of menstruation, will be positive. Inspection and palpation of the breasts is also mandatory.

COMPLEMENTARY EXAMINATIONS

Indispensable imaging techniques are the mammography (plus ultrasound scanning) and pelvic ultrasonography with a vaginal probe. Blood tests must include, in addition to a complete blood and platelet count, some tests of coagulation, fasting insulin and glucose, thyroid-stimulating hormone (TSH) and free thyroxin, [the sulphate ester of dehydroepiandrosterone (DHEAS) hydroxiprogesterone and testosterone, total and free, if there are signs of androgenism], urine analysis, and those carried out as routine. One can thus discard coagulation disorders, thyroid dysfunctions, insulin resistance and/or diabetes. A Pap smear test is essential, and an endometrial biopsy may be necessary.

CONTRACEPTION

If a woman is taking an oral contraceptive and complains of cycle irregularities then the chances are very high that she has a concomitant organic disease, either uterine or hematologic. The same may be the case if she has an intrauterine contraceptive device (IUCD) inserted. Therefore, in both cases, it is mandatory to exclude by all means available such possibilities.

However, many women do not take the Pill or have an IUCD fitted. For these women the onset of perimenopausal menstrual irregularities becomes more of a problem.

The beginning, or continuation, of low dose oral contraception is not necessarily contraindicated (in the absence of well-known contraindications) and may have the advantage, in addition to the contraceptive efficacy, to correct the underlying pituitary–ovarian dysfunction, to relieve symptoms, and protect the endometrium and breasts from hyperestrogenism. Furthermore, oral contraception may also be beneficial in protecting the vessel walls from atherogenesis when the menopause is reached. It is likely that there is still a good endothelium that will be protected by estrogens. However, in practical terms, the problem will be to decide when to stop the Pill if one does not want to go beyond an underlying occult menopause.

The suspension of oral contraception at a later age, e.g. 50 years, followed by FSH and estradiol assays to ascertain if physiologic primary ovarian failure has already occurred is not a safe guarantee. If this option is chosen then local contraception must be started because it is not unusual for a quiescent ovary to later become spontaneously reactivated and even ovulate.

An alternative method of contraception can be a progesterone-medicated IUCD. Besides having good efficacy it protects the endometrium from hyperplasia and does not interfere with ovarian function, thus allowing one to know when the menopause is reached. In addition, when it becomes necessary to treat the postmenopausal symptoms with estrogens its protection of the endometrium permits a much better estrogen-only treatment.

TREATMENT

Assuming that no other cause has been found for the premenstrual cycle anomalies, other than the premenopause in itself, treatment must be aimed at the correction of the symptoms and the prevention of breast and uterine pathology.

If no systemic contraception is required the objective is to correct luteal insufficiency and relative (or absolute) hyperestrogenism. This can be done with a cyclic (12–13 days/month) substitution with a progestogen. If the symptoms are also alleviated with this treatment one should go on every month until there is no more uterine bleeding, which means that the woman has become hypoestrogenic and has probably entered the menopause. Then is the time to start estrogen replacement therapy (ERT), without or with systemic or intrauterine progesterone depending on each case, but this is no longer the objective of present review.

Vasomotor symptoms can also be alleviated with serotonin reuptake inhibitors (e.g. fluoxetine) that have the additional advantages of improving mood and counteracting weight gain. Night sweats may also respond to gabapentin and vagolytic agents.

Last, but not least, the onset of premenopause cycle anomalies offer a very important opportunity to inform a woman about her upcoming menopause. Proper and timely education is the best way to avoid misconceptions that may be very traumatic in a woman's life.

It must be strongly emphasized that there is no reason to be afraid of a loss of libido and a poorer sex life. One should explain that, contrary to general belief, it is not breast cancer but heart disease that is the major cause of death in older women. Whereas breast cancer can be cured this is not the case with atherosclerosis, the consequent events of which can only be attenuated, hopefully, to a more or less steady state. Woman must be informed in depth about the importance of proper nutrition, cessation of smoking moderate alcohol consumption and aerobic exercise. Much to many women's surprise these measures and strategies, sometimes more than medications, have a profound influence on health maintenance and disease prevention.

Premenstrual cycle disturbances are no doubt important clinical problems that must be duly investigated and treated, usually for a short time. But what comes next, the postmenopause, is certainly far more important for a much longer time. Therefore, premenstrual cycle disturbances provide an important opportunity for the development of the woman–doctor relationship.

REFERENCES

Further reading

1. Bastian LA, Smith CM, Nanda K. Is this woman perimenopausal? *J Am Med Ass* 2003; **289:** 895–902.
2. French L. Approach to the perimenopausal patient. *J Family Practice* 2002; **51:** 271–6.
3. Neves-e-Castro M. Los últimos años de la Premenopausia. In: (Pérez-López FR, ed) *Climaterio Y Envejecimiento.* (Seisge, Zaragoza, 1999) 1–46.
4. Seifer DB, Naftolin F. Moving toward an earlier and better understanding of perimenopause. *Fertil Steril* 1998; **69:** 387–8.
5. Soares CN, Cohen LS. The perimenopause, depressive disorders, and hormonal variability. *Sao Paulo Med J* 2001; **119:** 78–83.
6. Taffe JR, Dennerstein L. Menstrual patterns leading to the final menstrual period. *Menopause* 2002; **9:** 32–40.

Scientific paper

1. Prior JC. Perimenopause: the complex endocrinology of the menopausal transition. *Endocr Rev* 1998; **19:** 397–428.

5

History of estrogen–progestogen replacement therapy

H Rozenbaum

Introduction • Discovery of endocrine activity of the ovaries • Menopause • Concept of hormone replacement therapy (HRT) • References

INTRODUCTION

Hormone replacement therapy (HRT) has been widely used during the last few decades. However, the idea of using hormones to treat women (or men) is linked to the physician's knowledge of the endocrine activity of the genital glands.

The first paper dealing especially with climacteric disorders appeared in 1776 and the first appearance of the term *menopause* occurred in 1821. The idea of using a 'substance' found in the testis first appeared in 1775, followed by the first human experimentation on humans in 1889. Opotherapy for women was first used in 1893 and the discovery of the chemical structure of estrogens occurred in the 1930s.

HRT as now understood began in the 1940s with the use of conjugated estrogens in the USA.

DISCOVERY OF ENDOCRINE ACTIVITY OF THE OVARIES

The relationship between menstruation and ovarian function was established in 1840 by Négrier d'Angers:

> Le flux menstruel est directement lié à une fonction des ovaires amenant tous les mois une vésicule de De Graaf à maturation.

Menstrual flow is directly linked to an ovarian function leading each month to the ripening of a De Graaf vesicle.

Halban (1870–1937), a Viennese gynecologist, showed that the menstruation in primates is dependent on ovarian function. In 1905, the word *oestrus* was used to describe the anatomical alterations induced by rutting in animals in *The Sexual Season of Mammals and the Relation of the Proestrum to Menstruation*, published by Walter Heape (Cambridge).

In 1912, Adier (Austria), and Fellner, Herrmann and Iscovesco (France), using organic solvents to prepare a fairly pure extract from sow ovaries, induced growth of rabbit and guinea-pig uteri.

Isolation and identification of estrogens

In 1923, Allen (1892–1943), a zoologist and anatomist, and Doisy (1893–1986), a biochemist, both from the Washington University School in St Louis (USA), induced a vaginal oestrus by injecting follicular fluid into castrated mice.[1] They called the active substance *folliculin*. The term *estrogen* was thereafter used to refer to any substance able to induce an oestrus in castrated animals.

In 1929, Allen et al isolated estrone, called

folliculin, from the follicular fluid of pigs, human placentae and urine of pregnant women. At the same time, Butenandt (Göttingen), in cooperation with Schoeller (Berlin), produced a raw oil extract (progynon) from sow ovaries.

In 1932 Butenandt discovered estrone's chemical structure. The same year, equilin and equilenin were isolated from the urine of pregnant mares and isolated from sow ovaries by McCorquodale et al.

Estriol was crystalized from the urine of pregnant women in 1929 by Marrian (London) and Doisy et al. Following the proposition of the Marrian group, the estrogenic hormones were given the trivial names of estradiol, estrone and estriol.

Production and synthesis of estrogens

In 1932, Girard and Sandulesco discovered how to extract estrone from urine.

Estradiol was obtained by Schwenk and Hildebrandt by estrone reduction in 1933. In 1935, Doisy obtained 11 mg of estradiol from 4 tons of sow's ovaries and considered it the main ovarian secretion. The partial synthesis of estradiol and estrone from cholesterol and dehydroepiandrosterone was performed by Inhoffen and Hohlweg (Berlin) in 1940. The total synthesis was achieved by Anner and Miescher (Basel) in 1948.

The synthesis of ethinylestradiol, the first orally effective estrogen, was realized by Inhoffen and Hohlweg in 1938: this estrogen is used mainly for oral contraception. Equilin and equilenin, conjugated estrogens, were extracted from the urine of pregnant mares in the 1930s (Zondek 1934; Girard et al 1932). Their use was approved by the American Food and Drug Administration (FDA) in 1942.

As estradiol was not orally active at this time, several derivatives active parenterally with a protracted effect were synthesized: estradiolbenzoate by Schwenk and Hildebrandt in 1933 and estradiolpropionate by Laqueur et al in 1948 and a crystaline depot preparation by Miescher.

In 1957, estradiol valerate was prepared, which was orally active and injectable with protacted effectiveness. Later, micronized estradiol, orally effective, was also available. Per- and transcutaneous methods of administration were in use by the 1970s.

Isolation and identification of progesterone

In 1889, Brown-Séquard showed that animals' ovaries secretion may be useful in therapy. Schokke (Zurich), a veterinary surgeon, observed that the persistence of the corpus luteum inhibited follicle development and ovulation in the cow.

In 1903, Fraenkel observed that removal of the corpus luteum inhibited the implantation of the ovum in the endometrium. Leo Leb (Philadelphia) observed that after removal of the corpus luteum ovulation occurred earlier in the guinea-pig. In 1910, Ancel and Bouin discovered the effect of the corpus luteum on the endometrium. In 1928, Corner and Allen maintained implantation of the ovum and gestation by corpus luteum extracts.

Production and synthesis of progesterone and progestogens

A crystaline preparation from lipid extract of corpus luteum was obtained for the first time in 1931 by Von Ruschig and Slotta (Breslau).

Isolation of progesterone was realized by four teams of chemists: Von Butenandt and Westphal (Schering), Slotta (IG Farber), Allen and Wintersteiner (Squibb) and Wettstein (Ciba). The name *progesterone* was chosen. At this time, progesterone was made from the ovaries of sows: 625 kg of ovaries from 50,000 sows were necessary to obtain 20 mg of pure progesterone. In 1940, Russel Marker (USA) discovered how to synthesize progesterone from diosgenine, a steroid contained in a Mexican tuberous herb named cabeza de negro.

Ethisterone, the first orally effective progestagen, was synthesized by Inhoffen and Hohlweg in 1938. *Norethisterone*, a progestogen still used worldwide, was synthesized by Djerassi in 1951. But this progestogen was not used immediately and in 1953 Colton discovered norethynodrel, used by Pincus in the first oral contraceptive. In fact, this progestogen was a prohormone converted in vivo to norethisterone. Numerous other progestogens were subsequently synthesized, e.g. lynestrenol and ethynodiol diacetate, which were, in fact, prohormones converted in vivo to norethisterone. All these progestogens were also able to induce androgenic effects when high doses were used.

More potent progestogens were synthesized in the 1960s, e.g. norgestrel, norgestrienone. These progestogens were also more androgenic.

At the same time, progestogens directly related to progesterone were discovered, e.g. dydrogesterone, a progesterone isomer, and the pregnane derivatives, e.g. chlormadinone acetate, medroxyprogesterone acetate, medrogestone. All of these progestogens were practically devoid of any androgenic effects.

In the 1970s, the removal of the methyl group at C19 resulted in the use of more potent progestogens also devoid of androgenic properties, the so-called norpregnane derivatives, e.g. promegestone, nomegestrol acetate and trimegestone. In addition, as for estradiol, a micronization process allowed the use of progesterone orally.

MENOPAUSE

Birth of a name

The term *menopause* made its first appearance in the French medical literature in 1821, in the preface of Gardanne's book *De la ménopause, ou de l'âge critique des femmes*.[2] Menopause was called 'cessatio menstruorum' by SD Titius in 1710, translated into French as 'la cessation des menstrues'. During the eighteenth century, the term *climacteric* was used both for men and women, as cited by Wilbush in 1981:

> The climacteric years are certain observable years which are supposed to be attended with some considerable change in the body; as the 7th year: the 21st, made of three times seven; the 49th made of seven times seven and so on: i.e. septennia. (Quincy J. 1730), Lexicon physico-medicum or a new medical dictionary explaining the difficult terms used

in several branches of the profession ... It is very probable that this came from Pythagoras who was very fond of the number seven.

Marshall Hall was apparently the first in England to apply this term to women in 1827.

The terminology used in English to describe the various stages of the cessation of menstruation was obviously borrowed from popular usage: 'dodging time' for the perimenopause, 'change of life' or 'turn of life' for the menopause. The terminology used in France during the late eighteenth and early nineteenth centuries was: 'la cessation des menstrues', 'le temps critique' or 'l'âge critique'.

In 1816, Gardanne introduced the term *menespausie*, which became menopause in 1821.[2] By the early 1840s the name menopause was known in England too, though it was not included in English medical dictionaries until the late 1880s.

Birth of a syndrome

Hippocrates believed that at the time of cessation of menstruation the moving of the uterus through the body toward the heart induced dizziness and suffocation, and that by moving to the head it could induce headache and hysteria. Hoffmann (1660–1742) a physician and chemist, described women of around 50 years of age to be inactive, becoming overweight, to be experiencing cardiac pain, and feelings heat on the back and the legs.

The first paper dealing especially with climacteric disorders appeared in 1776 in *The London Medical Observations and Inquiries*. Exerting a durable and wide influence, the paper by Fothergill presented the revolutionary idea that, far from being due to retained corrupt matter, the symptoms of the climacteric were mild ones due to plethora apart, largely iatrogenic, caused by 'use of improper medicines ... the bark administered very freely ... to no good purpose', emmenagogues, aloes, or other 'heating' purgatives, which caused piles, strangury, excessive uterine hemorrhage and 'pain in the loins'.

In the early nineteenth century the female climacteric received widespread attention in France. More than 30 doctoral theses dealing with the menopause were presented at the University of Paris between 1802 and 1830. In addition, four were presented in Montpellier and the same number in Strasbourg.

During the twentieth century several theories were proposed to explain the menopause syndrome. According to 'the blood theory of diseases of the change of life', disturbances of the climacteric were believed to be due to the retention of the blood otherwise lost in the menses. Some held that it caused a general plethora while others ascribed these disorders to local congestion of various organs.

Until the end of the eighteenth century, the catamenial flow was classically believed to serve as a venue for the excretion of 'peccant matter and morbid humour, sometimes acrimonious and malignant . . . whose retention never fails to be extremely injurious . . . to the constitution'. Well aware of their patients' self-indulgent licentious ways, doctors had long regarded many of the latters climacteric complaints as the result of their sybaritic lifestyle. Unable, to compete with beliefs which incriminated failure of excretion of poisons, previously 'purged' by the menses, accusations of 'de mauvais emploi de la vie' received but scant attention. High living, 'la profusion des mets', 'l'habitude de la bonne chère . . . (et) l'abus du vin', were the most frequent, almost routine, objects of medical disapproval and censure.

In the 1850s, Tilt rejected the 'blood theory' and offered instead a 'nervous theory'.[3,4] According to this English gynecologist, climacteric disturbances were due to an 'increased ovarian irritability previous to the subsidence of specific ovarian functions'. 'Diseases of the change of life', he later expounded, 'should be thought of as having their fons et origo in the ovaries whether their power be their own, or borrowed from the spinal cord. While involution is taking place, the ovaries disturb the viscera with which they have worked harmoniously for 30 years . . . I do not pretend to know the nature of this disturbing influence, but I suppose it is similar to that made manifest by the coming into power of the ovaries at puberty.'

In 1857, Tilt published the first epidemiological study ever performed on menopausal women.[3] He analyzed 500 climacteric women. Tilt vigorously advocated the use of sedative drugs instead of the abuse of alcohol. He pointed out the importance of many disturbances to the environment of the climacteric. Moreover, Tilt's ascription of many disturbances to the environment of the climacteric, when 'one by one snap the cords which anchor (a woman) to life. At 50 parents may have been gathered to the dust, children may have deserted the parental roof . . . (and) doubts rise whether with faded charms . . . she can possibly retain possession of her husband's affection', has since occupied many a sociologist.

During the last quarter of the nineteenth century, climacteric symptoms acquired a notoriety of not only 'having only a subjective existence' but of usually being trivial. Nonetheless, while identification of climacteric disturbances as but 'neurotic' disorders might not have been considered by many as misdiagnoses, failure to establish freedom from possible concurrent organic, at times ominous, disease had long been considered indefensible.

The influence of the intellectual revolution, wrought by objective studies of individual and group behavior, in the understanding of human mental processes and conduct had inadvertently also stimulated a number of aberrant views about menopause. The new interpretations offered by psychology and psychiatry as increasingly guided by environmental, social and cultural considerations, imperceptively, served to emphasize the duality of body and mind. Female ills became, inevitably, psychological ills, their organic aspects forgotten.

Concentrating attention on the emotional, social and behavioral facets of the climacteric has tended to divorce it from the life events of the menopausal transition. The menopausal syndrome, in this its latest form, has become just a disorder of middle life, with catamenial irregularities, not surprisingly, seldom if ever mentioned.

In 1869 gynecological study on menstruation

was reported by Krieger. Among this data, some observations were related with the cessation of the menses: genital atrophy, circulatory troubles, headache. Fat women were supposed to be less prone to these troubles than thin women. The menopause occurred earlier in women living in southern countries than in northern ones, and in women belonging to the lower social classes. These observations are still valid.

CONCEPT OF HORMONE REPLACEMENT THERAPY (HRT)

HRT for men

The concept of HRT was first imagined for men in 1775, when Théophile de Bordieu wrote: 'The specific substance found in the testis passes through the circulatory system. It may be possible in the future to compensate this substance insufficiency'.

In 1849, Arnold A Berthold, a physiologist, carried out the first testis transplantation in a castrated rooster. In 1889, Charles-Edouard Brown-Séquard, a well-known French doctor and physiologist, carried out the first human experimentation: he administered to himself, by the use of subcutaneous injections, a liquid extracted from the testes of guinea-pigs and dogs.

In 1920, Eugen Steinach, director of the Department of Experimental Biology at the Vienna Academy of Science, promoted the idea of rejuvenation of people through an operation of the puberty glands. In fact, he actually performed a vasectomy. Steinach was dismissed under the Nazi regime.

HRT for women

Opotherapy
The first opotherapy, using ovarian extracts, was used by Régis de Bordeaux in 1893 to treat 'madness induced by castration'.

Several opotherapy techniques were used during the following years: hatched fresh ovaries, ovarian powder obtained by desiccation, ovarian liquid. In 1896, Mond and Mainzer from Germany and Chrobak from Austria treated the climacteric complaints of castrated women with ovarian extracts.

Modern times
Modern HRT began with the discovery and the synthesis of estrogens. The idea of prevention of the climacteric syndrome by the administration of estrogens was first mentioned by Geist and Spielman in 1932. In 1948, Albright and Reifenstein hinted at the idea of osteoporosis prevention by the administration of sex hormones. However, it was Wilson et al[5] who recognized, in 1963, that the decrease in ovarian function leads not only to climacteric complaints but also to a whole series of degenerative processes which can be prevented by administration of estrogens. Robert Wilson later expanded on his ideas in a book for lay people, *Feminine Forever*, published in the UK and the USA in 1966.[6] The publication was warmly received by women's magazines, firstly in the USA and later in Europe, and in particular in Germany.

The first medical meeting on HRT was held by the International Health Foundation in Geneva in 1971. During the following years, HRT was already regarded as a regular part of medical practice. In continental Europe, there was a positive attitude towards the treatment of the menopause syndrome. Developments in the UK followed those on the continent but with a certain delay. In 1975, the publication of *No Change* by W Cooper, a book for lay readers, stimulated interest in HRT.

The International Menopause Society was founded in 1978 in Jerusalem. The French Menopause Society – Association Française pour l'Etude de la Ménopause (AFEM) – founded in 1979, was the first national menopause society. The European Menopause Society was founded in 1990, in Nice, France. The Federation of European Menopause Societies was founded in 1999 in Paris.

REFERENCES

1. Allen E, Doisy E. An ovarian hormone: preliminary report on its localization, extraction and

partial purification and action in test animals. *J Am Med Ass* 1923; **81:** 819–21.

2. Gardanne de CPL. (ed) De la ménopause ou de l'âge critique des femmes, 2nd edn. (Méquignon-Marvis: Paris, 1821.)

3. Tilt EJ. *The Change of Life in Health and Disease. A Practical Treatise on the Nervous and Other Affections Incidental to Women at the Decline of Life*, 2nd ed. (John Churchill: London, 1857.)

4. Tilt EJ. Reflections on a late discussion. *Lancet* 1850; **II:** 466–9.

5. Wilson RA, Brevetti RE, Wilson TA. Specific procedures for the elimination of the menopause. *West J Surg Obstet Gynecol* 1963; **71:** 110–21.

6. Wilson RA. *Feminine Forever*. (WH Allen: London, 1966.)

7. Djerassi C. Progestins in therapy. In: (Benagiano, ed) *Historical Developments in Progestogens in Therapy, Volume 1*. (Raven Press: New York, 1983.)

8. Fothergill L. Of the management proper at the cessation of the menses. *Med Observ Inquiries* 1776; **5:** 160–86.

9. Geist SH, Spielman F. The therapeutic value of amniotin in the menopause. *Am J Obstet Gynecol* 1932; **23:** 697.

10. Rozenbaum H, Peumery JJ. Histoire Illustrée de la ménopause. (Dacosta édit: Paris, 1990.)

11. Wilbush J. La menespausle: the birth of a syndrome. *Maturitas* 1979; **1:** 145–51.

12. Wilbush J. What's in a name? Some linguistic aspects of the climateric. *Maturitas* 1981; **3:** 1–9.

13. Wilbush J. Menorrhagia and menopause: a historical review. *Maturitas* 1988; **10:** 5–26.

14. Wilbush J. Menopause and menorrhagia: a historical exploration. *Maturitas* 1988; **10:** 83–108.

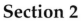

Section 2

The Patient's Perspective

Chapter 6   The awareness of the menopausal woman concerning the menopausal transition

Chapter 7   The considerations, hopes and fears of the menopausal woman

6

The awareness of the menopausal woman concerning the menopausal transition

S Palacios

Introduction • Cultural views of menopause • Patient information • Role of the physician • Compliance • References

INTRODUCTION

Menopause is a normal developmental process for women, in which a psychologic adjustment as well as physical and anatomic changes occur. Hormone replacement therapy (HRT) deserves consideration as a component of preventive health care for older women, and its use after menopause can effectively reduce climacteric-related symptoms and therefore increase the quality of life.[1] Nevertheless surveys generally show that only a small proportion of post-menopausal women use HRT and that long-term compliance to treatment is particularly low.[2] The decrease in optimal prevention due to low compliance remains unknown and the reasons why patients do not pursue their treatment in the long run remain unclear.

This evident reluctance to prescribe and use HRT, so-called poor compliance, is without doubt not only due to a misunderstanding of the beneficial effects of HRT but also (and mainly) due to a discordance between expectations and treatment available.

CULTURAL VIEWS OF MENOPAUSE

Every woman lives her climacteric in a very individual and personal way, in part influenced by the views of her culture.

Menopause is thought to represent a major cultural, psychological and physiological milestone for women during the middle years. It signifies the end of reproduction and is a prominent biological marker for an aging process in a world that prefers youthfulness. Through the ages, menopause has been viewed as a sign of decay, psychological loss and, more recently, as a deficiency disease. This negative view of menopause, however, is not shared across all cultures or among all women. Menopause is often viewed as a positive event in women's lives in non-Western cultures, where menopause removes constraints and prohibitions imposed upon menstruating women. In Western societies, where women are valued for sexual attractiveness and do not face restrictions found in other cultures, aging is not revered but rather is viewed quite negatively. In these societies menopause takes on a very different meaning. This negative view of menopause, however, is found more among society as a whole than among menopausal women themselves.[3]

The question arises, why if menopause brings similar physical and mental manifestations are there cross-cultural variations in attitudes toward it? Though menopause is experienced differently by women in different cultures, it may not always be due to genetic or lifestyle differences. Some investigators insist that Japanese menopausal women have far fewer hot flushes because of their high intake of soybean, but Koreans eat as much soy as Japanese and their incidence of hot flushes is more than double.

Lumbago or low back pain in Taiwan and hand joint pain in Korea are the most common climacteric symptoms. Yucatan women experience fewer hot flushes and have low fracture rates despite a high rate of osteoporosis. How can this be explained? Their lifestyle, diet, exercise, length of long bones and weather may be the factors influencing these differences. But these are not enough to explain everything.

In the Muslim culture menopause is regarded as a blessing because women are no longer prohibited from performing religious rituals, probably due to better social position and being freed from menstruation and pregnancy. In India, the menopause is a crisis of middle age but for the Rajput caste it is regarded as a reward, because women are now allowed to participate in men's activities.

Depending on the cultural setting, menopause can result in an increase or a decrease of social status. In some cultures, the loss of regular bleeding is linked to a social gain because menopause means the end of regularly returning days of impurity, whereas in other, more procreation-minded societies, menopause is seen mainly in a negative way because it means the end of fertility and the end of youth. Cross-cultural comparisons demonstrate that reported symptoms vary significantly among countries and among ethnic and religious groups within countries. Therefore, incidence and acceptance of menopausal symptoms is determined by the cultural region as well as by the social situation within a certain cultural region.

However, a major obstacle in comparing data from different cultures is the local variation in alimentation and other lifestyle factors making it difficult to distinguish cultural from biologic causes of symptom expression. Furthermore, there are differences in the language and the terms used to describe climacteric symptoms. In the Papago culture, menopause may be completely ignored, to the extent that the language contains no word for menopause. In Japan there is no word to describe hot flushes.[3] While the stereotypical view is that women view menopause quite negatively, research on women's attitudes toward menopause, conducted across a wide range of populations and cultures, has not found such negativity among middle-aged women.[3]

PATIENT INFORMATION

Women receive information about menopause from many sources, including health care providers, friends and mothers, but the primary source is women's magazines (76%).[4] Although women seem to have a basic understanding of the symptoms of menopause, their knowledge of the long-term health risks affected by menopause is poor.[4] Women who were undecided about HRT cited scientific confusion in the media as contributing to their reticence about making a decision. Many women think that menopause itself (independent of aging) increases the risk of breast cancer.

Over half of the women surveyed about menopause said they had left health care appointments with unanswered questions about menopause and HRT.[4] The level of information given to the patient varies from country to country but, in general, most of the information on the climacteric and HRT does not come from the doctor, and can therefore mislead about the actual treatment. Many women refrain from therapy because of fear and misconceptions.

Women who suffer premature menopause find themselves facing physiological, psychosocial and sociological challenges which leave them feeling alienated from not only the wider community but also from health professionals; they also feel that their diagnosis is often delayed. The establishment of a dedicated early menopause service in addition to the establishment of a support group has been requested.[5] In general, women who had a surgical menopause were more likely to have negative attitudes regarding the menopause experience.[3] Women consistently report that they are glad to no longer deal with menstruation, accompanying premenstrual syndrome or menstrual cramps, fear of pregnancy, or purchase of feminine products. Thus, the end of menstruation, rather than bringing on a sense of psychological loss, is often met with relief.[3]

While the medical community has often viewed menopause as a deficiency disease or condition requiring treatment, women in general view menopause as a normal life transition and are often relieved at the cessation of menses. It is clear that better education about menopause needs to be accomplished regarding the long-term risk associated with menopause and the pros and cons of HRT. Strategies for improving education and interactions with healthcare providers are suggested.[4]

Questionnaire studies in Europe show that women's concerns at the menopause are more related to their self-image and sexual identity than to medical consequences such as osteoporosis or coronary heart disease. Women long for help with menopausal problems, yet are concerned about the potential side-effects of HRT and often perceive the information they receive from their doctors to be inadequate. Adverse effects of menopausal estrogen deprivation on sexual and psychological function occur via two main mechanisms. Firstly, the physical changes that occur at menopause affect body image, sexual function and a woman's relationship with her partners. Secondly, there are changes in neuroendocrine and psychological function, affecting ego and self-perception.[6]

A study with 40 women between the ages of 45 and 55 was undertaken to investigate perception and experience of menopause, HRT, osteoporosis and doctor–patient relationships.[7] Most women thought that these topics were not widely or freely discussed in the community. Lack of reliable, accessible and current information on menopause and related topics was identified as a problem. Hysterectomy and osteoporosis were identified as specific areas in which information was inadequate and not readily accessible. Solutions suggested by the women included distributing information pamphlets with contact numbers for further information to nonhealth-related settings. The

need to foster open discussion between women and their doctors was highlighted, with contributions required from both parties to develop a more equal partnership. They found focus groups a useful method for accessing women's experiences and perceptions. Small group size and an emphasis on confidentiality were helpful strategies in encouraging discussion of intimate topics.

The Women's Health Initiative[8] was a randomized trial to assess risk and benefits of intervention strategies in a postmenopausal population. The arm of the study in which participants received conjugated equine estrogens and medroxyprogesterone acetate or placebo was halted after 5.2 years due to health risks exceeding health benefits. The way this information is given to patients is important. One way is to use estimated hazard ratios – coronary heart disease 1.29, breast cancer 1.26, stroke 1.41, pulmonary embolism 2.13, colorectal cancer 0.63, endometrial cancer 0.83, hip fracture 0.66. Another way is to use absolute excess risk – for 10,000 women taking HRT each year compared with those not taking it, there would be an additional eight cases of invasive breast cancer, seven heart attacks, eight strokes, and eight pulmonary embolisms. This is a relatively small annual increase in risk for an individual woman; however, there would also be six fewer bowel cancers and five fewer hip fractures. Overall, mortality was not increased with therapy. Yet another way is using the study findings – 41% increase in strokes, 29% increase in heart attacks, double the rate of venous tromboembolism, 22% increase in total cardiovascular disease, 26% increase in breast cancer, 37% reduction in cases of colorectal cancer, 33% reduction in hip fracture rates, 24% reduction in total fractures, and no difference in total mortality (of all causes). Women must know that the risk of breast cancer is not appreciably increased during the first 4 years, which is why the way a patient receives this information will help her to decide on the use or not of this specific combination of HRT.

HRT side-effects

Fear of cancer and drug-related side-effects, such as unacceptable bleeding, have been among the most frequently mentioned causes of low compliance. Thus, individual information for patients regarding HRT seems to be a crucial issue.

Vaginal bleeding is the most important parameter and should be examined individually, since the woman's acceptance of it or not is a key factor for treatment compliance. Generally speaking, pre- or perimenopausal women accept monthly bleeding from cyclic treatment. It should be noted that during this period most women worry about irregular cycles. Before initiation of HRT, it is essential to discuss with patients the possibility of bleeding. Women may accept the occurrence of bleeding if they are informed about it.[1]

Some surveys have documented that bleeding was a negative experience and contributed to poors compliance.[1] Rozenberg et al[1] found that women had rated bleeding as the most negative of a list of factors influencing their decision to use HRT. Among women who stop taking HRT, 10–50% mention bleeding as a reason for treatment discontinuation.

HRT-related risk of developing breast cancer is a very controversial issue which regularly frightens many women and physicians, and is a frequently reported reason for stopping therapy. It has been reported, in a survey of 2500 women, that over half of those to whom HRT had been prescribed (70%) either never used the prescription or stopped taking the medication because of fear of cancer.[1]

ROLE OF THE PHYSICIAN

The doctor–patient relationship is of utmost importance, since an atmosphere of confidence and trust is the basis of mutual comprehension. By understanding the patient's needs, her desires and her ways of coping with the situation, the physician will enable her to accept the proposed prescription. The controversies that appear in medical journals about HRT produce confusion between doctors not directly involved with menopause.

Ideally, education for doctors on menopause should begin at undergraduate level. Most doctors have not had training in menopause and so it is hardly surprising that many have little or no knowledge of the subject. Clearly, continuing education is required, and there is a need for dialogue between different specialties to avoid ignorance of important research and education in parallel disciplines – cross-disciplinary cooperation and research will improve the integrated approach to the management of menopausal women. Health systems must examine models of education for both providers and patients to ensure that women have access to information that will help them make informed decisions.

In Europe, osteoporosis has become more common over the last 45 years and with current demographic changes this will increase dramatically. It is unfortunate that much of the knowledge available is not being utilized in clinical practice. To overcome this, doctors must be adequately trained in menopause and its management.

When it comes to decisions about starting and continuing on HRT, it is important that women are treated with understanding, that their concerns are taken seriously, and they are given time to air their views and ask questions.[9] That is why the decision to continue HRT over the long term should be made according to each woman's needs and risks.

The mode of administration of HRT should be proposed and not imposed, and should take into account the lifestyle of the particular woman, allowing her a true role in the decision-making process. Observance and compliance will therefore naturally follow, with the woman feeling she has been listened to and understood as a mature adult by the physician.

HRT is a treatment not exempt from secondary effects, and the doctor is obligated to inform the patient of both benefits and risks. Correctly indicated HRT is based on the understanding of the woman's needs by the doctor, and the woman being fully informed.

In one study, women from France, Germany, Spain, and the UK were interviewed about their use of HRT.[10] It was found that only one-third of perimenopausal and 13% of postmenopausal women were taking HRT, but about 25% of postmenopausal women reported having taken HRT at some time. The proportion of perimenopausal women using HRT varied by country, ranging from 18% in Spain to 55% in France. Importantly, about half (range across countries, 38–61%) of the women interviewed had not discussed menopause or its symptoms with their doctors. While levels of HRT knowledge varied by country, two-thirds of respondents believed that they needed more information about HRT. Decisions about beginning HRT and choosing a formulation were viewed by most women as matters of personal choice, to be made with advice from a physician. In summary, despite the benefits of HRT and available choices among drug delivery options, a fairly small proportion of European women use it, largely because most remain poorly informed about the therapy. Increased physician–patient communication and public education programs are needed to provide women with the information they need to make judicious decisions concerning HRT.

Doctors must know that health status is not the same as quality of life, which is defined by the World Health Organization as an individuals perception of their situation in life in relation to their culture, objectives and interests.

A Canadian menopause study found that the importance of perceived health benefits of HRT and perceived social support for HRT may be substantially underestimated.[11] Conversely, the importance of perceived negative side-effects of HRT may be substantially overestimated. This information helps in understanding women's HRT decision-making and in counseling women about initiation or maintenance of therapy.

In a survey with Moroccan physicians, it was found that the majority of those interviewed were positively inclined towards the notion of prevention of disease and were therefore in favor of hormonal treatment, and approximately half reported that they had prescribed hormone therapy.[12] Gynecologists and male physicians prescribe hormones more frequently, as well as physicians in private practice.[12]

A study in Vermont, of 428 women between the ages of 50 and 70, found an overall prevalence of HRT use of 40%.[13] HRT use was significantly higher among women whose physicians had encouraged its use (58%) as opposed to those who received ambivalent recommendations from their physicians (20%). A recommendation by a health care provider is a powerful predictor of HRT use, but disparities in use exist by socioeconomic status.

The most important thing a clinician can offer to the perimenopausal woman is the education she needs to make therapeutic choices.

COMPLIANCE

It is essential to discuss with patients, before initiation of HRT, the possibility of bleeding. Women may accept the occurrence of bleeding if they are informed about it.

Compliance is a paradoxical phenomenon, because despite well-documented and widely known effects of HRT, only a small percentage of postmenopausal women actually use it. Some of this reluctance may stem from concerns about the medicalization of menopause and the labeling of menopause as a state of failure, or a disease that needs to be treated.

Two factors that influence compliance with HRT are education and motivation of patients, and the population characteristic. Motivation of the patient means that the patient should be involved in the decision-making process. When a woman receives a prescription and does not even start medication, this reflects a low level of communication between the patient and her physician.

Rozenberg et al[1] found that women who ceased HRT treatment more often had a lower level of education than current users.[1] It has also been observed that prevalence and compliance to HRT is higher in women who have had a hysterectomy, and women with a surgical menopause were about five times as likely to report current use of estrogen (compared with never users).[1]

In a study in Spain it was found that the use of HRT in that country was 5–10%, and that poor compliance was 39%. When compared with the results of the Women's Health Initiative, over a 9-month period HRT use was 20% but there was poor compliance in 60% of cases.[2]

Even in women who start HRT, treatment may be discontinued for a number of reasons:[2,14]

- if climacteric symptoms resolve, the need for continued treatment may not be fully understood;
- some women may experience side-effects associated with the components of the HRT;
- failure of treatment to meet expectations;
- fear of cancer;
- for some women on sequential therapy, the regular bleed may affect their quality of life;
- for women on continuous combined therapy, breakthrough bleeding may be troublesome.

As bleeding is one of the main reasons for discontinuation of HRT, achieving better bleeding control could see an improvement in compliance.

In a Spanish questionnaire attempting to determine what information women had received about HRT, it was found that 43% of women who had received HRT had stopped taking it, and that 40.4% of these women stopped because of secondary effects.[2]

It is possible that compliance can be improved by following an educational program. Surveys have found that only a minority of women start therapy for prophylaxis but that women who are on therapy are more informed about menopause and its consequences than women who are not treated.[1]

Studies have shown that the uptake of HRT varies from country to country. Ambivalence from those health professionals that women turn to for advice may play a part; here, education may be the key. Irresponsible reporting from the media has added to women's concerns. The physician is in an important position to influence health behaviors, to assess risk factors and to provide medical interventions which will prevent illness.

A study to assess whether results of bone density measurements affect a woman's decision to take HRT as a preventive measure

against osteoporosis was make by Rubin and Cummings.[15] It was found that women who reported their bone mass density to be below normal were much more likely to begin some type of fracture prevention than women with normal results (94 versus 56%; $P < 0.01$), to start HRT (38 versus 8%; $P < 0.01$) and to take precautions to avoid falling (50 versus 9%; $P < 0.01$).[1] In summary, the value of bone mass measurements to increase compliance is not well established but some studies suggest that it has a favorable role in this respect.[1]

Strategies to improve compliance

The best way to improve compliance is to correct the information that influences negativity. Information about menopause and HRT needs to be clearly understood and presented as benefits to a given culture. This would avoid confusion, alarm and lack of relevant information. Doctors should inform directly through the various methods of communication available, and help the mass media to give reliable information. As regards the economic point of view, it must be made clear that prevention is better and cheaper than cure, and therefore governments must also play a role in informing the public about HRT. As for HRT itself, treatment should be tailored to individual needs and scientific findings kept abreast of so that patients remain informed of changes in risks of benefits. If improvement in compliance is the key issue of HRT, women have to be viewed as decision-makers and treatment should meet their expectations. Informed decision-making about HRT use should consider the individual's perception of her menopausal stage. Education and behavioral strategies may be of use. Improved communication between patients and physicians, therefore establishing a confidential relationship, involving the woman in the decision-making process, explaining benefits and risk with clarity, providing time and an appropiate location for discussions, and provision of nursing counseling are all strategies which may improve compliance.

The decision to prescribe HRT should be made after a careful evaluation of the individual risks and benefits expected from the use of this therapy, and according to the needs, health risks and preferences of each woman.

Many women are reluctant to initiate HRT or to use it over a long-term period because of fear of cancer or because of vaginal bleeding among other reasons. Therefore, there is a real need for alternative treatments for postmenopausal women that could offer the benefits of estrogens without increasing the risk of cancer and the other risks associated with this therapy. Moreover, the preferences of the women, on problems like vaginal bleeding, method of and schedule of administration, should be taken into account in order to improve compliance and thus long-term adherence to HRT.

REFERENCES

1. Rozenberg S, Vandromme J, Kroll M et al. Compliance to hormone replacement therapy. *Int J Fertil* 1995; **40** (Suppl 1): 23–32.
2. Asociación Española para el estudio de la Menopausia (AEEM). In: (Cano A, González de merlo G, eds) *Medicina basada en la evidencia en menopausia.* (Runiprint: Madrid, 2002.)
3. Avis NE, Women's perceptions of the menopause. *Eur Menopause J* 1996; **3**: 80–4.
4. Clinkingbeard C, Minton BA, Davis J et al. Women's knowledge about menopause, hormone replacement therapy (HRT), and interactions with healthcare providers: an exploratory study. *J Womens Health Gender Based Med* 1999; **8**: 1097–102.
5. Pasquali EA. The impact of premature menopause on women's experience of self. *J Holist Nurs* 1999; **17**: 346–64.
6. Graziottin A. HRT: the woman's perspective. *Int Gynaecol Obstet* 1996; **52** (Suppl 1): S11–S16.
7. Fox-Young S, Sheehan M, O'Connor V et al. Women's perceptions and experience of menopause: a focus group study. *J Psychosom Obstet Gynaecol* 1995; **16**: 215–21.
8. Women's Health Initiative Investigators. Risk and benefits of estrogen plus progestin in healthy postmenopausal women. *J Am Med Ass* 2002; **288**: 321–33.
9. Graziottin A. Strategies for effectively addressing women's concerns about the menopause and HRT. *Maturitas* 1999; **33** (Suppl 1): S15–S23.
10. Schneider HPG. Cross-national study of women's use of hormone replacement therapy (HRT) in Europe. *Int J Fertil Womens Med* 1997; **42** (Suppl 2): 365–75.
11. Fisher WA, Sand M, Lewis W et al. Canadian menopause study-I: understanding women's intentions to utilise hormone replacement therapy. *Maturitas* 2000; **37**: 1–14.
12. Obermeyer CM, Sahel A, Hajji N et al. Physicians perceptions of menopause and prescribing practices in Morocco. *Int J Gynaecol Obstet* 2001; **73**: 47–55.
13. Finley C, Gregg EW, Solomon LJ et al. Disparities in hormone replacement therapy use by socioeconomic status in a primary care population. *J Comm Health* 2001; **26**: 39–50.
14. The North American Menopause Society. Achieving long-term continuance of menopausal ERT/HRT: consensus opinion of the North American Menopause Society. *Menopause* 1998; **5**: 69–76.
15. Rubins SM, Cummings SR. Results of bone densitometry affect women's decisions about taking measures to prevent fractures. *Ann Inter Med* 1992; **116**: 990–5,

7

The considerations, hopes and fears of the menopausal woman

G Zelinsky

Climacteric complaints? I must confess that I had never dealt with this phenomenon when I was younger. I thought that this was a subject for hysterical women who had no meaningful and satisfying work to do, who felt sorry for themselves, were unstable, who used their time to reflect about themselves and proclaim their suffering to everybody. I was sure that I would never suffer from climacteric complaints because I am working, I have a large family to care for, I care for a garden that gives me much pleasure, I engage in social matters, I have many good friends and pets to look after.

However, when I was 52, I felt miserable physically and psychologically. Sitting down to coffee with my friends of similar ages, I asked them how they felt because I felt miserable and exhausted without knowing why. 'What is the matter with you?' they asked. 'You have never been so negative.' I regretted telling them of my complaints, but when I noticed one or the other of them opening the top button of their blouse and wiping the sweat away from their forehead, I knew what was happening and no longer felt so isolated.

It is now 16 years since I first heard of hormone replacement therapy (HRT) for the woman in the climacteric. I was told of the benefit of HRT in treating complaints caused by the

hormonal change. I began to develop an interest in the subject, even though I was not affected at that time. I learned, however, that many women felt alone with their sorrows concerning the change of life. What happened was said to be natural and had to be accepted. Young and attractive women were the center of interest, not postmenopausal ones. Nobody wants to concern themselves with women who are aging, who complain, who are depressed, who develop the figure of a matronly woman and look back to lost beauty and attractiveness. In most cases these women disappeared behind the cooker, the ironing board, the knitting needles and as babysitters for their grandchildren. At that age the males often started a new life, seeking younger girlfriends.

Regrettably, these attitudes are not consigned to the past. However, the menopausal woman has a new trump card available, one capable of bringing her zest and quality of life to a new flourishing.

In the summer of 1986 I was sitting with my girlfriend on a terrace in the south of France. Our husbands were on a sailing turn and we were enjoying time to ourselves to discuss women's problems. I confessed that I had changed in the last few years and could scarcely recognize myself. I reported unmotivated crying, depressive moods, reluctance of everything that claimed discipline. The friend I was talking to was astonished when I told her of circulatory complaints, dry eyes, dry vagina, hot flushes, sleepless nights and existential fears.

My friend was astonished. 'Aren't you a modern, progressive woman? You are in the change of life. Your hormones are crazy. Did you not see your gynecologist? You can counteract your complaints: you do not have to accept these unpleasant symptoms. Besides, you are blonde, you are slim, you are disposed to osteoporosis.'

What my friend said seemed encouraging. On the other hand: osteoporosis, that sounded dangerous. She explained to me what the loss of bone mass and the risk of bone fractures caused by estrogen deficiency meant. I decided that I had to do something against this risk. Moreover, I wanted to regain the personality and the wellbeing I had enjoyed during the years before. Depressions, sleeplessness, vertebral and femoral fractures, circulatory complaints, a body which feels ablaze, a dry vagina, no pleasure in sex – no thank you. I promised my friend to see my doctor as soon as I returned home, and I confirmed my decision by wiping away the sweat of my hot flush.

The day came when I had an appointment with my gynecologist. Whilst at home I had written down all the questions I wanted to ask him because I knew from earlier visits that after entering the office I would forget everything that I had intended to discuss. At first I did not disclose my real requests but I put forward the neutral question of whether or not I was at risk of osteoporosis. He looked at my card, I presume to check my date of birth. Thereafter, looking at me, he said 'You are indeed at the age to think about preventing osteoporosis.' 'This is why I am here,' I answered. 'Have you any complaints that are indicative for a climacteric, symptomatology like hot flushes and sweating? When was your last menstrual bleeding?' I told him, that this event had come last time 11 months ago.

With this question, however, he had given me the cue and now I told him everything that was worrying me, how I felt, the loss of

autonomous balance, the change in my natural character and my desire to be on top of my life. The doctor proved to be a good listener and demonstrated understanding by asking the right questions in between. He explained to me clearly what was happening to my body, what hormones were, how they worked and what they could achieve. The decrease in ovarian hormones would not endanger my life but would increase the risk for many diseases such as osteoporosis, which could be prevented by estrogen medication. As life expectancy is now 30 years post-menopause, the lack of estrogens, which have governed many important metabolic processes for such a long time, must have grave consequences for many processes, which characterize aging.

The doctor also checked the family history concerning cancer and thrombosis. There was no case of these diseases in my ancestry. After this fruitful conversation I had a medical examination to exclude any physical contraindications against hormone medication. Everything was in order. The doctor concluded that, as far as it was possible to judge, there would be only a low risk in my taking estrogens together with a suitable progestogen to prevent bleeding problems. A hormone determination would not be necessary, he said, as age, amenorrhea and complaints were all typical for estrogen deprivation.

Thereafter a prescription was written for an estrogen–progestogen preparation. After he handed it to me, he explained possible risks like thrombosis and cancer and how to avoid them, and he gave me some important recommendations for a healthy lifestyle. The regular bleeding caused by the preparation, I told him, was no problem for me, it meant a piece of youth. The doctor admonished me to come for regular 6-monthly check-ups and to discuss a new prescription or a necessary change of preparation or method of administration. A mammography was recommended and scheduled.

I took my leave and was determined to try the HRT. I felt easy and cheerful and looked forward to the time when I would feel as well balanced and powerful as before. I took correctly what had been prescribed, and reverted back to my bright, calm and dynamic self. I felt great! No more of those embarrassing feelings that had dragged me down. All complaints disappeared within 8 weeks. The withdrawal bleeding did not bother me. I had my life back both physically and psychologically. My being a woman was no longer troublesome but gave me pleasure again. I did not put on weight as I had feared.

After 16 years of uninterrupted intake of hormones, still convinced of the considerable benefits of HRT, I decided, at 65 years of age, to allow my body to grow old. The discussion about the break–off of the estrogen–medroxyprogesterone acetate (MPA) arm of the Women's Health Initiative (WHI) facilitated my decision. Thus, some time ago I dismissed the hormone tablets. The fear of mammary cancer and the occurrence of this disease in some of my friends also played a role, although I am convinced that genes, environmental poisons, lifestyle and individual disposition play a decisive role in the genesis of mammary cancer.

My courageous decision to quit the benefits of HRT was not a success. Within a few days I noticed a strange change in my physical and psychological state of health, it began with troublesome sleep disturbances, a loss of concentration and circulatory problems. The former feeling of being an aging women occurred again. I was not willing to bear that. Therefore, I went to see my doctor and explained to him why I had dropped out of HRT. He informed me that the main problem of the WHI study was an unsuitable progestogen and the daily combined uninterrupted medication, plus some other problems of experimental design in this study. He offered me a preparation that had, in one tablet, an estrogenic, progestogenic and mild androgenic effect, and which did not stimulate the endometrium and the epithelium of the breast. My gynecologist convinced me. The daily tablet is routine again, with the return of my usual positive outlook cessation of my complaints.

My positive experience with HRT encouraged me to write a book called *No Reason for Panic*, dealing with the problems of climacteric women and of HRT, which is in its fourth edition and for which Professor Lauritzen wrote an introduction.

I believe that with regard to the climacteric and hormone substitution there is no reason for panic, and that the solution is to see a gynecologist experienced in the prescription of correct, competent and individually tailored HRT. The responsibility of the climacteric woman is to secure regular preventive check-ups, to trust science and your doctor, to secure your own information and to maintain a healthy lifestyle. That is my wish for every postmenopausal woman.

REFERENCE

1. Zelinski G. *Kein Grund zur Panik* (Nymphenburger Verlag: München, 1989).

Hormone Therapy and Replacement

Chapter 8 The climacteric syndrome

Chapter 9 Practice of hormone substitution

Chapter 10 Mechanisms of action of sex steroid hormones and their analogs

Chapter 11 Estrogens, progestogens and the endometrium

Chapter 12 Estrogen deprivation and hormone replacement therapy: effects on glucose and insulin metabolism and the metabolic syndrome

Chapter 13 Possible side-effects of sexual hormones

8

The climacteric syndrome

GA Hauser

Causes and symptoms of the climacteric syndrome • The Blatt Menopause index • The Kupperman Index • The Utian Menopause Quality of Life Score • The Menopause Rating Scale I (MRS I) • The Self-assessment Menopause Rating Scale II (MRS II) • References

CAUSES AND SYMPTOMS OF THE CLIMACTERIC SYNDROME

It is established that climacteric complaints are caused by the decline of ovarian function, i.e. by the decrease of estradiol and the cessation of progesterone production. The oophoropause is the consequence of burn out of the follicles and their hormone-producing cells and of early atherosclerotic changes of the ovarian vessels.[1-3]

The fact that castration of a sexually mature woman causes symptoms comparable to a spontaneous menopause, but which occur more rapidly, more intensively and for longer, is dramatic proof of the ovarian cause of the process. The oophorectomy model is also widely used as verification of the source of climacteric symptoms[4-6] and for the evaluation of therapeutic substances.

The withdrawal of estradiol and progesterone, which if present exert profound effects on mitosis, proliferation, metabolism, organ perfusion and other endocrine gland functions, leads to adaptory changes of the hormonal regulatory system and dependent metabolic events in a frustrated attempt to correct the loss. The ovary is the only endocrine gland (except for the placenta and thymus) which ceases to function long before the end of life. These events cause typical early symptoms of imbalance of the autonomous nervous system and late symptoms of hormone deficit, affecting the primary and secondary target organs of estrogens and progesterone. Climacteric changes are partly superimposed on other symptoms of aging. Individual psychological problems, such as self-esteem, sensibility, reception and tolerance of complaints, of coping, of body constitution, sociocultural circumstances, lifestyle and nutrition, all play a part in the qualitative and quantitative expression of the syndrome.

The great variety of symptoms, personal character and existing intercultural differences demand the diagnostic application of a reliable qualitative and quantitative assessment of the symptoms presented by the individual client to secure the diagnosis or differential diagnosis of climacteric complaints. In particular, therapeutic interventional studies, if they are to be compared with other similar studies, require comparable rating scales.

Frequency of climacteric complaints

Data concerning the frequency of climacteric complaints vary widely according to definition, to populations, and to different regions and cultures of the world.[7] Most data relate to specific age groups; indeed, data may vary in the different phases of the climacteric from perimenopause, to menopause to postmenopause. These changes may be related to the level and the rapidity of decreases in the estrogen level.

Flushes and sweating, for instance, increase in frequency and severity from premenopause to about 3 years after menopause and thereafter usually decrease. In contrast, irritability, nervousness and tension are highest during the premenopause.[8-11] From a Swiss population of 23,388 women with amenorrhea, menopausal complaints and high levels of follicle-stimulating hormone (FSH) and very low estrogens, Hauser[7,12] found 79% to have hot flushes, 75% nervousness, 74% sleep disorders, 69% articular and muscular disorders, 63% depression, 61% tiredness and loss of energy, 53% sexual dysfunction, 50% vaginal dryness, 43% urological symptoms and 42% dysfunctional heart disorders. Twenty per cent of women in the Western world may have no complaints during the climacteric change, 30% have severe complaints, 30% moderate complaints and 39% weak complaints. About 5% are unable to do their work for some months or years.[8]

Sociocultural factors

Women do not experience climacteric complaints with equal frequency. Racial, cultural, religious, sociological and nutritional factors modify the quality and incidence of menopausal symptoms. For instance, certain castes in India, such as large-scale land owners in Rajput, were free of menopausal symptoms, probably because these women experience a rise in social status after the menopause.[13] In Pakistan the frequency of typical symptoms is low, and is lowest among the low socioeconomic groups.[14] Arabian women in the postmenopause who emigrate to Israel are also reported not to complain of menopausal symptoms because they also experience an improvement in their social situation.[15] Malaysian women are reported never to experience climacteric symptoms,[16] and the same was found in the Maya population.[17] The Thai experience is that only 5.7% of women exhibit vasomotor

symptoms and only 15–22% psychosomatic disorders.[18]

The lower incidence of climacteric complaints in Japanese women – where no word exists for hot flushes – is presumed to result from their high intake of soya products.[19,20] This aspect is at present under discussion with respect to a treatment of climacteric complaints with soya.

In contrast, women in the Western world or those living a Western lifestyle, report a high incidence of typical climacteric complaints such as hot flushes and sweating. In Germany, a frequency of climacteric complaints of 80% is reported,[21] in the USA 75%,[22] 70–80% in Austria,[23] 80% in The Netherlands[24] and 80% in the UK.[25,26]

In the Western world, women who work full or part time, who experience fulfilment in their tasks and are not unnecessarily stressed, experience fewer climacteric disorders than 'housewives' with no other aspirations. Additional strain, such as the 'empty-nest syndrome' (also referred to as 'isolement a deux'[27]) or the care for and the death of close relatives, also affect symptomatology.[28]

The menopause is, after all, a phase of general loss of fertility and youth,[1,29] and of farewell and retirement, thus changes of life roles and of expectations are also to be coped with.[30,31]

The domino effect

Some researchers have assumed that hot flushes might be the cause of other climacteric symptoms such as sleep disorders, nervousness, depressive mood, tiredness, sexual dysfunction and poor memory.[32-35] These symptoms were accordingly supposed to be secondary consequences of hot flushes, or of that disorder of the autonomic nervous system that causes hot flushes.

However, more in-depth investigations of women with the menopausal syndrome, but without the symptom of hot flushes, identified domino symptoms as primary symptoms in their own right, each responding to estrogen medication.[36,37] On the other hand, the general feeling of wellbeing and the perceived state of health can be profoundly negatively influenced by suffering from severe climacteric complaints.

Placebo effects

For proof of the effectiveness of a treatment, there must be verification against a placebo in a double-blind trial. This is necessary because of the occurrence of a high percentage of positive effects of placebos in open investigations upon symptoms which are greatly influenced by psychic factors from the side of the probands. The expectations of the probands, but also the care, attention, engagement and the involuntary suggestions given by the therapeut or the investigator, play a prominent role in this regard.

The first double-blind trials against placebo were performed by Greenblatt et al,[38] Wied[39] and Hauser. Surprisingly good results of placebos were found for instance upon hot flushes, vaginal dryness, urinary frequency and poor memory by Campbell[40] and Utian[5] in up to 40% of cases after 6–12 weeks of placebo medication. On the other hand, in trials where psychological influences were excluded as far as possible, placebo effects of between only 12 and 30% were registered.[41,42]

The placebo effect can be minimized if the medication is begun with the placebo in both groups and after 4 weeks the change is made to treatment in one of the groups. In this case the placebo effect will vanish after a few weeks, symptoms will recur and the effect of treatment will become more pronounced in the treated group.[43] Moreover, the placebo effect is seldom of long duration and symptoms will mostly recur after 2–3 months in spite of continuing placebo medication.

Controlled trials have indisputably demonstrated that estrogens exert significant and reliable effects on symptoms clearly caused by estrogen deficiency, e.g. hot flushes, poor memory, sweating, nervousness, depressive mood, vaginal atrophy and dryness, and urologic atrophic complaints.

Hot flushes

The symptom of hot flushes is the earliest, and most prominent and characteristic, symptom of estrogen deficiency and accordingly of the climacteric syndrome. Some authors distinguish between hot flushes and flashes. Hot flush means the flush, accompanied with a visible hyperemia of the skin, hot flash means the subjective cortical perception of flash without hyperemia. Flashes are usually more frequent than flushes.

Hot flushes do not occur in all women during the climacteric but 65–85% do experience them. The flushes start with symptoms such as dizziness, a feeling of congestion to the head and a local sense of heat. The flush then begins in the face, thereafter including the neck, breast and back. Up to 4 minutes may pass until an increase in skin temperature can be measured, which occurs in about 75% of cases in the forehead, upper part of the body, fingers and toes. This becomes visible by a reddening of the skin. The flushes often induce feelings of nausea, suffocation, formication, burning, lack of concentration, heart pounding and arrhythmia.

According to Strecker and Lauritzen,[3] the flush normally lasts for 3.3±5.48 minutes (0.5–60 minutes). It is followed by sweating, tachycardia and, in some cases, by a brief increase in blood pressure. The loss of sweat amounts to 3–8 g per flush. The sweat induces a small decrease in skin temperature, which is followed by an increase. Caused by the dilatation of blood vessels and radiant heat, the temperature of the inner body decreases by about 0.2°C and skin resistance increases (see Figs 8.1 and 8.2). The frequency of flushes varies from one to more than 100/day in extreme cases. Voda[44] reported a mean of 55 flushes/day, i.e. two flushes/hour. About 80% of flushes occur during the day and 20% at night, the latter usually causing awakening.

The period of time over which hot flushes occur is 1 year in 80% of cases, more than 5 years in 50% and more than 10 years in 10%. The prevalence of hot flushes increases from the premenopause, is maximal 2–3 years after the menopause and decreases thereafter.

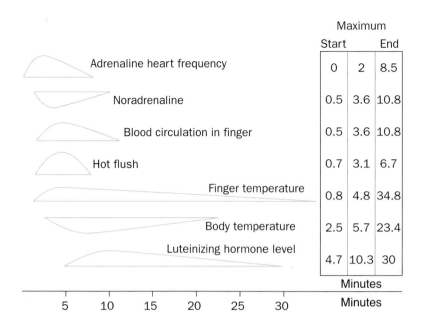

		Maximum	
	Start		End
Adrenaline heart frequency	0	2	8.5
Noradrenaline	0.5	3.6	10.8
Blood circulation in finger	0.5	3.6	10.8
Hot flush	0.7	3.1	6.7
Finger temperature	0.8	4.8	34.8
Body temperature	2.5	5.7	23.4
Luteinizing hormone level	4.7	10.3	30
			Minutes

Figure 8.1 Changes in various physiological parameters during a hot flush related to time (after Kuhl and Taubert[80]).

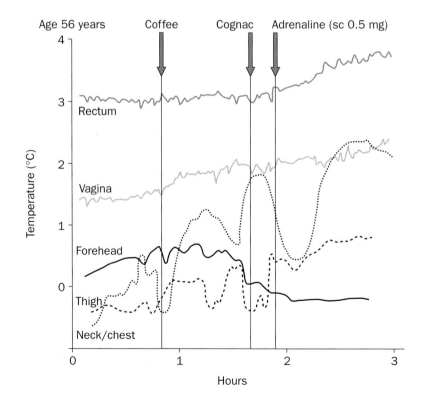

Figure 8.2 Objectivization of hot flushes by continuous measurement of temperature (after Hauser et al)[81]. Hot flushes were also triggered by black coffee, alcohol and adrenaline. s.c., subcutaneous injection.

Flushes are particularly vehement following oophorectomy, occurring after the fifth postoperative day. Following radiological castration the flushes start after 2–4 weeks.

Hot flushes occur much less frequently in Asiatic countries, which has been explained by the fact that, in some cultures, the menopause is accompanied by an improved social status. Alternatively, the higher consumption of soya estrogens may attenuate the flushes.

Biochemical causes of hot flushes

Whether flushes occur or not is dependent on psychosomatic problems of the stability of the autonomous nervous system, especially of hypothalamic regulation, the production and the metabolism of catecholamines in the brain, and the periphery. Furthermore, the production of androgens and their conversion to estrogens in the subcutaneous fat tissue is also a factor. However, the absolute level of estradiol is not the determinant for the occurrence of flushes, but the relative decrease is. This fact is evidenced by the experience of patients with gonadal agenesia or dysgenesia in whom no flushes occur. However, after administration of estrogens flushes occur following withdrawal of the hormone. Also, during treatment with antiestrogens and gonadotropin-releasing hormone (GnRH), causing inhibition of gonadotrophins and accordingly of estrogen production, flushes recur.

Emotional factors, like excitation, fear and tension, can cause or strengthen flushes. The partly psychic causation is evidenced by the high effectivity of placebo to mitigate flushes. A hot surrounding, or the intake of coffee and Cognac, can trigger flushes. Flushes are accompanied by an increase in adrenalin in the central nervous system (CNS) and the periphery, and an increase in β-endorphin. It is assumed that the release of endorphins is the cause of flushes: GnRH, luteinizing hormone (LH), β-lipoprotein, growth adrenocorticotropic hormone (ACTH), cortisol, dehydroepiandrosterone (DHEA) and thyroid-stimulating hormone (TSH) increase following a hot flush. The reason for the automonous and hormonal 'thunderstorm' is the narrow connection between the hypothalamic centers of regulation. It is to be interpreted as a frustrated attempt to restore the disturbed balance between the ovaries and the hypopthalamic–anterior pituitary system.

Differential diagnosis

Causes such as hyperthyroidism, pheochromocytoma, mastocytoma and paraneoplastic syndrome must be excluded if menopause is uncertain. When hot flushes are missing and the women is still menstruating, the diagnosis of climacteric complaints can be difficult (larvate or concealed climacteric syndrome).

Systematic questioning with the help of the Menopause Rating Scale (MRS) will determine the climacteric syndrome and prevent treatment with sedatives, antidepressants or antirheumatics instead of hormone replacement therapy (HRT). Another possibility is the diagnosis ex juvantibus when HRT is given (Fig. 8.3).

Dysfunctional heart disorders

These are palpitations, rapid and irregular heart beats (Kupperman's palpitations), and angina pectoris. Symptoms of heart insufficiency such as breathlessness, cyanosis and edema are not included.

To ensure that heart complaints are recognized as part of the climacteric syndrome, systematic questioning according to the MRS offers great help for a correct diagnosis. Patients often do not mention these symptoms as they do not associate them with the climacteric.

Dysfunctional heart complaints are experienced in 42% of cases.[45,46] They may occur with or without flushes.[12,45,47] They are most alarming for sufferers, who often fear a life-threatening heart attack.

Dysfunctional climacteric heart disorders respond effectively to estrogen treatment. The effect occurs rapidly, usually within 2 weeks.[12] This effect is a positive benefit of HRT.

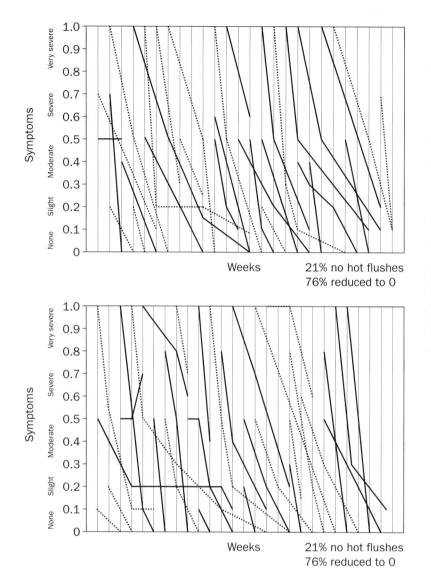

Weeks 21% no hot flushes
76% reduced to 0

Weeks 21% no hot flushes
76% reduced to 0

Figure 8.3 Effectiveness of hormone replacement therapy (HRT) on the hot flushes over time as indicated by the Menopause Rating Scale I (MRS I).[12] 1.0, Very severe symptoms; 0.5, moderate symptoms; 0.0, no symptoms; time between two vertical lines, 1 week; each case is represented by one line; all observed cases are recorded. Only one case shows no reaction, one other case deteriorates in the progestogen phase; one case only reacts after 1 week. As a rule, the positive effect occurs very rapidly and is sustained. (The bottom graph is a continuation of the top graph; showing similar additional cases, all improving in the scale from 1.0 or 0.5 to zero or near to zero.)

Sleep disorders

Sleep disorders may have many different causes. Within the menopausal syndrome the complaint registered in about 75% of cases and is the most common climacteric complaint. Both falling asleep and sleeping through the night are disturbed.

Some authors dismiss this symptom as non-specific, psychological or simply as a consequence of the nocturnal flushes, i.e. it was misinterpreted as a domino effect.

Surprisingly good results are achieved with estrogen medication together with progestogens, with a response in 96% of cases within 6 weeks. In the sleep laboratory it has been found that duration and quality of sleep are improved, especially the rapid-eye-movement (REM) sleep phase and dreaming, which is very important for recovery. Awakening episodes are also reduced. This success is registered by the patient as an important improvement to their quality of life.

Depressive mood

Within the climacteric syndrome depression is the most controversial symptom. Discrimination must be made between endogenous depression and depressive mood (melancholia) – the psychiatrist Kraepelin coined the term *involutional depression*. Psychiatrists mostly ignore the fact that depressive mood can be caused by estrogen withdrawal, as, for instance, in the puerperium.[48]

Depressive mood is marked by sadness, tearfulness, low spirit, lack of energy and lack of determination/concentration. The incidence of depressive mood in the menopausal syndrome is about 63%.[46,49]

Estrogens reduce the concentration of monoamino oxidase[50] which is responsible for the catabolism of catecholamines, which are increased in depression. Estrogens increase tryptophan by preventing indolamine from protein binding – tryptophan is a precursor of serotonin. A therapeutic effect of estrogen was shown in the Hamilton depression score.[51] Estrogens reduce the necessary dose of antidepressants. However, during the luteal phase an intensification of depression is not uncommon.[52,53] Estrogens in higher doses are also effective in real endogenous depression. The response to estrogen substitution is very high and becomes effective after 2 weeks of treatment in 81% or cases. Complete remission is seen after 1–3 months,[54] or after 4–5 cyles of estrogen replacement therapy (ERT).[55]

The social value of the success of ERT in depressive mood treatment cannot be overestimated, since not only the patient but also her partner and family may suffer considerably. The partner should be included in the consultations explaining the causes of the symptomatology, and the value of his understanding and help.

Nervousness, irritability and anxiety

The scope of nervousness includes conditions such as irritability, anxiety, tension and aggressiveness. Irritability occurs in about 65% of women during the premenopause, 49% during the menopause, 48% 1–3 years after the menopause and 17% more than 3 years after the menopause.[21]

Ninety-five per cent of patients complaining of irritability show an improvement of symptoms with treatment – 68% of cases within 2 weeks.[56] As irritability may be an important disturbing factor in a partnership, the therapeutic effect is highly regarded by those women affected and by their partners.

Tiredness, lack of energy and decline in memory

Tiredness is one of the nonspecific, but nevertheless important, symptoms of the climacteric syndrome. This symptom has occurred in 61% of the present author's cases. Often, tiredness is treated using stimulants or polyvitamins rather than realizing its association with the climacteric syndrome. For all women between 45 and 60 years of age a hormone deficiency should be considered as the primary etiology, including low values of DHEA. Tiredness does not respond to HRT as rapidly as other complaints, e.g. hot flushes. Two to 8 weeks of treatment are necessary to achieve significant positive result in 94% of cases.[12]

Lack of energy occurs in 48% of all postmenopausal women. In particular, apathy can be treated successfully by estrogen, DHEA or estrogen–testosterone combinations.

Decline of memory is very common (86%) during the postmenopause and senium. HRT during this period of life improves cognitive functions, particularly concentration, and recall of names and words.[57]

Impaired sexuality

Postmenopausally and with progressing age generally, sexual dysfunction, loss of libido and giving up sexual relations increases. Loss of libido is reported in about 30% of women and decrease of libido in another 30%.[58] More than half of women report impaired sexuality (78%,[59] 77%[60]). Impaired sexuality is not included in the Kupperman Index, which is another reason to abandon it and to use the MRS. Capability of orgasm is maintained up to a high age.

Causes of impaired sexuality are manifold, like a decrease of vaginal perfusion, proliferation and lubrication. Dryness and vulnerability of the vagina may cause discomfort, pain and even lesions. Vaginal dryness increases from 15% during early postmenopause to 50% during the late postmenopause and senium. Diseases of the woman or her partner, or lack of a partner, are other frequent reasons for disinterest in sex. Analysis of the causes of impaired sexuality may be difficult because of a lack of knowledge and for reasons of discretion between the doctor and patient.

HRT shows a positive effect on impaired sexuality in about 74% of cases, so long as atrophic changes are causal. The effect is often somewhat delayed because of the necessity of physical adaption to the changed situation.[61]

Estrogens do not increase libido but this aspect of treatment can be achieved by the administration of testosterone, by oral or transdermal application, or by injection or implants. However, possible unwanted androgenic side-effects must be considered.

Urological symptoms

Forty-three per cent of all postmenopausal women report urological symptoms.[12] The taking of the patient history is delicate because the questions concern a most intimate matter, but this is necessary to prepare an appropriate treatment.

Urological symptoms are mostly caused by atrophic changes of the urogenital organs and by a resulting inflammation because of a decreased resistance to bacterial infections, due to chronic estrogen deficiency. Ectropion urethrae, dysuria, stranguria, pollakiuria, urinary urge, and stress incontinence, and recurrent urethocystitis are the most frequent symptoms of postmenopausal estrogen deprivation. Because the real primary problem of estrogen deficiency is often not recognized, many women are treated with antibiotics or urinary disinfectants unsuccessfully for a long time. This syndrome is missing in the Kupperman Index.

A positive effect of ERT is derived from better blood perfusion, proliferation of the epithelium of bladder and urethra, as well as from strengthening of muscles and ligaments. Sixty-eight per cent of patients respond positively to estrogens within 2 weeks and 94% within 6 weeks. Addition of a progestogen (via an effect on metalloproteinases) and of testosterone improves the success rate of the treatment. The response rate is about 90%, with 60% within 2 weeks.[12]

In urodynamic tests, urethral length and urethral closing pressure can be improved, but subjective improvement may also be reported by the patient if objective changes of the urodynamics cannot be demonstrated.

Dryness of the vagina

This symptom is not included in the Kupperman Index. Van Keep and Kellerhals[62] and Utian[63] regard this symptom as one of the cardinal complaints of the postmenopause. Most women do not mention vaginal dryness spontanously but Hauser[12] found it to be present in 50% of postmenopausal women. The symptom responds in 90% of cases to a local, oral or parenteral estrogen treatment, 60% respond within 2 weeks. Further improvement in the remaining cases is thereafter slow but complete.

Muscular and articular complaints

Sixty-nine per cent of postmenopausal patients, complain of articular and muscular disorders. In 1924, Menge[64] coined the term *arthropathia and myalgia ovaripriva sive climacterica*, which was described especially following castration. Novak[65] called it *osteoarthritis deformans climacterica*. The syndrome had already been mentioned by Garrod and Charcot in 1890.[66]

Kupperman et al[67] listed 'athralgia' and 'myalgia' in their index as frequently occurring symptoms during the climacteric. These complaints received the low multiplication factor of 1, which is then calculated with the grade of severity. Mostly the small joints of the hands (carpo-metacarpal and intercarpal) and toes are affected, not always symmetrically, but also knees, elbows and the cervical spine. Sometimes Heberden's nodes are found at the finger joints and toes. Examination shows swelling and pain, and the woman reports pain and restriction of mobility.

Pathogenetically the syndrome is linked to a decrease in estrogen. In addition, dysfunctions of the thyroid and parathyroid glands are mentioned. Pathological findings are slackening of the synovial membrane, and thickening of the capsules of the joints and of the periarticular soft tissues. Initially no articular changes in the

X-ray image are found. Later on, arthritic changes are seen.

These complaints have received less attention in recent decades, since considerable progress has been made in the diagnosis and treatment of rheumatic diseases. However, rheumatoid factors are negative in the patient having climacteric myalgia and athralgia.

A positive effect of estrogen medication is obtained in 87% of cases, if organic changes are still not present. The effects begins within 2 weeks and are usually complete after 8 weeks (Fig. 8.4).[12]

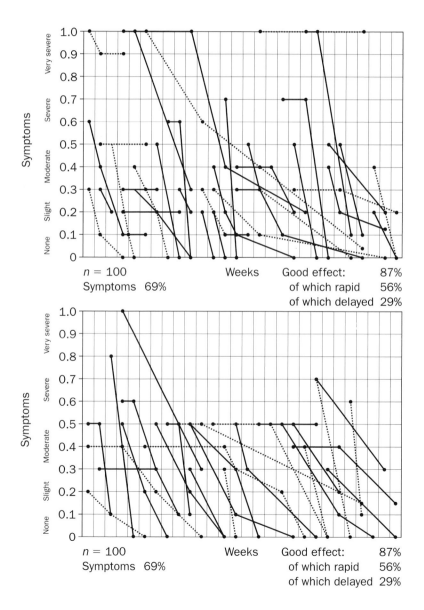

Figure 8.4 Effectiveness of hormone replacement therapy (HRT) on articular and muscular symptoms over time as indicated by the Menopause Rating Scale I (MRS I).[12] (Articular and muscular symptoms are taken together. Severity of complaints: 1.0–0.5.) Almost all articular-muscular complaints are improved by HRT.

In 13% of cases HRT had no effect on articular or muscular symptoms; only 56% showed a rapid effect, so for almost half the effect was delayed by several weeks or even months. The effect is much less sustained than for hot flushes, i.e. it takes longer to reach permanent or even temporary success.

Other symptoms during the climacteric

In both MRS I and II many symptoms are not found that appear in the literature and in the Kupperman Index, such as headache, giddiness (Kupperman's 'vertigo'), formication and paresthesia. These symptoms are of little specificity and significance for the climacteric syndrome. Instead of 'palpitations' the MRS lists 'functional heart disorders'.

How long does it take to improve the climacteric symptoms by HRT?

Knowledge of the time needed for treatment success is important for the counseling of the patient, for practical treatment and also for scientific investigations.

Most practitioners re-evaluate the symptoms from baseline after 6–8 weeks. However, different symptoms show disparate time responses under estrogen treatment. Foremost consideration is usually given to hot flushes because these are often the most prominent and typical symptom and respond effectively to estrogen administration. However, if the flushes have disappeared not everything has been done. In fact, most other symptoms, which may be more important in terms of quality of life, lag behind. Therefore, in accordance with the data of Hauser,[12] the time response of different complaints under HRT will be considered.

The most rapid response is that of hot flushes with about 90% of cases showing improvement within 4–14 days. Depressive mood is improved in 80% of cases within 14 days, but further progress may be very slow. About 10% of cases show no improvement, which may lead to diagnosis of real endogenous depression.

There is an immediate response of dysfunctional heart disorders within 1 week in 77% of cases. Slight sleep disorders, caused by awakening due to hot flushes during the night, will improve in 75% of cases within 1–2 weeks. Severe sleep disorders will take 6–8 weeks to improve and additional therapy, including profound changes of lifestyle, may be required.

Nervousness reacts relatively slow, usually after 2 weeks of treatment in about 60% of cases. Tiredness usually improves in 75% of cases within 1–2 weeks, and if this is not the case further diagnostics are indicated. Articular and muscular complaints respond in 65% of cases within 3–9 weeks. Urological symptoms usually required 2–3 weeks of treatment before improvement occurs. Vaginal dryness improves in 60% of cases within 2 weeks.

The slowest response is of sexual dysfunction, which responds in only about 40% of cases within 6–8 weeks, when vaginal dryness and atrophy or slight psychological problems are improved. Of course, sexual dysfunction can be multifaceted, and individual and partner problems may also be causal.

THE BLATT MENOPAUSE INDEX

To calculate this index 11 subjective climacteric complaints are taken into account. The severity of each complaint is expressed by numerals: 0, no complaint; 1, slight; 2, moderate; 3, marked or severe. The various complaints have been given a conversion factor: 4 for hot flushes, 2 for paresthesia, insomnia and nervousness, and 1 for seven other complaints – melancholia, vertigo, fatigue, arthralgia and/or myalgia, headaches, palpitations and tingling sensations. To calculate the Blatt Menopause Index one multiplies the conversion factor of each complaint by the severity score. A woman who suffers severely from all 11 complaints will show the maximum score of 51. Sexual problems are not included. The Blatt Menopause Index has not been used very often and not at all in more recent scientific publications. The index was further developed by Kupperman, so the Blatt Menopause Index is in fact the forerunner of the Kupperman Index.

THE KUPPERMAN INDEX

Although by 1934 Marañon[68] had written a monograph on the menopause (*L'âge critique*), it was only in 1953 that Kupperman et al[67] attempted quantification and qualification, and therefore naming and weighting of menopausal disorders. Subsequently, this index gained acceptance and for decades was widely recognized. The Kupperman Index had the following characteristics:

- a *list* of the symptoms classified as menopausal in order of their importance;
- a *weighting* of the individual symptom with a multiplication factor corresponding to their importance: e.g. the symptom 'vasomotor' (commonly referred to as hot flushes or sweating) was given a multiplication factor of 4; the symptoms 'paresthesia', 'insomnia' (sleep disorders) and 'nervousness' were given a multiplication factor of 2; a weighting of only 1 was assigned to the remaining symptoms of 'melancholia', 'vertigo', 'weakness', 'arthralgia' and 'myalgia', 'headaches', 'palpitations', and 'formication';
- for each symptom, the Kupperman Index assigned four degrees of *intensity*, which were also used as a multiplication factor when calculating the sum of the index: absence of symptoms received the factor 0, slight symptoms factor 1, moderate symptoms factor 2 and severe symptoms factor 3.

Criticisms of the Kupperman Index

After decades of validity and use, the Kupperman Index became increasingly problematical due to a wide range of issues.

1. *Change in libido*, which in the recent past has received steadily increasing attention, is completely absent from the Kupperman Index.
2. *Dryness of the vagina* is not included in the Kupperman Index and two important research groups have identified this as the second main menopausal symptom (see point 7).
3. *Urological disorders* are absent from the Kupperman Index.
4. Over time, *paresthesia*, assigned a multiplication factor of 2 by the Kupperman Index and ranked second in order of importance, has increasingly been ignored by most workers. Moreover, the term *paresthesia* may be practically identical to *formication*,

occupying the last position in the Kupperman Index.

5. *Giddiness* as an individual symptom is rarely mentioned by researchers any more, even though the Kupperman Index placed it sixth in order of importance.
6. *Headaches* were given ninth place in the Kupperman Index but subsequently proved to be of little significance.
7. A working group of the International Health Foundation, that included well-known authors such as van Keep and Jaszmann,[69] concluded, on the basis of very large and careful epidemiological studies, that all symptoms mentioned by Kupperman except hot flushes and vaginal atrophy are non specific. Somewhat later, the group, working with Utian,[5] reached the same conclusions as the Dutch researchers, but this time on the basis of biochemical data such as measurements of estrogen and gonadotropin in the blood. The intervention of these highly respected and competent research groups leads to hot flushes and genital atrophy being the only symptoms regarded as specifically menopausal for many years. In their opinion, all other symptoms were only the 'psychological consequences of the menopause'. Other authors referred to these further disorders as the so-called domino effect (see earlier section).

In this confused situation, at the conference of the Menopause Association of German-Speaking Countries in Dresden in 1989 the question of symptoms of the menopause was reopened and discussed. It was shown that not only do hot flushes and genital atrophy respond to appropriate hormone therapy, but that other symptoms such as sleep disorders, nervousness, depressed mood, heart disorders, lack of energy, sexual dysfunction do too.[70] In fact, it was even shown that a number of women at the climacteric have symptoms of a so-called menopausal nature but no hot flushes and that these ailments respond effectively to hormone therapy (see below). This was a valid indication that these symptoms are due to estrogen deficiency,[7] and were not due to psychological causes. It is these symptoms, dismissed by the two research groups mentioned above as psychological, that most influence the quality of life of women in the menopause.

For this reason, the Menopause Association of German-Speaking Countries commissioned a group of experts to design a new and more suitable means of assessing menopausal disorders. The members of the expert group (in alphabetical order) were GA Hauser (Lucerne), JC Huber (Vienna), PJ Keller (Zurich), C Lauritzen (Ulm) and HPG Schneider (Münster). The basis for the new assessment was a summary of the symptoms mentioned in the literature with their frequency of occurrence.[7] It soon became clear that it would not be possible to construct an index based on the 20 symptoms most frequently mentioned in the literature as attributable to the menopause, and therefore it was decided to form groups of symptoms. In addition, each group was given its own scale ranging from 0.0

(no symptoms) to 1.0 (very severe symptoms), without assigning weights to the individual symptoms themselves. A separate legend contained a fuller designation and description of the corresponding symptoms. The designations used were chosen to be those in general use so that patients would also understand them and possibly be able to complete the scale themselves. It is then left to the individual examiner to determine the average score (Figs. 8.5 and 8.6).

THE UTIAN MENOPAUSE QUALITY OF LIFE SCORE

A patient's perception of her quality of life may be critical for her willingness to see her doctor and to adhere to her prescribed health care. It would therefore be beneficial for health care providers to be able to measure this perception accurately and to incorporate it into a woman's care plan in order to meet her needs.

Menopause Rating Scale (MRS)	Disorders	None		Slight		Moderate		Severe		Very severe		
		0	0.1	0.2	0.3	0.4	0.5	0.6	0.7	0.8	0.9	1.0
Patient: MM	Hot flushes, sweating											
Age: 55 years	Heart disorders											
	Sleep disorders											
	Depressed mood											
	Nervousness, irritability											
Medication: Premarin Plus	General lack of energy, decline in memory											
Dosage: 0.625 mg once daily	Sexuality											
Uterus present: Yes	Urinary disorders											
Bleeding occurs: Yes	Dryness of the vagina											
Ovaries present: Yes	Articular and muscular disorders											
Date	⋯⋯⋯, 28.10.91 Average 0.85	——, 25.11.91 Average 0.36				- - - - -, 14.02.92 Average 0.05						

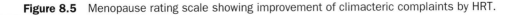

Figure 8.5 Menopause rating scale showing improvement of climacteric complaints by HRT.

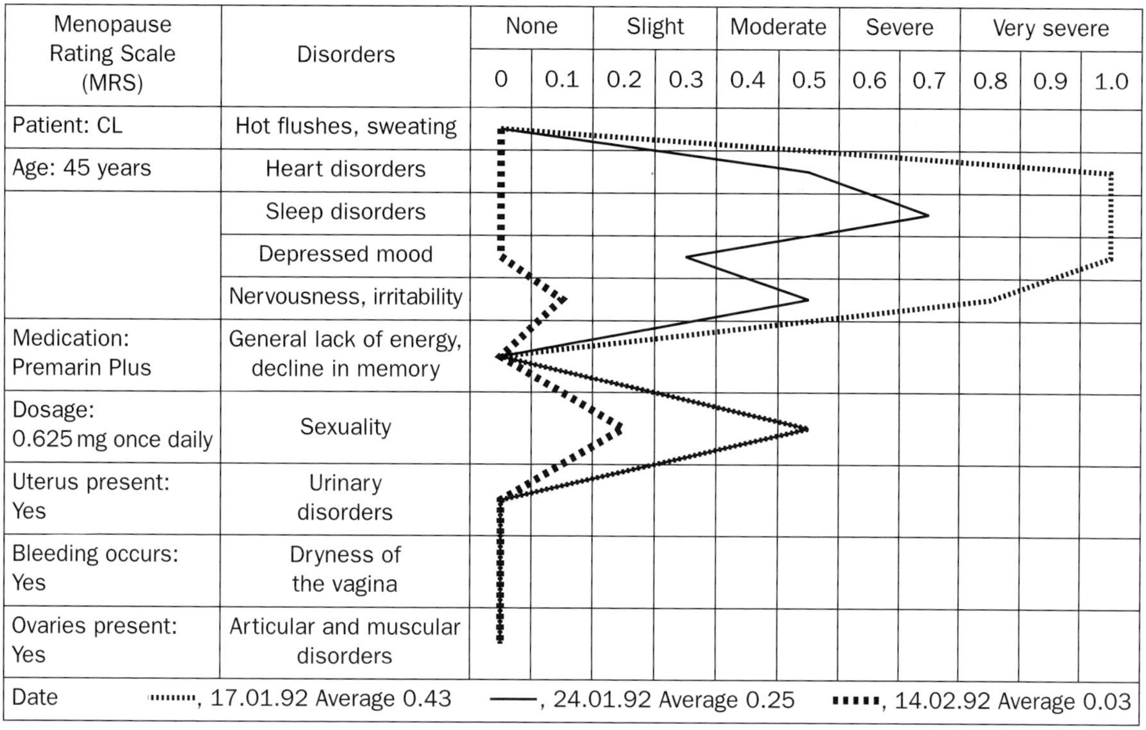

Menopause Rating Scale (MRS)	Disorders	None		Slight		Moderate		Severe		Very severe		
		0	0.1	0.2	0.3	0.4	0.5	0.6	0.7	0.8	0.9	1.0
Patient: CL	Hot flushes, sweating											
Age: 45 years	Heart disorders											
	Sleep disorders											
	Depressed mood											
	Nervousness, irritability											
Medication: Premarin Plus	General lack of energy, decline in memory											
Dosage: 0.625 mg once daily	Sexuality											
Uterus present: Yes	Urinary disorders											
Bleeding occurs: Yes	Dryness of the vagina											
Ovaries present: Yes	Articular and muscular disorders											
Date	·········, 17.01.92 Average 0.43			——, 24.01.92 Average 0.25				▪▪▪▪▪, 14.02.92 Average 0.03				

Figure 8.6 Improvement of climacteric complaints according to the Menopause Rating Scale I; from very severe to slight or no complaints during the duration of treatment for the period of 17.1.92 until 14.2.92.

Quality of life may be defined as a reflection of a person's belief about functioning and achievement in various aspects of their life.[71] Besides the patient's health status, several somatic, psychological and cognitive symptoms, sexual functioning, and social and life circumstances must be included.

A pool of questions was formulated by four senior clinicians with expertise in the psychological and medical aspects of the menopause. The following items were compiled, and are questioned and answered:

- *Factor 1 Occupational quality of life*
  I feel challenged by my work;
  I believe my work benefits society;

- *Factor 2 Health quality of life*
  my diet is nutritionally sound;
  I routinely engage in active exercise three or more times a week;
  I feel physically well;

- *Factor 3 Sexual quality of life*
  I am content with my romantic life;
  I am content with the frequency of my sexual interactions with a partner;

- *Factor 4 Emotional quality of life*
  my mood is generally depressed;
  I consider my life stimulating;
  most of the things that happen to me are out of my control.

An analysis of the answers using Crombach Alpha Analysis showed a good correlation of 0.834 with the perceived quality of life. Utian recommends a combination of his Quality of Life Questionnaire with the Green's Menopause Index,[72,73] which is a brief, precise and validated standard measure of core climacteric symptoms. The combination of the Utian Menopause Quality of Life Score in combination with the Green Score would seem to be a useful tool to capture both a woman's sense of wellbeing and its somatic context.

THE MENOPAUSE RATING SCALE I (MRS I)

A new assessment tool for the evaluation of climacteric complaints was elaborated by an ad hoc working group of experts. After some pilot tests, lasting for about 1 year, the expert group decided, on July 5 1992, on the final version, which was published in 1994 (Fig. 8.7).

During the menopause individual symptoms do not occur simultaneously. However, rating scales must record both early and late occurring symptoms. Only if early symptoms are correctly recognized as climacteric can possible later symptoms be avoided, thus allowing proper prevention.

Disturbances of the menstrual cycle are, in most cases, the earliest symptom of the

Name:	Disorders										
Age:	None		Slight		Moderate		Severe		Very severe		
	0	0.1	0.2	0.3	0.4	0.5	0.6	0.7	0.8	0.9	1.0
1. Hot flushes, sweating											
2. Functional heart disorders											
3. Sleep disorders											
4. Depressed mood											
5. Nervousness, irritability											
6. General lack of energy, decline in memory											
7. Impaired sexuality											
8. Urological disorders											
9. Dryness of the vagina											
10. Articular and muscular disorders											
Date:											
Average score:											

Medication:
Dosage:
Uterus present: Yes/No
Bleeding occurs: Yes/No
Ovaries present: Yes/No

Explanations of the menopausal symptoms:

1. Upward-spreading hotness, sweating (frequency/intensity per 24 hours)
2. Palpitations, racing heart, irregular heartbeat, heart tightness
3. Difficulty going to sleep, waking in the night, waking too early
4. Low spirits, sadness, tearfulness, lack of energy, fluctuating moods
5. Nervousness, inner tension, aggressiveness
6. Physical and mental exhaustion, poor concentration, forgetfulness
7. Reduced sexual desire, activity or satisfaction
8. Problems with urination, frequent need to urinate, involuntary urination
9. Feeling of dryness in the vagina, difficulties with sexual intercourse
10. Pains mainly in the area of the finger joints, rheumatism-like ailments, tingling

Figure 8.7 Menopause Rating Scale I (MRS I).

premenopause. However, these are not specific and they can only be classified as pre-menopausal if they are associated with other more or less specific symptoms.

Late changes of the postmenopause, which are at least partly estrogen dependent, like atherosclerosis and its sequelae and osteo-porosis and its consequences, are not included in MRS I.

Individual MRS I symptoms

Hot flushes

This symptom appears in the Kupperman Index under 'vasomotor' complaints (Kupperman lists 'paresthesia' and 'formica-tion' separately).

In the patient's legend to MRS I, 'hot flush and sweating' is used and is further defined as 'upward-spreading hotness', a term frequently used by patients. 'Sweating' is listed by many authors separately to hot flushes (this symptom is given a multiplication factor of 4 in the Kupperman Index).

Functional heart disorders

Disturbing heart sensations cause more fear in patient than do hot flushes. In the patient's leg-end of MRS I the expression 'heart disorders' is explained as palpitation, cardiac irregularity, quickening of the pulse (tachycardia) and angina pectoris. All of these symptoms corre-spond to Kupperman's 'palpitations' and 'vaso-motor' complaints.

Sleep disorders

Kupperman listed sleep disorders in third place. Some authors regard this symptom as a consequence of the nocturnal hot flushes which may cause awakening and difficulty in falling asleep again, classifying it as a domino effect. There are, however, some women who do not experience hot flushes but nevertheless still report sleep disorders; however estrogen sub-stitution will mostly free these patients from complaint (Fig 8.6).

Depressive mood

Kupperman termed this symptom 'melancho-lia'. It probably has the greatest effect on the quality of life of the women affected. Depressive mood has to be discriminated from real endogenous depression. The patient's leg-end of MRS I contains the terms 'low spirits', 'sadness', 'tearfulness' and 'lack of energy'. It is advisable to offer all these terms to the patient when taking the case history.

Nervousness, irritability, anxiety

This group of symptoms probably presents the highest difficulty in defining a boundary, and there are many similarities to depressed mood. The Kupperman Index uses the term 'nervous-ness'. In the legend of MRS I this group of symptoms is expanded to 'nervousness', 'inner tension' and 'aggressiveness'.

General lack of energy, decline in memory

In the MRS I legend, the terms 'general lack of energy' and 'decline in memory' are expanded to 'physical and mental exhaustion', 'poor con-centration' and 'forgetfulness' (these include tiredness and fainting). The Kupperman Index used the terms 'weakness' and 'fatigue'.

Not infrequently, the patient will mention these symptoms during the consultation with-out being asked. It is then for the doctor to explore for a menopausal symptom by ques-tioning for other signs of illness such as, for example, hot flushes, sleep disorders or heart symptoms.

Sexuality

The Kupperman Index did not mention this symptom. The legend to MRS I defines and describes it as follows: 'changes in sexual desire, sexual activity and satisfaction'.

Urological disorders

The collective syndrome of urological disorders is described more precisely in the legend of MRS I as 'problems with urination', 'frequent need to urinate' and 'involuntary urination'. As for the other collective syndromes, not all symptoms need occur, one symptom is suffi-cient.

Dryness of the vagina

The symptom 'dryness of the vagina' usually occurs relatively late in the climacteric. The legend to MRS I includes another aspect of this symptom – 'painful intercourse'. It is remarkable that this symptom was not mentioned in the Kupperman Index, whereas researchers working with van Keep[33] and Utian[63] presented dryness of the vagina next to hot flushes as the only clear and specific symptoms, and in double-blind tests it responded well to estrogen therapy.

Articular and muscular disorders

This syndrome is not listed last because it is the least important but because, in recent literature and in the group of experts, it generates the most controversial opinions, even though Greenblatt[74] had drawn attention to it in 1963. Although the Kupperman Index pointed the way clearly with the terms 'Arthralgia' and 'Myalgia', these symptoms increasingly disappeared from examiners' assessments. In the legend of MRS I they are described more fully with the expressions 'pains mainly in the area of the finger joints' 'rheumatic-type disorders' and 'tingling', corresponding to 'formication' and 'paresthesia' in the Kupperman Index.

However, pains in the joints are not limited to the fingers (arthrosis digitalis),[75] a fact which is rarely mentioned spontaneously by patients. Not infrequently, the elbows, shoulders and/or back are affected.

Discussion of MRS I

In contrast to the Kupperman Index, which greatly overemphasized important symptoms and gave hot flushes, for example, a multiplication factor of 4, MRS I dispenses with weighting of individual symptoms with their differing frequencies and intensities. As a result, each case gives an individual profile of the symptomatology. Nonspecific symptoms such as 'giddiness' and 'headache' are excluded from MRS I. On the other hand, the symptoms 'sexual dysfunction', 'dryness of the vagina' and 'urinary disorders' are taken into account. Contrary to the group of researchers working with van Keep[33]

and Utian[63], MRS I retains the so-called psychological symptoms, as well as the articular and muscular disorders already recognized in the Kupperman Index. These subjective symptoms are significantly responsible for the patient's quality of life.

In MRS I, the weighting of the individual symptoms is more finely differentiated with a scale ranging in each case from 0.0 (no symptoms) to 1.0 (very severe symptoms). This gives a refined profile of the patient which is not only numerically but also visually elegant (see Fig. 8.7). Under therapy, progress along the individual scales makes the effects not only numerically measurable but also immediately visible (see Figs 8.5 and 8.6). A similar methodology is used by the Hamilton Rating Scale and the Hospital Rating Scale. At the same time, it can quickly be seen which symptoms change. If the scale for individual symptom groups remains unchanged, it indicates either that the symptom is not estrogen dependent or that the dosage is far too low. Our experience is that it becomes apparent after 7–10 days of treatment whether the initiated therapy is having an effect (see Figs 8.5 and 8.6).

Specifically, interested examiners can determine an average value from the individual scales (see Figs 8.5 and 8.6). A lower average value would imply improvement (e.g. in Fig. 8.6, from 0.43 to 0.03 in 8 weeks).

Experience with MRS I shows it to be simple and effective. It is left to the examiner to decide at which intervals to make check-ups. It is, however, advisable to state clearly whether the check-up took place before, during or after taking progestogen, and whether in a purely estrogen phase or even in a hormone phase in the sense of a 'cycle record'.

THE SELF-ASSESSMENT MENOPAUSE RATING SCALE II (MRS II)

MRS II allows women to draw up an account of their symptoms before they visit their doctor, for example, and to describe their condition exactly. This assists the doctor with taking the patient's case history and later with checking progress (Fig. 8.8).

Which of the following symptoms do you have at present?

Please mark each symptom with a cross to show how severely you suffer from it. If a symptom does not affect you, please cross 'None'.

	Symptoms				
	None	Slight	Moderate	Severe	Very severe
Points	0	1	2	3	4
Hot flushes, sweating (upward-spreading hotness, sweating attacks)	☐	☐	☐	☐	☐
Functional heart disorders (palpitations, racing heart, irregular heartbeat, heart tightness)	☐	☐	☐	☐	☐
Sleep disorders (difficulty going to sleep, waking in the night, waking too early)	☐	☐	☐	☐	☐
Depressed mood (low spirits, sadness, tearfulness, lack of energy, fluctuating moods)	☐	☐	☐	☐	☐
Irritability (nervousness, inner tension, aggressiveness)	☐	☐	☐	☐	☐
Anxiety (inner agitation, panic)	☐	☐	☐	☐	☐
Physical and mental exhaustion (general lack of energy, poor concentration, forgetfulness)	☐	☐	☐	☐	☐
Sexual problems (reduced sexual desire, activity or satisfaction)	☐	☐	☐	☐	☐
Urinary disorders (problems with urination, frequent need to urinate, involuntary urination)	☐	☐	☐	☐	☐
Vaginal dryness (feeling of dryness in the vagina, difficulties with sexual intercourse)	☐	☐	☐	☐	☐
Articular and muscular disorders (pains mainly in the area of the finger joints, rheumatism-like ailments)	☐	☐	☐	☐	☐

Figure 8.8 Menopause Rating Scale II (MRS II).

Published in 1999, MRS II uses the same basic structure as MRS I, except that the additional symptom 'anxiety' was added and the scores range from 0 to 5.[76] The legend contained in MRS I – which for many laypersons is essential for understanding – is now placed immediately below the main designations. As part of the validation process, by reference to 479 women in Germany, the advantages relative to the Kupperman Index were demonstrated (Fig. 8.9) and a good correspondence with quality of life was proved (Fig. 8.10) and the frequency of individual symptoms was investigated for moderate to severe disorders. These show a different picture than when all symptoms are considered, in that articular and muscular

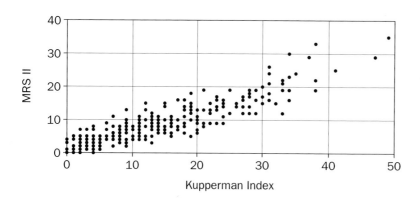

Figure 8.9 Correlation between Kupperman Index and MRS II.[12]

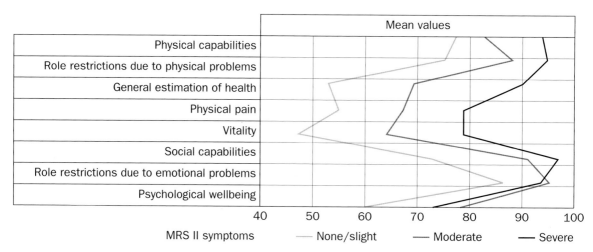

Figure 8.10 Health-related quality of life under HRT.

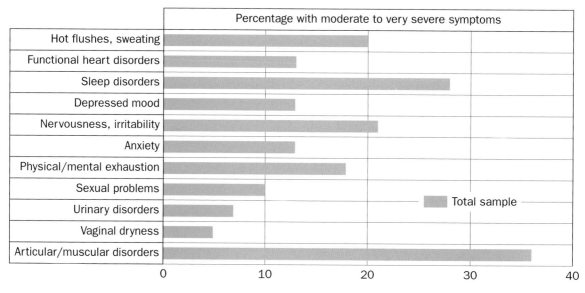

Figure 8.11 Frequency of climacteric complaints in 479 women.[12]

complaints top the list, with sleep disorders in second place, followed by nervousness and only then hot flushes (Fig. 8.11). Further substantiation of the validation and meaningfulness of MRS II is contained in the publications of Schneider et al[77,78] and Potthoff et al.[79]

The woman's preparatory work of completing the self-assessment scale makes the doctor's consultation less time consuming and more efficient. The woman can also complete the scale before each further check-up, thereby providing the doctor with information of specific importance.

REFERENCES

1. Hauser GA, Wenner R. Das Klimakterium der Frau. In: (Heilmier L, Schoen R, de Rudder B, eds) *Ergebnisse der inneren Medizin und Kinderheilkunde*. Berlin: Springer-Verlag, 1961: 125–97.
2. Voest RV. End organ respond to estrogen deprivation. In: (Buchsbaum HJ, ed) *The Menopause*. Springer, 1983: 9–22.
3. Strecker JR, Lauritzen C. *Praxis der Hormonbehandlung im Klimakterium*. Enke, 1989.
4. Rauramo L, Lagerspetz K, Engblom P, Punnonen R. The effect of castration and peroral estrogen therapy on some psychological function. In: (van Keep P, Lauritzen C, eds) *Estrogens in the Post-Menopause*. (Karger: Basel 1976) 94–104.
5. Utian WH. The mental tonic effect of oestrogens administered to oophorectomized females. *S Afr Med J* 1972; **46:** 1079–83.
6. Campell S. Double blind psychometric studies on the effect of natural estrogens. In: menopausal and postmenopausal years. In: (Campbell S) *Management of the Menopause and Postmenopausal Years*. (MTP Press: Lancaster, 1976) 149–68.
7. Hauser GA. Häufigkeit klimakterischer Symptome. In: (Lauritzen C, ed) *Menopause. Hormonsubstitution heute*. (Stabil Verlag: München, 1992) Bd 5, 18–21.
8. Lauritzen C. *Das Klimakterium der Frau*. (Schering: Berlin, 1982).
9. van Keep P, Utian WH, Vermeulen A. *The Controversial Climacteric*. (MTP Press: Lancaster, 1981).
10. Frick-Bruder V. *Klimakterium der Frau*. Berlin: Schering, 1983: 21–37.
11. Metka M, Fischl FH. Der Stellenwert der extragenitalen Symptomatik in der Menopause. In:

(Fischl FH, Huber JC, eds) *Menopause*. (Krause und Pachernegg: Gablitz, 1995) 151–60.
12. Hauser A. Die Häufigkeit der einzelnen klimakterischen Symptome und ihre unterschiedliche Ansprechbarkeit auf Hormontherapie. *J Menopause* 1999; **4:** 44–50.
13. Flint M, Surapti SR. Cultural and subcultural meanings of the menopause. In: (Flint M, Kronenberg F, Utian W, eds) *Multidisciplinary Perspectives on Menopause*. Ann NY Acad Sci 1990; **592:** 134–8.
14. Wasti S, Kamak RF, Robinson SC. Characteristics and perception of the menopause in a Pakistani community. In: (Berg G, Hammar M, eds) *The Modern Management of the Menopause*. (Parthenon: London, 1994).
15. Maoz B. The perception of menopause in five ethnic groups in Israel. In: (Haspels AA, Mustaf H), *Psychosomatics in Perimenopause*. Thesis. Leiden, 1970.
16. Payer L. The menopause in various cultures. In: (Burger H, Boulet M, eds) *Portrait of the Menopause*. Parthenon, 1991: 3–22.
17. Beyene Y. Cultural significance and physiological manifestations of menopause: a biocultural analysis. *Cult Med Psychiatry* 1986; **5:** 1047–71.
18. Dusitsin and Snidvongs. 1994.
19. Locke M, Kaufert P, Gilbert P. Cultural construction of the menopausal syndrome. *Maturitas* 1988; **10:** 317–31.
20. Adlercreutz H, Honjo H, Higashi A et al. Urinary excretion of lignane and isoflavonoid phytoestrogens in Japanese men and women consuming traditional Japanese diet. *Am J Clin Nutr* 1991; **540:** 1093–100.
21. Lauritzen C. *Klimakterium der Frau*. Berlin: Schering, 1982.
22a. Boulet MJ, Oddens BJ, Lehert P et al. Climacteric and menopause in seven south-east Asian countries. *Maturitas* 1994; **19:** 157–76.
22b. Neugarten BL, Kraines RJ. Menopausal symptoms in women at various ages. *Psychosom Med* 1965; **27:** 266–73.
23. Burger HG, Hailes J, Menelaus M et al. The management of persistant menopausal symptoms with estradiol-testosterone implants: clinical, lipid and hormonal results. *Maturitas* 1984; **6:** 351–8.
24. Oldenhave A, Jaszman LJB. The climacteric: absence or presence of hot flushes and their relation to other complaints. In: (Schonbaum E, ed) *Progress in Basic Clinical Pharmacology 6, The climateric hot flush*. Karger, 1991: 6–39.

25. Barret CW, Fairfield L, Nicholson W et al. An investigation of the menopause in one thousand women. *Lancet* 1973; **1:** 106–8.

26. Wilbush J. Climacteric expression and social context. *Maturitas* 1982; **4:** 195–205.

27. Perrault M, Klotz B, Widlocher D. *Traitement des troubles de la menopause climacteric.* (Doin: Paris, 1961).

28. Greene JG. *The social and psychological origin of the climacteric syndrome.* (Gower Publ Comp: Aldershot, 1984).

29. Kielholz P. Diagnostik und Therapie der sogenannten klimakterischen Depression. *Geburtsh Frauenheilk* 1960; **20:** 614–17.

30. Rosemeier HP, Schultz-Zehden B. Psychologische Aspekte des Klimateriums. In: (Fischl FH, Huber JC, eds) *Menopause.* (Krause und Pachernegg: Gablitz, 1995) 23–33.

31. Schulz-Zehden B. *Frauengesundheit in und nach den Wechseljahren. Die 1000-Frauen-Studie.* (Kempkes: Gladenbach, 1998).

32. Cambell S, Whitehead M. The endometrium in the menopause. In: (van Keep PA, Serr DM, Greenblatt RB, eds) *Female and male Climacteric. Current Opinion.* MTP, 1979: 111–20.

33. van Keep PA. *The Menopause, a Study of Women in Belgium, France, Great Britain, Italy and West-Germany* (International Health Foundation: Geneva, 1970.)

34. Townsend AT, Whitehead MJ, McQueen J et al. Double blind studies on the estrogens in postmenopausal women. A follow up report. In: (Pasetto N, Paoletti R, Ambrus J, eds) *The menopause and Postmenopause.* MTP, 1979: 75–84.

35. Parsons AD. Psychological aspect. In: (Page ML, ed) *Current Approaches in Hormone Replacement Therapy.* Duphar, 1990: 29–36.

36. Dennerstein L, Burrows G. Effects of estrogens and progestins on mood and behavior. In: (Christiansen C, ed) *Osteoporosis 1987.* International Symposium Osteoporosis. Osteopress, 1987: 52–64.

37. Hauser GA, Huber JC, Keller PJ et al. Evaluation der klimakterischen Beschwerden (Menopause Rating-Scale (MRS)). *Zentralb Gynaekol* 1994; **116:** 16–23.

38. Greenblatt RB, Barfield WE, Garner JF et al. Evaluation of estrogen, androgen–estrogen combination and a placebo in the treatment of the menopoause. *J Clin Endocr Metab* 1950; **10:** 1547–52.

39. Wied GL. Über die Bedeutung der Suggestion in der Therapie klimakterischer Anfallsbeschwerden. *Ärztl Wschr* 1953; **8:** 623.

40. Campbell S. Double blind psychometric studies on the effects of natural estrogens on post-menopausal women. In: (Campbell, ed), *The Management of the Menopause and Post-menopausal Years.* (MTP Press; Lancaster, 1976) 149.

41. Lauritzen C. The management of the premenopausal and postmenopausal patient. In: (van Keep PA, Lauritzen C, eds) *Aging and Estrogens.* Karger Basel, 1973.

42. Wolf A. Beschwerden der Wechseljahre und Altersveräbderungen an Urogenitale und Mammae. In: (Lauritzen C, ed) *Altergynäkologie.* New York: Thieme, 1997: 89–111.

43. Herrmann WL. *Hormontherapie Klimakterischer Beschwerden.* Berlin: Schering, 1983: 41–52.

44. Voda AM. Climacteric hot flash. *Maturitas* 1981; **3:** 73–90.

45. Hauser GA, Qualifizierung und Quantifizierung der klimakterischen Beschwerden mit der Menopause Rating Scale (MRS). In: (Lauritzen C, ed) *Menopause Hormonsubstitution heute. Bd 8.* (Pia Verlag: Nürnberg, 1996) 121–45.

46. Frick-Bruder V. *Klimakterium der Frau.* Berlin: Schering, 1983.

47. Hauser GA. Das larvierte klimakterische Syndrom. *J Menopause* 1997; **4:** 7–15.

48. Studd JWW. The menopause: biological sabotage. In: (Page ML, ed) *Current Hormone Replacement Therapy*, 1990: 1–4.

49. Lauritzen C. *Keine Angst vor den Wechsejahren.* Ullstein, 1996.

50. Klaiber EL, Broverman DM, Vogel W, Kobayashi Y. The use of steroid hormones in depression. In: (Itil TM, Laudahn G, Hermann WM, eds) *Psychotropic Action of Hormones.* (Spectrum: New York, 1976) 135.

51. Aylward M. Plasma tryptophan levels and mental depression in postmenopausal subjects. Effects of oral piperazine-oestrone-sulphate. *Med Sci* 1973; **1:** 30.

52. Studd JWW, Panay N. Estrogens in the treatment of climacteric depression, premenstrual depression, postnatal depression and chronic fatigue syndrome. In; (Wren B, ed) *Progress in the Management of the Menopause.* (Parthenon: London, 1997), 385–92.

53. Haspels AA, Coelingh-Bennink HJT, Keep PA, Schreurs WPH. Disturbance of tryptophane metabolism and its correction during oestrogen treatment in postmenopausal women. *Maturitas* 1978; **1:** 15–19.

54. Kerr D. Psychohormonal approach to the menopause. *Med Treatment* 1968; **53:** 587–91.

55. Moore B, Gustafson R, Studd J. Experience of a national health service menopause clinic. *Curr Med Res Opin* **3** (Suppl. 3): 42.

56. Hauser GA. Häufigkeit klimakterischer Symptome (Eine Literaturübersicht). In: (L Lauritzen C, ed) *Menopause. Hormonsubstitution heute.* Bd 5, Stabel-Verlag, 1992: 18–21.

57. Sherwin BB. Estrogen and/or androgen replacement therapy and cognitive functioning in surgically postmenopausal women. *Psychology* 1988; **13:** 345–57.

58. Wenderlein JM. Postmenopausale Östrogentherapie der Harninkontinenz. In: (Lauritzen C, ed) *Menopoause. Hormonsubstitution heute, Volume 2.* (Edition Ionformed: München, 1989) 56–65.

59. Baron J. *Klimakterium i senium Pamietnik XVII Zjadzu Polskiego Towarzystwa Ginekogocznego.* (Poznan Univ, 1968) 15–41.

60. Sarrell PM. Effects of transdermal estradiol on sensation, bloodflow and sexual function. In: (Whitehead MI, Schenkel I, eds) *Transdermal Hormone Replacement.* Parthenon, 1990: 23–33.

61. Hauser GA. Häufigkeit der einzelnen klimakterischen Symptome und ihre unterschiedliche Ansprechbarkeit auf Hormontherapie. *J Menopause* 1999; **2:** 44–50.

62. van Keep PA, Kellerhals J. The impact of sociocultural factors on symptom formation. *Psycho Ter Psychosomat* 1974; **23:** 251.

63. Utian WH. Definitive symptoms of postmenopause – incorporating use of vaginal parabasal cell index. In: (van Keep P, Lauritzen C, eds) *Estrogen in the Postmenopause, Volume 3. Front Hormone Res.* (Karger: Basel, 1975) 74–89.

64. Menge. Arthropatia ovaripriva. In: (Metka M, Fischl F) *Der Stellenwert der 'extragenbitalen Symptome' in der menopause.* In: (Fischl F, Huber JC) *Menopause.* Krause und Pachernegg 1995, 1924: 154.

65. Novak J. Über Arthropathia ovaripriva. *Zbl Gynäkol* 1924; **47:** 2218–21.

66. Garrod J. Arthropathia, neuralgia and myalgia ovaripriva, 1890. In: (Kehrer E) *Endokrinologie für den Frauenarzt.* (F Enke: Stuttgart, 1937).

67. Kupperman HS, Blatt HG, Wiesbaden H, Filler W. Comparative clinical evaluation of estrogen preparations by the menopausal and amenorrhea indices. *J Clin Endocr* 1953; **13:** 88–92.

68. Maranon G. *Gynecologia endocrina.* Espaso-Calpe: Madrid, 1935.

69. Jaszman L. Epidemiology of climacteric and post-climacteric complaints. In: (van Keep P, Lauritzen C, eds) *Ageing and Estrogens. Front. Hormone Res.* vol. 2 (Karger: Basel, 1973) 23–31.

70. Hauser GA. Einßluss der Oestrogene auf die Psyche der Frau in der Postmenopause. In: (Lauritzen C, ed) *Menopause. Hormonsubstitution heute.* Informed Bd. 3 1990, Stabel-Verlag, 1990: 46–58.

71. Utian WH, Janata JW, Kingsberg SA et al. Determinants and quantification of quality of life after the menopause: the Utian Menopause Quality of Life score. In: (Aso T, Yanaihara T, Fujimoto S eds) *The Menopause at the Millenium.* (Parthenon: London, 2000) 141–4.

72. Greene JG. *The Social and Psychological Origin of the Climacteric Syndrome.* (Gower Publ Comp: Aldershot, UK, 1984).

73. Greene JG. *Guide to the Greene Climacteric Scale.* (University of Glasgow Publishers: Glasgow, 1991).

74. Greenblatt RB. Menopause and its management. In: (Dorfman R, Castro M, eds) *Pitituary and Ovarian Endocrinology.* San Francisco: Holden Day, 1963: 159.

75. Perrault M, Klotz B, Widlocher D. *Traitement des Trouples de la Ménopause Climactérique.* Doin, 1961.

76. Hauser GA, Schneider HPG, Rosemeier, HP et al. *Die Selbstbeurteilungs-Skala für Klimakterische Beschwerden.* (Menopause Rating Scale I). *J Menopause* 1999; **4:** 12–15.

77. Schneider HPG, Heinemann LA, Rosemeier HP et al. The Menopause Rating Scale (MRS). Comparison with Kupperman Index and quality-of-life scale SF-36. *Climacteric* 2000; **3:** 50–8.

78. Schneider HPG, Heinemann LA, Rosemeier HP et al. The Menopause Rating Scale (MRS). Reliability of score of menopausal complaints. *Climacteric* 2000; **3:** 59–64.

79. Potthoff P, Heinemann LAJ, Schneider HPG et al. Menopause rating scale (MRS II) Methodische Standartisierung in der deutschen Bevölkerung. *Zentralb Gynäkol* 2000; **122:** 280–6.

80. Kuhl H, Taubert HD. *Das Klimakterium. Pathophysiologie-Klinik-Therapie.* Thieme Verlag, 1987.

81. Hauser. 1999.

83. Chompootweep M, Tankeyoon, YP et al. The menopausal age and climacteric complaints in Thai women in Bangkok. *Maturitas* 1993; **17:** 63–71.

84. Coope J. Double-blind cross-over study of estrogen replacement therapy. In: (Campbell S,

ed) *The Management of Menopause and Post-menopausal Years*. (MTP Press: Lancaster, 1976) 159.

85. Fedor-Freybergh P. The influence of oestrogens on well being and mental performance in climacteric and postmenopausal women. *Acta Obstet Gynecol Scand* 1977; Suppl 64.

86. Gray RH. The menopause – epidemiological and demographical considerations. In: (Beard RJ, ed) *The Menopause*. (University Park Press: Baltimore, 1976; 11–16.)

87. Hauser GA, Dahinden U, Samartzis S, Wenner R. Effects and side-effects of estrogen therapy on the climacteric syndrome. In: (van Keep P, Lauritzen C, eds) *Ageing and Estrogens. Front. Hormone Res.* vol. 2 (Karger: Basel, 1973) 35–42.

88. Hauser GA. Erfahrungen mit der Erstfassung der Menopause Rating Scale (MRS). In: (Lauritzen C, ed) *Menopause. Hormonsubstitution heute, Bd 6.* (Aesopus: Basel, 1993) 103–10.

89. Hauser GA, Huber JC, Keller PJ et al. Evaluation der klimakterischen Beschwerden, Menopause Rating Scale (MRS). *Zbl Gynäkologie* 1994; **116:** 16–23.

90. Haines CJ, Chung THK, Leung DHY. A prospective study of the frequency of acute menopausal symptoms in Hong Kong Chinese women. *Maturitas* 1994; **18:** 75–81.

91. Ismael NN. A study of the menopause in Malaysia. *Maturitas* 1994; **19:** 205–9.

92. van Keep PA, Humphrey M. Psychosocial aspects of the climacteric. In: (van Keep PA, Greenblatt RD, Albeaux-Fernet M, eds) *Consensus on Menopause Research.* (MTP Press: Lancaster, 1976).

93. Kielholz P. Diagnostik und Therapie der depressiven Zustandsbilder. *Schweiz Med Wschr* 1957; **87:** 109–22.

94. Kopera H. Estrogens and psychic functions. In: (van Keep A, Lauritzen C, eds) *Ageing and Estrogens.* (Karger: Basel, 1973) 118.

95. Lauritzen C, Mueller, P. Pathology and involution of the genitals in the aging female. In: (Money I, Musaph H, eds). *Handbook of Sexology.* (Exc. Medica: Amsterdam, 1977), 846.

96. Lock M. Culture and the menopause. In: (Aso T, Yanaihara T, Fajimoto S, eds) *The Menopause at the Millennium.* (Parthenon: New York, 2000) 29–35.

97. Martin M, Block J, Sanchez S et al. Menopause without symptoms: the endocrinology of menopause among rural Mayan Indians. *Am J Obstet Gynecol* 1993; **168:** 1839–454.

98. McCarthy T. The prevalence of symptoms in menopausal women in the Far East Singapore Segment. *Maturitas* 1994; **19:** 199–204.

99. Prill HJ, Lauritzen C. Das Klimakterium. In: (Schwalm H, Doederlein G, eds) *Klinik der Frauenheilkunde und Geburtshilfe, Volume 8,* (Urban u Schwarzenberg: München, 1970) 339.

100. Saletu B, Brandstätter N, Metka M et al. Double-blind placebo controlled, hormonal, syndromal and EEG-mapping studies with transdermal oestradiol therapy in menopausal depression. *Psychopharmacology* 1995; **122:** 321–9.

101. Shea J. *Revolutionary women at middle age: an ethnographic survey of menopause and midlife aging in China.* Thesis Harvard University, 1989.

102. Sherwin BB. The impact of different doses of estrogen and progestin on mood and sexual behaviour in postmenopausal women. *J Clin Endocr, Metab* 1991; **72:** 336–43.

103. Yeh A. *The experience of menopause among Taiwanese women.* Thesis, Harvard University, 1989.

9

Practice of hormone substitution

C Lauritzen

Basic considerations • Expectation: hopes and fears of the patients • Contraindications • Indications for hormone replacement therapy (HRT) • Basis of medical recommendations • Selection of preparations • Success rate of hormone replacement therapy (HRT) • Indications for long-term therapy • Preconditions of long-term therapy • Duration of treatment • Adherence to therapy • Handling of risk factors • Forms of application • Side-effects • Alternatives to conventional hormone replacement therapy (HRT) • Nonhormonal medicaments • Conclusions • Recommended reading

BASIC CONSIDERATIONS

The art and success of hormone replacement therapy (HRT) is primarily based on the creation of good social contact and on mutual sympathy between doctor and patient. The feelings, fears, doubts and wishes of the patient should be sensibly and empathically discussed before HRT is prescribed (Box 9.1). A careful search for and exclusion of possible contraindications and risks will secure the justification and safety of the hormone prescription. These efforts will create an atmosphere of trust between patient and physician.

The application of a critical controlled therapeutical experience of the physician, together with a thorough knowledge of preparations and of the modes of application available, will lead to a prudent selection of the optimal individual treatment. The course of treatment must always be accompanied by alertness of the consulting therapist for his/her personal professional responsibility, which should give the patient an impression of reliability, and will secure cooperation and adherence to the therapy by the patient.

The patient will leave the practice satisfied only if she has the feeling that all her fears and all problems of treatment have been discussed, that all uncertainties have been removed, that her wishes have been appropriately taken into account and that she can leave the management of her complaints calmly to the competence of her doctor, who will secure for her the benefits of treatment and keep away any possible harm. The motivation for adherence to therapy is determined by the severity of complaints, the quality of medical advice, the symptomatic success of treatment, the absence of side-effects and the conviction of overall positive effects of HRT concerning prevention of diseases and safeguarding quality of life.

EXPECTATION: HOPES AND FEARS OF THE PATIENTS

Many climacteric women have negative expectations as concerns the change of life in the years to follow (Table 9.1). If this is the case, it is important to assure the woman at menopause that climacteric is not a disease, that her symptoms are not threatening and to convince her that this change of life can be a chance for a

---

Box 9.1 Indications for estrogen–progestogen substitution in menopausal and postmenopausal women with climacteric complaints

---

Early spontaneous menopause

Early castration (before the age of 48)

Heavy climacteric complaints

Reactive depressive emotional symptoms

Complaints due to urogenital atrophy (senile colpitis, dry vagina, urethrocystitis, dys-stranguria, urinary stress incontinence)

Atrophy of skin and mucous membranes (including conjunctiva) causing complaints

Hirsutism, virilism, alopecia caused by estrogen deficiency and hyperandrogenism – preferential oral medication; addition of an antiandrogenic progestogen

Multiple risk factors for osteoporosis; beginning of manifestation of osteoporosis – calcium and vitamin D supplementation

Elevated low-density lipoprotein, decreased high-density lipoprotein, hyperhomocysteinaemia, elevated protein C, risk factors for coronary disease – only early use of primary prevention with estrogen will be effective; not suited as only indication of estrogen substitution; no secondary prevention in case of preceding cardiovascular event and manifest atherosclerosis

Cognitive disturbances – only early prevention will be effective

Morbus Alzheimer(?) – only early prevention may be effective, not suited as only indication for estrogen substitution

---

new beginning, for additional sources of freedom, for the fulfillment of secret wishes, and a possibility to strive for calmness, new knowledge and equanimos wisdom.

All these possibilities of self-fulfillment can however only be utilized by those women whose wellbeing is not restricted by severe climacteric complaints, pain, depression, lack of determination and loss of physical and psychological activity. This is how estrogens can help to fulfill wishes and to support the realization of plans for the third phase of life of a woman.

If a good patient–doctor relationship has been built up, adherence to therapy will be stable and all uprising problems and doubts concerning hormones will be immediately and trustfully discussed between them, and the patient will reliably come to regular check-ups.

Some climacteric women may have no complaints and so do not need estrogens. About 30% of climacteric women with complaints would prefer the use of so-called natural methods, meaning plant extracts, homeopathy

or a change of lifestyle. There is no sense in persuading such a patient to have hormonal treatment that she does not want. Experience shows that the course of treatment in such cases is characterized by accumulation of dissatisfaction and manifold problems. Adherence to treatment will accordingly be poor. Possible alternatives to conventional hormonal treatment, if asked for, should therefore be explained to such patients.

CONTRAINDICATIONS

Before an indication is realized by the prescription given, all contraindications have to be excluded (Box 9.2). Absolute contraindications exclude the use of estrogen replacement therapy (ERT) and HRT. If relative contraindications have been found, these can possibly be bypassed by lower doses of hormones, by parenteral application (patch, gel, injection, nasal, oromucosal rectal, vaginal), by an additional safeguarding treatment or elimination of risk

Table 9.1 Worries and fears of climacteric women (Outpatients Clinic *n* = 262; 48–65 years of age; University of Ulm, Department of Gynaecology and Obstetrics, 1990)	Frequency (%)
Fear of cancer	78
long-lasting illness with pain and suffering	62
operations	41
osteoporosis	14
Worry about illness or death of the partner	40*
Not being able to get along in old age	39
Being permanently disabled	17
Financial and housing problems	27
Marriage problems, loss of libido, loss of attractiveness, loss of femininity	32
Problems with the family	
death of parents	32†
needing to care for parents or relatives	17‡
Worries about children	25§
Fears of menopause	
weight gain	63
loss of wellbeing and joy of life	16
loss of energy and efficiency	–
loss of memory and concentration	–
Fear of or objections to hormone treatment	44

* Partner had already died in 3% of case; † parents already dead in 21% of cases; ‡ patients already in need of care in 3% of cases; § no children in 8% of cases.

factors (e.g. of varicosis), by specific medicaments or lifestyle counseling (e.g. weight decrease, age-adapted gymnastics).

A secondary prevention of cardiovascular diseases (following myocardial infarction or stroke) is not indicated or relatively contraindicated. Apparently, statins show fewer side-effects and give better therapeutical results, and can possibly be combined with estrogens.

The meticulous consideration of contraindications and of risk factors will prevent unnecessary side-effects and complications as seen in some randomized controlled studies. If contraindications against estrogens are present in patients with severe complaints then, alternatives have to be considered, e.g. designer hormones, selective estrogen receptor modulators (SERM), phytoestrogens, medicaments covering the most embarrassing main symptoms, gymnastics, yoga or changes of lifestyle. For instance, serotonin reuptake inhibitors (e.g. fluoxetine) will mitigate vasomotor symptoms and may at the same time improve mood.

INDICATIONS FOR HORMONE REPLACEMENT THERAPY (HRT)

Complaints may in some cases have a dimension which attains the character of an illness. Moreover, estrogen deficiency can, after several

---

Box 9.2   Contraindications against estrogens

Absolute contraindications

Acute deep venous thrombosis, pulmonary embolism

APC resistance, factor V mutation Leiden – Parenteral estrogen medication with low doses of estrogen and progestogen can be considered in the absence of genetic anomalies of coagulation; treat risk factors and prevent thrombosis-triggering events; substitution at earliest 6 months after the event as long as no residual symptoms are present; local application of estriol in low doses is always possible

Genetic anomaly of control of cell growth (BRCa1 and 2)

Family history of multiple breast, genital and intestinal cancer; status short after breast cancer, if tamoxifen, SERM or aromatase inhibitors are indicated – thereafter treatment of severe climacteric symptomatology by low-dose estrogens, phytoestrogens or designer hormones(?)

Status short after stroke and myocardial infarction

Hematoporphyria; severe acute liver diseases, acute hepatitis; Dubin–Johnson syndrome, Rotor's syndrome (very rare) – low doses of transdermal estradiol could be tried; minimal liver load by estriol

Relative contraindications

The decision not to treat, to withdraw or to treat is dependent on the weight of the indication for hormone substitution. Special considerations are necessary concerning doses and mode of application (parenteral). Addition of an appropriate progestogen. Local application of estriol. Consider tibolone, SERM, phytoestrogens. Careful advice and supervision. If meaningful: internistic consilium. Additional advice and treatment of risk factors with the aim of risk reduction. Informed consent of the patient.

Severe climacteric symptoms

Status after breast, endometrial and ovarian cancer, but not if patient is doubtful

Severe fixed hypertension. Severe diabetes with vascular damages

Status some years after stroke and myocardial infarction. Internistic consilium. Statins, secondarily combined with parenteral estrogen

Genetically caused anomalies of lipid status, hypertriglyceridemia – internistic consilium; low parenteral estrogens; some gestagens and tibolone decrease trigylcerides

Pancreatitis, cholecystitis, cholelithiasis – refrain from alcohol; low-fat diet; low dose of parenteral estrogen and/or parenteral progesterone (lipid-neutral progestogen)

Cardiogenic and nephrogenic edemas – treatment of causes. Thereafter low estrogen doses, progesterone or a progestogen with diuretic activity (drospirenon)

Trauma or status after major operations; long-lasting immobilization – parenteral treatment with low doses if possible; treatment allowed during medication of heparin or coumarins; early mobilization

Severe epilepsy or migraine after receiving estrogen and progestogen – change of preparation; continuous low estrogen plus progestogen medication

Fast growing myomas, severe endometriosis, proliferating mastopathia – remove myoma, if possible, by minimal invasive operation; low parenteral estrogen; progesterone with no estrogenic but antiestrogenic activity; SERM, tibolone, phytoestrogens

---

SERM, Selective estrogen receptor modulators.
BRCa1 and 2, Breast cancer genes.
APC, Activated Protein C.

years postmenopause, lead to the development of real diseases such as osteoporosis and atherosclerosis and its sequelae, which require prevention or early intervention. This would necessitate early menopausal substitution. Co-operation with collegues of internal medicine is recommended in such cases. For the absolute and relative indication for ERT and HRT see Box 9.1.

The treatment of climacteric complaints and of urogenital atrophic changes by estrogens are highly effective (near 100%) and undisputed. Osteoporosis and bone fractures are the only well-secured indication for a primary prevention of a postmenopausal disease by estrogens. This primary prevention goes together with ERT and HRT treatment of climacteric symptoms for more than 5 years. The substitution must be long-term to achieve a full prevention. After withdrawal of the substitution the effect on bone density and fractures will regress within a few years.

The primary prevention of cardiovascular complaints seems to be effective so long as a good estrogenic effect is not blocked by addition of an inadequate progestogen. Primary prevention of cardiovascular diseases should not be the only indication for ERT or HRT; however, it is accepted as an additional beneficial effect of symptomatic long-term treatment of climacteric complaints. Primary cardiovascular prevention by estrogen is possible if it is begun at menopause and maintained long-term. The effect on reduction of cardiovascular events will last for some years after withdrawal of hormones.

BASIS OF MEDICAL RECOMMENDATIONS

The accumulation of medical experience over more than 60 years with estrogen treatment has led to the possibility of relatively safe predictions of effectivity and of well-tried or even proven rules of treatment. However, experience and statistics can only give general information about a positive influence of estrogen intake on the incidence of typical complaints and of reduction of the incidence of postmenopausal diseases in large population groups. They do not give accurate and safe insights into a possible effect of estrogens in a specific case. Therefore, when an indication is made, only predictions of a certain probability are possible in an individual case. This means that the physician's recommendations for a hormonal substitution will accordingly only be based on assumptions and probabilities with varying degrees of certainty. This is however true for all treatments with hormones.

Because this is so, HRT may cause, in some cases, side-effects during the first weeks of intake. Mostly, an overdosage of estrogen or poor tolerance of the progestogen are the cause of side-effects. It is therefore important to make an appointment to see the patient within 6 weeks after the start of treatment for a possible adaption of dose, preparation or mode of application.

SELECTION OF PREPARATIONS

Advantages and disadvantages of the different hormones and of the forms of estrogen-progesterone application are shown in Box 9.3. Estradiol and progesterone are the genuine ovarian hormones. They should therefore be preferentially used as estradiol or estradiol valerate (1 and 2 mg) and as oral progesterone (200 mg capsules), or as vaginal applicable progesterone gel. Most investigations on ERT and HRT have been performed in the USA with conjugated estrogens and the progestogen medroxyprogesterone acetate (MPA), a combination that seems not to be optimal. As new oral active estradiol and progesterone are available, I prefer the human estrogens to the equine ones, and genuine progesterone to artificial progestogens. In particular, MPA is not an ideal progestogen. There are however special indications for antiandrogenic progestogens (e.g cyproterone acetate, chlormadininacetate, dienogest), as in cases of postmenopausal hyperandrogenic syndromes. In view of the rather unphysiologic levels of estrone following oral estradiol, the question arises whether oral medication is indeed the gold standard in all cases. Transdermal application of estradiol as patch or gel creates lower and more steady

---

Box 9.3   Advantages and disadvantages of different forms of application of estradiol and progesterone

---

Estradiol

Oral medication

Advantages (mostly because of the first liver passage from the intestine into the circulation)

Strong favorable effect on lipids [HDL, LDL, homocystein, Lp(a), Apo A]

Primary preventive effect against atherosclerosis and consecutive cardiovascular events

Strong increase in SHBG; favourably used in cases of hirsutism and virilism, because of binding of
free androgens

Disadvantages (mostly because of the first liver passage)

Increase of triglycerides, renin substrate, renin and hepatic coagulation factors

Parenteral application (transdermal, lingual, nasal, intramuscular, rectal, vaginal)

Advantages (bypass of the first liver passage)

No significant influence on coagulation, triglycerides, renin substrate, renin

Favorable for patients at risk for thromboembolism, hypertension, stroke,
diseases of the liver, gallbladder stomach and intestine, and diabetes

Disadvantages [lower increase of HDL and lower decrease of LDL than with oral medication; increase in
IGF; no increase of SHBG (less antiandrogenic effect of the estrogen)]

With patches, allergic reactions of the skin are possible

Local application (ointment, ovula, suppositories)

Advantages [no load of metabolic organs (stomach, intestine, liver and gallbladder)

No other metabolic and target organ effects, if not desired; low doses effective

Target close to organ, organ-selective effect

Progesterone

Oral medication

Advantages   Natural ovarian hormone; orally effective

Disadvantages   Rapid metabolization in the liver on first liver passage, therefore high doses required

Vaginal application (vaginal gel, suppositories)

Advantages   Effective resorption and tolerance; predominant flow to the endometrium; no first pass
through the liver, therefore less hepatic metabolization

Local application

Advantages   Application directly to the target organ; effective local resorption; short distance; low
dose, high concentration. When applied to the breast there is a significant antimitotic effect. Low
local metabolization rate; no general effects in the organism

---

Apo A, apolipoprotein A; HDL, high-density lipoprotein; IGF, insulin-like growth factor; LDL, low-density lipoprotein; Lp(a),
lipoprotein (a); SHBG, sex hormone-binding globulin.

levels of estradiol, less estrone and less binding to sex hormone-binding globulin (SHBG) than oral medication. Effects on liver factors influencing coagulation are less. This pattern is much nearer to the blood levels and estradiol/estrone relations during normal ovarian secretion. Special indications for an oromucosal, nasal or vaginal application is a contraindication against oral or transdermal treatment.

Oral progesterone (200 mg in capsules) is given for an optimum of 14 days during the second half of the cycle, securing a regular bleeding pattern. I prefer to give progesterone in the evening, which has the advantage that any side-effects (e.g. tiredness) will fall into the sleep phase and the estrogen effect will act unmodified during the day. Vaginal progesterone gel and rectal or vaginal progesterone suppositories allow an individualization of treatment. The tolerability of this mode of application is, in my experience, better than with oral medication.

An interesting possibility is the use of an intrauterine contraceptive device (IUCD), securing perimenopausal contraception for more than 5 years by secreting small amounts of levonorgestrel to the endometrium, thus leading to endometrial atrophy, even during estrogen substitution. Oral progestogen medication is then not necessary.

Local application of progesterone gel over the breast will significantly reduce the rate of mitoses in the mammary gland epithelium induced by estrogen.

SUCCESS RATE OF HORMONE REPLACEMENT THERAPY (HRT)

The treatment of climacteric complaints has a very high success rate in randomized double-blind studies against placebo of about 85–95% as concerns hot flushes and sweating. This effect of improvement begins within 10 days and is complete within 4–6 weeks. Sleeping disturbances and depressive moods, which are often multicausal, show a lower rate of improvement and may sometimes take more time to disappear (Table 9.2). Atrophic urogenital complaints may take weeks to disappear.

Local, oral and parenteral medication in urogenital indications are equally successful. In local application, estriol in low doses can be used, which will not proliferate the endometrium.

INDICATIONS FOR LONG-TERM THERAPY

About 20–25% of all estrogen takers will choose long-term therapy, i.e. medication for longer periods than 5 years. The preconditions and indications are shown in Box 9.4.

PRECONDITIONS OF LONG-TERM THERAPY

The most important precondition for a long-term therapy is that complaints persist and that the treatment is well tolerated and is without severe side-effects. Of course, the patient must wish to continue the treatment. A sound additional indication could be given, for example, risk of osteoporosis.

DURATION OF TREATMENT

Climacteric complaints will last a mean of 3–5 years and this is how long a symptomatic treatment should last. If in later years atrophic urogenital complaints occur, oral or parenteral estrogen treatment is in most cases not necessary and local application of estriol is usually sufficient.

If, together with the treatment of climacteric complaints, a prevention of osteoporosis or of atherosclerosis is intended, treatment should be maintained for as long as possible, as most fractures and cardiovascular events occur after the age of 70. The drop-out in later years is mostly conditioned by severe diseases and the necessity of taking many other medicaments. In old age the estrogen dose can be reduced in most cases. Parenteral medication (patches, gel or local application) is to be preferred to oral intake, at least if a primary treatment is begun in old age.

ADHERENCE TO THERAPY

The adherence to medical prescription is highly dependent on the patient's motivation, which is

Table 9.2 Success of an oral estrogen–progestogen substitution for typical climacteric symptoms (225 patients, 50–65 years of age; 2 mg estradiol valerate, 1.25 mg conjugated estrogens plus different progestogens; University of Ulm, Department of Gynaecology and Obstetrics, 1991)

Complaints	Women free of complaints or clear signs of improvement	
	After 2 weeks	After 6 weeks after initiation of treatment (%)
Hot flushes, sweating	89	98
Heart palpitations, irregular heart beats	78	93
Nervousness, irritability, anxiety	72	95
Tiredness, inefficiency	74	97
Sleeplessness	77	92
Depressive moods, lack of drive	62	87
Muscle and joint complaints	66	83
Dry vagina, cohabitation problems	61	100
Complaints of urinary tract	54	89
Urinary incontinence (subjective improvement)	12	74

determined by the severity of the climacteric complaints, on the fast reduction of the complaints by the preparation, on absence of side-effects and on the insight into the overall positive effects of estrogens on vitality and quality of life. Misinformation by friends or the press often cause fears and disturb motivation. Therefore, a good patient–doctor relationship is important because it will lead to a rapidly clarifying discussion of all problems. The knowledge of the reason for drop-outs may make it possible for the therapist to improve adherence by avoidance of those reasons (Table 9.3).

HANDLING OF RISK FACTORS

Of all the factors, those for mammary cancer and thrombotic diseases in relation to estrogen–progestogen medication are the most impor-

tant. They do however concern only a small percentage of the population treated and must not be taken as real or unchangeable for all patients. When risk factors are present, the decision must be taken as to whether the treatment is contraindicated or can be allowed under certain conditions.

There are risk factors which can be changed and those that cannot. Family history of cancer, BRCa mutation, childlessness, late first pregnancy and not having breastfed are cancer risks that are unchangeable because they concern the past. Reduction of calories and of weight, stopping alcohol and nicotine, and an increase in physical activity are possible measures to possibly delay or to reduce the risk of manifestation of cancer. Whether and under what conditions this is true must be further tested by appropriate trials.

Box 9.4   Indications for long-term substitution (> 5 years) with estrogen–progestogen

Preconditions

So far well-tolerated substitution without any side-effects and with good effectiveness; no new risk factors; continuing climacteric complaints or atrophic urogenital changes; freely expressed wishes and informed consent of the patient. A primary start of estrogen treatment after the age of 60 should be initiated with low doses of estrogens, preferably transdermal or possibly local estriol.

Osteoporosis

High-risk factors are: osteoporosis in a first-degree relative; hints from the patient's history, e.g. late menarche, pubertas tarda, amenorrheic episodes without substitution; underweight; status after bone fracture without plausible reason; bone density less than one standard deviation below the mean age-related value – consider calcium, vitamin D substitution, bisphosphonates, age-adapted gymnastics, hip protectors

Cardiovascular diseases

High risk for angina pectoris, ST; depression on electrocardiogram, hyperlipidemia [high LDL, high Lp(a), low HDL, hyperhomocysteinaemia, high protein C]; myocardial infarction in a first-degree relative; NB: If indications for existing severe atherosclerosis are recommended; first-line statin therapy; thereafter, low doses of transdermal estradiol

Atrophic changes caused by estrogen deficiency of the urogenital system, skin, mucous membranes and conjunctiva of the eyes, hirsutism, virilization

Atrophy of the vulva, colpitis atrophicans, dry vagina, chronic urethrocystitis, cystalgia, pollakis-stranguria, urge incontinence and mixed forms; atrophy of the skin and mucous membranes, keratoconjunctivitis sicca; increased levels of androgens: hirsutism; acne, seborrhea, alopecia – oral estrogens in combination with antiandrogenic progestogens; local application of estriol ointment or vaginal suppositories, estradiol eye drops 0.025%

Deterioration of cerebral performance (under discussion)

Morbus Alzheimer in a first-degree relative; deterioration of attention, vigilance, concentration, short-term memory, word finding, recall of names, mental fatiguability; postmenopausal dysphoria, depressive mood, climacteric sleep disturbances – so far experience mostly with oral estrogens; consider combination with

---

HDL, High-density lipoprotein; LDL, low-density lipoprotein; Lp(a), lipoprotein (a).

FORMS OF APPLICATION

For advantages and disadvantages of different forms of application see Box 9.3. The most often used form of treatment is oral intake. However, investigation of hormone levels suggest that the oral application is not optimal and far from the pattern of physiological ovarian secretion. The primary passage through the intestine produces high rapidly changing estradiol levels and high estrone levels. The passage through the liver causes early metabolism, high stimulation of SHBG levels and, accordingly, strong steroid hormone binding. The production of coagulation products by the liver is stimulated by oral medication.

Transdermal application will bring unmetabolized estradiol directly into the circulation and will cause more constant low levels of estradiol without excessive estrone. The relatively lower

Table 9.3 Reasons given by postmenopausal women for discontinuation of an estrogen–progestogen substitution within the first year of treatment (225 patients, 50–60 years of age; University of Ulm, Department of Gynaecology and Obstetrics, 1991)

	Women discontinuing estrogen–progestogen substitution (%)		
Reason	Oral sequential estrogen–progestogen	Estrogen patches oral progestogen	Estrogen–progestogen combined continuously
Instruction leaflet induced fears	23	16	10
Strong or prolonged bleedings, premenstrual syndrome	8	8	0
Intermenstrual bleedings	4	5	21
Breast complaints	2	6	14
Edema, heavy legs, varicosis	2	3	8
Headache	2	4	4
Nausea	2	4	6
Free of complaints	47	15	11
Too many medications	3	6	9
Negative press reports	6	7	5
Discontinuation by the physician; side-effects	5	6	11
Change to other medication	4	8	0
Skin irritation by patches	–	13	–

estradiol levels are equally as effective as the higher levels following oral therapy, because the binding to SHBG is low and the estradiol is therefore more bio-available.

In addition to transdermal patches and gel, parenteral treatment is possible by oromucosal application (estradiol valerate in alcoholic solution), nasal sprays, vaginal rings and intramuscular injections. Locally effective application is possible by estriol ointment and suppositories.

Application of progesterone is performed orally by capsules, parenterally or by vaginal gel rectal and vaginal application of progesterone suppositories, or by intramuscular injection and locally over the breast by proges-terone ointment. This application over the breast will alter resorption of the progesterone through the skin and reduce the rate of mitoses in the breast epithelium. This effect should perhaps be used more often in a HRT that stimulates the mitoses of the breast epithelium.

SIDE-EFFECTS

Subjective side-effects such as soreness of the breast and extracellular water inbalance must not occur. They are mostly consequences of too high doses of estrogens, or sometimes of poor tolerance of a progestogen. Lowering of the dose, changing the mode of application, or changing the progestogen and time of medication may remove the side-effects.

Breast symptoms can mostly be improved by local application of progesterone gel to the breasts. Weight increase, as feared by many women, is not a conseqence of estrogen intake. This fact has been shown in many controlled studies. A small increase in weight in the first month of treatment may be caused by water retention and will be regulated within a short time. A lowering of the estrogen dose and the prescription of a diuretic progestogen may help to overcome such symptoms.

ALTERNATIVES TO CONVENTIONAL HORMONE REPLACEMENT THERAPY (HRT)

Alternatives may be steroid or designer hormones, nonhormonal medicaments, and relaxing and gymnastic methods such as yoga and lifestyle changes. Designer hormones offer new possibilities of an organ-specific application of hormonoid substances (Table 9.4).

Testosterone is a steroid hormone that can be administered as a depot injection or orally in combination with an estradiol ester. Indications are low testosterone levels following castration, loss of drive, apathic melancholia, loss of libido and anorgasmia.

Tibolone is a designer hormone. The parent compound is metabolized by 3α- and 3β-hydroxylation and Δ 4–5 isomerization in the organism to an estrogen, a progestogenic and a weak androgenic compound. Endometrium and epithelium of the breast are not, or only scarcely, stimulated by tibolone. Therefore, uterine bleeding and proliferation of the breast epithelium will usually not occur. The beneficial influence on lipids is however less than that of estradiol. A slight sexual stimulation by tibolone was reported in some cases.

Whether tibolone can preferentially be used in cases where there is a risk of breast cancer or after treatment, breast cancer must be clarified by further investigations.

17α-estradiol also does not stimulate the endometrium but will, when given orally, influence climacteric complaints favorably. This compound is so far only available in hair tinctures.

Dehydroepiandrosterone (DHEA) is an adrenal C19 steroid which is normally secreted from the adrenal gland together with cortisol. Production rate and blood level of this compound decrease with advancing age. Levels below the normal range for age will produce chronic fatigue. Part of the parent compound is metabolized in the organism to estrone–estradiol and to androstenedione–testosterone. Doses of 5, 10, 20 and 50 mg per tablet or capsule are freely available without prescription. Indication is so far only for patients with a level of DHEA below the normal range for age showing fatigue.

Phytoestrogens (e.g. genistein) are triterpenes, rather similar to the steroid or SERM molecule. They mostly stimulate the β-estrogen receptors, less so the α ones. As the endometrium and breast tissue contain mostly α-estrogen receptors, the endometrium and breast will not be stimulated and so uterine bleeding will not occur. All other effects of estrogens are exerted by genistein, albeit with a relatively weak effect, for instance on climacteric complaints, lipids and bone. Whether the hypothesis is true, that phytoestrogens could prevent mammary cancer by occupying the estrogen receptors, must be investigated in further studies.

NONHORMONAL MEDICAMENTS

Sedatives (such as diazepames) or antidepressants (such as fluoxetin) can be given in low doses for a short time if estrogens are contraindicated or not desired by the patient. They will cover prominent symptoms, e.g. unrest, anxiety and depressive moods.

Psychological and physical measures including: walking, jogging, anaerobic exercise – all age-adapted – and yoga, as well as respiration therapy can improve climacteric symptoms such as hot flushes and sweating, and other symptoms of an imbalance of the autonomous nervous system and the psyche. The avoidance of trigger substances for hot flushes, e.g. curries, concentrated alcohol and coffee, can be recommended so as not to worsen symptoms.

Of course, real estrogen-deficiency syndromes can only be cured by estrogen.

Table 9.4 New possibilities of organ-specific hormone therapy and substitution (designer estrogens, selective estrogen receptor modulators (SERM) and scavestrogens) as compared to the natural hormones estradiol and estriol

Classification	Endometrial proliferation	Breast stimulation	Heart protection	Decreased LDL Lp(a)	Osteoporosis protection	Neuro protection	Improvement in climacteric complaints
Agonist – estradiol	yes	yes	yes	yes	yes	yes	yes
Agonist – estriol	no*	little	no	no	no	no	weak
Partial antagonist – tamoxifen	yes, atypical	no, inhibitory	yes	yes	yes	no	no, intensification
Pure antiestrogen – toremifene	no	no, inhibitory	yes	?	yes	no	no
SERM – raloxifene	no	no, inhibitory	yes	yes	yes	no	no
Designer hormone – tibolone	weak	no	yes	no	yes	?	yes
Scavestrogen – 17α-estradiol	no	no	yes	?	no	yes	no

* When administered once a day.
LDL, Low-density lipoprotein; Lp(a), lipoprotein (a).

CONCLUSIONS

Estrogen–progestogen substitution during menopause and postmenopause is an attempt to prolong the euhormonal state of the midlife phase, to maintain endocrine autonomous equilibrium. This treatment is extremely effective, well tolerated and, if properly indicated and performed, a low-risk procedure. As long as natural human estrogens and progesterone are used parenterally, a pharmacodynamic pattern is attained which is near to that of ovarian secretion. The treatment can then rightly be called natural.

The aim is to prevent or to remove severe, and indeed senseless and unnecessary, climacteric complaints as well as the embarrassing postmenopausal regressive changes of the urogenital organs. Hormone therapy will thus prevent climacteric complaints dominating the life of the postmenopausal woman.

In a long-term substitution, bone and cardiovascular diseases can be partly prevented, provided they are caused mainly by estrogen deficiency and are begun at menopause. Therefore, such treatment will improve both psychological and physical life conditions compared to untreated controls. This goes together with a compression of morbidity to the end of life, thus securing as far as possible social competence and human dignity in old age.

For this aim to be realized, the substitution of estrogen–progesterone should, I repeat, be as near as possible to normal ovarian hormone secretion, which is possible with modern parenteral medication. On the other hand, modern pharmacodesign has created hormone-like substances which exert estrogenic effects without unwanted side-effects such as endometrial proliferation, uterine bleeding and cancer of the breast. Such designer hormones, and perhaps the phytoestrogens, offer new possibilities of prevention and treatment in patients with risk factors for, for example, breast cancer.

Prevention of diseases in the third phase of life will be the main task of medicine in the future. The possibilities of such an undertaking have been expanded in the last decades and will probably lead to new highly interesting and effective medicaments with low risks of side-effects.

Beneficial effects on cerebral functions, anti-aging and esthetic medicine, for the time being still of questionable use, will probably increase in significance and may contribute to the motivation of postmenopausal women to practice and to maintain hormone substitution. Changes in lifestyle are also effective in the prevention of postmenopausal diseases and should always accompany hormonal treatment.

RECOMMENDED READING

Goldstein SR. Individualizing HRT with lower dose regimens: Clinical trial review: Menopausal symptoms and bleeding profile. In: (Fischl FH, ed) *Menopause. Andropause. Hormone Replacement Therapy through the Ages. New Cognition and Concepts.* Krause & Pachernegg: Gablitz, 2001).

Kenemans P, Barendsen R, van der Weyer P. *Practical HRT.* Medicum, Bussum, 1995.

Lauritzen C. Management of the patient at risk. In: (Lauritzen C, van Keep PA, eds) *Estrogen therapy. Benefits and risks* Karger: Basel, 1978; 230–4.

Lauritzen C. Clinical use of estrogens and progestogens. *Mauritas* 1990; 199–214.

Lauritzen C. *Hormone replacement therapy. Practical guidelines for general practitioners.* Excerpta Medica; Amsterdam, 1995.

Lauritzen C. Hormone substitution before, during and after the menopause. In: (Fisch FH, ed) *Menopause. Andropause.* Krause & Pachernegg: Gablitz, 2001; 67–88.

Lobo RA. *Treatment of the postmenopausal woman. Basic and clinical aspects.* Raven Press: New York, 1944.

Recommendations of the American College of Preventive Medicine. *Am J Prev Med* 1999; **17**: 249–53.

10

Mechanisms of action of sex steroid hormones and their analogs

C Ibanez and EE Baulieu

Hormone action: general • Sex steroid hormones: cellular modes of action • Sex steroid hormones, receptors and specific receptor modulators • Physiologic aspects • References

HORMONE ACTION: GENERAL

Hormonal communication is an essential physiological process for the development, survival and reproduction of individuals. Hormones are messenger molecules responsible in part for gender characteristics, the regulation of vital biological constants (glycemia, calcemia, blood protein level, plasma and cellular pH, etc.), and important behavioral components (sexual behavior, reaction to stress, psychological states, etc.). Produced by hormone-synthesizing cells, they reach target cells according to three different modes. Distant cellular communication via general bloodstream is designated as endocrine. Paracrine refers to transfer to neighboring cells. Autocrine means that cells can produce molecules acting within themselves. We do not deal here with pheromones, which establish communication between separate organisms (for instance, some pregnene steroids are secreted into water by female fishes and influence male behavior).

Hormones may be classified as water- or lipid-soluble molecules. Hypophyseal glycoproteins such as luteinizing hormone (LH), follicle-stimulating hormone (FSH) and gonadal peptides (inhibin, follistatin) are examples of the water-soluble family. The lipid-soluble hormones are represented mainly by thyroid hormones and steroids.

Hormonal steroids originate from the same precursor molecule – cholesterol. The limiting step for entry into the hormonal pathway is the cleavage of the cholesterol side-chain by the P450scc enzyme (scc, side-chain cleavage) leading to the formation of pregnenolone. Then, specific enzyme activities catalyze the synthesis of glucocorticosteroids (such as cortisol and corticosterone), mineralocorticosteroids (aldosterone), estrogens (estradiol), progestogens (progesterone) and androgens (testosterone) (Fig. 10.1). The sex steroids, estrogens, progestogens and androgens are directly implicated in reproductive functions. Their activities are mainly conveyed by nuclear receptors leading to activation of specific gene expression but several other modes of action, designated as nongenomic, will also be mentioned.

SEX STEROID HORMONES: CELLULAR MODES OF ACTION

Gene expression and the nuclear receptor superfamily

Steroid hormone nuclear receptors are soluble proteins responsible for specific hormonal

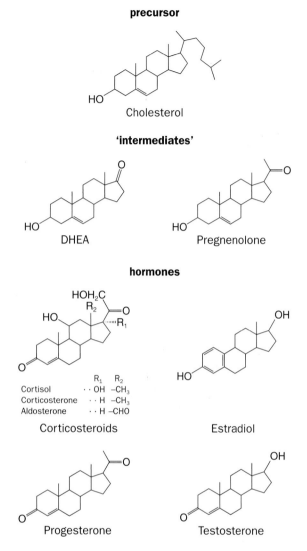

precursor

Cholesterol

'intermediates'

DHEA

Pregnenolone

hormones

	R_1	R_2
Cortisol	· · OH	–CH₃
Corticosterone	· · H	–CH₃
Aldosterone	· · H	–CHO

Corticosteroids

Estradiol

Progesterone

Testosterone

Figure 10.1 Chemical structures of the most representative steroids taken from the five classical classes of steroids: glucocorticosteroids, mineralocorticosteroids, estrogens, progestogens and androgens. Corticosterone is the most important glucocorticosteroid in rodents, cortisol is the most important in humans.

message transduction.[1,2] High affinity, a relatively small number of hormone-binding sites per target cell (usually a few thousand per cell) and specificity for hormonal ligands are the main characteristics of this receptor family (their structure is reported below). Hormonal specificity is indicated by the high affinity of a

group of molecules, whether they have agonist or antagonist activity, for a specific receptor which does not bind compounds with other physiological activities. However, this may not always be the case and, for instance, progesterone is also able to bind the glucocorticosteroid receptor and, in so doing, interestingly displays anticorticosteroid activity.

Receptor modular structure
The structure of sex steroid nuclear receptor protein (molecular weight 60–110 kDa) is modular and thus includes several domains demonstrating each characteristic functions. Two of them are very similar in all receptors, even bearing the features determining much of the functional specificity. One binds specifically the hormone and is named the ligand-binding domain (LBD), and the other binds DNA at specific promoter regions of hormone-regulated genes and is termed the DNA-binding domain (DBD) (Fig. 10.2).

The LBD (approximately 250 amino acids) is constituted of 12 α-helices. Transactivation takes place once the ligand is bound to the receptor involving the displacement of the twelfth helix and the subsequent binding of transcription coactivators (see Brzozowski et al. Fig. 3).[2a] Some details have been obtained by crystallization and X-ray analysis of both agonist- and antagonist-binding LBD.[3] In addition to its role in transactivation, due to the presence of the transactivation domain TAF-2 and because of the interaction of helix 12 with other nuclear proteins, the LBD also displays activity for binding the chaperone molecule – the 90 KDa heat-shock protein (hsp 90) – in the nonactivated heteropolymeric form of the receptor, and is involved in the receptor nuclear localization sequence (NLS: nuclear localization sequence) and dimerization of the receptor (Fig. 10.2). Hence, this LBD domain appears as a complex protein with different biochemical activities and, indeed, this module has been used to construct chimeric proteins responding to hormonal ligand. It has been observed that the binding itself and the subsequent transconformation induced by antagonist differs from those of the agonist ligand. Hence, this domain appears as a real molecular trigger.

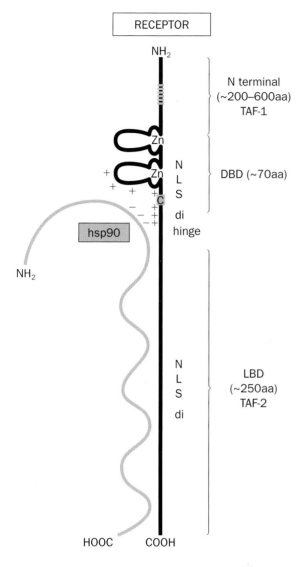

RECEPTOR

NH₂

N terminal
(~200–600aa)
TAF-1

Zn

Zn

+
+   +
+
N
L
S

DBD (~70aa)

C
+
−   +
−   +
−   +

hsp90

di
hinge

NH₂

N
L
S
di

LBD
(~250aa)
TAF-2

HOOC   COOH

Figure 10.2 A representation of the modular structure of steroid receptor. The different functional domains are represented DBD, DNA-binding domain with the characteristic zinc fingers motifs; LBD, ligand-binding domain; TAF-1 and -2, transactivation domains 1 and 2, respectively; NLS, nuclear localization sequence; di, dimerization sequence; aa, amino acid. The chaperone molecule the 90 kDa heat-shock protein (hsp90) is also indicated.

The DBD (approximately 70 amino acids) is the central part of the receptor (C region) and is responsible for the positioning of the receptor on the target gene promoter. It is characterized

by the presence of two zinc finger structures. Each of these two loops contains four cysteines stabilized by coordination bonds with Zn^{2+} ions (Fig. 10.3). Site-directed mutagenesis experiments revealed the existence of specific amino acid residues within these zinc finger motifs. In the first finger, the amino acids of the so-called P-box (Fig. 10.3) dictate the specificity of DNA recognition on specific DNA sequences called hormone response elements (HRE) (described in a later chapter). For instance, the P-box is responsible for the distinction between an estrogen or progestogen response element (ERE and PRE, respectively). In the second zinc finger, there is a D-box (Fig. 10.3) influencing the dimerization process of steroid nuclear receptors. Details of these structures and the interactions that they mediate have been obtained using nuclear magnetic resonance (NMR) spectroscopy and crystallographic methods. The hinge between the LBD and the DBD is involved in hsp90 binding and it is thought to be important for the spatial configuration of the protein.

Another important domain of the receptor is its amino terminal extremity, much more variable in amino acid composition and length according to receptor than the LBD and the DBD. It has a role in transactivation because of the presence of the transactivation domain TAF-1 (Fig. 10.2). This extremity is the most immunogenic part of the protein and many antibodies against it have been obtained.

The transactivation domains (TAF) allow interactions between steroid nuclear receptors and transcription coactivators, and thus subsequently activation of target gene expression. TAF-1, situated in the N-terminal extremity of the protein, works constitutively, whereas TAF-2, located in the LBD, is a hormone-dependent transactivation domain. They both stimulate transcription but differently according to cellular type, target gene promoter and hormonal ligand.

NLS are responsible for the shuttle of steroid nuclear receptors from the cytoplasm to the nucleus particularly after hormone binding. They are constituted by small sequences of basic amino acids located in the hinge and the LBD.

present in target tissues as a hetero-oligomer. This large receptor form contains at least two different proteins: the ligand-binding subunit (i.e. the receptor itself) and a chaperone molecule (hsp90), which is present as a dimer explaining the resulting hetero-oligomeric structure (Fig. 10.4). Indeed, additional proteins can also be associated with the native receptor, principally the FKBP52 immunophilin, hsp70 and p23. Exposure to the ligand at physiologic temperatures leads to the transformation of the native receptor into the active form of the receptor. This process is associated with funda-

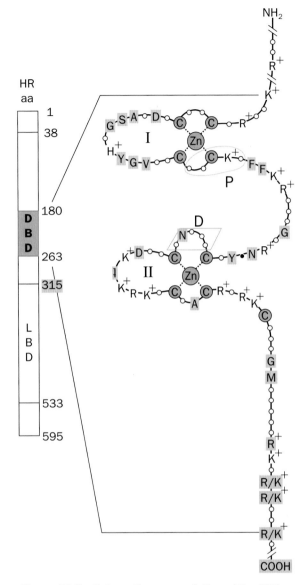

Figure 10.3 Schematic representation of the DNA-binding domain (DBD). The two zinc fingers are indicated; their coordination bonds with four cysteine residues attach to the zinc atoms. Conserved amino acids are shown, and the proximal (P) and distal (D) domains involved in the DNA sequence recognition and nuclear receptor dimerization, respectively, are boxed.

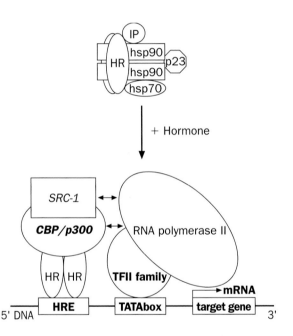

Figure 10.4 A simplified representation of the activation of steroid receptors. The native receptor is present as a heterodimer associated with the chaperone molecule the 90 kDa heat-shock protein (hsp90), an immunophilin (IP), and hsp70 and p23. After hormone binding, the native receptor undergoes structural changes, releases the hsp90/IP/hsp70 complex and forms a homodimer which is able to interact with DNA on hormone-response elements (HRE) and with the coactivator complex. This complex includes RNA polymerase II, coactivators of the TFII family, and the proteins CREB-binding protein/p300 (CBP/p300) and steroid receptor coactivator 1 (SRC-1), which are thought to possess a histone acetyltransferase activity facilitating target gene transcription.

Activation of the receptor, the first hormonal effect and transcriptional activity

In the absence of hormone, the unliganded steroid receptor, designated 'native receptor', is

mental changes in the receptor subcellular distribution and physicochemical properties: the dissociation of the hsp90 chaperone molecule leads to a conformational change, to translocation of the receptor in the nucleus, to receptor dimerization and interaction with DNA. Recent evidence has revealed that native receptors are already, although weakly, associated with the nuclear compartment and hsp90 may modulate the transcriptional response.[4] The observed subcellular receptor distribution reflects the existence of a nucleocytoplasmic transfer which may also be part of the intracellular recycling of steroid nuclear receptors between the nucleus and cytoplasm. The dissociation of hsp90 from receptor protein remains a necessary condition for activation of specific gene expression.

The classical, and the most important physiologically, manner to activate steroid receptors follows the binding of an agonist ligand. The steroid induces important changes in the receptor spatial structure and more precisely in the structure of the LBD (the twelfth α-helix). These changes cause the dissociation of the other constituents of the hetero-oligomeric complex (hsp90 and others) from the native receptor. At the same time, the transactivation domains become operational. Apart from natural activation by agonist ligands, several steroid nuclear receptors can be activated by phosphorylation. For example, signalling pathways triggered by peptide growth factors like insulin growth factor-1 (IGF-1), epidermal growth factor (EGF), transforming growth factor-α (TGF-α) via serine–threonine protein kinases (PKA, PKC) can lead to activation of the transactivation domains of progesterone and estradiol receptors.[5,6] Effects mediated by natural ligand binding and kinase-mediated signals are additive and can be inhibited by antagonist ligands.

The next step toward modulation of target gene expression is the interaction of receptor homodimers with DNA on HRE (Fig. 10.4).[7] These are palindromic sequences of 10–15 base pairs present in steroid target gene promoters and divided into two hemipalindromes of six base pairs each interacting with one molecule of receptor and participating actively in the dimer-

ization of the receptor. These palindromes are constituted by a consensus sequence, and a sequence has been described for each steroidal category: estrogens, progestogens and androgens. Nevertheless, receptor specificity for HRE is less restricted than that of the ligand–receptor interaction. Dimer formation is essential for transcriptional activation of gene expression. Several receptors are already dimeric before binding to DNA, such as the estrogen receptor but, generally, association with DNA favors the formation and stability of receptor dimers.

To ensure correct regulation of gene expression, mechanisms other than the simple HRE–receptor interaction are involved. These mechanisms rely on the presence of cellular proteins that modulate transcriptional activation by steroid nuclear receptors. Indeed, in eukaryotic cells, promoter-specific initiation of mRNA synthesis requires the assembly of RNA polymerase II and a set of general transcription initiation factors (TF).[8] These factors are located at the core promoter and are members of the TFII family (Fig. 10.4). Different subclasses are designated by the letter TFIIA, B, D, E, F and H. However, these interactions between steroid nuclear receptors and general transcription factors are not sufficient for effective mediation of the transcriptional activity. Hence, other additive factors are intervening.[9]

Among them are found general transcription factors such as steroid receptor coactivator 1 (SRC-1), the first described coactivator, and CREB binding protein (CBP)/p300 that can both bind steroid nuclear receptors and interact with each other (Fig. 10.4). Other SRC have been discovered, leading to the formation of a whole family of SRC. Other transcription factors are represented by chromatin factors that appear as crucial components since their acetyltransferase activity has an important consequence on the three-dimensional chromatin organization of the promoter region. Indeed, histone acetylation leads to a modification of the chromatin structure and a subsequent facilitated access for general transcription factors. SRC-1 and CBP/p300 have been shown to possess intrinsic histone acetyltransferase activity.

Lack of transcription occurs in the absence of

hormone or in the presence of antihormone.[9] Evidence is growing that co-repressors are involved in the inhibitory action of antagonist-bound steroid receptors. Some are also thought to possess a histone deacetylase activity that leads to the restoration of a nonaccessible three-dimensional conformation for other transcription coactivators.

Another interesting feature is the capacity of steroid nuclear receptors to exercise other modes of transcriptional regulation. The gluco-corticosteroid receptor (GR) can interact with the proteins c-jun and c-fos, binding the activating protein-1 (AP-1) site and thus inhibit the expression of stress-responsive genes [such as interleukin IL-1, IL-2 and tumor/necrosis factor (TNF)]. There is mutual inhibitory activity due to a direct protein–protein interaction between c-jun and the GR that prevents subsequent DNA binding by either transcription factors.[10] The estrogen and progesterone receptors may also have some activity through the nonclassical AP-1 pathway.[11,12]

Nongenomic actions of steroids

Apart from the classical steroid mode of action via nuclear receptors, rapid effects, that do not rely on protein synthesis, have been observed with hormonal steroids. Membrane-binding sites were revealed using estradiol and progesterone coupled with bovine serum albumin or other polymers that preclude the steroids penetrating into the cells.[13] Progesterone induces meiosis in *Xenopus* oocytes[14] and provokes the spermatozoid acrosomal reaction[15] after binding to sites on the plasma membrane. But these proteins remain largely unidentified, although some experiments have shown the existence of a 30 kDa protein that binds progesterone on *Xenopus* oocyte membranes and others have suggested, that the classical progesterone receptor may be situated in part at the plasma membrane level. More recently, the existence of a proper 'membrane receptor' has been suggested, but not yet proved, by the discovery of a membrane-associated progesterone-binding protein called 25-Dx in brain regions involved in female reproductive behavior.[16] Experiments

using nuclear estrogen receptor antibodies have revealed the presence of an immunoreactive protein on dendrites and axons.[17]

Steroids reaching the brain from classical steroidogenic glands, as well as neurosteroids synthesized in the central and peripheral nervous systems (CNS and PNS, respectively) can act differently. This is the case for pregnenolone, dehydroepiandrosterone (DHEA) and their sulfates (PREGS and DHEAS), and progesterone and its reduced metabolites (Fig. 10.5). Some of these have neuromodulatory effects on receptors for neurotrasmitters, e.g. gamma-aminobutyric acid (GABA), N-methyl D-Aspartate (NMDA), $\sigma 1$, nicotinic acetylcholine receptor.[18] Steroid-opposite effects can be observed on the same receptor, e.g. the $GABA_A$ receptor: pregnenolone sulfate has a negative modulatory effect whereas $3\alpha5\alpha$ tetrahydroprogesterone enhances GABA-evoked currents. Very recently, the binding of preg-nenolone to microtubule-associated protein 2 (MAP2) has been shown to provoke polymerization of microtubules, designating MAP2 as a new type of steroid receptor (Fig. 10.6).[19] Interestingly, two metabolites of pregnenolone – pregnenolone sulfate and progesterone – bind to the same site and are antagonists.

Genomic and nongenomic actions of steroids have frequently been opposed or seen as

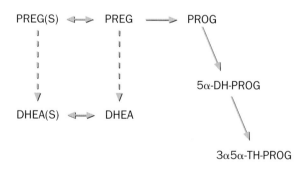

Figure 10.5 The main neuroactive neurosteroids and some of their metabolic sequences. PREG(S), pregnenolone (sulfate); DHEA(S), dehydroepiandrosterone (sulfate); PROG, progesterone; 5α-DH-PROG, 5α-dihydroprogesterone; 3α5α-TH-PROG, 3α5α-tetrahydroprogesterone.

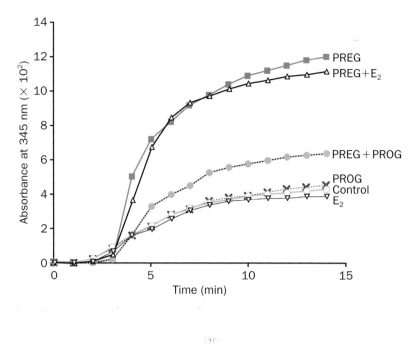

Figure 10.6 In vitro assay of the steroid effect on polymerization of microtubules. Purified tubulin and microtubule-associated protein 2 (MAP2) were incubated with steroids. Pregnenolone (PREG) is the most potent molecule in increasing polymerization of microtubules, progesterone (PROG) is a competitor of PREG, estradiol (E_2) has no effect on polymerization but in contrast to PROG, it does not compete with the effect of PREG. These results indicate that PREG and PROG may be competing for the same MAP2 sites but display opposite effects. (Tubulin 1 mg/ml; MAP2, 0.05 mg/ml; steroid, 500 nM; 37°C.)

competing phenomena. However, it has recently been shown that these two different modes of action can synergize. For instance, using a two-pulse estradiol administration, it has been observed that a first pulse with estradiol–bovine serum albumine (BSA) activating membrane-signaling pathways potentiates the later transcriptional actions via nuclear receptors of the second estradiol pulse in a nerve cell line.[20]

SEX STEROID HORMONES, RECEPTORS AND SPECIFIC RECEPTOR MODULATORS

Estrogen, selective estrogen receptor modulators (SERM) and phytoestrogen activities

α and β receptors

Estrogen actions are mediated by two different nuclear receptors: estrogen receptor-alpha and -beta (ERα and ERβ). These receptors are coded by separate genes, localized on two different chromosomes: 6q25–1 for ERα and 14q22–24 for ERβ in humans.

The ER is the only receptor to contain an additional F region at the C-terminal extremity. ERβ has been cloned more recently than ERα, but they share similar structures. ERα and ERβ can form both homo- and heterodimers.[21] They have different binding specificities and finally are involved in differential responses of the same ligands. Hence, cellular responses are dependent on the relative abundance of the two forms.

ERα and ERβ are expressed, in particular, in reproductive tissues in women (i.e. ovaries, endometrium, breast) and men (prostate), and also in skin, blood vessels, bones and brain. As mentioned above, some of the differential effects of estrogens are explained, in part, by the differential expressions of either ERα or ERβ. For instance, both isoforms are equally expressed in ovaries, but ERβ is predominant in granulosa cells. On the other hand, ERα is predominant in the endometrium. In brain, there is an almost ubiquitous immunohistochemical localization of ERβ, with the exception of the hippocampus which stains positively and exclusively for ERα.

Estrogen physiologic activities

Estrogens, in particular estradiol, are responsible for the growth of female secondary organs. In mammary glands, estrogens are responsible for the preparation of the glands for lactogenesis, even if this process will then be controlled by other hormones, in particular by prolactin. The CNS is another target of estrogens, where they are responsible for the modulation of LH and FSH secretion by the hypothalamic–hypophyseal system. According to the estrogen plasma concentration and the phase of the menstrual cycle, estrogens are involved in a negative-feedback control, reducing the secretion of LH and FSH, or in a positive-feedback control, stimulating their secretion. They also influence sexual behavior. In the skeleton, estrogens have a crucial role on bone metabolism: they reduce bone resorption by inhibiting the expression of IL-6, which is a stimulator of osteolysis.[22] Estrogens are also thought to be beneficial for the cardiovascular system since they can tilt the cholesterol physiologic balance in favor of the high-density lipoprotein (HDL) component.

SERM and phytoestrogens

Compounds other than endogenous estrogens also have the capacity to modulate ER actions. Among them are the antiestrogens, which have been divided into two classes. Pure antiestrogens, such as ICI 182780 (Fig. 10.7), are believed to alter the receptor binding to estrogen response elements (ERE). The second class is represented by partial antiestrogens, termed SERM.[23] These molecules can bind to the ER, modulate its action, and activate or inhibit transcription of specific genes, probably because transconformation of the receptor induced by SERM leads to interactions of the receptor with different coactivators and co-repressors according to the SERM and the target cell type. As these molecules exhibit tissue-specific estrogen agonist or antagonist activities, the goal is to develop molecules that can have estrogenic action on extrareproductive tissues such as bones and on the cardiovascular system, and that are antiestrogenic on breast and uterus tissues for example. This latter property is crucial in the prevention and/or treatment of breast cancer. These molecules may also be useful in substitutive estrogenic treatment on bones

(osteoporosis), the cardiovascular system, urogenital tract and CNS without increasing the risk of breast cancer.

The two most available SERM are tamoxifen and raloxifene (Fig. 10.7). On the skeleton, raloxifene acts as an estrogen agonist, preventing bone loss; it also exhibits estrogen-like effects on cholesterol metabolism and cardiovascular endothelial tissue. In contrast, raloxifene exhibits estrogen-blocking effects in reproductive tissues (uterus and mammary tissue), whereas tamoxifen has a partial agonist profile in uterus. Among the different hypotheses on the mechanism of action of raloxifene, one proposal is that ER binds to a specific DNA element, called the raloxifene response element (REE), and the agonist–antagonist activity of raloxifene depends on the relative presence of the different ER subtypes (i.e. ERα and/or ERβ).

Recent works have detected several natural compounds with similar properties to SERM, which are designated phytoestrogens.[23] This term is used to define classes of compounds that are of plant origin or derived from the in vivo metabolism of precursors present in several plants eaten by humans. The two main classes of these compounds are the isoflavones [genistein, daidzein (Fig. 10.7)] and lignans (enterodiol). Soybeans and flaxseed are particularly abundant sources of phytoestrogens. As with synthetic SERM, phytoestrogens appear to have both estrogenic and antiestrogenic effects depending on the concentration of circulating endogenous estrogens and ER subtypes. It has been suggested that they could protect against hormone-dependent cancer (breast and prostate cancer), cardiovascular diseases (by modulating the metabolism of cholesterol) and osteoporosis, and reduce postmenopausal symptoms (e.g. hot flushes, vaginal dryness). In particular, genistein has been shown to inhibit cancer cell proliferation in vitro.[24] This effect is mediated by a competitive inhibition of ER[25] and also by inhibition of tyrosine kinases which may be involved in control of cell proliferation and carcinogenesis.[26] Much more work has to be done to ascertain both beneficial and potentially deleterious effects.

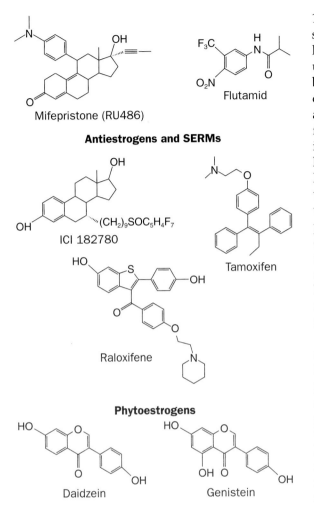

Mifepristone (RU486)

Flutamid

Antiestrogens and SERMs

ICI 182780

Tamoxifen

Raloxifene

Phytoestrogens

Daidzein

Genistein

Figure 10.7 Chemical structure of some sex steroid hormone antagonists, specific estrogen receptor modulators (SERM) and phytoestrogens. RU486 is an antagonist of both the progesterone and glucocorticosteroid receptors. Flutamid is an anti-androgen. Among the antiestrogens and SERM are ICI 182780, a pure antiestrogen, and two estrogen receptor modulators, tamoxifen and raloxifene. Phytoestrogens are represented by two molecules of the isoflavone family, daidzein and genistein.

Progestogen activities

A and B receptors

A single gene encodes two isoforms (A and B) of the progestogen receptor (PR). In humans, the PR gene is located on chromosome 11q22–23. PR-B is larger than PR-A because some of the mRNA produced by the PR gene lacks the 5′ region that encodes the portion unique to PR-B. The shorter PR-A is produced by initiation of transcription at an internal AUG codon,[27] hence this form lacks the first 164 amino acids of PR-B. Nevertheless, the two forms have identical LBD and DBD. The localization of a nuclear localization sequence in the hinge is responsible for the constitutive nuclear localization of the PR.[28] An additional transactivation domain, TAF-3, is located in the region which is unique to PR-B. PR is expressed particularly in reproductive tissues (e.g. ovaries, uterus) and the nervous system. In the uterus and in reproductive regions of the brain, such as the hypothalamus, the PR is inducible by estrogens. Nevertheless, the molecular mechanism of this modulation is not clearly understood.

Progestogen physiologic activities

Progestogen actions are mainly mediated by progesterone. This hormone is responsible for cellular differentiation in the uterus. For example, its action on the endometrium prepares the uterus for the implantation of a blastocyst. Progesterone exerts a relaxing effect on the myometrium. Progesterone blockade leads to myometrial contraction and then to pregnancy interruption or parturition. These effects can be obtained with a synthetic antagonist of the PR RU486 [mifepristone (Fig. 10.7)] – its additional antiglucocorticosteroid property is not involved in pregnancy interruption – which binds the PR in the LBD but on a different site to progesterone. RU486 keeps the receptor in a spatial configuration that prevents transcription coactivators interacting with it,[29] leading to an inhibition of progesterone's biological effects. Progesterone is also involved in the control of the mammary gland, as are estrogens. It exerts an inhibitory effect on lactogenesis and it participates in the differentiation of alveoli. Progesterone has an influence on the respiratory system: it is now accepted that women hyperventilate during the luteal phase of the menstrual cycle and during pregnancy. It has been shown that the respiratory stimulation in response to progesterone is mediated through a PR mechanism of action whose expression can be enhanced by estrogens at hypothalamic sites.[30] It is also important to note that progesterone is not only a sex steroid – it can also be synthesized in the CNS and PNS, and local progesterone administration has been shown to increase the myelin sheath thickness of the regenerating mouse sciatic nerve after cryolesion.[31] Progesterone might also participate in CNS remyelination.

Androgen activities

Androgen receptor (AR)

AR is specified by a single gene located at Xq11–12 in humans. AR is among the larger members of the nuclear receptor family, owing to its large N-terminal extremity.[32] The function of this large N-terminal domain is required for full activity and its structure influences both hormone and DNA binding of the receptor. It contains repeated segments that affect the receptor function, in particular glutamine repeats (glutamine homopolymeric segment) that are the most polymorphic. Alterations in the length of the glutamine repeat have been linked to the pathogenesis of the X-linked spinal and bulbar muscular atrophy. AR is expressed in reproductive tissues such as testis and prostate, and also in brain, skin, muscles and bones.

Androgen physiologic activities

Testosterone and its 5α-reduced metabolite, dihydrotestosterone (5α-DHT) that displays a higher affinity for AR than testosterone, are the two main active androgens. But, testosterone can also be metabolized in estradiol by aromatase enzyme activity. Androgens exert a trophic effect on male secondary sexual organs (e.g. prostate, seminal vesicles). Testosterone has a stimulatory action on spermatogenesis in seminiferous tubules. During development, androgens are responsible for the sexual differentiation of the hypothalamus. They also have a stimulatory effect on erythropoiesis and an anabolic effect on muscles and bones. Among anti-androgens acting at a higher level, the most

active are nonsteroidal such as flutamid (Fig. 10.7). However, recently some compounds, such as 7α-methyl-19nor-testosterone, have been considered to be potential selective androgen receptor modulators (SARM), since they have both androgenic and anti-androgenic activities and could be used to supplement androgen deficiency in aging males without effects on the prostate and the associated risks.

PHYSIOLOGIC ASPECTS

In organisms, estrogens, progestogens and androgens coexist in both men and women, but in different relative concentrations (Table 10.1). In fact, many cells express two or even three classes of sex steroid receptors. It is well known that if estrogens and progestogens are the main circulating hormones in blood in women before menopause, a non-negligible concentration of androgens can also be measured. At the same time, in men, androgens are predominant but small amounts of progesterone and estradiol are also synthesized and circulate in the blood. After menopause, hormone levels dramatically decrease in a woman's plasma; at the same age, elderly men have higher estradiol plasma concentrations than elderly women. Another important physiologic condition concerns the synthesis of a nonsexual steroid by the adrenal glands – DHEA(S). Its secretion reaches a maximum around 25 years of age and then decreases progressively, paralleling the aging process in both men and women (Table 10.1). Daily supplementation with DHEA in elderly women (70–80 years of age) has a beneficial effect on bone density, skin hydration and libido.[33] A large part of the effects of DHEA is due to partial conversion to estrogens and androgens.

Steroid hormones can have complementary or opposite effects according to the nature of the target. For example, in women, estrogen secretion reaches its maximum in the first part of the cycle, concomitant with the pick of LH and FSH triggering ovulation, whereas progesterone ovarian synthesis increases progressively after ovulation and prepares the uterus for pregnancy. In men, the physiologic situation

Table 10.1 Sex steroid and dehydroepiandrosterone sulfate (DHEAS) plasma concentrations in men and women (order of magnitude)

	Men		Women		
	Young (24–35 years)	Old (64–75 years)	Before menopause FP	LP	After menopause*
E_2 (pg/ml)	25	25	20–90	70–250	5–25
PROG (ng/ml)	< 0.8	< 0.8	0.05–1.5	5–25	0.5
Testo (ng/ml)	6	3	0.5		0.2
DHEAS (µg/ml)	3.6	1	2.6		0.8

* With no hormone replacement therapy.
FP, Follicular phase (first week); LP, luteal phase; E_2, estradiol; PROG, progesterone; Testo, testosterone.

is different since the secretion of testosterone is constant through life after puberty and decreases progressively in aging men. When steroids are synthesized in the nervous system by glial cells or neurons, the so-called neurosteroids, the sexual dimorphism inherent to sex steroids disappears, i.e. after castration and adrenalectomy both male and female rats exhibit the same concentrations of remaining neurosteroids in the brain.

It appears that, in vivo, physiological processes dependent on steroid hormones are very often regulated by the combined actions of several steroids. Each sex steroid hormone has multiple targets, not only in reproductive tissues but also skin, skeleton and brain cells. The three categories of sex steroid hormones – estrogens, progestogens and androgens – frequently act together, simultaneously or successively, on these targets. As mentioned earlier, one of the archetypal examples of cooperation between sex steroids is observed when estrogens are priming progesterone action by inducing PR expression in reproductive tissues and brain. This phenomenon is controlled by the negative-feedback regulation operated by progesterone on ER expression. There is no doubt that steroid hormones are essential molecules for the function and reproduction of individuals.

REFERENCES

1. Baulieu EE, Alberga A, Jung I et al. Metabolism and protein binding of sex steroids in target organs: an approach to the mechanism of hormone action. *Rec Prog Horm Res* 1971; **27**: 351–419.
2. Jensen EV, DeSombre ER. Mechanism of action of the female sex hormones. *Ann Rev Biochem* 1972; **41**: 203–30.
2a. Brzozowski AM, Pike AC et al. Molecular basis of agonism and antagonism in the oestrogen receptor. *Nature* 1997; **389**: 753–8.
3. Moras D, Gronemeyer H. The nuclear receptor ligand-binding domain: structure and function. *Curr Opin Cell Biol* 1998; **10**: 384–91.
4. Kang KI, Meng X, Devin-Leclerc J et al. The molecular chaperone Hsp90 can negatively regulate the activity of a glucocorticosteroid-dependent promoter. *Proc Natl Acad Sci USA* 1999; **96**: 1439–44.
5. Ignar-Trowbridge DM, Pimentel M, Teng CT et al. Cross talk between peptide growth factor and estrogen receptor signaling systems. *Environ Health Perspect* 1995; **103 (Suppl 7)**: 35–8.
6. Power RF, Conneely OM, O'Malley BW. New insights into activation of the steroid hormone receptor superfamily. *Trends Pharmacol Sci* 1992; **13**: 318–23.
7. Truss M, Beato M. Steroid hormone receptors: interaction with deoxyribonucleic acid and transcription factors. *Endocr Rev* 1993; **14**: 459–79.
8. Roeder RG. The role of general initiation factors

in transcription by RNA polymerase II. *Trends Biochem Sci* 1996; **21**: 327–35.

9. Freedman LP. Multimeric coactivator complexes for steroid/nuclear receptors. *Trends Endocr Metab* 1999; **10**: 403–7.

10. Schule R, Rangarajan P, Kliewer S et al. Functional antagonism between oncoprotein c-Jun and the glucocorticoid receptor. *Cell* 1990; **62**: 1217–26.

11. Kushner PJ, Agard DA, Greene GL et al. Estrogen receptor pathways to AP-1. *J Steroid Biochem Molec Biol* 2000; **74**: 311–17.

12. Savouret JF, Rauch M, Redeuilh G et al. Interplay between estrogens, progestins, retinoic acid and AP-1 on a single regulatory site in the progesterone receptor gene. *J Biol Chem* 1994; **269**: 28,955–62.

13. Godeau JF, Schorderet-Slatkine S, Hubert P, Baulieu EE. Induction of maturation in *Xenopus laevis* oocytes by a steroid linked to a polymer. *Proc Natl Acad Sci USA* 1978; **75**: 2353–7.

14. Baulieu EE, Godeau F, Schorderet M, Schorderet-Slatkine S. Steroid-induced meiotic division in *Xenopus laevis* oocytes: surface and calcium. *Nature* 1978; **275**: 593–8.

15. Cheng FP, Gadella BM, Voorhout WF et al. Progesterone-induced acrosome reaction in stallion spermatozoa is mediated by a plasma membrane progesterone receptor. *Biol Reprod* 1998; **59**: 733–42.

16. Krebs CJ, Jarvis ED, Chan J et al. A membrane-associated progesterone-binding protein, 25-Dx, is regulated by progesterone in brain regions involved in female reproductive behaviors. *Proc Natl Acad Sci USA* 2000; **97**: 12,816–21.

17. Collins P, Webb C. Estrogen hits the surface. *Nat Med* 1999; **5**: 1130–1.

18. Baulieu EE. Neurosteroids: a novel function of the brain. *Psychoneuroendocrinology* 1998; **23**: 963–87.

19. Murakami K, Fellous A, Baulieu EE, Robel P. Pregnenolone binds to microtubule-associated protein 2 and stimulates microtubule assembly. *Proc Natl Acad Sci USA* 2000; **97**: 3579–84.

20. Vasudevan N, Kow LM, Pfaff DW. Early membrane estrogenic effects required for full expression of slower genomic actions in a nerve cell line. *Proc Natl Acad Sci USA* 2001; **98**: 12,267–71.

21. Pettersson K, Grandien K, Kuiper GG, Gustafsson JA. Mouse estrogen receptor beta forms estrogen response element-binding heterodimers with estrogen receptor alpha. *Molec Endocr* 1997; **11**: 1486–96.

22. Jilka RL, Hangoc G, Girasole G et al. Increased osteoclast development after estrogen loss: mediation by interleukin-6. *Science* 1992; **257**: 88–91.

23. Krishnan V, Heath H, Bryant HU. Mechanism of action of estrogens and selective estrogen receptor modulators. *Vitamin Horm* 2000; **60**: 123–47.

24. Peterson G, Barnes S. Genistein inhibition of the growth of human breast cancer cells: independence from estrogen receptors and the multidrug resistance gene. *Biochem Biophys Res Commun* 1991; **179**: 661–7.

25. Martin PM, Horwitz KB, Ryan DS, McGuire WL. Phytoestrogen interaction with estrogen receptors in human breast cancer cells. *Endocrinology* 1978; **103**: 1860–7.

26. Markovits J, Linassier C, Fosse P et al. Inhibitory effects of the tyrosine kinase inhibitor genistein on mammalian DNA topoisomerase II. *Cancer Res* 1989; **49**: 5111–17.

27. Conneely OM, Kettelberger DM, Tsai MJ et al. The chicken progesterone receptor A and B isoforms are products of an alternate translation initiation event. *J Biol Chem* 1989; **264**: 14,062–4.

28. Guiochon-Mantel A, Loosfelt H, Lescop P et al. Mechanisms of nuclear localization of the progesterone receptor: evidence for interaction between monomers. *Cell* 1989; **57**: 1147–54.

29. Vegeto E, Allan GF, Schrader WT et al. The mechanism of RU486 antagonism is dependent on the conformation of the carboxy-terminal tail of the human progesterone receptor. *Cell* 1992; **69**: 703–13.

30. Bayliss DA, Millhorn DE. Central neural mechanisms of progesterone action: application to the respiratory system. *J Appl Physiol* 1992; **73**: 393–404.

31. Koenig HL, Schumacher M, Ferzaz B et al. Progesterone synthesis and myelin formation by Schwann cells. *Science* 1995; **268**: 1500–3.

32. Lubahn DB, Joseph DR, Sar M et al. The human androgen receptor: complementary deoxyribonucleic acid cloning, sequence analysis and gene expression in prostate. *Molec Endocr* 1988; **2**: 1265–75.

33. Baulieu EE, Thomas G, Legrain S et al. Dehydroepiandrosterone (DHEA), DHEA sulfate, and aging: contribution of the DHEAge Study to a sociobiomedical issue. *Proc Natl Acad Sci USA* 2000; **97**: 4279–84.

11

Estrogens, progestogens and the endometrium

DW Sturdee

Introduction • Unopposed estrogen • Endometrial response to sequential estrogen–progestogen hormone replacement therapy (HRT) • Malignant potential of endometrial hyperplasia • Long-cycle therapy • Continuous combined therapy (CCT) • Conclusions • References

INTRODUCTION

During the fertile premenopausal years, the endometrium is uniquely endowed with a complex monthly cycle of periodic proliferation, differentiation, breakdown and regeneration. This high cellular turnover, conditioned by ovarian hormones and growth factors, has many opportunities of losing its regulatory controls, such as during the menopausal transition when cycles are frequently irregular and anovulatory, but despite this significant endometrial disease is uncommon in premenopausal women. After the menopause and in the absence of exogenous hormone stimulation, the endometrium will generally become thin and atrophic, though still retaining the ability to respond to estrogen and progestogen. Sequential regimens of estrogen and progestogen hormone replacement therapy (HRT) are intended to mimic the cyclic stimulation of the endometrium and will usually produce a similar response with proliferative and secretory changes.

The ideal HRT will not only provide relief from menopausal symptoms, prevention of osteoporosis and possibly reduction in cardiovascular disease, but will also protect the endometrium from endometrial hyperplasia or carcinoma. In postmenopausal women who have not been taking estrogen therapy, the incidence of endometrial cancer is relatively low at about one per 1000 women per year.[1] One of the recognized risk factors for endometrial cancer is a delayed or late menopause, and because HRT effectively prolongs the menopausal age, HRT can be an additional risk factor. So, despite our increasing knowledge of the effect of hormones on the endometrium, endometrial cancer remains a significant risk for postmenopausal women taking HRT.

UNOPPOSED ESTROGEN

Unopposed oestrogen therapy causes endometrial proliferation initially but a gradually increasing incidence of hyperplasia with prolonged unopposed stimulation. A study of 596 postmenopausal women who were randomized to placebo, unopposed estrogen, continuous or sequential HRT over 36 months found that those receiving estrogen alone – 0.625 mg conjugated equine estrogen (CEE) – were significantly more likely to develop simple (27.7%), complex (22.7%) or atypical (11.7%) hyperplasia than the placebo group (simple 0.8%, complex 0.8%, atypical 0.7%; $P > 0.001$).[2] More recently the Cochrane review of all the appropriate studies found that after 6 months of unopposed estrogen, the odds ratio (OR) was 5.4 [95% confidence interval (CI) 1.4–20.9] and after 36 months was 16.0 (95% CI 9.3–27.5).[3]

One might expect that lower dose unopposed estrogen therapy would be associated with less risk of hyperplasia, and Notelowitz et al[4] reported a 1.7% rate of hyperplasia in women receiving 0.3 mg unopposed esterified estrogen for 2 years, which was similar to that in the control women. However, a further case control study found a fivefold higher risk of developing endometrial cancer in women taking 0.3 mg unopposed CEE daily compared with untreated women.[5]

There is no evidence that use of the weaker estrogen estriol, either vaginally or orally, has any less effect on the risk of endometrial hyperplasia.[6]

For over 25 years it has also been recognized that unopposed estrogen is associated with a significant increased risk of endometrial cancer, with relative risks (RR) ranging from 1.4 to 12.0,[7,8] and that this increases with the duration of unopposed therapy up to a RR of 15.0 (Table 11.1).[9] A cohort study in California of 5160 women reported a RR of 10 in women who had taken unopposed estrogen,[10] equivalent to an absolute risk of endometrial cancer of 1 per 100 women per year. Furthermore, it is not widely recognized that the risk of endometrial cancer remains increased for many years after stopping unopposed estrogen therapy.[11] Even after 15 years or more without therapy, there is still a significantly increased RR of 5.8 (95% CI 2.0–17).[10] To counteract this risk, progestogen has been added to estrogen replacement therapy in a sequential regimen for (usually) 10–14 days in each cycle, with the intention of imitating the normal premenopausal ovarian cycle. This form of HRT should also produce a regular bleed, which for older women in particular is unsatisfactory. For this reason, continuous combined regimens have been developed which contain estrogen and progestogen every day, and by avoiding a cycle there is no period-type bleed.

Estrogen causes endometrial proliferation by increasing the number of estrogen/progesterone receptors, and also increasing the mitotic rate in the glandular cells of the endometrium. The administration of progestogen during estrogen therapy causes downregulation of the receptors and induction of 17β-estradiol dehydrogenase, which converts estradiol to the less active estrone, thereby reducing the estrogenic stimulus.[12] The histological evidence of a progestogenic effect is a change from a proliferative to a secretory endometrium from which hyperplasia is less likely to develop.

Table 11.1   Endometrial cancer risk with unopposed estrogens: case control studies

Study (ref)	Year	Relative Risk	
		Ever use	Long-term
Smith et al[54]	1975	4.5	–
Ziel and Finkle[55]	1975	7.6	13.9
Gray et al[56]	1977	3.1	11.6
Horowitz and Feinstein[8]	1978	12.0	5.2
Antunes et al[9]	1979	6.0	15.0
Weiss et al[1]	1979	7.5	8.2
Shapiro et al[57]	1980	3.9	6.0
Kelsey et al[58]	1982	1.4	3.1

ENDOMETRIAL RESPONSE TO SEQUENTIAL ESTROGEN–PROGESTOGEN HORMONE REPLACEMENT THERAPY (HRT)

The addition of progestogen in sequential regimens of HRT will reduce the incidence of hyperplasia. In 1985 Varma and colleagues reported on 398 patients and found that the addition of progestogen for 7 days in each cycle did not prevent hyperplasia.[13] Paterson et al[14] found that after 7 days of progestogen in each month, the incidence of hyperplasia was reduced to 3–4%, after 10 days of progestogen it was 2%; the maximum protective effect was achieved with 12–13 days of progestogen.[15,16] As a result, there has been some complacency about the protective effect of sequential HRT regimens. However, these early studies were of relatively short duration with biopsies being taken after usually 6–9 months of therapy. More recent studies with longer duration HRT have raised concerns about protection of the endometrium. In the largest published study of this type, 1192 women who were taking standard sequential regimens of HRT for a mean of 3.29 years (median 2.56 years; 5–95th centile; 0.77–8.49 years) had endometrial aspiration biopsies taken by Pipelle® during the progestogen phase of cycle (Table 11.2). As expected, a large proportion (47.4%) had a secretory endometrium, but complex hyperplasia (Fig. 11.1) was found in 5.5% and atypical hyperplasia (Fig. 11.2) in 0.7%.[17,18] There were no significant differences in the prevalence of hyperplasia between regimens containing 10 or 12 days of progestogen in each cycle.

A prospective cohort follow-up study of 23,244 women for a mean of 5.7 years did not, however, show an increase in the risk of endometrial carcinoma associated with sequential estrogen and progestogen regimens.[19] But a more recent case control study of women between the ages of 45 and 74.[20] found that, among women who were taking sequential HRT regimens with at least 10 days of progestogen in each cycle, the RR of endometrial cancer was not increased with up to 5 years of use, but with more than 5 years of use there was a RR of endometrial cancer of 2.5 (95% CI 1.1–5.5).

Table 11.2 Endometrial histology during sequential estrogen–progestogen replacement therapy for a mean of 3.29 years (reproduced with permission)[27]

Endometrial histology	No women	%
Unassessable	214	18.0
Inactive/atrophic	90	7.6
Proliferative	180	15.1
Secretory	565	47.4
Menstrual	32	2.7
Pseudodecidual	11	0.9
Complex hyperplasia	65	5.5
Atypical hyperplasia	8	0.7
Carcinoma	0	0.0
Other	27	2.3
Total	1192	100.0

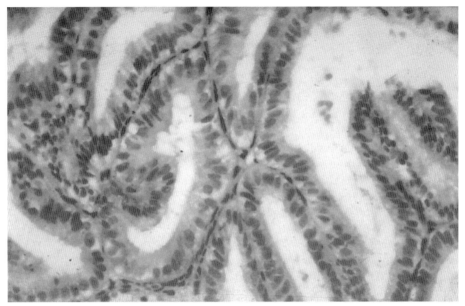

Figure 11.1 Complex endometrial hyperplasia during sequential estrogen–progestogen hormone replacement therapy showing crowded and irregular branched glands.

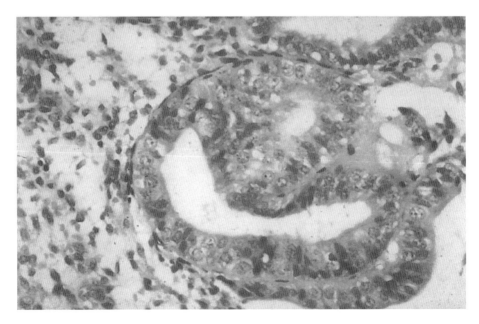

Figure 11.2 Atypical endometrial hyperplasia during sequential estrogen–progestogen hormone replacement therapy showing crowded and irregular glands and atypical epithelial cells.

MALIGNANT POTENTIAL OF ENDOMETRIAL HYPERPLASIA

There is continued debate about the implications of endometrial hyperplasia and the potential for progressing to carcinoma. In the clinical situation, the finding of endometrial hyperplasia will usually prompt the clinician to take some action such as treatment with progestogen or surgery. There are, therefore, few data on the natural history of untreated hyperplasia. In a prospective study of 51 patients with endometrial hyperplasia followed for 6 months, Terakawa et al[21] found that in 69% (35 of 51) of the patients the endometrium became normal during the observation period, but the findings persisted in 17% (six of 35) of those with simple hyperplasia, in 25% (one of four) of those with complex hyperplasia, in one of seven with simple atypical hyperplasia and four of five with complex atypical hyperplasia. In the remaining three patients with simple hyperplasia, there was progression to complex atypical hyperplasia at the end of 6 months. However, although evidence on the long-term outcome is limited, the general consensus is that endometrial hyperplasia without atypia has a low potential for malignant progression, but the presence of cytological atypia increases the risk considerably.[22]

In addition, there is a low background prevalence of endometrial hyperplasia and carcinoma in postmenopausal women. In a study of 801 asymptomatic peri-and postmenopausal women, Archer et al[23] found a 5.2% prevalence of hyperplasia, with atypia in 0.6%. There was one case of endometrial adenocarcinoma. A further study of endometrial biopsy specimens from 2964 women before taking HRT found that 68.7% were atrophic, 23.5% were proliferative, 0.5% were secretory, 0.6% had hyperplasia, 0.07% had adenocarcinoma and 6.6% were insufficient for classification.[24] It is from data such as these that clinical management guidelines for HRT suggest that it is not obligatory to perform an endometrial biopsy in every women prior to starting HRT.

Bleeding during sequential estrogen–progestogen HRT

Sequential regimens of estrogen and progestogen are intended to produce a regular and predictable bleed, similar to menstruation, and this is so for at least 77% of postmenopausal women.[25] While most women will accept this as a small price to pay for the benefits of HRT, bleeding remains one of the commonest causes for patient dissatisfaction and poor long-term adherence to therapy, particularly if it is irregular, as may happen in about 8% of women on such therapy.[25] Clinicians would also wish that the timing of the bleed during sequential therapy might provide some guide to the state of the endometrium. This was suggested by Padwick et al[26] in 1986, who considered that bleeding on or after day 11 from the start of the progestogen phase was indicative of an adequate progestogenic effect and endometrial protection. However, that study was based on only 96 women, none of whom presented with endometrial hyperplasia; moreover, it was assumed that hyperplasia develops from a proliferative endometrium and that secretory transformation indicates adequate progestogenic protection of the endometrium. A large UK multicenter study investigated the timing of the bleed in 413 postmenopausal women who had been taking standard sequential regimens of HRT with 10 or 12 days of progestogen per cycle for a mean of 2.7 years.[27] For most women, bleeding started around day 13 after starting progestogen, and there was no correlation between endometrial histology and the time of onset of bleeding. In particular, with continuation of the study, 37 of 65 cases with complex hyperplasia and four of eight with atypia had regular bleeds after day 11. It is therefore quite clear that regular bleeding during sequential HRT is not a helpful guide to the state of the endometrium or the presence of hyperplasia (Fig. 11.3).[28]

LONG-CYCLE THERAPY

As monthly sequential therapy results in a cyclical bleed, which is inconvenient in some

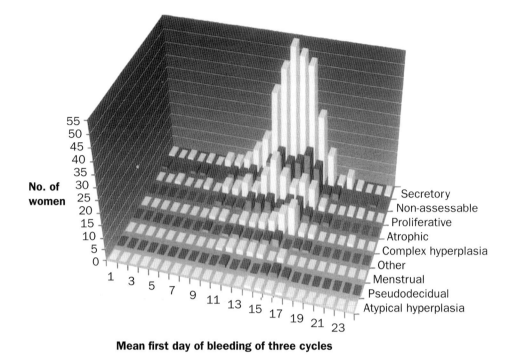

No. of women

Secretory
Non-assessable
Proliferative
Atrophic
Complex hyperplasia
Other
Menstrual
Pseudodecidual
Atypical hyperplasia

Mean first day of bleeding of three cycles

Figure 11.3 Endometrial histology in postmenopausal women taking sequential estrogen–progestogen and the mean first day of bleeding over three cycles from the start of the progestogen phase (from Sturdee,[59] with permission).

patients and may reduce compliance, attempts have been made to limit the frequency of bleeding by longer sequential cycles ranging from 3 to 6 months. However, David et al[29] demonstrated that simple hyperplasia of the endometrium develops after three cycles of unopposed estrogen (Table 11.3). Ettinger et al[30] reported on 214 women using CEE and medroxyprogesterone acetate (MPA) to see whether the progestogen could be given quarterly instead of monthly without increasing the risk of endometrial hyperplasia. Hyperplasia was found in 1.5% of 199 women completing follow-up, which was similar to the 0.9% prevalence found as a baseline risk. The quarterly MPA resulted in longer bleeds (7.7 ± 2.9 versus 5.4 ± 2.0 days), more reports of heavy bleeds (31.1 versus 8.0%) and unscheduled bleeding (15.5 versus 16.8%). Nevertheless, the women reported a preference for the quarterly regimen compared with a monthly sequential regimen by 4:1.

A randomized prospective controlled trial with a quarterly sequential HRT regimen reported that simple hyperplasia without cytological atypia developed at the end of the estrogen phase, which was independent of the estrogen dose but was converted to an inactive or atrophic endometrium by the addition of gestodene for 12 days.[31] The authors claimed that this combination offered good cycle control, but no statistical analysis of the results was offered and only 30 women were studied.

Thus, 3 months is generally considered to be the maximum interval for adding the progestogen.[29,30,32] The Scandinavian Long Cycle Study Group reported a 4-year study of 240 early postmenopausal women.[33] They found that the incidence of endometrial pathology (simple, complex or atypical hyperplasia, or carcinoma) was significantly higher in the 12-week cycle group ($P = 0.0003$), with an annual incidence of 5.6% as compared to 1% in the monthly cycle

Table 11.3   Risk of endometrial cancer with sequential estrogen–progestogen (E+P) and continuous combined therapy (adapted from Weiderpass,[6] with permission)

Duration	Sequential E+P OR (95% CI)	Continuous combined OR (95% CI)
< 5 years	1.5 (1.0–2.2)	0.8 (0.5–1.3)
> 5 years	2.9 (1.8–4.6)	0.2 (0.1–0.8)
Per year	1.1 (1.06–1.15)	0.86 (0.77–0.97)

OR, Odds ratio; CI, confidence interval.

group. They further confirmed that long-cycle therapy resulted in more irregular bleeding but reported no improved compliance. Another study from Finland found that long-cycle HRT was associated with a higher RR of endometrial pathology than monthly cycle HRT, with a standardized incidence ratio (SIR) for the quarterly cycle of 2.0 (95% CI 1.6–2.6), compared to a SIR for the monthly cycle of 1.3 (95% CI 1.1–1.6),[34] giving further support to the previous studies.

All these data indicate that progestogens will reduce the risk of endometrial hyperplasia and carcinoma, but the duration of progestogen in each cycle is important and should be for at least 10 days. Furthermore, there may still be a risk with long-term use of monthly sequential HRT and more so with long-cycle regimens.

CONTINUOUS COMBINED THERAPY (CCT)

The biochemical and morphological changes in the endometrium induced by progestogen are maintained so long as progestogen is administered.[35] If this is continuous, the proliferative effect of estrogen will be prevented and the endometrium should become atrophic. This was the rationale for the introduction of CCT, since without any cycle or a progestogen phase, and with no tissue to be shed, there should not

be any bleeding,[36] whereas the benefits should be the same as for sequential therapy.[37]

Although the main aim of CCT is to avoid cyclical bleeding, all studies of CCT have found a high incidence of bleeds, particularly in the first 3 months, varying from 50 to 80%. This occurs more often in women who are within 1 year of the menopause rather than postmenopausal, probably as a result of some residual ovarian activity.

Several studies have confirmed that an atrophic endometrium is achieved with CCT in 90–100% of women, even after only 3 months of treatment with daily doses of progestogen as low as 0.25 mg/day norethisterone acetate or 2.5 mg/day MPA. After 1 year of treatment with CEE 0.625 mg/day and MPA 2.5 or 5.0 mg/day, Woodruff and Pickar[38] found endometrial hyperplasia without atypia in < 1% of women, which is lower than the background rate in postmenopausal women. The Cochrane data[3] reported that endometrial hyperplasia may be less likely with CCT than a sequential regimen, in particular with long duration of therapy; OR 0.3 (95% CI 0.1–0.97). Endometrial cancer has also only rarely been reported in women taking continuous combined regimens, and most of these cases had other risk factors.[39–42] Hill et al[43] assessed the risk of endometrial cancer in 969 women taking CCT. They found a RR of 0.6 (95% CI 0.3–1.3), concluding that there was no increased risk for endometrial cancer over the baseline and that there may even be a decreased risk. Archer et al[44] reported a randomized trial of 625 women using a transdermal CCT regimen of estradiol and norethisterone acetate that also prevented endometrial hyperplasia. However, both of these studies were of relatively short duration (72 and 12 months, respectively, so the long-term effects are not known.

In the PEPI trial,[2] conducted over 3 years, there were no recorded cases of complex hyperplasia in women on CCT, compared with 1.7% of 118 women treated with sequential HRT and 0.8% of women taking a placebo. Another study of CCT using estrone sulphate and MPA over a 2-year period also reported no cases of endometrial hyperplasia.[45]

In the UK, a multicenter study reported on 751 women who had previously been taking sequential HRT and 445 untreated post-

menopausal women (total 1196) who completed 9 months of CCT with estradiol 2 mg/day and norethisterone acetate 1 mg/day. There were no cases of endometrial hyperplasia and the endometrium was atrophic in more than two-thirds of the women. Furthermore, all the women with complex hyperplasia during the previous sequential HRT and who completed the study (n = 42) reverted to normal endometrial patterns (Fig. 11.4). Continuation of this study for 5 years confirmed the protective effect of this CCT regimen in 387 women, with > 70% having an atrophic endometrium and the remainder having other normal histology and no hyperplasia or carcinoma.[46] These data indicate the protective effect of the continuous progestogen of CCT regimens not only in preventing hyperplasia but also the correction of pre-existing hyperplasia.

There is further evidence for the protective effect of CCT regimens from a population-based case control study from Sweden.[6]

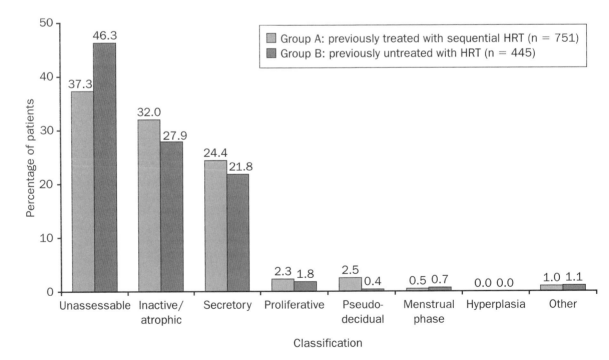

Figure 11.4 Histological results of endometrial biopsies after treatment with continuous combined hormone replacement therapy (estradiol 2 mg/day and norethisterone acetate 1 mg/day) for 9 months (reproduced from Sturdee et al,[17] with permission).

Table 11.4   Endometrial histology before and after one, two and three cycles of unopposed 17β-estradiol 2 mg/day for 21 days, and after the fourth cycle consisting of 17β-estradiol 2 mg/day for 21 days with additional norethisterone acetate (NETA) 1 mg/day for the last 10 days[59]

	Atrophic	No tissue	Proliferative	Secretory	Simple hyperplasia
Before HRT	44	52	4	0	0
After month 1	71	11	18	0	0
After month 2	13	3	84	0	0
After month 3	4	1	80	0	15
After month 4 + NETA for 10 days	3	16	3	78	0

With < 5 years use of CCT, the observed risk of developing endometrial carcinoma was 0.8 (95% CI 0.5–1.3) and with > 5 years use it was 0.2 (95% CI 0.1–0.8). This was in marked contrast to the risk with sequential estrogen–progestogen where the risk after > 5 years use was 2.9 (95% CI 1.8–4.6) (Table 11.4).

The Women's Health Initiative report, following the premature termination of the continuous combined arm of the randomized controlled trial found that after a mean of 5.3 years of CEE 0.625 mg/day with MPA 2.5 mg/day in 8506 women, there was no change in the risk of endometrial cancer.[47] The hazard ratio (HR) was 0.63 (95% CI 0.47–1.47).

Tibolone is a synthetic hormone that has similar effects to CCT.[48] In the endometrium it is converted to a Δ-4 metabolite, which has no estrogenic activity, so the endometrium is not stimulated. As with CCT, the endometrium is mainly kept in an atrophic state but there are few long-term data.[49]

Raloxifene is a selective estrogen receptor modulator (SERM) which is licensed for the treatment and prevention of osteoporosis. It has anti-estrogenic effects on both breast and endometrial tissue, and estrogenic benefits on bone and lipid metabolism. A randomized double-blind trial of 7705 women over 4 years compared raloxifene to placebo.[50] This confirmed no endometrial stimulation and suggested that there may be a reduction in the risk

of endometrial cancer in those taking raloxifene (*P* = 0.23). A randomized controlled trial of 136 women compared the effects of raloxifene and CCT on the endometrium.[51] From the women taking raloxifene, endometrial biopsies revealed a normal atrophic endometrium in 94.4% and benign stimulatory endometrium in 5.6%; whereas, from the women taking CCT, there was an atrophic endometrium in 78.7%, benign stimulated endometrium in 19.1% and 2.1% of biopsy specimens showed benign abnormal endometrium. Overall, there was no endometrial proliferation found with raloxifene.

Postmenopausal women who have had a hysterectomy can have unopposed estrogen replacement therapy, as there is no evidence of any benefit from additional progestogen other than to protect the endometrium. It is logical therefore to deliver the progestogen directly into the endometrial cavity, which will give a high local concentration in the endometrium but with lower circulating levels than following systemic administration. An intrauterine system that delivers levonorgestrel (LNG) has been available for contraception and the treatment of menorrhagia for several years (Mirena®), but many studies have also demonstrated the merits of using this route of progestogen delivery for continuous combined HRT. Since 1991, 16 studies of intrauterine LNG in combination with different types and routes of estrogen in 809 women have all reported no

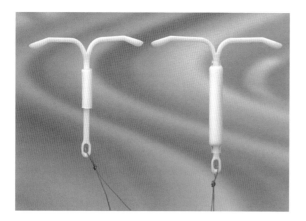

Figure 11.5 The levonorgestrel (LNG)-releasing Mirena intrauterine system and the smaller menopausal LNG system (MLS). (Photograph courtesy of Professor F Riphagen of Leiras, Turku, Finland.)

cases of endometrial hyperplasia.[52] A smaller intrauterine system that delivers 10 µg LNG/day, compared to 20 µg LNG/day with Mirena, is more suitable for postmenopausal woman, and has also been shown to be acceptable and to protect the endometrium (Fig. 11.5).[53]

CONCLUSIONS

- Unopposed estrogen therapy is associated with a significantly increased risk of developing endometrial hyperplasia and, with continued use, of carcinoma. This risk remains for many years after cessation of therapy.
- The addition of progestogen reduces the risk of endometrial disease but regimens should include at least 10 days in each monthly cycle. After 5 years there is probably less protection of the endometrium. Postmenopausal women who have been taking sequential estrogen–progestogen therapy for > 5 years are at increased risk of endometrial carcinoma and should be advised to change to a CCT regimen.
- During sequential estrogen–progestogen therapy, the timing of the bleed does not give any guide to the state of the endometrium or the possible presence of hyperplasia.

- Long-cycle regimens with a progestogen at less than monthly intervals may not provide adequate endometrial protection.
- For women taking long-term HRT a continuous combined estrogen and progestogen regimen should be recommended for endometrial safety.
- SERM therapy such as raloxifene may provide a suitable alternative to long-term HRT.
- Intrauterine delivery of progestogen causes fewer progestogenic effects outside the uterine cavity than systemic therapy, while providing long-term protection of the endometrium.

REFERENCES

1. Weiss NS, Szekely DR, English DR et al. Endometrial cancer in relation to patterns of menopausal estrogen use. *J Am Med Ass* 1979; **242:** 261–4.
2. Writing Group for the PEPI Trial. Effects of hormone replacement therapy on endometrial histology in postmenopausal women. The Postmenopausal Estrogen/Progestin Interventions (PEPI) Trial. *J Am Med Ass* 1996; **275:** 370–5.
3. Lethaby A, Farquhar C, Sarkis A et al. The association of oestrogen, oestrogen–progestogen and placebo with endometrial hyperplasia and irregular bleeding in menopausal women. *The Cochrane Library 4*. Oxford: Update Software.
4. Notelowitz M, Varner RE, Rebar RW et al. Minimal endometrial proliferation over a two-year period in taking 0.3 mg of unopposed esterified estrogens. *Menopause* 1997; **4:** 80–8.
5. Cushing KL, Weiss NS, Voigt LF et al. Risk of endometrial cancer in relation to use of low-dose unopposed estrogens. *Obstet Gynecol* 1995; **91:** 35–9.
6. Wiederpass E. Risk of endometrial cancer following estrogen replacement with and without progestins. *J Nat Cancer Inst* 1999; **91:** 1131–7.
7. Henderson BE, Casagrande JT, Pike MC et al. The epidemiology of endometrial cancer in young women. *Br J Cancer* 1983; **47:** 749–56.
8. Horowitz R, Feinstein AR. Alternative analytic methods for case control studies of estrogens and endometrial cancer. *N Engl J Med* 1978; **299:** 1089–94.
9. Antunes CMF, Stolley PD, Rosenstein MB et al. Endometrial cancer and estrogen use. Report of

a large case control study. *N Engl J Med* 1979; **300:** 9–13.

10. Paganini-Hill, Ross RK, Henderson BE. Endometrial cancer and patterns of use of oestrogen replacement therapy: a cohort study. *Br J Cancer* 1989; **59:** 445–7.

11. Green PK, Weiss NS, McKnight B et al. Risk of endometrial cancer following cessation of menopausal hormone use. *Cancer Causes Control* 1996; **7:** 575–80.

12. Casper RF. Regulation of estrogen/progestogen receptors in the endometrium. *Int J Fertil Menop Studies* 1996; **41:** 16–21.

13. Varma TR. Effect of long-term therapy with estrogen and progesterone on the endometrium of post-menopausal women. *Acta Obstet Gynecol Scand* 1985; **64:** 40–6.

14. Paterson MEL, Wade-Evans T, Sturdee DW et al. Endometrial disease after treatment with oestrogens and progestogens in the climacteric. *BMJ* 1980; **280:** 822–4.

15. Whitehead MI, McQueen J, Beard RJ et al. The effects of cyclical oestrogen therapy and sequential oestrogen therapy on the endometrium of post-menopausal women. *Acta Obstet Gynecol Scand* 1977; **65:** 91–101.

16. Sturdee DW, Wade-Evans T, Paterson ME et al. Relations between bleeding pattern, endometrial histology and oestrogen treatment in post-menopausal women. *BMJ* 1978; **I:** 1575–7.

17. Sturdee DW, Ulrich LG, Barlow DH et al. The endometrial response to sequential and continuous combined oestrogen–progestogen replacement therapy. *Br J Obstet Gynaecol* 2000; **107:** 1392–400.

18. Bergeron C, Nogales F, Masseroli M et al. A multi-centric European study testing the reproducibility of the WHO classification of endometrial hyperplasias with a proposal of a simplified working classification for biopsy and curettage specimens. *Am J Surg Pathol* 1999; **23:** 1102–8.

19. Persson I, Adami HO, Bergkvist L et al. Risk of endometrial cancer after treatment with oestrogens alone or in conjunction with progestogens: results of a prospective study. *BMJ* 1989; **298:** 147–51.

20. Beresford JAA, Weiss NS, Voigt LF, McKnight B. Risk of endometrial cancer in relation to use of oestrogen combined with cyclic progestogen therapy in post-menopausal women. *Lancet* 1997; **349:** 458–61.

21. Terakawa N, Kigawa J, Taketani Y et al. The behaviour of endometrial hyperplasia: a prospective study. *J Obstet Gynaecol Res* 1997; **28:** 223–30.

22. Kurman RJ. The behaviour of endometrial hyperplasia. A long term study of 'untreated' hyperplasia in 170 patients. *Cancer* 1985; **56:** 403–12.

23. Archer DF, McIntyre-Seltman K, Wilborn WW et al. Endometrial morphology in asymptomatic postmenopausal women. *Am J Obstet Gynecol* 1991; **165:** 317–22.

24. Korhonen MO, Symons JP, Hyde BM et al. Histologic classification and pathologic findings for endometrial biopsy specimens obtained from 2,964 perimenopausal and postmenopausal women undergoing treatment with continuous hormones as replacement therapy (CHART 2 STUDY). *Am J Obstet Gynecol* 1997; **176:** 377–80.

25. Archer DF, Pickar JH, Bottiglioni F. Bleeding patterns in postmenopausal women taking continuous combined or sequential regimens of conjugated estrogens with medroxyprogesterone acetate. *Obstet Gynecol* 1994; **83:** 686–92.

26. Padwick ML, Pryse-Davies J, Whitehead MI. A simple method for determining the optimal dosage of progestin in postmenopausal women receiving estrogens. *N Engl J Med* 1986; **315:** 930–4.

27. Sturdee DW, Barlow DH, Ulrich LG et al. Is the timing of withdrawal bleeding a guide to endometrial safety during sequential oestrogen–progestogen replacement therapy? *Lancet* 1994; **344:** 979–82.

28. Utian WH. Predicting endometrial pathology by timing of withdrawal bleeding to sequential HRT. *Menop Management* 1994; **3:** 6 (editorial).

29. David A, Czernobilsky B, Weisglass L. Long cyclic hormonal cycle therapy in post-menopausal women. In: (Berg G, Hammar M, eds) *The Modern Management of the Menopause. Proceedings of the VII International Congress on the Menopause.* (Parthenon Publishing: London, 1994) 463–70.

30. Ettinger B, Selby J, Citron JT, Vangessel A. Cyclic HRT using quarterly progestin. *Obstet Gynecol* 1994; **83:** 693–700.

31. Boerrigter PJ, Baak JPA, Fox H. Endometrial response in estrogen replacement therapy quarterly combined with a progestogen. *Maturitas* 1996; **24:** 63–71.

32. Hirvonen E, Salmi, Puolakka J et al. Can progestin be limited to every third month only in postmenopausal women taking oestrogen? *Maturitas* 1995; **21:** 39–44.

33. Bjarnason K, Cerin A, Lindgren R, Weber T. The Scandinavian Long Cycle Study Group. Adverse

endometrial effects during long cycle hormone replacement therapy. *Maturitas* 1999; **32:** 161–70.

34. Pukkala E, Tulenheimo-Silfvast A, Leminem A. Incidence of cancer among women using long versus monthly cycle HRT, Finland 1994–1997. *Cancer Causes Control* 2001; **12:** 111–15.

35. Whitehead ML, Townsend PT, Pryse-Davies J et al. Effects of estrogens and progestins on the biochemistry and morphology of the post-menopausal endometrium. *N Engl J Med* 1981; **305:** 1599–605.

36. Mattsson LA, Cullberg G, Samsioe G. Evaluation of a continuous combined oestrogen/progestogen regimen for climacteric complaints. *Maturitas* 1982; **4:** 95–102.

37. Hillard, TC. Period-free HRT. In: (Sturdee DW, Oláh K, Keane D, eds) *The Yearbook of Obstetrics and Gynaecology.* (RCOG Press: London, 2001) 98–118.

38. Woodruff JD, Pickar JH. Incidence of endometrial hyperplasia in postmenopausal women taking conjugated estrogens alone. *Am J Obstet Gynecol* 1994; **170:** 1213–23.

39. Leather AT, Savvas M, Studd JWW. Endometrial histology and bleeding patterns after 8 years of continuous combined oestrogen and progestogen therapy in post-menopausal women. *Obstet Gynecol* 1991; **78:** 1008–10.

40. McGonigle KF. Development of endometrial cancer in women on oestrogen and progestin hormone replacement therapy. *Gynecol Oncol* 1994; **55:** 126–32.

41. Ulrich LG. Accumulated knowledge of Kliogest® safety aspects. *Br J Obstet Gynaecol* 1993; **103:** 99–103.

42. Comerci JT, Fields AL, Runowicz CD, Goldberg GL. Continuous low dose combined hormone replacement therapy and the risk of endometrial cancer. *Gynecol Oncol* 1997; **64:** 425–30.

43. Hill DA, Weiss NS, Beresford SA et al. Continuous combined hormone replacement therapy and risk of endometrial cancer. *Am J Obstet Gynecol* 2000; **183:** 1456–61.

44. Archer DF, Furst K, Tipping D et al (Combipatch Study Group). A randomised comparison of continuous combined transdermal delivery of estradiol–norethindrone acetate and estradiol alone for menopause. *Obstet Gynecol* 1999; **94:** 498–503.

45. Nand SL, Webster MA, Baber R, O'Connor V, for the Ogen/Provera Study Group. Bleeding pattern and endometrial changes on continuous combined hormone replacement therapy for 2 years. *Obstet Gynecol* 1998; **91:** 678–84.

46. Wells M, Ulrich LG, Sturdee DW et al. Effect on endometrium of long term treatment with continuous combined oestrogen–progestogen replacement therapy: follow up study. *BMJ* 2002; **325:** 239–42.

47. Writing Group for the Women's Health Initiative. Risks and benefits of estrogen plus progestin in healthy postmenopausal women. *J Am Med Ass* 2002; **288:** 321–33.

48. Moore RA. Livial: a review of clinical studies. *Br J Obstet Gynaecol* 1999; **106:** 1–21.

49. Völker W, Coelingh Bennink HJT, Helmond FA. Effects of tibolone on the endometrium. *Climacteric* 2001; **4:** 203–8.

50. Delmas PD, Bjarnason NH, Mitlak et al. Effects of raloxifene on bone mineral density, serum cholesterol concentrations, and uterine endometrium in postmenopausal women. *N Engl J Med* 1997; **337:** 1641–7.

51. Fugene P, Scheele WH, Shah A et al. Uterine effects of raloxifene in comparison with continuous-combined HRT in post-menopausal women. *Am J Obstet Gynecol* 2000; **182:** 568–74.

52. Riphagen FE. Intrauterine application of progestins in hormone replacement therapy. *Climacteric* 2000; **3:** 199–211.

53. Raudaskoski T, Tapanainen J, Tomás E et al. Intrauterine 10 µg and 20µg levonorgestrel systems in postmenopausal women receiving oral oestrogen replacement therapy: clinical, endometrial and metabolic response. *Br J Obstet Gyndecol* 2002; **109:** 136–44.

54. Smith DC, Prentice R, Thompson D, Herman W. Association of exogenous estrogens and endometrial carcinoma. *N Engl J Med* 1975; **293:** 1164–7.

55. Ziel H, Finkle W. Increased risk of endometrial carcinoma among users of conjugated estrogens. *N Engl J Med* 1975; **293:** 1167–70.

56. Gray Sr La, Christopherson WM, Hoover RN. Estrogens and endometrial cancer. *Obstet Gynecol* 1977; **49:** 385–9.

57. Shapiro S, Kaufman DW, Slone D et al. Recent and past use of conjugated estrogens in relation to adenocarcinoma of the endometrium. *N Engl J Med* 1980; **303:** 485–9.

58. Kelsey JL, LiVolsi VA, Holford TR et al. A case-control study of cancer of the endometrium. *Am J Epidemiol* 1982; **116:** 333–42.

59. Sturdee DW. HRT, the endometrium and bleeding. In: (Barlow DH, Sturdee DW, Miles A, eds) *The Effective Management of the Menopause. UK Key Advances in Clinical Practice.* (Aesculapius Medical Press: London, 2002) 49–59.

12

Estrogen deprivation and hormone replacement therapy: effects on glucose and insulin metabolism and the metabolic syndrome

IF Godsland

Introduction • Metabolic syndrome • Diabetes and cardiovascular disease • Estrogen deficiency and carbohydrate metabolism • Estrogen replacement and carbohydrate metabolism • Combined hormone replacement therapy (HRT) and carbohydrate metabolism • Hormone replacement therapy (HRT) in postmenopausal women with diabetes • Conclusions • References

INTRODUCTION

In general, the clinical condition of diabetes arises in one of two ways. Type 1 diabetes appears in childhood, with a sudden and potentially catastrophic decline in the ability of the pancreas to secrete insulin. Type 2 diabetes, on the other hand, emerges later in life out of a continuum of metabolic disturbances that may have been present for many years before the pancreatic insulin response to glucose begins to decline and symptoms of diabetes appear. This continuum of metabolic disturbances has been a topic of growing interest since 1988 when Reaven[1] brought its features together in the unifying concept of an insulin resistance or metabolic syndrome.

The metabolic profile from which Type 2 diabetes emerges has amongst its principal features: insulin resistance, hyperinsulinemia, hypertriglyceridemia, excessive centrally located body fat, hypertension, low levels of high density lipoprotein (HDL) cholesterol, high levels of plasminogen activator inhibitor-1, increased uric acid concentrations and low sex hormone-binding globulin (SHBG) levels. The origins, interrelationships and implications of these disturbances are worth considering in some detail since estrogen deprivation and replacement can affect them all.

METABOLIC SYNDROME

In a continuum of metabolic disturbances, tendencies may be distinguished without all characteristic features necessarily being present at once. Nevertheless, in the development of the metabolic syndrome concept, insulin resistance has been taken as a defining characteristic, since virtually all the other features of the syndrome can derive from it.

Consequences of insulin resistance

As shown in Fig. 12.1 insulin action depends on

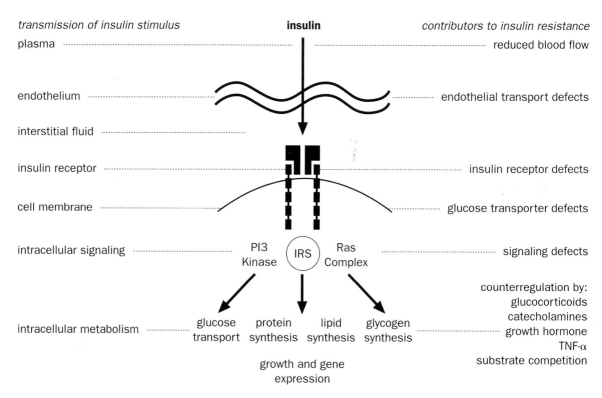

Figure 12.1 Steps involved in the transmission of the insulin stimulus in the blood to the intracellular or nuclear response. Defects in any one of these steps can induce insulin resistance.

a number of steps which mediate the link between insulin circulating in the plasma and insulin acting at the cellular or nuclear level. Defects or inhibition at any one of these steps can lead to a situation in which a given concentration of insulin in the plasma leads to less than the expected physiological or biochemical effect, i.e. a state of insulin resistance.

The effects of insulin resistance may be inferred from the manifold effects that insulin has in promoting an anabolic or energy-saving metabolic profile. Primarily, insulin stimulates glucose elimination from the blood and suppresses hepatic glucose production. Therefore, when there is insulin resistance, blood glucose concentrations might be expected to rise. However, providing the pancreatic beta cell can still respond normally to rising glucose concentrations, pancreatic insulin output increases in states of insulin resistance to maintain normal basal glucose levels. Thus, although some deterioration in glucose tolerance may be seen, glucose homeostasis is generally maintained, but at the expense of higher insulin concentrations.

Insulin suppresses adipose tissue lipolysis and therefore reduces the supply of nonesterified fatty acids to the liver.[2] Since this supply is the primary determinant of hepatic triglyceride synthesis and very low density lipoprotein (VLDL) secretion, insulin suppresses serum triglyceride and VLDL concentrations. Insulin can also directly suppress hepatic release of VLDL and can stimulate the synthesis of one of the principal enzymes responsible for the metabolism of VLDL, lipoprotein lipase. Therefore, where there is insulin resistance nonesterified fatty acid turnover is increased, and triglyceride and VLDL levels are consistently increased. The reduction in lipoprotein lipase activity associated with insulin resistance may have further potentially adverse consequences, including diminished assembly of anti-atherogenic HDL particles and reduced elimination of atherogenic cholesterol-enriched remnants of VLDL metabolism.

Whether increased central fat deposition is a cause or a consequence of insulin resistance is controversial, although the weight of evidence is tending to favor it as a cause.[3] Central, visceral or android fat is characterized by a relatively high lipolytic rate, which combines a heightened sensitivity to lipolytic stimuli – primarily catecholamines – and a reduced sensitivity to antilipolytic stimuli – primarily insulin. Increased central fat deposition is, therefore, associated with increased supply of nonesterified fatty acids, which may promote insulin resistance by acting as a competitor for fuel metabolism with glucose.[4] Most recently, adipose tissue has come to be recognized as an important endocrine tissue in its own right, intimately involved in the regulation of energy metabolism and in the secretion of various cytokines.[5,6] Leptin, resistin, tumor necrosis factor-alpha (TNF-α) and interleukin (IL)-6 are amongst its secretory products, each of which may act to increase insulin resistance.

Resistance to insulin action has also been linked to hypertension. Although the hyperinsulinemia associated with insulin resistance could contribute to this association (see below), a well-characterized feature of insulin resistance is an impairment in insulin-stimulated vasodilation, which could have a role in elevating blood pressure.[7] Other effects of insulin resistance include hyperuricemia, which could result from the diversion of metabolic intermediates from the glycolytic pathway following inhibition of downstream insulin-sensitive enzymes.[8] A further area potentially related to insulin resistance, but still relatively under-researched, is hepatic uptake of newly secreted insulin. This is reduced in states of insulin resistance and may contribute to lower HDL concentrations.[9]

Consequences of hyperinsulinemia

The consequences of insulin resistance may themselves have consequences which contribute further to the development of the metabolic syndrome. With regard to the vasculature, chronically elevated insulin levels may increase smooth muscle cell proliferation and arterial lipid deposition,[10] and may also increase sympathetic tone and stimulate renal sodium reabsorption, thus further contributing to a tendency to hypertension.[11] Insulin may also stimulate the production of several hepatic proteins. Principal amongst these is the antifibrinolytic factor, plasminogen activator inhibitor (PAI)-1,[12] but there is also evidence for significant associations between insulin and procoagulatory factors, including factors VII and X.[13]

Consequences of hypertriglyceridemia

The increased synthesis and release of triglycerides and VLDL that accompanies insulin resistance has additional consequences for lipoprotein metabolism.[14] Increased provision of triglyceride substrate can lead to increased activity of cholesterol ester transfer protein (CETP). Increased CETP activity then results in more triglyceride enrichment of HDL particles.[15] This makes HDL a better substrate for the triglyceride lipase action of the enzyme hepatic lipase and therefore more likely to undergo catabolism.[16] In consequence, high triglyceride concentrations are often associated with low HDL cholesterol levels. Increased VLDL triglyceride enrichment could also contribute to an increase in the proportion of low-density lipoprotein (LDL) particles in the small, dense subfraction, which may be particularly atherogenic on account of their increased tendency to undergo oxidation.

DIABETES AND CARDIOVASCULAR DISEASE

The various manifestations of the metabolic syndrome are listed in Box 12.1. Each of these manifestations has been independently related to risk of coronary heart disease (CHD),[17–19] and it is as a CHD risk factor that the metabolic syndrome has been of most interest. But many of these features have also been linked with increased risk of developing Type 2 diabetes, in particular insulin resistance and increased central fat. There is then the possibility that both CHD and Type 2 diabetes can represent alternative clinical consequences of prolonged exposure to the disturbances of the metabolic syndrome, which emerge at a stage dependent on whether damage to the pancreas or the

---

Box 12.1   Metabolic and physiologic disturbances associated with insulin resistance that are independently associated with increased risk of cardiovascular disease

---

Hyperinsulinemia

Hypertriglyceridemia

Low high-density lipoprotein (HDL)
   concentrations

Increased small dense low-density lipoprotein
   (LDL)

Decreased sex hormone-binding globulin
   (SHBG)

Increased uric acid concentrations

Increased fibrinogen and factor VII

Decreased fibrinolysis

Decreased postprandial fat elimination

Hypertension

Central obesity

---

vasculature exceeds the threshold for diagnostic features to appear.

Interestingly, several studies have shown that it is possible to derive a continuous quantitative measure of the severity of the correlated disturbances of the metabolic syndrome,[20–22] and such a measure can predict the development of CHD[23] or Type 2 diabetes.[24] The predictive power of the syndrome measure for Type 2 diabetes was particularly strong, those in the top quintile of the measure's distribution having a tenfold greater risk of diabetes than those in the lower quintiles.[24]

It should be noted that, in the context of the metabolic syndrome, the distinction between CHD and Type 2 diabetes may be more apparent than real. Those with vascular disease are at increased risk of having Type 2 diabetes[25] and, reciprocally, Type 2 diabetes is a well-established risk factor for vascular disease, which carries with it its own additional contributions to vascular risk. Thus, the elevated glucose levels seen in diabetes may adversely affect the vasculature, either directly by protein glycosylation[26] or by increasing free-radical damage to the vessel wall.[27] Moreover, the deficiency in

insulin secretion in Type 2 diabetes may augment the disturbances of the metabolic syndrome, particularly with regard to lipid metabolism.[28] It is noteworthy that these lipid and lipoprotein changes are particularly marked in women with Type 2 diabetes[29] and such women are also at particular risk of developing cardiovascular disease.[30] This raises the question of how estrogen deficiency and replacement affects the complex association of the metabolic syndrome, Type 2 diabetes and CHD.

ESTROGEN DEFICIENCY AND CARBOHYDRATE METABOLISM

Menopause is not associated with any immediate change in glucose or insulin levels but there are underlying changes which may have clinical implications and which may become apparent with increasing time since menopause. Pancreatic insulin secretion falls with the decline in estrogen concentrations, although insulin levels are maintained by an increase in the plasma insulin half-life.[31] Insulin resistance may not change immediately following menopause but there is a progressive increase in insulin resistance and in insulin concentrations that relates to time since menopause rather than chronologial age.[32,33] Thus postmenopausal women are generally more insulin resistant than would be expected from the effects of age alone. There is also a progressive decrease in the amount of newly secreted insulin taken up by the liver.[33]

Postmenopausal women exhibit many of the characteristics associated with the metabolic syndrome, including increased triglyceride and decreased HDL cholesterol levels, decreased triglyceride elimination and increased uric acid concentrations, an increased proportion of centrally distributed fat, increased uric acid levels and decreased SHBG.[34] Whilst estrogen deficiency is likely to be the principal contributing factor, increasing insulin resistance may also provide an added metabolic burden, the effects of the two combining to generate a characteristic menopausal metabolic syndrome.

Whilst in general the decline in pancreatic insulin secretion at menopause may be compensated for by an increase in insulin half-life, this decline in secretion could lead, in certain susceptible or borderline individuals, to the emergence of frank diabetes. In accord with earlier observations,[35] the US National Health and Nutrition Examination Survey has established that incidence of diabetes increases more rapidy in middle-aged women than it does in middle-aged men.[36] Moreover, there is evidence that if the onset of diabetes is related to time since menopause rather than chronologic age, a very strong relationship may emerge between menopause and the development of diabetes.[37]

ESTROGEN REPLACEMENT AND CARBOHYDRATE METABOLISM

It is well established that estrogen replacement can reverse many of the adverse clinical and metabolic effects of menopause, including effects on carbohydrate metabolism. In the past, there has been some confusion over this on account of the adverse effects reported in association with oral contraceptive use. These stem from use of potent alkylated estrogens, including ethinylestradiol, which the majority of studies have shown to cause deterioration in glucose tolerance and insulin resistance.[38] This is also the case in postmenopausal women taking higher doses (≥ 1.25 mg/day) of conjugated equine estrogens; however, with lower doses (0.625 mg/day) studies are equally divided between those showing no effect and those showing an improvement in insulin sensitivity.

With the native estrogen, estradiol, administered orally or transdermally, the majority of studies are consistent with an improvement in insulin sensitivity.[38] The simplest interpretation of these findings is that physiologic estrogen replacement in postmenopausal women improves insulin sensitivity, whereas estrogen in excess is associated with an adverse effect. Such an adverse effect could result from secondary effects of high estrogen exposure, increased glucocorticoid activity being the most likely candidate.[38] In support of the proposition that the underlying physiologic effect of estrogens is an improvement in insulin sensitivity, it is noteworthy that both muscle and adipose tissue isolated from animals given estrogens show improved responses to insulin (Fig. 12.2).[39,40]

In addition to insulin resistance, the great majority of other disturbances of menopausal metabolic syndrome are reversed by estrogen replacement (Table 12.1). Of particular note is the increase in triglyceride concentrations seen after menopause. The expected effect of estrogen replacement would be a fall in triglycerides, but oral administration of estrogen results in a pharmacologic increase in triglyceride levels as a result of the stimulation of hepatic triglyceride synthesis by estrogen.[41] However, with parenteral administration of estrogen, e.g. with transdermally administered 17β-estradiol there is the expected fall in triglyceride levels.[42] The physiologic effect of estrogen most likely relates to changes in VLDL elimination, which deteriorates after the

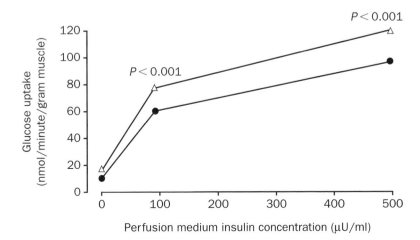

Figure 12.2 Estrogen-induced improvement in the sensitivity of glucose uptake to insulin in isolated muscle from the rat. ●, Untreated controls; △, treated with estradiol benzoate (0.005 mg/day) for 21 days. (From Rushakoff and Kalkhoff,[40] with permission.)

Table 12.1   Features of the menopausal metabolic syndrome and the effects of physiologic estrogen replacement (from Spencer et al,[34] with permission)

Effects of menopause	Effects of physiologic estrogen replacement
Increased total cholesterol	Reduced total cholesterol
Increased triglycerides	Reduced triglycerides
Decreased HDL-C	Increased HDL-C
Reduced insulin sensitivity	Increased insulin sensitivity
Increased android fat distribution	Increased gynoid fat distribution
Increased small, dense LDL-C	Reduced LDL-C
Increased HDL_3:HDL_2	Reduced HDL_3:HDL_2
Increased Lp(a)	Reduced Lp(a)
Reduced insulin elimination	Increased insulin elimination
Reduced insulin secretion	Increased insulin secretion
Impaired vascular function	Reduced vascular resistance
Increased Factor VII	Reduced Factor VII
Increased fibrinogen	Reduced fibrinogen
Increased oxidative stress	Reduced oxidative stress
? Increased BP	Reduced/no change in BP

BP, Blood pressure; HDL, high-density lipoprotein; LDL, low-density lipoprotein; Lp(a), Lipoprotein (a).

menopause[43] but improves in response to estrogen.[44,45]

Estrogen replacement could theoretically reverse the menopause-associated decline in insulin secretion. The effects of estrogens on insulin secretion were most strikingly demonstrated many years ago in experiments in which administration of estrogens diminished the development of diabetes in subtotally pancreatectomized animals (Fig. 12.3).[46] This effect is associated with hypertrophy and hyperplasia of the remaining pancreatic tissue, and, in accord with these findings, increased pancreatic insulin output has been demonstrated in perfused pancreas preparations exposed to estrogen[47] and in isolated pancreatic islets from estrogen-treated animals.[48] These experimental findings contrast with expectations generated by the effects of oral contraceptive use, i.e. that estrogen replacement in post-menopausal women might increase the incidence of diabetes. Interestingly, detailed analysis of data from an earlier study of insulin secretion patterns in oral contraceptive users[49] showed that the age-related decline in pancreatic insulin release was eliminated in these individuals.[50] Evidence for an influence of postmenopausal estrogen use on the development of Type 2 diabetes is, however, equivocal. One study suggested that women who took estrogens were less likely to develop diabetes than those who did not,[51] but another found no such association.[52]

One additional effect of estrogens on carbohydrate metabolism that could relate to a reduced risk of Type 2 diabetes is estrogen-induced resistance to glucagon action. This resistance extends to both the effects of glucagon on glucose homeostasis and the stimulation of glucagon release by glucose.[53,54]

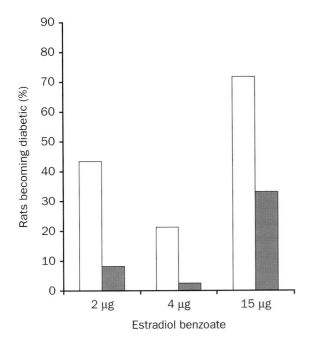

Figure 12.3 Prevention of diabetes in the partially pancreatectomized rat by daily administration of estradiol benzoate for 6 months at the doses shown. Open bars, untreated controls; filled bars, treated. (From Foglia et al,[46] reproduced with permission. © The Endocrine Society)

These effects are seen primarily in the fasted state in which effects on gluconeogenesis are most apparent. Significant reductions in both fasting glucose and fasting insulin may then be seen, particularly with high potency estrogens.

COMBINED HORMONE REPLACEMENT THERAPY (HRT) AND CARBOHYDRATE METABOLISM

The effects of progesterone and progestogens alone have not been studied in postmenopausal women, although there have been a number of studies in premenopausal women using progestogen-only oral contraceptives. The weight of evidence suggests that progesterone alone is probably neutral; although at levels equivalent to those seen in pregnancy some deterioration in carbohydrate metabolism may be seen.[38] The majority of studies of medroxyprogesterone

acetate and levonorgestrel provide evidence for induction of insulin resistance. With medroxyprogesterone acetate this may be expected since this steroid has some glucocorticoid-like activity.[55] Amongst the other progestogens that have been employed in HRT, norethisterone acetate has generally been found to be neutral with regard to carbohydrate metabolism, whereas dydrogesterone alone does not appear to have been studied in this respect.[38]

Given the variety of regimens employed in combined HRT and the relative lack of studies of their effects on carbohydrate metabolism, it is difficult to draw general conclusions. Studies are therefore best considered separately according to the type of progestogen employed. Increased insulin resistance has been described during the estrogen plus progestogen phase of the treatment cycle with those progestogens – medroxyprogesterone acetate and levonorgestrel – which when given alone are associated with increased insulin resistance (Fig. 12.4).[56–58] With regimens containing these progestogens, the weight of evidence favors deterioration in glucose tolerance as the predominant effect of the combination.[58–61]

One feature that has emerged as a possible contributing factor to this deterioration in glucose tolerance is a reduction in the initial insulin output in response to glucose. This was seen in modeling studies of intravenous glucose tolerance test (IVGTT) glucose and insulin concentration profiles in women taking a combination of conjugated equine estrogens and levonorgestrel.[58] Interestingly, in the study of Lobo et al,[60] of women taking conjugated equine estrogens alone and with varying doses of medroxyprogesterone acetate, the oral glucose tolerance test (OGTT) glucose response was significantly increased during at least one of the three cycles studied (cycles 3, 6 and 13) in the combination users, but not in the users of estrogen alone, and, in accord with a reduction in the initial insulin response to glucose, OGTT insulin response was reduced, primarily during the early part of the OGTT.

A combination containing estradiol and norethisterone has been reported to improve glucose tolerance in women with impaired

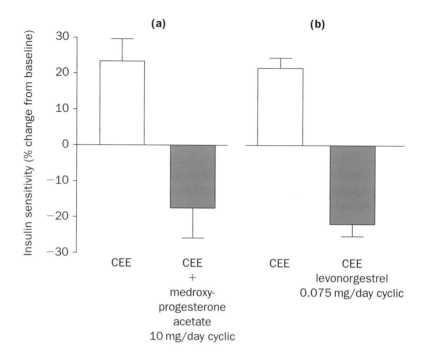

Figure 12.4 Induction of insulin resistance by inclusion of medroxyprogesterone acetate or levonorgestrel as progestogens in combined postmenopausal hormone replacement therapy. (From Godsland,[38] with permission.) (**a**) Percentage change in insulin sensitivity, measured as the glucose elimination constant following insulin injection, in five women given conjugated equine estrogens (CEE: 0.625 mg/day: open bar) and five women given the same dose of estrogen plus cyclical medroxyprogesterone acetate (10 mg/day: closed bar) for 2 months. (From Lindheim et al,[57] with permission.) (**b**) Percentage change in insulin sensitivity, measured by modeling analysis of intravenous glucose tolerance test glucose and insulin concentrations, in 30 women taking CEE (0.625 mg/day) and cyclic levonorgestrel (0.075 mg/day), tested during the estrogen only phase (open bar) and the estrogen plus progestogen combined phase (closed bar) of the third treatment cycle. (From Godsland et al,[58] with permission.)

glucose tolerance, but was without effect on either OGTT glucose or insulin levels in diabetic women or women with normal glucose tolerance.[62] A similar lack of effect on IVGTT glucose and insulin levels was seen when norethisterone acetate was administered transdermally in a cyclic regime with transdermally administered estradiol.[58] Neither insulin resistance nor any other measure of insulin metabolism was affected. This was also the case when variables, including insulin resistance, were compared in the estrogen alone phase and the estrogen plus progestogen phase during the third cycle of treatment.

This was confirmed in a subsequent study in which norethisterone acetate was administered

orally with transdermal estradiol: no effect on insulin sensitivity was apparent during either phase.[63] However, this study also included a group in which both norethisterone acetate and estradiol were given orally, and in this group the expected improvement in insulin sensitivity was seen during the estrogen alone phase. It is also noteworthy that, in this study, improvements in both pancreatic insulin secretion and hepatic insulin elimination were apparent in both treatment groups.

These findings suggest that norethisterone does not oppose estrogen-induced improvements in insulin secretion and hepatic insulin elimination, but, as suggested by the between-phase comparisons, may oppose the favorable effects of estradiol. This opposition may nevertheless be overcome by the more powerful stimulus – possibly to the liver – provided by the oral route of administration.

Cyclically administered dydrogesterone has been studied at high dose (20 mg/day) in combination with conjugated equine estrogens (0.625 mg/day).[64] No effect on OGTT glucose or insulin levels was apparent. However, when a lower dose was employed (10 mg/day) with estradiol (2 mg/day) the beneficial effects of estradiol on insulin action and metabolism appeared to be preserved.[65] In 29 women followed for 24 months, fasting glucose levels were unchanged but there was a steep decline in insulin levels and some increase in fasting C-peptide. A similar, albeit nonsignificant trend, was apparent with OGTT insulin responses. Similar trends with this combination have also been reported in other studies.[66,67]

HORMONE REPLACEMENT THERAPY (HRT) IN POSTMENOPAUSAL WOMEN WITH DIABETES

Given that estrogen replacement in postmenopausal women has the potential for restoring menopause-associated disturbances in glucose and insulin homeostasis, there is good theoretic justification for its use in postmenopausal women with Type 2 diabetes, and no apparent contraindication with regard to Type 1 diabetes. Such a justification would seem particularly strong with regard to Type 2 diabetes since physiologic estrogen replacement could also have favorable effects on the dyslipidemia typical of this form of diabetes. Add to this the favorable effects of estrogen replacement on vascular function, and its reported antioxidant properties, and the case becomes very strong. Moreover, there is evidence from observational studies that, like nondiabetic women, women with diabetes who take HRT have lower risk of CHD compared with those who do not.[68,69]

Estrogen replacement has, however, been widely equated in the past with oral contraceptive therapy. Use of contraceptive formulations containing the potent synthetic estrogen ethinylestradiol is associated with deterioration in glucose tolerance and insulin resistance.[49] However, oral contraceptive therapy represents a state of estrogen excess, in contrast to postmenopausal estrogen replacement therapy that represents restoration of physiologic estrogen levels. As mentioned previously, too little or too much estrogen has adverse effects on carbohydrate metabolism, but restoration of normal physiologic levels is associated with an improvement. Several recent surveys have shown that HRT use amongst women with diabetes remains about half that of women without diabetes,[70–72] suggesting that the potential benefits are not widely appreciated and that inappropriate comparisons with the effects of oral contraceptives still influence prescribing.

To date, there have been surprisingly few studies of the effects of HRT on glucose homeostasis and features of the metabolic syndrome in women with diabetes. Published studies have been reviewed in detail by Cefalu.[73] In summary, the weight of evidence indicates an improvement in glycemic control. Of particular note, an in-depth study by Brussard et al[74] of glucose homeostasis in women with Type 2 diabetes demonstrated improvements in fasting glucose levels, glycosylated hemoglobin levels and insulin sensitivity in response to 17β-estradiol. A reduction in hepatic gluconeogenesis was also apparent, in accord with the glucagon insensitivity induced by estrogen therapy. This reduction was not apparent in women with hypertriglycemia. Possibly, in these women, there was an increased flux of nonesterified fatty acids to the liver. This might have overcome the glucagon insensitivity, since nonesterified fatty acids are a powerful stimulus to hepatic gluconeogenesis.

Other potentially beneficial effects of HRT that have been reported in postmenopausal women with diabetes include improvements in body fat distribution,[75] decreased carotid artery intima media thickness,[76] decreased inflammatory indices[77] and potential improvements in fibrinolytic activity.[78] The expected improvement in vasodilatory response may, nevertheless, be attenuated in diabetics.[79]

Findings with regard to lipid and lipoprotein

levels in women with diabetes taking HRT will be highly dependent on the combination of estrogen and progestogen employed. As mentioned above, orally and parenterally administered estrogens have opposite effects on triglycerides, although both raise HDL cholesterol levels. So-called androgenic progestogens, such as levonorgestrel or norethisterone acetate, oppose the oral estrogen-induced increase in triglycerides but also oppose the increase in HDL cholesterol, and may even cause a net lowering of HDL cholesterol.[42] Other progestogens, such as dydrogesterone, natural progesterone or medrogestone, exert much less opposition, and medroxyprogesterone acetate has intermediate effects. All formulations lower total and LDL cholesterol to a similar extent.[42]

These relative differences in effects of different HRT regimens on lipid and lipoprotein levels have been identified in healthy women but are also apparent in women with diabetes, although there is evidence for an exaggerated increase in triglyceride levels in response to oral estrogen.[73] According to our current understanding of the clinical significance of changes in lipid and lipoprotein levels, the optimum HRT combination for use in women with diabetes would therefore be one that preserves the beneficial effects of estrogen replacement without raising triglycerides or lowering HDL. Such a combination could include transdermally admistered 17β-estradiol with a neutral progestogen such as dydrogesterone or natural progesterone. However, with the recent elucidation of key steps in HDL metabolism there is now the possibility that pharmacologically induced reductions in HDL cholesterol may not be as potentially detrimental as previously supposed.[80] A combination of orally administered estradiol and an 'androgenic' progestogen, such as norethisterone acetate or levonorgestrel, or the single-steroid formulation tibolone, might also be considered, since with these formulations the increase in triglycerides is minimized or reversed.[42]

CONCLUSIONS

Contrary to previous expectations, based on the

effects of oral contraceptive therapy, postmenopausal estrogen replacement has the potential for improving carbohydrate metabolism. These changes would be expected to contribute to improvements in the cardiovascular risk profile that have already been established for estrogen replacement. Both reductions in insulin resistance and indirect effects mediated through improvements in the diabetes risk profile could contribute. Reductions in insulin resistance have been most clearly demonstrated in relation to unopposed therapy with the native estrogen estradiol. Other estrogen regimens may be relatively neutral and this effect may be opposed when a progestogen is included in the treatment. Experimental studies of the effects of progestogens on pancreatic insulin release suggest that there may be similar improvements to those seen with estrogens. It is therefore possible that improvements in the diabetes risk profile may be a more general effect of postmenopausal hormone replacement. These possibilities still remain relatively unexplored, but it should be apparent that further investigation would be worthwhile given the potential benefits that could be confirmed.

REFERENCES

1. Reaven G. Banting Lecture 1988: role of insulin resistance in human disease. *Diabetes* 1988; **37:** 1595–607.
2. Frayn K. Insulin resistance and lipid metabolism. *Curr Opin Lipidol* 1993; **4:** 197–204.
3. Bergman RN, Van Citters GW, Mittelman SD et al. Central role of the adipocyte in the metabolic syndrome. *J Invest Med* 2001; **49:** 119–26.
4. Randle P, Garland P, Hales C, Newsholme E. The glucose fatty-acid cycle. Its role in insulin sensitivity and the metabolic disturbances of diabetes mellitus. *Lancet* 1963; **i:** 785–9.
5. Yudkin JS, Kumari M, Humphries SE, Mohamed-Ali V. Inflammation, obesity, stress and coronary heart disease: is interleukin-6 the link? *Atherosclerosis* 2000; **148:** 209–14.
6. Shuldiner AR, Yang R, Gong D-W. Resistin, obesity and insulin resistance – the emerging role of the adipocyte as an endocrine organ. *N Engl J Med* 2001; **345:** 1345–6.
7. Baron AD. Hemodynamic actions of insulin. *Am J Physiol* 1994; **267:** E187–E202.

8. Leyva F, Wingrove CS, Godsland IF, Stevenson JC. The glycolytic pathway to coronary heart disease. *Metabolism* 1998; **47**: 657–62.

9. Godsland IF, Crook D, Walton C et al. Influence of insulin resistance, secretion, and clearance on serum cholesterol, triglycerides, lipoprotein cholesterol, and blood pressure in healthy men. *Arterioscler Thromb* 1992; **12**: 1030–5.

10. Stout R. Insulin and atheroma: 20-yr perspective. *Diabetes Care* 1990; **13**: 631–54.

11. Reaven GM, Lithell H, Landsberg L. Hypertension and associated metabolic abnormalities – the role of insulin resistance and the sympoathoadrenal system. *N Engl J Med* 1996; **334**: 374–81.

12. Kooistra T, Bosma P, Töns H et al. Plasminogen activator inhibitor 1: biosynthesis and mRNA level are increased by insulin in cultured human hepatocytes. *Thromb Haemostas* 1989; **62**: 723–8.

13. Godsland IF, Sidhu M, Crook D, Stevenson JC. Coagulation and fibrinolytic factors, insulin resistance and the metabolic syndrome of coronary heart disease risk. *Eur Heart J* 1996; **17**: 331.

14. Ginsberg HN, Huang LS. The insulin resistance syndrome: impact on lipoprotein metabolism and atherothrombosis. *J Cardiovasc Risk* 2000; **7**: 325–31.

15. Murakami T, Michelagnoli S, Longhi R et al. Triglycerides are major determinants of cholesterol esterification/transfer and HDL remodeling in human plasma. *Arterioscler Thromb Vasc Biol* 1995; **15**: 1819–28.

16. Brinton E, Eisenberg S, Breslow J. Increased apo A-I and apo A-II fractional catabolic rate in patients with low high density lipoprotein-cholesterol levels with or without hypertriglyceridaemia. *J Clin Invest* 1991; **87**: 536–44.

17. Després J-P, Marette A. Relation of components of insulin resistance syndrome to coronary disease risk. *Curr Opin Lipidol* 1994; **5**: 274–89.

18. Godsland IF, Stevenson JC. Insulin resistance: syndrome or tendency? *Lancet* 1995; **346**: 100–3.

19. Ginsberg HN. Insulin resistance and cardiovascular disease. *J Clin Invest* 2000; **106**: 453–8.

20. Leyva F, Godsland IF, Walton C et al. Factors of the metabolic syndrome – baseline interrelationships in the first follow-up cohort of the HDDRISC Study (HDDRISC-1). *Arterioscler Thromb Vasc Biol* 1998; **18**: 208–14.

21. Edward KL, Burchfiel CM, Sharp DS et al. Factors of the insulin resistance syndrome in nondiabetic and diabetic elderly Japanese American men. *Am J Epidemiol* 1998; **147**: 441–7.

22. Gray RS, Fabsitz RR, Cowan LD et al. Risk factor clustering in the insulin resistance syndrome. The Strong Heart Study. *Am J Epidemiol* 1998; **148**: 869–78.

23. Pyörälä M, Miettinen H, Halonen P et al. Insulin resistance syndrome predicts the risk of coronary heart disease and stroke in healthy middle-aged men – the 22-year follow-up of the Helsinki Policemen Study. *Arterioscler Thromb Vasc Biol* 2000; **20**: 538–44.

24. Godsland IF, Leyva F, Bruce R et al. The metabolic syndrome predicts development of diabetes in the first follow-up cohort of the RISC Study (RISC-1): an application of factor analysis. *Diabetic Med* 1997; **14 (suppl 1)**: S18.

25. Oswald GA, Corcoran S, Yudkin JS. Prevalence and risks of hyperglycaemia and undiagnosed diabetes in patients with acute infarction. *Lancet* 1984; **i**: 1264–7.

26. Cerami A, Vlassara H, Brownlee M. Role of advanced glycosylation products in complications of diabetes. *Diabetes Care* 1988; **11 (suppl 1)**: 73–9.

27. Wolff SP. Diabetes mellitus and free radicals. *Br Med Bull* 1993; **49**: 642–52.

28. Howard B. Lipoprotein metabolism in diabetes mellitus. *J Lipid Res* 1987; **28**: 613–28.

29. Walden C, Knopp R, Wahl P. Sex differences in the effect of diabetes mellitus on lipoprotein triglyceride and cholesterol concentrations. *N Engl J Med* 1984; **311**: 953–9.

30. Barrett-Connor EL, Cohn BA, Wingard DL, Edelstein SL. Why is diabetes mellitus a stronger risk factor for fatal ischaemic heart disease in women than in men? The Rancho Bernardo Study. *JAMA* 1991; **265**: 627–31.

31. Walton C, Godsland I, Proudler A et al. The effects of the menopause on insulin sensitivity, secretion and elimination in non-obese, healthy women. *Eur J Clin Invest* 1993; **23**: 466–73.

32. Proudler A, Felton C, Stevenson J. Ageing and the response of plasma insulin, glucose and C-peptide concentrations to intravenous glucose in postmenopausal women. *Clin Sci* 1992; **83**: 489–94.

33. Godsland IF, Walton C, Stevenson JC. Impact of menopause on metabolism. In: (Diamond MP, Naftolin F, eds) *Metabolism in the Female Life Cycle*. (Ares Serono Symposia: Rome, 1993) 171–89.

34. Spencer CP, Godsland IF, Stevenson JC. Is there a menopausal metabolic syndrome? *Gynecol Endocr* 1997; **11**: 341–55.

35. Pyke DA. Parity and the incidence of diabetes. *Lancet* 1956; **i:** 818–21.

36. Harris MI, Hadden WC, Knowler WC, Bennett PH. Prevalence of diabetes and impaired glucose tolerance and plasma glucose levels in US population aged 20–74 yr. *Diabetes* 1987; **36:** 523–34.

37. Seige K, Hevelke G. The effect of female gonadal function on the manifestation and frequency of diabetes mellitus. Proceedings of the Sixth Symposium of the German Endocrinological Society: *Modern Developments in Progestagenic Hormones in Veterinary Medicine.* (Springer Verlag: Keil, 1959) 274–9.

38. Godsland IF. The influence of female sex steroids on glucose metabolism and insulin action. *J Int Med* 1996; **240 (Suppl 738):** 1–65.

39. Gilmour K, McKerns K. Insulin and estrogen regulation of lipid synthesis in adipose tissue. *Biochim Biophys Acta* 1966; **116:** 220–8.

40. Rushakoff R, Kalkhoff R. Effects of pregnancy and sex steroid administration on skeletal muscle metabolism in the rat. *Diabetes* 1981; **30:** 545–50.

41. Walsh BW, Schiff I, Rosner B et al. Effects of postmenopausal estrogen replacement on the concentrations and metabolism of plasma lipoproteins. *N Engl J Med* 1991; **325:** 1196–204.

42. Godsland IF. Effects of postmenopausal hormone replacement therapy on lipid, lipoprotein and apolipoprotein (a) concentrations: summary analysis of studies published between 1974 and 2000. *Fertil Steril* 2001; **75:** 898–915.

43. Tollin C, Ericsson M, Johnson O, Backman C. Clearance of triglycerides from the circulation and its relationship to serum lipoproteins: influence of age and sex. *Scand J Clin Lab Invest* 1985; **45:** 679–84.

44. Westerveld HT, Kock LAW, van Rijn JM et al. 17β-estradiol improves postprandial lipid metabolism in postmenopausal women. *J Clin Endocr Metab* 1995; **80:** 249–53.

45. Tilly-Kiesi M, Kahri J, Pyörälä T et al. Responses of HDL subclasses, Lp(AI) and Lp(AI:AII) levels and lipolytic enzyme activities to continuous oral estrogen-progestin and transdermal estrogen with cyclic progestin regimens in postmenopausal women. *Atherosclerosis* 1997; **129:** 249–59.

46. Foglia V, Schuster N, Rodriguez R. Sex and diabetes. *Endocrinology* 1947; **41:** 428–34.

47. Sutter-Dub M-T. Preliminary report: effects of female sex hormones on insulin secretion by the perfused rat pancreas. *J Physiol (Paris)* 1976; **72:** 795–800.

48. Costrini N, Kalkhoff R. Relative effects of pregnancy, estradiol and progesterone on plasma insulin and pancreatic islet insulin secretion. *J Clin Invest* 1971; **50:** 992–99.

49. Godsland IF, Walton C, Felton C et al. Insulin resistance, secretion and metabolism in users of oral contraceptives. *J Clin Endocr Metab* 1992; **74:** 64–70.

50. Godsland IF. Interactions of oral contraceptive use with the effects of age, exercise habit and other cardiovascular risk modifiers on metabolic risk markers. *Contraception* 1996; **53:** 9–16.

51. Manson JE, Rimm EB, Colditz GA et al. A prospective study of postmenopausal estrogen therapy and subsequent incidence of non-insulin-dependent diabetes mellitus. *Ann Epidemiol* 1992; **2:** 665–73.

52. Gabal LL, Goodman-Gruen D, Barrett-Connor E. The effect of postmenopausal estrogen therapy on the risk of non-insulin-dependent diabetes mellitus. *Am J Public Health* 1997; **87:** 443–5.

53. Thomas J. Modification of glucagon-induced hyperglycaemia by various steroidal agents. *Metabolism* 1963; **12:** 207–12.

54. Mandour T, Kissebah A, Wynn V. Mechanism of oestrogen and progesterone effects on lipid and carbohydrate metabolism: alteration in the insulin:glucagon molar ratio and hepatic enzyme activity. *Eur J Clin Invest* 1977; **7:** 181–7.

55. Siminoski K, Goss P, Drucker DJ. The Cushing Syndrome induced by medroxyprogesterone acetate. *Ann Intern Med* 1989; **111:** 758–60.

56. Elkind-Hirsch K, Sherman L, Malinak R. Hormone replacement therapy alters insulin sensitivity in young women with premature ovarian failure. *J Clin Endocr Metab* 1993; **76:** 472–5.

57. Lindheim SR, Presser SC, Ditkoff EC et al. A possible bimodal effect of estrogen on insulin sensitivity in postmenopausal women and the attenuating effect of added progestin. *Fertil Steril* 1993; **60:** 664–7.

58. Godsland I, Gangar K, Walton C et al. Insulin resistance, secretion and elimination in postmenopausal women receiving oral or transdermal hormone replacement therapy. *Metabolism* 1993; **42:** 846–53.

59. Barrett-Connor E, Laakso M. Ischaemic heart disease risk in postmenopausal women: effects of estrogen use on glucose and insulin levels. *Arteriosclerosis* 1990; **10:** 531–4.

60. Lobo RA, Pickar JH, Wild RA et al. Metabolic impact of adding medroxyprogesterone acetate to conjugated estrogen therapy in post-

menopausal women. *Obstet Gynecol* 1994; **84:** 987–95.

61. The Writing Group for the PEPI Trial. Effects of estrogen or estrogen/progestin regimens on heart disease risk factors in postmenopausal women: the Postmenopausal Estrogen/Progestin Interventions (PEPI) Trial. *J Am Med Ass* 1995; **273:** 199–208.

62. Luotola H, Pyörälä T, Loikkanen M. Effects of natural oestrogen/progestogen substitution therapy on carbohydrate and lipid metabolism in post-menopausal women. *Maturitas* 1986; **8:** 245–53.

63. Spencer CP, Godsland IF, Cooper AJ et al. Effects of oral and transdermal 17 beta estradiol with cyclical norethindrone acetate on insulin sensitivity, secretion and elimination in post-menopausal women. *Metabolism* 2000; **49:** 742–7.

64. DeCleyn K, Buytaert P, Coppens M. Carbohydrate metabolism during hormonal substitution therapy. *Maturitas* 1989; **11:** 235–42.

65. Crook D, Godsland IF, Hull J, Stevenson JC. Hormone replacement therapy with dydrogesterone progestin and estradiol-17β: effects on serum lipoproteins and on glucose tolerance during 24 month follow-up. *Br J Obstet Gynaecol* 1997; **104:** 298–304.

66. Gaspard UJ, Wery O, Herman P et al. Carbohydrate metabolism in postmenopausal women using oral oestradiol and dydrogesterone. *Int J Gynecol Obstet* 1994; **46 (Suppl 1):** P020.17.

67. Cucinelli F, Paparella P, Soranna L et al. Differential effect of transdermal estrogen plus progestagen replacement therapy on insulin metabolism in postmenopausal women: relation to their insulinemic secretion. *Eur J Endocr* 1999; **140:** 215–23.

68. Psaty BM, Heckbert SR, Atkins D et al. The risk of myocardial infarction associated with the combined use of estrogens and progestins in postmenopausal women. *Arch Intern Med* 1994; **154:** 1333–9.

69. Kaplan RC, Heckbert SR, Weiss NS et al. Postmenopausal estrogens and risk of myocardial infarction in diabetic women. *Diabetes Care* 1998; **21:** 1117–21.

70. Feher MD, Isaacs AJ. Is hormone replacement therapy prescribed for postmenopausal diabetic women? *Br J Clin Pract* 1996; **50:** 431–2.

71. Troisi RJ, Cowie CC, Harris MI. Hormone replacement therapy and glucose metabolism. *Obstet Gynecol* 2000; **96:** 665–70.

72. Palin SL, Kumar S, Sturdee DW, Barnett AH. Hormone replacement therapy for post-menopausal women with diabetes. *Diabetic Obestet Metab* 2001; **3:** 187–93.

73. Cefalu WT. The use of hormone replacement therapy in postmenopausal women with Type 2 diabetes. *J Womens Health Gender Based Med* 2001; **10:** 241–55.

74. Brussard HE, Gevers-Leuven JA, Frolich M et al. Short-term oestrogen replacement therapy improves insulin resistance, lipids and fibrinolysis in postmenopausal women with NIDDM. *Diabetologia* 1997; **40:** 843–9.

75. Samaras K, Hayward CS, Sullivan D et al. Effects of postmenopausal hormone replacement therapy on central abdominal fat, glycemic control, lipid metabolism, and vascular factors in type 2 diabetes: a prospective study. *Diabetes Care* 1999; **22:** 1401–7.

76. Dubuisson JT, Wagenknecht LE, D'Agostino RBJ et al. Association of hormone replacement therapy and carotid wall thickness in women with and without diabetes. *Diabetes Care* 1998; **21:** 1790–6.

77. Sattar N, Perera M, Small M, Lumsden MA. Hormone replacement therapy and sensitive C-reactive protein concentrations in women with type-2 diabetes. *Lancet* 1999; **354:** 487–8.

78. Hahn L, Mattsson L-Å, Andersson B, Tengborn L. The effects of oestrogen replacement therapy on haemostatic variables in postmenopausal women with non-insulin-dependent diabetes mellitus. *Blood Coagul Fibrinol* 1999; **10:** 81–6.

79. Lim SC, Caballero AE, Arora S et al. The effect of hormonal replacement therapy on the vascular reactivity and endothelial function of healthy individuals and individuals with type 2 diabetes. *J Clin Endocr Metab* 1999; **84:** 4159–64.

80. von Eckardstein A, Nofer J-R, Assmann G. High density lipoproteins and atherosclerosis: role of cholesterol efflux and reverse cholesterol transport. *Arterioscler Thromb Vasc Biol* 2001; **21:** 13–27.

13

Possible side-effects of sexual hormones

G Creatsas

Introduction • Weight gain and water retention • Vaginal bleeding • Breast tenderness • Mood and emotional wellbeing • Gastrointestinal, liver and gallbladder diseases • Other symptoms • Androgens – subjective side-effects • Selective estrogen receptor modulators (SERM) and phytoestrogens • Consultation and examinations • Conclusion • References

INTRODUCTION

The benefits and risks of hormone therapy (HT) are well documented in recent reports and meeting proceedings. However, there are still controversies related to the effect of HT on the breast and cardiovascular disease (CVD).[1-5] several ambiguities induce confusion among the female population and physicians, having a direct effect on the compliance of HT. Users are very sensitive to information provided by the media and are more concerned about the symptoms of menopause such as vasomotor symptoms, skin or vaginal dryness and psychological intolerance as compared to the essential results of estrogen depletion, i.e. osteoporosis, CVD and mental health.

The results of HT are correlated to the HT formulations and their components, the route of administration and the dose and duration of treatment. The development of new products, such as selective estrogen receptor modulators (SERM), phytoestrogens and others, based on a tissue-specific approach to menopause, has led to a better tailoring of therapy to a woman's needs at the beginning of the new millennium.

However, compliance and discontinuation remain major concerns for a woman's post-menopausal health. The above are directly related to the subjective side-effects of sexual hormones used during HT. In a recent study, the side-effects of HT were found to be the number one reason for discontinuation of treatment, accounting for 31.8% of all reasons. Weight gain accounts for another 30.7%,[6] while unexpected bleeding has also been considered a major reason for discontinuation of HT.[7]

Sex hormones are used alone or in combination. Subjective side-effects can be reported either from the use of the estrogenic or progestogenic compounds separately or during continuous combined and sequential therapy. Although there are many regimens in use, subjective side-effects are more or less similar during the use of the various treatments. In addition, the subjective effects of other products such as tibolone and SERM should be considered as they are currently used by a significant number of women.

WEIGHT GAIN AND WATER RETENTION

Weight gain is one reason for discontinuation of HT. Menopausal women often complain of increased body weight, considering it to be a serious symptom for cosmetic reasons. Until now there have been insufficient data showing

Table 13.1   Mean change in body weight and waist:hip ratio over a 3-year period in postmenopausal women enrolled in the Postmenopausal Estrogen/Progestin Intervention (PEPI) study[8]

	Placebo	CEE alone	CEE+MPA (cyclic)	CEE+MPA (continuous)	CEE+MP (cyclic)
Body weight (kg)	+1.3	+0.4	+0.8	+0.6	+0.6
Waist:hip ratio	+0.010	+0.003	+0.010	0.007	0.007

CEE, Conjugated equine estrogens: MPA, medroxyprogesterone acetate; MP, micronized progesterone.

that women on HT present with weight gain. On the other hand, the Postmenopausal Estrogen/Progestin Intervention (PEPI) study has shown that a weight gain after 3 years of treatment was more obvious in the placebo group than in the estrogen-replacement group (Table 13.1). Similar results have been reported by previous studies in women on similar diets and long-term HT.[8–11] Recently, another study has shown that continuous 17β-estradiol 2 mg/day combined treatment with sequential dydrogesterone 10 mg/day for 14 days per cycle compared to tibolone and transdermal estradiol/dydrogesterone prevented increased body weight and the redistribution of body fat mass that occur at menopause.[12]

The age-related weight distribution and waist:hip ratio, changes in lifestyle, a decrease in physical activity and changes in dietary habits should be discussed with the HT users as causes of weight gain independent of HT. Since weight gain is correlated with an increased risk of CVD, and is also related to the appearance of the woman, it should be suggested that menopausal women remain physically active and match their calorie intake to their requirements. On the other hand, physicians should monitor the estrogen dose to minimize water retention, since edema in relation to weight gain accounts for 15–16.7/1000 person years of the causes of discontinuation of HT.[13] Finally no change in migraine was noted in women on HT among 451 female patients.[14]

VAGINAL BLEEDING

Vaginal bleeding and spotting causes discomfort and is considered a major reason for discontinuation of HT (29.4 and 51.7% for ages 50–55 and ≥ 65, respectively).[15] This symptom may be seen under almost any kind of treatment but mainly among women using unopposed estrogens. Ultrasonography and endometrial histology evaluate the significance of the problem and will rule out endometrial hyperplasia and neoplasia. As endometrial safety is related to the progestogenic compound of HT, proper monitoring and tailoring will assist in the management of this side-effect. The use of continuous combined HT, tibolone[16] or raloxifene are alternatives to previous treatments. The possibilities of using vaginal estrogenic preparations, cosmetic creams or exposure to xenoestrogens should be ruled out before any modification of treatment is suggested.

BREAST TENDERNESS

Breast tenderness is considered a frequent cause of discontinuation of HT (3.3 and 18.4% for ages 50–55 and ≥ 65, respectively).[15] Younger women having the experience of premenstrual syndrome (PMS) correlate the syndrome with this discomfort. Older women are more sensitive and are aware of the possibility of breast malignancy. Breast tenderness is mainly related to the estrogenic compound but is also an adverse effect of progestogens.[17] An increased incidence of breast tenderness has been reported in postmenopausal women receiving a combination of estradiol valerate and cyproterone acetate or medroxyprogesterone acetate.[18] On the other hand, Prior et al[19] reported no breast tenderness (symptom score = 0) in women treated with medroxyprogesterone accetate 10 mg/day alone as compared to placebo treatment. Estrogens cause breast tenderness depending on the dose of treatment and the route of administration. Adding a progestogen per os or as a cream applied directly to the breast reduces breast tenderness. Another suggestion for the relief of the symptom is the use of danazol 50–100 mg or the addition of an androgenic compound, usually 5 mg of fluoxymesterone or testosterone 2–5 mg. If, however, mastodynia persists the estrogen dose should be reduced. The group of symptoms including edema, bloating, breast tenderness and PMS-like symptoms may also be relieved if a mild diuretic is given for 7–10 days before menstruation.[20]

MOOD AND EMOTIONAL WELLBEING

Both mood and emotional wellbeing are impaired during menopause. HT is used to improve mental status and mood. It is therefore important to use the various HT products to improve these symptoms, or at least to anticipate subjective side-effects related to the psychological status of the woman. Finally, there are various reports presenting the progestogenic negative effects related to the psychology of the woman (Box 13.1).[21]

It seems that estrogen therapy (ET) alone has better results on mood as compared to HT. Women with a long duration of menopause and higher treatment serum estradiol levels had significantly more dysphoria when receiving both estrogens and progestogens as compared to women with short duration of menopause and lower serum estradiol levels.[22] In the same study it was also reported that both short and long duration menopausal groups presented improvement in mood when estrogens were given alone. Progestogens may cause unfavorable effects on mental status, mood and wellbeing. As different progestogens may differ in their effect on mood (i.e. 19 nor-steroids have been reported as provoking mood changes),[23] the decrease in dose or changing the progestogenic compound usually improves mental status.

Box 13.1 Psychologic effects of progestogens (modified from Panay and Studd)[21]

Anxiety
Depression
Emotional lability
Forgetfulness
Irritability
Lethargy
Panic attacks
Poor concentration
Restlessness

GASTROINTESTINAL, LIVER AND GALLBLADDER DISEASES

HT, especially ET, causes only minimal gastrointestinal symptoms which do not seem to significantly impair the compliance rate. It is also reported that oral contraceptives and non-contraceptive estrogens are unlikely to have an important influence in the etiology of gallbladder disease.[24] On the other hand, others report that oral estradiol has an adverse influence on biliary cholesterol saturation and biliary bile acid composition in the subgroup of women with a high increase in serum estrogen levels following oral administration.[25] Avoidance of hepatic first-pass metabolism, using transdermal systems and gels for HT, produce fewer adverse effects on the gastrointestinal system, liver and gallbladder.

The effect of oral androgens in liver dysfunction depends on the dose and duration of treatment. Long-term high-dose methyltestosterone therapy may be associated with pathologic changes in the liver.[26] On the contrary, a meta-analysis of eight clinical trials has not shown hepatic biochemical changes in women treated with a combined estrogen–androgen preparation as compared to estrogen treatment alone.[27] Finally, transient jaundice and hepatic dysfunction have been reported 1 week after a single dose of dehydroepiandrosterone 150 mg.[28]

OTHER SYMPTOMS

In addition to the above-mentioned adverse effects, women on HT (estradiol patches) report skin reactions in the form of hyperemia, blistering and discoloration that occur in up to 20% of patients.[29] The substitution of these patches with the new matrix delivery systems or a decrease in the dose alleviate the symptoms. If the symptoms persist another route of HT is recommended.

Occasionally ocular symptoms such as photophobia, visual fluctuation and deep ocular pain may be seen.[30]

ANDROGENS – SUBJECTIVE SIDE-EFFECTS

In recent years there has been an increased interest in the potential role of androgen use in the aging male and female. Dehydroepiandrosterone is being sold over-the-counter to enhance wellbeing and retard the aging process. The beneficial and negative effects of androgens as menopausal supplementation have been well documented.[31] Most studies on the side-effects of androgen replacement emphasize the potential virilizing effects of the products. There are only a few reports on the effect of androgens on the liver or the induction of neoplastic disease as previously reported.

Barett-Connor et al[26] reported no difference in the side-effects (headache, breast pain, weight increase, vaginitis and hirsutism) between two groups of women treated with esterified estrogen 0.625 mg plus methyltestosterone 1.25 mg and esterified estrogen 1.25 mg plus methyltestosterone 2.5 mg with esterified estrogen alone in respective doses in 291 surgically menopausal women. Only four estrogen–androgen women developed hirsutism and the Feriman–Gallway index showed

increased hair growth in 14–22% of the women tested in each treatment group.

Acne is another side-effect accounting for 38% of methyltestosterone-treated women, while other studies suggest a lower incidence.[32] Other studies reported adverse effects such as deepening of the voice and clitoromegaly. The above symptoms are typically dose and duration dependent, and reversible when the dose is modified.[33]

SELECTIVE ESTROGEN RECEPTOR MODULATORS (SERM) AND PHYTOESTROGENS

SERM are promising new products. Raloxifene exerts several beneficial effects while at the same time presents no adverse effects on the endometrium, thus reducing the possibility of bleeding and breast discomfort. The Multiple Outcomes of Raloxifene Evaluation (MORE) study has shown 7.0 and 3.7% leg cramps in women treated with raloxifene hydrocloride and placebo, respectively. Hot flushes were found in 9.7 and 6.4% in the same groups of patients.[34] Another study has shown that although the incidence of leg cramps is higher in women treated with raloxifene as compared to placebo, this symptom does not cause discontinuation of therapy.[35]

Phytoestrogens exert minimal estrogenic activities and have no side-effects as compared to estradiol. However, as they have not yet been studied in detail, and may have unknown toxic effects, it is suggested that more data are required before deciding the beneficial or negative effects of these products.

CONSULTATION AND EXAMINATIONS

Compliance and discontinuation are very much related to subjective side-effects of HT. The first consultation is very important and a frank explanation should be given to the woman so that she understands both the beneficial effects of HT and possible side-effects.

Pretreatment hormonal profiles and basic endometrial biopsies should be avoided. Mammographic breast screening and tests for evaluating bone mass have a place during the basic consultation. Attention should be given to the medical history, a gynecological examination, cervical cytology and breast palpation. Unnecessary biochemical tests should be avoided.

As most side-effects occur within the first 8 weeks of starting HT, the woman should be informed that a second visit is necessary to adjust the dose of treatment and tailor the appropriate preparation. At the same time reassurance should be given and questions should be answered to overcome any fears about HT.

CONCLUSION

HT is an important advance in preventive medicine. Subjective side-effects can usually be avoided by monitoring the dose or changing the regimen. Among ET/HT users the main reasons for discontinuation of treatment are the presence of side-effects such as uterine bleeding, breast tenderness and weight gain. Proper education will improve compliance and will assist the menopausal women in enjoying the beneficial effects of HT.

REFERENCES

1. Schairer C. Menopausal estrogen and estrogen progestin replacement therapy and breast cancer risk. *JAMA* 2000; **283**: 485–91.
2. Ross R, Paganini-Hill A, Wan PC, Pike MC. Effect of HRT on breast cancer risk, estrogen versus estrogen plus progestin. *J Nat Cancer Inst* 2000; **92**: 328–32.
3. Hulley S, Grady D, Busch T et al. Randomized trial of estrogen plus progestin for secondary prevention of coronary heart disease in post-menopausal women. *J Am Med Ass* 1998; **280**: 605–13.
4. Herington DM, Reboussin DM, Brosnihan B et al. Effects of estrogen replacement on progression of coronary artery atherosclerosis. *N Engl J Med* 2000; **343**: 522–9.
5. Larkin M. Up and downs for HRT and heart disease. *Lancet* 2000; **355**: 1338.
6. Den Tonkelaar I, Oddens BJ. Determinants of long-term hormone replacement therapy and reasons for early discontinuation. *Obstet Gynecol* 2000; **95**: 507–12.
7. Karakoc B, Erenus M. Compliance considerations with hormone replacement therapy. *Menopause* 1998; **5**: 102–6.
8. The Writing Group for the PEPI Trial. Effects of estrogen in estrogen/progestin regimens in the heart disease. Risk factors in postmenopausal women. *JAMA* 1995; **273**: 199–208.
9. Nachtigall LE. Enhancing patient compliance with HRT at menopause. *Obstet Gynecol* 1990; **75**: 77S–80S.
10. Graziottin A. Strategies for effectively addressing women's concern about the menopause and HRT. *Maturitas* 1999; **33**: 15S–23S.
11. Crawford SL, Casey VA, Avis NE, McKinlay SM. A longitudinal study of weight and the menopause transition results from the Massachusetts Women's Health Study. *Menopause* 200; **7**: 96–104.
12. Espeland MA, Stefanick MC, Silvrstein D et al. Effects of postmenopausal hormone therapy on body weight and waist and hip girths. Postmenopausal Estrogen–Progestin Investigation study investigators *J Clin Endocr Metab* 1997; **82**: 1549–56.
13. Vestergaard P, Hermann AP, Gram J et al. Improving compliance with hormonal replacement therapy in primary osteoporosis prevention. *Maturitas* 1997; **28**: 137–45.
14. Mueller L. Predictability of exogenous hormone effect on subgroups of migrainers. *Headache* 2000; **40**: 189–93.
15. Ettinger B, Pressman A, Silver P. Effect of age on reasons of initiation and discontinuation of hormone replacement therapy. *Menopause* 1999; **6**: 282–9.
16. Doeren M. Hormonal replacement regimens and bleeding. *Maturitas* 2000; **34**: S17–S23.
17. Smith RNJ, Holland EFN, Studd JWW. The symptomatology of progestogen intolerance. *Maturitas* 1994; **18**: 87–91.
18. Marslew V, Riis B, Christiansen C. Progestogens therapeutic and adverse effects in early post-menopausal women. *Maturitas* 1991; **13**: 7–16.
19. Prior JC, Alojado N, McKay DW, Vigna YM. No adverse effects of medroxyprogesterone treatment without estrogen in postmenopause women: double-blind, placebo-controlled crossover trial. *Obstet Gynecol* 1994; **83**: 24–8.
20. Don Gambrell R. Progestogens in estrogen replacement therapy. *Clin Obstet Gynecol* 1995; **38**: 890–901.
21. Panay N, Studd J. Progesterone intolerance and compliance with hormone replacement therapy

in menopausal women. *Hum Reprod Update* 1997; **3**: 159–71.

22. Klaider EL, Broverman DM, Vogel W et al. Relationships of serum estradiol levels, menopausal duration and mood during hormonal replacement therapy. *Psychoneuroendocrinology* 1997; **27**: 549–58.

23. Hammarback S, Backstrom T, Holst J et al. Cyclical mood changes as in the estrogen–progestogen postmenopausal replacement therapy. *Acta Obstet Gynecol Scand* 1985; **64**: 393–7.

24. La Vecchia C, Negri E, d'Avanzo B et al. Oral contraceptives and non-contraceptive oestrogens in the risk of gallstone disease requiring surgery. *J Epid Commun* Health 1992; **46**: 234–6.

25. Van Eprecum KJ, Van Berge Henegouwen GP, Verschoor L et al. Different hepatobiliary effects of oral and transdermal estradiol, in post-menopausal women. *Gastroenterology* 1991; **100**: 482–8.

26. Barett-Connor E, Timmons C, Young R, Wiita B and the Estratest Working Group. Interim safety analysis of a 2-year study comparing oral estrogen–androgen and conjugated estrogens in surgically menopause women. *J Womens Health* 1996; **5**: 593–602.

27. Gitlin N, Korner P, Yang HM. Liver function in postmenopausal women on estrogen-analysis of eight clinical trials. *Menopause* 1999; **6**: 216–24.

28. Katz S, Morales AJ. Dehydroepiandrosterone (DHEA) and DHEA-sulfate (DS) as therapeutic options in menopause. *Semin Reprod Endocr* 1998; **16**: 161–70.

29. Studd J. Complications in hormone replacement therapy in post-menopausal women. *J Roy Soc Med* 1992; **85**: 376–8.

30. Gurwood AS, Gurwood I, Gubman D, Brzezicki L. Idiosyncratic ocular symptoms associated with the estradiol transdermal estrogen replacement patch system. *Optom Vis Sci* 1995; **72**: 29–33.

31. Hoeber KM, Guzick DS. The use of androgens in menopause. *Clin Obstet Gynecol* 1999; **42**: 883–94.

32. Slayden SM. Risks of menopausal androgen supplementation. *Semin Reprod Endocr* 1998; **16**: 145–52.

33. Sherwin B. Affective changes with estrogen and androgen replacement therapy in surgically menopausal women. *J Affect Disord* 1998; **14**: 177–87.

34. Ettinger B, Black DM, Mitlak BH et al. Reduction of vertebral fracture risk in postmenopausal women with osteoporosis treated with raloxifene: results from a 3-year randomized clinical trial. *JAMA* 1999; **282**: 637–45.

35. Davies GC, Huster WJ, Lu Y et al. Adverse events reported by postmenopausal women in controlled trials with raloxifene. *Obstet Gynecol* 1999; **93**: 558–65.

Role of Hormones in Preventive Gynecology

Chapter 14 Osteoporosis

Chapter 15 Hormone replacement therapy and atherosclerotic vascular disease

Chapter 16 Direct vascular actions of estrogens

Chapter 17 Neurotropic and psychotropic action of estrogens: implications for Alzheimer's disease

Chapter 18 Sexuality in postmenopause and senium

Chapter 19 Estrogens and urogenital atrophy

Chapter 20 Estrogens in the treatment of premenstrual, postnatal and perimenopausal depression

Chapter 21 Anti-aging and esthetic endocrinology

Chapter 22 Skin and connective tissue

Chapter 23 Lifestyle counseling

Chapter 24 Phytoestrogens

Chapter 25 Possible risks of hormone replacement therapy (HRT): venous thromoembolism (VTE)

Chapter 26 Gallbladder, liver, pancreas

Chapter 27 Carcinogenesis and the role of hormones: promotion and prevention

Chapter 28 Strategies for the prevention of breast and gynecologic cancer

Chapter 29 Benefits, risks and costs of estrogen and hormone replacement therapies

14

Osteoporosis

NH Bjarnason and C Christiansen

Introduction • **Estrogen deficiency and pathogenesis of osteoporosis** • **Importance of risk markers in preventive strategies** • **Prevention and treatment of osteoporosis** • **Antiresorptive therapies** • **Formation stimulating therapies** • **Monitoring** • **Perspectives – individualizing therapy** • **References**

INTRODUCTION

Osteoporosis is a metabolic bone disease characterized by a low bone mass and microarchitectural deterioration of bone tissue followed by enhanced bone fragility and a consequent increase in fracture risk.[1] From epidemiological surveys, osteoporosis may be estimated to be the most prevalent metabolic bone disease in Europe.[2] It is the level of the peak bone mass obtained in young adults and the bone loss subsequent to menopause that additively contributes to the development of osteoporosis, and the measurement methods used in diagnosis, prognosis and monitoring aim to assess these two factors.[1] All currently available therapies focus on the inhibition or reversal of bone loss, since no intervention has so far demonstrated the potential to manipulate peak bone mass.

ESTROGEN DEFICIENCY AND PATHOGENESIS OF OSTEOPOROSIS

Bone loss occurs in postmenopausal women as a result of the increase in the level of bone resorption as compared to the level of bone formation. Bone remodeling takes place at discrete sites within the skeleton with osteoclast activity (bone resorption) always being followed by osteoblast activity (bone formation), a sequence of processes known as coupling. If the level of bone resorption exceeds the bone formation capacity, a remodeling imbalance occurs, which results in irreversible bone loss.[3] This is the scenario induced by estrogen deficiency and together with age both are very important risk factors for postmenopausal bone loss. Thus, in the first 5 years after menopause, bone loss is accelerated to about 1–5% per year, thereafter the loss stabilizes at about 0.5% per year.[4] There is a gradient of fracture risk with declining levels of bone mass, with a lower bone mass an exponential higher risk of fracture.[5]

IMPORTANCE OF RISK MARKERS IN PREVENTIVE STRATEGIES

Peak bone mass and bone loss are osteoporosis risk markers requiring technical equipment to assess them. A list of clinically evaluable factors which may affect peak bone mass, bone loss and fracture risk is given in Table 14.1.

A preventive strategy should ideally be initiated before the occurrence of fractures. Although there is no universally accepted algorithm for the evaluation of individuals with or at risk for osteoporosis, the aims of the assessment of menopausal women should be to:

Table 14.1   Risk factors for the development of low peak bone mass, of fast/large bone loss and of fractures

Genetic	Hormonal	Pathology	Environmental
Risk factors for the development of a low peak bone mass			
White or Asian ethnicity	Late menarche	Disease*	Malnutrition/leanness
Family history	Gonadal insufficiency	Medication†	Smoking
Risk factors for the development of a fast/large bone loss			
Age	Early menopause	Disease*	Malnutrition/leanness
Family history	Oophorectomy	Medication†	Smoking
Additional risk factors for the development of fractures			
Hip geometry		Disease‡	Frequent falls
Family history		Medication§	Low sunlight exposure

* Hyperparathyroidism, hyperthyroidism and Cushing's syndrome, as well as neoplasia, rheumatoid arthritis and malabsorption, but a poor health particularly when concomitant with weight loss is associated with increased risk.
† Corticosteroids, cytotoxic chemotherapy, heparin and anticonvulsants.
‡ Decreased visual acuity, impaired neuromuscular function, previous fractures and a poor health in general.
§ Hypnotic or sedative medication.

- identify women with or at high risk of osteo-porosis and fractures;
- establish the correct diagnosis and identify correctable causes of bone loss;
- determine the severity, extent and activity of the disease;
- select and monitor therapy.

The bone mass measurement has a pivotal role in the assessment of diagnosis and prognosis of osteoporosis due to the well-established relationship between bone mass and breaking strength.[6] A low bone mass as a predictor of fracture is equivalent to that of high blood pressure of stroke and may be superior to the value of cholesterol in the prediction of myocardial infarction.[3] The World Health Organization (WHO) has defined diagnostic criteria for osteoporosis based on bone mass (Table 14.2). There are both strengths and limitations of this definition. The strengths comprise a straightforward result for the busy practitioner and the possibility to diagnose before fractures occur. Limitations concern the dependency of the instruments' accuracies as well as the reference population utilized (largely Caucasian women). Additionally, the implication of a threshold rather than a gradient of fracture risk, the misinterpretation of the diagnostic cut-offs as therapeutic thresholds and the potential misuse to deny reimbursement may be problematic. A working group is currently discussing updating the diagnostic criteria in order to include risk factors other than bone mass. Bone mass can be measured in sites known to be particularly prone to osteoporotic fracture (spine, hip and forearm), in sites being preferential because of a relatively small amount of soft tissue (calcaneus and finger) and in the total body, which allows assessment of body composition. Because of the universal nature of bone loss, a measurement at any site predicts all clinical fractures equally well.[7] The preferred site of measurement is the hip if only one assessment is possible. This is a compromise based on the importance of hip fracture, the relative inadequacy of a spine measurement for diagnosis in the elderly and the well-established response to various therapies in the hip. There are large numbers of techniques available, but dual energy X-ray absorp-

Table 14.2 World Health Organization (WHO) criteria for the diagnosis of osteoporosis based on bone mineral density (BMD)	
Category	**Criteria**
Normal	BMD ≥ –1 SD of average peak young normal
Osteopenia	–1 SD ≥ BMD ≥ –2.5 SD of average peak young normal
Osteoporosis	–2.5 SD ≥ BMD of average peak young normal
Severe osteoporosis	–2.5 SD ≥ BMD of average peak young normal in addition to a fragile fracture

SD, Standard deviation.

tiometry (DEXA) has gained widespread use due to its improved spatial resolution, faster scan and optimized precision. Therefore, most of the available data are obtained using DEXA. However, new methods such as ultrasound and quantitative computed tomography (QCT) are promising. Ultrasound because of the lack of radiation and possible information about bone structure, QCT because of its ability to differentiate between cancellous and trabecular bone. The radiation dose of QCT is, however, significantly higher than that of absorptiometry.

Currently, it is not recommended to perform a bone mass measurement in all menopausal women. The most important reason is the lack of evidence for cost-effectiveness of screening. A set of specific criteria leading to a bone mass measurement is under discussion, but there seems to be consensus that a bone mass measurement is not cost-effective in women over the age of 60–65 with a prevalent vertebral fracture. Such women should be treated regardless of bone mass and other risk factors. In otherwise healthy postmenopausal women under 65 years of age, indications for a bone mass measurement include a history of osteoporotic fracture, low body weight, smoking or a family history. For women with a well-established cause of osteoporosis other than estrogen deficiency (diseases and medications mentioned in Table 14.1), a measurement is also recom-

mended if the result will influence treatment decision. A thorough medical history and clinical evaluation including assessment of the body mass index (BMI), height loss, smoking history, age at menopause, prior fracture and back pain is compulsory. Studies of biochemical markers of bone turnover have indicated that, particularly high bone resorption marker levels are associated with both increased future bone loss and fracture, but specific cut-offs have not yet been agreed upon.[8] Biochemical markers will most likely be used as a supplement to evaluation of bone mass.[8]

PREVENTION AND TREATMENT OF OSTEOPOROSIS

The operational definition of osteoporosis given in Table 14.2 is less helpful when considering osteoporosis intervention. Because almost all available therapies can only arrest progression of disease, it may be too late to treat a person with osteoporosis based on such criteria, if the patient is relatively young. On the other hand, there may be reasons to decide to monitor or treat a person with a normal bone mass if a strong genetic disposition exists, or if a concomitant medication that adversely affects bone is prescribed. Thus, risk factors other than bone mass play an important role in the decision to treat. Moreover, evidence level and therapeutic efficacy, as well as extraskeletal and adverse effects of the various treatments, differ. For example, the most important clinical feature of osteoporosis is fracture, but evidence for fracture protection during intervention is not available for all therapies and is in these circumstances based on the assumption that prevention of a decline in bone mass may reduce fracture risk. In addition, not all therapies are equally efficacious and some have additional benefits/adverse effects, which affect choice of therapy and regimen. For these reasons, there is at present no consensus on how to classify patients in need of treatment, when the diagnosis is based on bone mineral density (BMD). Most opinion leaders agree, however, that in the case of strong risk factors such as prior hip or vertebral fracture, treatment should be given. At the other end of the spectrum, they agree that for all postmenopausal women it is important to identify and discuss lifestyle factors which increase the risk. Thus, women should be encouraged to stop smoking, improve level of physical activity and ensure an adequate intake of calcium (~ 1200 mg/day) and vitamin D (~400–800 IU/day). In the case of a BMD low relative to age (for example a Z-score less than −1) a pharmacological therapy should be initiated in most cases and in the case of (BMD) lower than premenopausal women – osteopenia or osteoporosis as diagnosed in Table 14.2 – an individual approach should be undertaken. This should include an evaluation of additional risk factors, benefits/adverse effects of the different treatment options, as well as the woman's own concerns.

ANTIRESORPTIVE THERAPIES

Antiresorptive therapies act by decreasing bone resorption and efficacious regimens lower resorption markers to the level seen in premenopausal women. The effect on bone resorption markers is significant after 1 month and fully expressed after 3–6 months. As a coupled decrease in bone formation occurs secondarily and more slowy (fully expressed at 12 months), bone mass may temporarily increase over the following 2 years and this new level in bone mass will be maintained for as long as treatment is continued.

Hormone replacement therapy (HRT) and its alternatives

The influence of estrogen and combinations of estrogen and progestogen on bone mass have been evaluated in numerous studies (Fig. 14.1). All types of estrogens have been found to be efficacious, thus both estradiol,[9,10] conjugated equine estrogens,[10,11] ethinyl estradiol[12] and piperazine estrone sulfate[13] increase bone mass. In addition, the response seems to be independent of administration form – if estrogen reaches the circulation, it has an effect on bone.[14,15] In hysterectomized women, estrogen can be given alone. The question of dose depends on the presence of risk factors. For example, recent data have shown that in early postmenopausal women, the response to oral estradiol 2 mg is independent of smoking, whereas the response to oral estradiol 1 mg is influenced by smoking such that smoking women only gain half the amount of bone as do nonsmokers.[16] In the same study, the response to therapy with estradiol 1 and 2 mg was independent of BMI. Additionally, other (as yet unidentified) confounders for the response may exist, and these confounders may depend on administration form. A conservative conclusion may be that doses lower than oral estradiol 1 mg may not be effective in all women. In women with an intact uterus, it is necessary to add a progestogen to the estrogen therapy to ensure endometrial transformation and shedding. Most progestogens do not seem to influence bone, neither with regard to type nor to regimen, but this is not very well studied. However, one progestogen – norethisterone acetate – seems to have an influence on bone that is additional to that of estrogen (Fig. 14.1).[10,12,13]

From observational studies there is evidence that estrogen therapy protects against fractures.[17,18] Post hoc analyses from two small randomized, controlled trials found estrogen to be efficacious in vertebral fracture prevention,[19,20] but in HERS – a study of 2763 women with

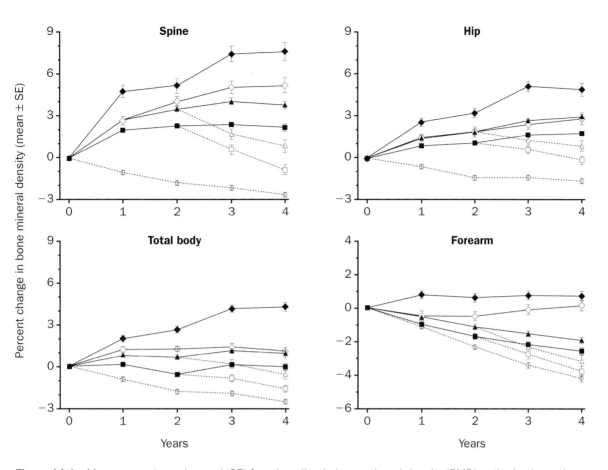

Figure 14.1 Mean percentage change (±SE) from baseline in bone mineral density (BMD) at the lumbar spine, total hip, total body and one-third distal forearm. ▲, Women who received 4 years of alendronate 5 mg/day; ■, women who received 4 years of alendronate 2.5 mg/day; ○–○, women who received 4 years of placebo; ◇, women who received 4 years of estrogen–medroxyprogesterone acetate; ◆, women who received 4 years of estradiol–norethisterone acetate; △–△, women who received 2 years of alendronate 5 mg/day followed by 2 years of placebo; □–□, women who received 2 years of alendronate 2.5 mg/day followed by 2 years of placebo. For graphical presentation, results from groups that received the same dosage of alendronate during the first 2 years of the study were pooled during this period for the two strata combined. (Reproduced from Ravn et al,[10] with permission.)

ischemic heart disease – designed to study the influence of HRT upon heart disease, no preventive influence of conjugated equine estrogen in combination with medroxyprogesterone acetate on nonvertebral fracture could be identified.[21] Recently, 22 randomized HRT studies of > 12 months duration, having collected nonvertebral fracture data, was pooled in a meta-analysis.[22] The overall reduction in nonvertebral fractures was 27% [relative risk (RR) 0.73

(0.56–0.94)]. Further details of this analysis are shown in Table 14.3. Although the literature lacks a study designed to investigate the influence of HRT upon fractures, the result of this well-conducted meta-analysis indicates significant protection.

Based on observational evidence, estrogen has been thought to have anti-atherosclerotic properties;[23,24] however, recent randomized trials have not been able to confirm this.[21,25] The

Table 14.3   Prevention of nonvertebral fracture during hormone replacement therapy according to the meta-analysis by Torgerson and Bell-Eeyer[22]

Analysis	RR (95% CI)
Total reduction in nonvertebral fracture	0.73 (0.56–0.94)
Age < 60 years	0.67 (0.46–0.98)
Age ≥ 60 years	0.88 (0.71–1.08)
Total reduction in hip and wrist fracture alone	0.60 (0.40–0.91)
Age < 60 years	0.45 (0.26–0.79)
Age ≥ 60 years	0.88 (0.47–1.59)

RR, Relative risk; CI, confidence interval.

background for this inconsistency is unknown, but is under discussion.[26,27] There seem to be essential elements of atherosclerosis and estrogen properties which are not yet fully elucidated. Alternatives to HRT include tibolone (a synthetic steroid with estrogenic, progestogenic and androgenic activities) and raloxifene (a benzothiophene with mixed estrogen agonist – antagonist properties). Traditionally used regimens of tibolone are slightly stimulatory on the endometrium, with 20% of those treated experiencing spotting.[28] Raloxifene dose not influence the endometrium. Tibolone has been found to influence bone mass similarly to HRT (Fig. 14.2),[28] whereas raloxifene seem to be somewhat less efficacious (Fig. 14.3).[29] Raloxifene reduces vertebral fracture incidence by 30%, whereas no effect has been found on nonvertebral fractures.[30] In addition, raloxifene lowers the risk of newly diagnosed estrogen-receptor-positive breast cancer by 90% in osteoporotic women.[31] A possible antifracture efficacy of tibolone remains to be investigated.

Bisphosphonates

Bisphosphonates are pyrophosphate analogs that inhibit bone resorption but have no extraskeletal effects. Cyclical etidronate therapy is used in Europe, but concerns have been raised because of findings of impaired mineralization, first in patients with Paget's disease, who received continuous therapy, but also during cyclical therapy, although rarely.[32] The most comprehensively studied bisphosphonate is alendronate. Like other bisphosphonates, alendronate is poorly absorbed and must be taken without food. Alendronate decreases bone turnover, increases bone mass (Fig. 14.1), and decreases the risk of vertebral, hip and forearm fracture.[33] New data indicate that another bisphosphonate, risedronate, has a comparable efficacy, both with regard to bone turnover, bone mass and fracture protection.[34,35] A new bisphosphonate, ibandronate, has an effect on bone mass and bone turnover equivalent to those of alendronate and risedronate,[36] and preliminary data suggest prevention of fractures as well.

Calcium and vitamin D

Based on bone mass assessments, calcium seems to increase its efficacy with increasing age. Thus, only very little effect is seen in early postmenopausal women, where the decrease in endogenous estrogen production is driving bone loss.[37] In elderly women, calcium seems to become increasingly efficacious. In elderly, institutionalized individuals, a combination of calcium and vitamin D has been found to reduce the risk of hip fracture.[38] Interestingly, vitamin D given alone does not seem to influence bone mass.[39] Calcium and vitamin D may

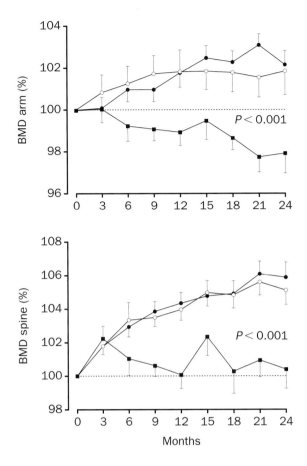

Figure 14.2 Densitometric measurements at 3-month intervals, expressed as percentages of initial values (mean ± SEM). ○, tibolone 2.5 mg; ●, tibolone 1.25 mg; ■, placebo, BMD spine, bone mineral density (BMD) of the spine (L2–L4); BMD arm, BMD of the distal forearm. (Reproduced from Bjarnason et al,[28] with permission.)

be regarded as a baseline therapy before adding pharmacological treatment in women who have passed early menopause. This is underlined by the fact that all fracture studies are conducted based on this principle.

FORMATION STIMULATING THERAPIES

Fluoride

Fluoride stimulates bone formation but questions remain regarding its optimum pharma-

ceutical formulation and dose. This is because sodium fluoride in a high dose has been associated with fluorosis and other adverse effects. Interestingly, a study combining a low dose of sodium monofluorophosphate with HRT demonstrated an uncoupling of bone resorption and formation with a consequent large increase in bone mass (Fig. 14.4).[40] Similar results have been seen with a combination of fluoride and tibolone,[41] but a fracture study with a combination has not been conducted.

Parathyroid hormone

Recent studies have shown that daily subcutaneous injections of relatively low doses of parathyroid hormone stimulate bone formation in osteopenic animals and osteoporotic women and men.[42] New data from a fracture trial in 1700 osteoporotic women suggest that 1.5 years of therapy reduces vertebral and nonvertebral fractures by 70%.[43]

MONITORING

The larger the decrease in bone turnover, the larger the increase in bone mass during HRT. Post hoc analyses have shown that there is a highly significant association between a short-term change in bone turnover and a long-term response in bone mass for both estradiol,[44,45] tibolone,[46] ibandronate[47] and alendronate.[48,49] Interestingly, recently an association between short-term decrease in bone turnover and long-term vertebral risk reduction during raloxifene treatment has been demonstrated.[50] In these analyses, all associations remained significant after adjustment for age, baseline BMD and fracture status.[50] These results may indicate that fracture protection during antiresorptive therapies can be mechanistically understood from bone turnover decrease over bone mass increase to bone strength increase, thereby providing fracture prevention. This theory is supported by the demonstration of a positive relationship between the increase in bone mass and reduction in vertebral fracture risk during alendronate therapy.[51] Such results indicate that biochemical markers of bone turnover may be

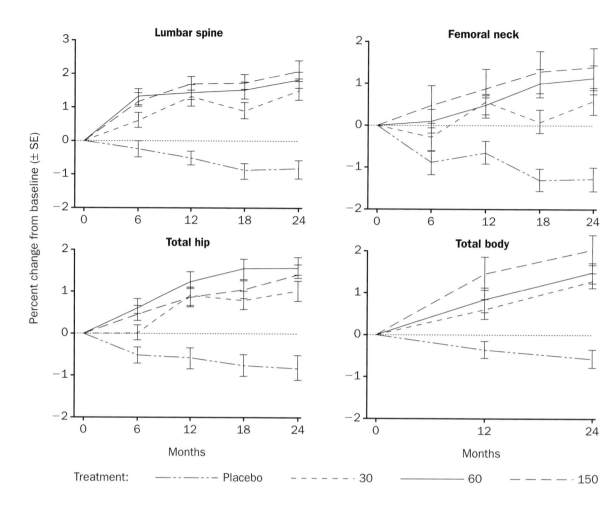

Figure 14.3 Mean percentage change in bone mineral density (BMD) in postmenopausal women given raloxifene or placebo for 2 years. (Reproduced from Delmas et al,[29] with permission.)

used for monitoring individuals during therapy, and a recent consensus panel suggested cut-offs as given in Table 14.4.[8]

PERSPECTIVES – INDIVIDUALIZING THERAPY

Ideally, osteoporosis should be treated as individually as the treatment of endocrinologic diseases such as hypothyroidism and diabetes, where dose and treatment regimens are based on biochemical and clinical evaluations. Thus, the choice of therapy and dose should depend on the severity of the disease and the response of the target organ. The severity of the disease depends on diagnostic and prognostic methods; the response in the target organ depends on the therapy and maybe on some of the risk factors influencing this target organ. Individualizing therapy is an important goal for future investigations.

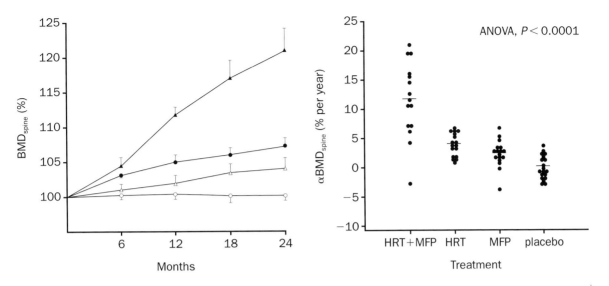

Figure 14.4 The time-related changes in the percentage of bone mineral density (BMD) of the lumbar spine (left). Values are mean ± SEM. The average change per year (%) is also shown (right). Horizontal lines indicate the mean. ANOVA, $P < 0.0001$ applies for both sites. ▲, Hormone replacement therapy (HRT) + monofluorophosphate (MFP); ●, HRT; △, MFP; ○, placebo. (Reproduced from Alexandersen et al,[40] with permission.)

Table 14.4 Cut-offs to predict a positive bone mineral density (BMD) response (+3%) with a specificity of 90% expressed as a percentage decrease from baseline and based on data with hormone replacement therapy (HRT) or alendronate. (Adapted from Delmas,[8] with permission.)

	HRT (%)	Alendronate (%)
Urinary fragments of collagen-1 degradation (C- or N-terminal)	−45	−65
Urinary deoxypyridinoline	−20	−30
Serum C-telopeptide fragments of collagen-1 degradation	−35	−55
Serum osteocalcin or bone alkaline phosphatase	−20	−40

For a 90% sensitivity, the cut-offs are, in general, 20% higher, e.g. −25% cf −45% for HRT and alendronate, respectively, for urinary fragments of collagen-1 degradation (C- or N-terminal). A 90% specificity leads to ≤ 10% false-positive results, a 90% sensitivity leads to ≤ 10% false-negative results. Thus, if the concern is to classify nonresponders, the specificity criteria should be chosen. The suggested time point to measure is before initiation of therapy and again 3–6 months later. If the results are equivocal, a third measurement 3 months later is likely to correctly classify 50% of misclassified individuals.[8]

REFERENCES

1. Consensus Development Statement. Who are candidates for prevention and treatment for osteoporosis? *Osteoporosis Int* 1997; **7**: 1–6.
2. O'Neill TW, Felsenberg D, Varlow J et al. The prevalence of vertebral deformity in European men and women: the European Vertebral Osteoporosis Study. *J Bone Miner Res* 1996; **11**: 1010–18.
3. Kanis JA. *Osteoporosis*. (Blackwell Science Ltd: London, 1994.)
4. Bjarnason NH, Alexandersen P, Christiansen C. Number of years since menopause: spontaneous bone loss is dependent, but response to HRT is independent. *Bone* 2002; **30**: 637–42.
5. Melton 3rd LJ, Kan SH, Frye MA et al. Epidemiology of vertebral fractures in women. *Am J Epidemiol* 1989; **129**: 1000–11.
6. Genant HK, Engelke K, Fuerst T et al. Noninvasive assessment of bone mineral and structure: state of the art. *J Bone Miner Res* 1996; **11**: 707–30.
7. Marshall D, Johnell O, Wedel H. Meta-analysis of how well measures of bone mineral density predict occurrence of osteoporotic fractures. *BMJ* 1996; **312**: 1254–9.
8. Delmas PD. The use of biochemical markers of bone turnover in the management of post-menopausal osteoporosis. *Osteoporosis Int* 2000; **11** (Suppl 6): S1–S76.
9. Bjarnason NH, Byrjalsen I, Hassager C et al. Low dose estradiol in combination with gestodene to prevent early postmenopausal bone loss. *Am J Obstet Gynecol* 2000; **183**: 550–60.
10. Ravn P, Bidstrup M, Wasnich RD et al. Alendronate and estrogen–progestin in the long-term prevention of bone loss: four-year results from the early postmenopausal intervention cohort. A randomized, controlled trial. *Ann Intern Med* 1999; **131**: 935–42.
11. The Writing Group for the PEPI trial. Effects of hormone therapy on bone mineral density: results from the Postmenopausal Estrogen/Progestin Interventions (PEPI) trial. *J Am Med Ass* 1996; **276**: 1389–96.
12. Speroff L, Rowan J, Symons J et al. The comparative effect on bone density, endometrium and lipids of continuous hormones as replacement therapy (CHART study). A randomized controlled trial. *JAMA* 1996; **276**: 1397–403.
13. Alexandersen P, Byrjalsen I, Christiansen C. Piperazine oestrone sulphate and interrupted norethisterone in postmenopausal women: effects on bone mass, lipoprotein, metabolism,

14. climacteric symptoms and adverse effects. *Br J Obstet Gynaecol* 2000; **107**: 356–64.
14. Cooper C, Stakkestad JA, Radowicki S et al. Matrix delivery transdermal 17beta-estradiol for the prevention of bone loss in postmenopausal women. The International Study Group. *Osteoporosis Int* 1999; **9**: 358–66.
15. Garnero P, Tsouderos Y, Marton I et al. Effects of intranasal 17beta-estradiol on bone turnover and serum insulin-like growth factor I in post-menopausal women. *J Clin Endocr Metab* 1999; **84**: 2390–7.
16. Bjarnason NH, Christiansen C. The influence of thinness and smoking on bone loss and response to HRT in early postmenopausal women. *J Clin Endocr Metab* 2000; **85**: 590–6.
17. Cauley JA, Seeley DG, Ensrud K et al. Estrogen replacement therapy and fractures in older women. *Ann Intern Med* 1995; **122**: 9–16.
18. Michaelsson K, Baron JA, Farahmand BY et al. Hormone replacement therapy and the risk of hip fracture: population-based case-control. *BMJ* 1998; **361**: 1858–63.
19. Lufkin EG, Wahner HW, O'Fallon WM et al. Treatment of postmenopausal osteoporosis with transdermal estrogen. *Ann Intern Med* 1992; **117**: 1–9.
20. Lindsay R, Hart DM, Forrest C, Baird C. Prevention of spinal osteoporosis in oophorec-tomized women. *Lancet* 1980; **2**: 1151–3.
21. Hulley S, Grady D, Bush T et al. Randomized trial of estrogen plus progestin for secondary prevention of coronary heart disease in post-menopausal women. *JAMA* 1998; **280**: 605–13.
22. Torgerson DJ, Bell-Syer SEM. Hormone replacement therapy and prevention of non-vertebral fractures. *JAMA* 2001; **285**: 2891–7.
23. Stampfer MJ, Colditz GA. Estrogen replacement therapy and coronary heart disease: a quantitative assessment of the epidemiologic evidence. *Prev Med* 1991; **20**: 47–63.
24. Grodstein F, Stampfer MJ, Manson JE et al. Postmenopausal estrogen and progestin use and the risk of cardiovascular disease. *N Engl J Med* 1996; **335**: 453–61.
25. Herrington DM, Reboussin DM, Brosnihan KB et al. Effects of estrogen replacement on the progression of coronary-artery atherosclerosis. *N Engl J Med* 2000; **343**: 522–9.
26. Herrington DM. The HERS trial results: paradigms lost? *Ann Intern Med* 1999; **131**: 463–6.
27. Crook D. The role of HRT in the prevention of coronary heart disease: contemplations in the

aftermath of HERS. *J Br Menopause Soc* 2000; **S2:** 4–7.

28. Bjarnason NH, Bjarnason K, Haarbo J et al. Tibolone: prevention of bone loss in late post-menopausal women. *J Clin Endocr Metab* 1996; **81:** 2419–22.

29. Delmas PD, Bjarnason NH, Mitlak BH et al. The effects of raloxifene on bone mineral density, serum cholesterol and uterine endometrium in postmenopausal women. *N Engl J Med* 1997; **337:** 1641–7.

30. Ettinger B, Black DM, Mitlak BH et al. Reduction of vertebral fracture risk in postmenopausal women with osteoporosis treated with raloxifene. *JAMA* 1999; **282:** 637–45.

31. Cummings SR, Eckert S, Krueger K et al. The effect of raloxifene on risk of breast cancer in postmenopausal women. Results from the MORE randomized trial. *JAMA* 1999; **281:** 2189–97.

32. Eyres KS, Marshall P, McCloskey E et al. Spontaneous fractures in a patient treated with low doses of etidronic acid (disodium etidronate). *Drug Safety* 1992; **7:** 162–5.

33. Black DM, Cummings SR, Karpf DB et al. Randomized trial of effect of alendronate on risk of fracture in women with existing vertebral fractures: Fracture Intervention Trial research group. *Lancet* 1996; **348:** 1535–41.

34. McClung MR, Geusens P, Miller PD et al. Effect of risedronate on the risk of hip fracture in elderly women. Hip Intervention Program Study Group. *N Engl J Med* 2001; **344:** 333–40.

35. Harris ST, Watts NB, Genant HK et al. Effects of risedronate treatment on vertebral and nonvertebral fractures in women with postmenopausal osteoporosis: a randomized controlled trial. Vertebral Efficacy With Risedronate Therapy (VERT) Study Group. *JAMA* 1999; **282:** 1344–52.

36. Ravn P, Clemmesen B, Riis BJ, Christiansen C. The effect on bone mass and bone markers of different doses of ibandronate: a new bisphosphonate for prevention and treatment of postmenopausal osteoporosis: a 1-year, randomized, double-blind, placebo-controlled dose-finding study. *Bone* 1996; **19:** 527–33.

37. Riis B, Thomsen K, Christiansen C. Does calcium supplementation prevent postmenopausal bone loss? A double-blind, controlled clinical study. *N Engl J Med* 1987; **316:** 173–7.

38. Chapuy MC, Arlot ME, Duboeuf F et al. Vitamin D3 and calcium to prevent hip fractures in the elderly women. *N Engl J Med* 1992; **327:** 1637–42.

39. Heikkinen AM, Parviainen M, Niskanen L et al. Biochemical bone markers and bone mineral density during postmenopausal hormone replacement therapy with and without vitamin D3: a prospective, controlled, randomized study. *J Clin Endocr Metab* 1997; **82:** 2476–82.

40. Alexandersen P, Riis BJ, Christiansen C. Monofluorophosphate combined with hormone replacement therapy induces a synergistic effect on bone mass by dissociating bone formation and resorption in postmenopausal women: a randomized study. *J Clin Endocr Metab* 1999; **84:** 3013–20.

41. Reginster JY, Agnusdei D, Gennari C, Kicovic PM. Association of tibolone and fluoride displays a pronounced effect on bone mineral density in postmenopausal osteoporotic women. *Gynecol Endocr* 1999; **13:** 361–8.

42. Cosman F, Nieves J, Woelfert L et al. Parathyroid hormone added to established hormone therapy: effects on vertebral fracture and maintenance of bone mass after parathyroid hormone withdrawal. *J Bone Miner Res* 2001; **16:** 925–31.

43. Neer RM, Arnaud CD, Zanchetta JR et al. Effect of parathyroid hormone (1–34) on fractures and bone mineral density in postmenopausal women with osteoporosis. *N Engl J Med* 2001; **344:** 1434–41.

44. Bjarnason NH, Christiansen C. Early response in biochemical markers predicts long-term response in bone mass during HRT in early postmenopausal women. *Bone* 2000; **26:** 561–9.

45. Delmas PD, Hardy P, Garnero P, Dain M. Monitoring individual response to hormone replacement therapy with bone markers. *Bone* 2000; **26:** 553–60.

46. Bjarnason NH, Bjarnason K, Hassager C, Christiansen C. The response in spinal bone mass to tibolone treatment is related to bone turnover in elderly women. *Bone* 1997; **20:** 151–5.

47. Ravn P, Christensen JO, Baumann M, Clemmesen B. Changes in biochemical markers and bone mass after withdrawal of ibandronate treatment: prediction of bone mass changes during treatment. *Bone* 1998; **22:** 559–64.

48. Ravn P, Hosking D, Thompson D et al. Monitoring of alendronate treatment and prediction of effect on bone mass by biochemical markers in the early postmenopausal intervention cohort study. *J Clin Endocr Metab* 1999; **84:** 2363–8.

49. Garnero P, Darte C, Delmas PD. A model to monitor the efficacy of alendronate treatment in

women with osteoporosis using a biochemical marker of bone turnover. *Bone* 1999; **24:** 603–9.

50. Bjarnason NH, Sarkar S, Duong T et al. 6 and 12 months changes in bone turnover are related to reduction in vertebral fracture risk during 3 years raloxifene treatment in postmenopausal osteoporosis. *Osteoporosis Int* 2001; **12:** 922–30.

51. Hochberg MC, Ross PD, Black D et al. Larger increases in bone mineral density during alendronate therapy are associated with a lower risk of new vertebral fracture in women with postmenopausal osteoporosis. *Arthritis Rheum* 1999; **42:** 1246–54.

15

Hormone replacement therapy and atherosclerotic vascular disease

E Windler and B-Chr Zyriax

Introduction • Risk factors • Hormone replacement therapy • Study results • Patients and clinical trials • Risk predictors • Genetic factors • Conclusion • References

INTRODUCTION

Arteriosclerotic cardio- and cerebrovascular disease emerged from being a rare disease to the main cause of death in women in the twentieth century. From menopause on, its morbidity plays an increasing role and eventually its mortality outnumbers severe illnesses and classical causes of death in women like breast, cervical, endometrial and ovarian cancer. Thus, in preventive medicine of women, arteriosclerotic vascular disease needs to be adequately considered. Hormone replacement therapy (HRT), or hormone therapy, in the peri- and post-menopause is one candidate in the array of possible preventive measures that has become a contentious and hotly debated issue.

Because of the insidious onset of the manifestation of arteriosclerotic disease with menopause it is conceivable that, on the one hand, the decrease of plasma estrogens plays a decisive role in the development of arteriosclerosis. On the other hand, the observed lower rate of cardiovascular events in women on HRT is thought to be linked to the effects of estrogens. However, no causal relationships can be derived from observational trials. Still, undoubtedly women who freely decide to use HRT have a significantly, in many trials 50%, lower risk of cardiovascular events and mortality.[1] Moreover, it is still a noteworthy fact that women develop arteriosclerotic vascular disease 10–15 years later than men and this has not changed despite an increase in incidence that is now similar to that of men.

RISK FACTORS

However, it should not be overlooked that many trials have found that classical risk factors play a similar major role for atherogenesis in women as they do in men.[2] In the recent CORA trial (Coronary Risk Factor for Atherosclerosis in Women) from Germany not a single woman with coronary artery disease was identified who was not affected by at least one of the major classical risk factors like hypertension, diabetes and insulin resistance, dyslipidemia or smoking (unpublished observations). Indeed, > 90% of the women were affected by a combination of two, three or even four of these risk factors. Two-thirds of the women met the criteria of a metabolic syndrome. Even smoking women with coronary artery disease, who are believed to develop arteriosclerosis through effects of the tobacco, were characterized by the metabolic syndrome in contrast to smoking women without coronary artery disease. In essence, deprivation of estrogen alone is not responsible for the increased risk for atherosclerotic artery disease in postmenopausal women. However, it is not excluded that estrogen, or rather the deprivation of it, has a significant influence on the development of these risk factors and therefore on the atherogenesis.

Still, in many women risk factors emerge long before menopause. The concentrations of risk factors like low-density lipoprotein (LDL) cholesterol and lipoprotein(a) (Lp(a)) or the incidence of hypertension and diabetes begin to rise clearly before menopause. The metabolic syndrome and its characteristic risk factors appear to have their origin long before menopause. Women with coronary artery disease typically have gained weight in early adulthood. The critical weight gain which will determine the cardiovascular risk in the postmenopause may even occur between the ages of 20 and 40. That means, though, that in the postmenopause cardiovascular prevention requires correction of the classical risk factors. Estrogens as HRT alone cannot be expected to be sufficient. Actually, a healthy diet and physical activity should be the backbone of preventive measures. Yet, in practical medicine the pharmacological treatment of the sequelae of weight gain – diabetes, hypertension and lipid disorders – prevail. Lifestyle changes to prevent their manifestation probably would have to be installed decades earlier, anyway, to be fully successful. It has been shown that a sufficient weight reduction to fully reverse the manifestation of diabetes is difficult to achieve in the postmenopause.

HORMONE REPLACEMENT THERAPY

Still, it appears not to be unreasonable to expect a certain benefit on cardiovascular disease when HRT is undertaken. For example, changes in the lipoprotein pattern should be favorable in terms of coronary and cerebral artery disease.[3] On the other hand, the effects of estrogens are numerous and diverse.[4,5] Due to the ubiquitous distribution of estrogen receptors in tissues and the vascular system, estrogen may affect any organ and cell type. Considering the pleiotropic effects on the vascular system, like endothelial-dependent and independent vasodilation, inhibition of inflammation, reduction of cell adhesion or platelet aggregation, it seems impossible to predict the overall harm or benefit of HRT on the vasculature.

The results of effects of estrogen may even vastly differ depending on the age of the patient and the stage of vascular disease.[6] For example, in the early stage of coronary artery disease, inhibited cell proliferation may slow the development of plaques and stenoses by reducing the proliferation of vascular smooth muscle cells. However, in the late phase of atherosclerosis, inhibition of cell proliferation may impede the healing of ruptured plaques. Additionally, in this stage even slight effects on the hemostasis, which may go unrecognized as long as the arteries are intact, may have deleterious consequences since a thrombus evolving from a ruptured plaque may grow larger and reach a critical size to occlude the artery. Thus, only clinical trials can tell us for which women at which age HRT is beneficial, likewise, results from trials on women of a certain age or stage of vascular disease cannot uncritically be generalized and transferred to women of different ages and vascular situations.

STUDY RESULTS

Considering this, the results of the Heart and Estrogen/progestin Replacement Study (HERS) were not predictable, so that the null-effect of HRT on cardiovascular and cerebrovascular events in this study may not be unexpected.[7] Also, the results of HERS obtained in women at advanced age cannot uncritically be transferred to HRT in the peri- and early postmenopause, since at this age women are typically still healthy and vascular disease is uncommon. The risk of myocardial infarction increases sharply in the late 50s and 60s, followed by the incidence of cerebrovascular disease a decade later. Thus, generally, women at menopause are still in what may be designated primary prevention for vascular disease. The overall results of HERS only apply to women with vascular disease; however, certain observations and subgroup analyses may provide information on problems and chances of HRT in general.

A particular issue is the increased risk of vascular and thromboembolic events during the first year of HRT observed in HERS. The relative risk for coronary events increased more than twofold but normalized within 2 years. Actually, this increase was most prominent within the first 4 months and after that appeared to normalize. Yet, the implications are not entirely clear. The report is based on only 19 additional cardiovascular events and nine thromboembolic events. In several secondary prevention studies of similar design this phenomenon was not observed.[3] One study considered the effects of HRT after stroke in women, a second study did so in coronary patients using quantitative angiography, and others measured the carotid intima media thickness by ultrasonography with and without HRT. A possible explanation is simply the smaller size of these studies. This would be in line with data from the Nurses' Health Study, which reported a similar finding to that in HERS.[8] In this large observational trial the cardiovascular risk was increased about twofold within the first year of starting HRT, but normalized within the second year and from then on decreased. After 5 and 10 years an overall benefit was reported. Although the results underscore the existence of this phenomenon, the interpretation is not straightforward due to the design of the study, since it is not known if these events may have hit only or preferentially women with clinical or even subclinical arteriosclerosis. This would be in agreement with a recent report on more than 24,000 diabetic patients that showed an increased rate of myocardial infarction only for women on HRT with a previous myocardial infarction and only within the first year of application.[9]

Less clear are the data of the Women's Health Initiative having applied a combination of estrogen and progestin. The cumulative hazard for cardiovascular events separates the two groups of treated and untreated women mostly within the first two years. Thereafter the incidence of cardiovascular events appears to be fairly similar and even merges within the last

year.[10] The estrogen arm of the same study did not yield any difference of cardiovascular events between women on estrogens or placebo.[11] Thus, some of the results of the arm using a combination of estrogens and medroxyprogesterone acetate may be due to chance. At least for the cardiovascular event rate within the first 2 years, no difference is apparent between the estrogen arm and the combination arm of the Women's Health Initiative. A more detailed analysis of individual cases and the time trend of risk might be worthwhile. Characterization of those patients who have experienced an early event as to atherosclerosis and concomitant risk factors will enable us to understand the impact of the findings. The assumption of healthy women as to their vasculature in the Women's Health Initiative is certainly inadequate, since among women at the age of 60 or higher, who comprised the majority of the study population, many will have silent atherosclerosis.

Meticulous analysis of the cases and well defined subgroups will provide the basis on which to decide which patients may benefit from HRT and those it might possibly harm. The low rate of events in HERS and especially in the Women's Health Initiative would allow a closer look at individual cases. The observation in the Women's Health Initiative of an increased risk for cardiovascular events persistent over years, however, is unique and has not been reproduced so far. Neither is it compatible with the results from other randomized intervention trials like HERS that showed a null-effect with the same medication in women at similar age and even higher coronary risk, nor with one of those large observational trials. Thus, it barely can sweep away the results of all other studies and should therefore be interpreted with caution.

An interesting view is provided by the idea that this transient effect is the result of changing estrogen blood level in the presence of freshly ruptured plaques. If so, those whose plaques have been stabilized before initiating HRT, should fare better. Statins are thought to stabilize plaques, an effect which may even appear within weeks.[12] It is noteworthy that those patients in HERS who were on a statin did not show any increased risk during the first year of HRT.[13] Likewise, in the Women's Health Initiative, women on a statin did not have an increased risk for cardiovascular events.[10] In other words, the transient risk may apply only to patients with existing coronary artery disease and a relatively recent plaque rupture who are not adequately treated for their heart disease before starting HRT. It may be noteworthy in this context that, in Germany, among women admitted to a university hospital for incident coronary artery disease over a 3-year period there was not a single case of a patient who had started HRT within the year preceding the event (unpublished observation). However, in healthy age-matched controls randomized to 200 of these women with coronary artery disease there were several HRT users. Since all emergency cases of a certain district are delivered to a certain hospital, there should be little selection bias unless women on HRT are at particular risk for sudden death and will not reach a hospital. No prospective study, including HERS and the Women's Health Initiative, has yet reported an elevated cardiovascular mortality. Thus, it may be concluded that the observation of an early rise in cardiovascular risk may not be a particular problem in regions with a high standard of public health care.

The concept of harm through changing estrogen levels would argue the case for not stopping estrogens when a woman on HRT develops an acute coronary syndrome. No prospective study, including HERS and the Women's Health Initiative, has yet reported an elevated cardiovascular mortality anyway. This is supported by a large recent observational trial on women admitted for myocardial infarction to various hospitals in the USA.[14] Those more than 6000 women, who were on HRT had a much lower hospital mortality, reduced by 60%. This may be due to HRT but also to other factors correlated with it. However, this observation clearly does not argue in favor of stopping HRT at the time of the development of an acute coronary syndrome. This view is in line with a recent study that reported women with a

myocardial infarction who were on HRT had a lower rate of reinfarction and cardiac death than those who were not on HRT.[15] Still, it may be appropriate to re-evaluate the indication for a long-term HRT on the occasion of the manifestation of vascular disease.

A recent subgroup analysis of the Women's Health Initiative seems to support this view. Though the assessment of cardiovascular risk in different age groups was not unambiguous, more importantly the hazard ratio for cardiovascular events was only elevated in women ten or more years past menopause, especially only in those being 20 or more years after menopause. In contrast, within the first 10 years after menopause the risk was even below one.[10] Thus, the interesting question if the data of the Women's Health Initiative really show an elevated cardiovascular risk for women that are in the peri- and early postmenopause and therefore may have an indication for hormone replacement therapy has to be negated. This is also supported by an analysis of those women that actually suffered from climacteric symptoms, although this important analysis is hampered by the fact that perimenopausal symptoms curiously were principally an exclusion criterion. However, those women that were included into the study despite hot flushes had a risk ratio below one. If hot flushes and night sweats were the criteria the risk ratio was 1.19 with the confidence intervals including one. In other words, the postulated increased risk in the Women's Health Initiative was due to those women that had no perimenopausal symptoms and were at old age or, in short, had no indication for hormone replacement therapy anyway.

Strikingly the results of the estrogen arm of the Women's Health Initiative indicate a 44% lower risk for women 50 to 59 years of age on estrogens versus placebo. This is in agreement with the observational studies indicating benefit from estrogen-containing HRT like the Nurses' Health Study. Thus, medroxyprogesterone acetate, at least in the tested dosage, may have some adverse effects, which, however, other progestins may not necessarily share. So far there are no data of endpoint studies as a solid basis for a clinical decision of a preference for one of the available progestins, which certainly differ in their pharmacologic characteristics. For now one may choose the progestin according to personal preference and experience, as well as measurable effects of known risk factors.

In contrast, the influence of the dose of estrogens appears to emerge from recent data. In HERS, overall there was no increase in stroke, however, in the Nurses' Health Study there appeared to be an elevated risk with the highest dose of conjugated estrogens (1.25 mg).[16,17] In the survey of Northern California Kaiser Permanente Diabetes Registry there was an apparent reduction of cardiovascular events with 0.3 mg conjugated estrogens, which was not obvious with higher doses and even turned into a slightly elevated rate using more than 0.6 mg.[9] Thus, the standard dose in HERS and the Women's Health Initiative of 0.6 mg conjugated estrogens is probably the highest acceptable dose and may be too high to show a positive long-term effect of HRT on vascular risk.

PATIENTS AND CLINICAL TRIALS

An important issue is the recruitment of patients for clinical trials. In the Women's Health Initiative the reported small number of responders to the invitation of < 5% makes a selection bias very probable. Preferential participation of women of a lower economic status who may see a chance to be provided with free medication would have a significant influence on outcome. Recent meta-analyses of observational trials of acceptable quality clearly indicates that the socioeconomic status has a decisive impact on cardiovascular risk and correlates with the use of HRT. In other words, much of the repeatedly shown lower cardiovascular risk associated with the use of HRT vanishes when controlled for socioeconomic differences between women using and not using estrogens. The most plausible explanation is better health status and care, including the use of HRT, in women of higher socioeconomic status. Thus, the most plausible explana-

tion for the lower vascular risk of women on HRT are the effects of a variety of healthy measures concomitant with the use of HRT. This certainly does not exclude a contribution from HRT.

The above may explain the differences in outcome in certain subgroups of HERS. In this trial only about half of the women received a statin, although as a rule a cholesterol-lowering agent is indicated after myocardial infarction.[18] Women on a statin did not experience elevated risks of cardiovascular events during the first year of the trial. They had a markedly lower rate of myocardial infarction and thromboembolic events, a slightly lower incidence of cerebral events and a reduced total mortality as compared to those not on a statin. These effects are probably not only, or at least in the case of thromboembolic events not even at all, the consequence of the statin therapy but rather the result of an overall better health status and medical treatment of those that can afford statins. Thus, statin use is probably a marker of a higher socioeconomic status and therefore better health care.

Thus, the results of HRT appear to depend decisively on the standard of medical care. Unless more detailed analyses of the results of HERS and the Women's Health Initiative are implemented, their outcomes are difficult to apply to other countries with different health care systems. However, at this point it appears clear from meta-analyses, and also from HERS, that women with coronary heart disease need to undergo consequent treatment with respect to their vascular risk before being put on HRT. On the other hand, HERS indicates no risk against starting HRT even after a myocardial infarction, provided that the woman is well treated as to her heart disease. Since atherosclerosis develops insidiously, it appears appropriate to have any woman checked as to her cardiovascular risk profile, possibly by an internist, before initiating HRT. By doing so the woman has a chance of lowering her vascular risk and receiving the benefits of HRT.

RISK PREDICTORS

Still, some 90% of myocardial infarctions and almost all strokes occur in women after menopause. However, atherosclerosis develops earlier in life, over decades. Thus, the risk can well be predicted at the time of menopause. Today, the global risk can easily be assessed using the Framingham or PROCAM algorithm (www.chd-taskforce.com). These consider the established risk factors together and give the risk for developing a major cardiovascular event for the following 10 years. The score includes lipid parameters, blood pressure, diabetes, smoking and family history, and age as major determinants of risk. It should be noted that an increased blood sugar level or raised blood pressure needs to be treated, but will only marginally or partly, respectively, correct the risk for coronary artery disease.[19,20] Treating hyperglycemia mostly prevents microvascular disease, and lowering blood pressure will mainly reduce stroke, heart and renal failure. Reduction of coronary risk is achieved mainly by lipid therapy and lifestyle changes. Treating hyperglycemia mostly prevents microvascular disease, and lowering blood pressure will mainly reduce stroke, heart and renal failure.

An evaluation of health status becomes of pivotal importance with increasing age, since the risk of myocardial infarction increases only marginally after menopause, but drastically so after the age of 60. For stroke this is even later. Since atherosclerotic vascular disease is the main cause of mortality and morbidity in women, which affects at least half of the population, with increasing age most women can be expected to develop some atherosclerotic disease. The overall findings of HERS and the Women's Health Initiative may apply to elderly women, but not to those in the perimenopause. Thus, in women for whom HRT is being considered for treating osteoporosis or urogenital problems at an age well beyond menopause, evaluation of vascular risk and if necessary, treatment of risk factors appears mandatory.

Consequently, it is probably advisable to ensure that any woman considered for HRT has been seen by her practitioner or internist for a vascular check-up. This is even more important in women with risk factors and in the elderly. In Germany, every third woman beyond the age of 55 can be expected to have impaired glucose tolerance or diabetes. This is a high-risk group, since the metabolic syndrome goes along with hypertension and dyslipidemia. A Danish study has shown that diabetic women on HRT have a ninefold increased cardiovascular risk.[21] Certainly, from these data no causal relationship with HRT can be derived. However, the report urges caution in a high-risk population. Still, the Northern California Kaiser Permanente Diabetes Registry has shown, in almost 20,000 diabetic women, that even in this group those on HRT have a cardiovascular risk that is 20% lower as compared to those not substituted.[9] Thus, again, the crucial point appears to be concomitant medical care.

This is also reflected for conditions in the recent German case-control study on women with incident coronary artery disease (the CORA study, unpublished observation). Fewer women with coronary artery disease than healthy controls were on HRT, indicating no principle health hazard due to HRT. It is noteworthy though, that the women on HRT had less vascular risk factors and a healthier lifestyle on average. However, those few women who were on HRT and developed a myocardial infarction comprised a subgroup that had the least healthy lifestyle and a markedly adverse risk profile. In essence, HRT can well be part of a healthy lifestyle, including good medical care, but HRT cannot compensate for deficits in individual health care. This, however, is closely linked to sociodemographic and socioeconomic factors and may be appreciably influenced by the health care system. Therefore, observations from one country may not be readily applicable to others.

GENETIC FACTORS

In some instances genetic factors may determine the effects of HRT. This may lead to positive effects but may also prevent positive effects of estrogens and provide an explanation for missing cardiovascular risk reduction. E.g. a polymorphic form of paroxonase, an enzyme on high-density lipoproteins (HDL), prohibits the rise of HDL cholesterol in response to HRT. It would be of interest if the common genetic variants of Lp(a) respond differently to estrogens. Lp(a) is found to be elevated above the conventional upper limit of normal of 25 mg/l in up to 40% of women with coronary artery disease. While estrogens lower the levels of Lp(a), subgroups on HRT that developed coronary heart disease were characterized by elevated levels. This raises the question of whether the polymorphic forms of Lp(a) of these patients respond adequately or not to HRT. This would be especially remarkable since, in general, those with elevated Lp(a) concentrations benefit from HRT with an above-average reduced cardiovascular risk. This has been shown in observational studies, but also in HERS and is compatible with findings of the Women's Health Initiative.[10,22] These are interesting examples that may draw our attention from the interpretations of recent studies, which are no more than a gross look at average values, to a more detailed analysis which may dissect subgroups with different responses to HRT. It might be worthwhile to identify subgroups of women that benefit from HRT as to cardiovascular disease, so that in those patients cardiovascular prevention may be an indication for HRT.

On the other hand, closer analysis will also lead to recognition of women who do not gain from HRT or may even be exposed to undue harm. Likewise, these might be worth being characterized in order to be able to exclude the woman at risk from HRT beforehand. The risk for thrombosis is certainly elevated in women on HRT. This applies especially to the first year when the rate of thromboembolic events is raised three- to fourfold,[23,24] but also in the succeeding year when the risk remains about double. However, the absolute risk is quite low. Thus, refraining from HRT for this reason would, in general, mean withholding HRT from > 99% of women despite no exceptional risk for thrombosis. This illustrates the need to be able to identify a high-risk group for possible side effects and exclude only these patients from HRT. Conceivably, screening for mutations like that of factor V Leiden gives information of elevated risk of thrombosis under HRT. Yet, the factor V Leiden mutation is much more frequent than for thromboembolic relevant gene polymorphisms, and there is no straightforward clinical test to detect thromboembolic predisposition under HRT, but for an obvious clinical history. For patients identified as being at risk an alternative would be to keep them under close observation, but still consider HRT as an option. This makes previous identification necessary.

CONCLUSION

In summary, initiation of HRT early in the perimenopause will prevent disproportionate fluctuations of estrogen concentrations, and thus premenopausal hormone status should be retained. There are no data indicating any added cardiovascular burdens following this procedure. Neither HERS nor the Women's Health Initiative has studied such women with perimenopausal discomfort; in fact, these cases were explicitly excluded from the Women's Health Initiative. However, HRT does not substitute for preventive medical care towards atherosclerotic vascular disease, rather, HRT can only be part of a healthy lifestyle. Caution should be exercised if women are to be put on HRT in the course of the postmenopause, though, as initiation of HRT appears to temporarily increase the cardiovascular and thromboembolic risk. However, this seems to be preventable by use of appropriate medical measures. Research is urgently needed as to the effects on vascular disease of HRT starting in the early perimenopause, since the published intervention trials do not address this question and a benefit is not yet excluded as harm has not been shown. Still, replacement of estrogens from early perimenopause on is an appropriate goal, with relief from perimenopausal symptoms as the principle indication.

REFERENCES

1. Humphrey LL, Chan BKS, Harold CS. Postmenopausal hormone replacement therapy and the primary prevention of cardiovascular disease. *Ann Intern Med* 2002; **137**: 272–84.
2. Stangl V, Baumann G, Stangl K. Coronary atherogenic risk factors in women. *Eur Heart J* 2002; **23**: 1738–52.
3. Windler E. Hormone rsatztherapie und kardiovaskuläre Prävention – Chance oder Risiko. *J Menopause* 2002; **10**: 32–40.
4. Mendelsohn ME, Karas RH. The protective effects of estrogen on the cardiovascular system. *N Engl J Med* 1999; **340**: 1801–11.
5. Finking G, Gohar MH, Lenz C, Hanke H. Die Wirkungen von Östrogen im kardiovaskulären System. *Z Kardiol* 2000; **89**: 442–53.
6. Cano A, van Baal WM. The mechanisms of thrombotic risk induced by hormone replacement therapy. *Maturitas* 2001; **40**: 17–38.
7. Hulley S, Grady D, Bush T et al. Randomized trial of estrogen plus progestin for secondary prevention of coronary heart disease in postmenopausal women. Heart and Estrogen/progestin Replacement Study (HERS) Research Group. *JAMA* 1998; **280**: 605–13.
8. Grodstein F, Manson JE, Stampfer MJ. Postmenopausal hormone use and secondary prevention of coronary events in the nurses' health study. a prospective, observational study. *Ann Intern Med* 2001; **135**: 1–8.
9. Ferrara A, Quesenberry CP, Karter AJ et al. Current use of unopposed estrogen and estrogen plus progestin and the risk of acute myocardial infarction among women with diabetes. The Northern California Kaiser Permanente Diabetes Registry, 1995–1998. *Circulation* 2003; **107**: 43–8.
10. Manson JE, Hsia J, Johnson KC et al. Women's Health Initiative Investigators. Estrogen plus progestin and the risk of coronary heart disease. *N Engl J Med* 2003; **349**: 523–34.
11. Anderson GL, Limacher M, Assaf AR et al. Women's Health Initiative Steering Committee. Effects of conjugated equine estrogen in postmenopausal women with hysterectomy: the Women's Health Initiative randomized controlled trial. *JAMA* 2004; **291**: 1701–12.
12. Schwartz GG, Olsson AG, Ezekowitz MD et al. Effects of atorvastatin on early recurrent ischemic events in acute coronary syndromes: the MIRACL study: a randomized controlled trial. *JAMA* 2001; **285**: 1711–8.
13. Herrington DM, Reboussin DM, Brosnihan KB, et al. Effects of estrogen replacement on the progression of coronary-artery atherosclerosis. *N Engl J Med* 2000; **343**: 522–9.
14. Shlipak MG, Angeja BG, Go AS et al. Hormone therapy and in-hospital survival after myocardial infarction in postmenopausal women. *Circulation* 2001; **104**: 2300–4.
15. Newton KM, LaCroix AZ, McKnight B et al. Estrogen replacement therapy and prognosis after first myocardial infarction. *Am J Epidemiol* 1997; **145**: 269–77.
16. Grodstein F, Manson JE, Colditz GA et al. A prospective, observational study of postmenopausal hormone therapy and primary prevention of cardiovascular disease. *Ann Intern Med* 2000; **133**: 933–41.
17. Simon JA, Hsia J, Cauley JA, et al. Postmenopausal hormone therapy and risk of stroke: the Heart and Estrogen-Progestin Replacement Study (HERS). *Circulation* 2001; **103**: 638–642.
18. Herrington DM, Vittinghoff E, Lin F et al. Statin therapy, cardiovascular events, and total mortality in the Heart and Estrogen/Progestin Replacement Study (HERS). *Circulation* 2002; **105**: 2962–7.
19. Collins R, Peto R, Godwin J, MacMahon S. Blood pressure and coronary heart disease. *Lancet* 1990; **336**: 370–1.
20. UK Prospective Diabetes Study (UKPDS) Group. Intensive blood-glucose control with sulphonylureas or insulin compared with conventional treatment and risk of complications in patients with type 2 diabetes (UKPDS 33). *Lancet* 1998; **352**: 837–53.
21. Løkkegaard E, Pedersen AT, Heitmann BL et al. Relation between hormone replacement therapy and ischaemic heart disease in women: prospective observational study. *BMJ* 2003; **326**: 1–5.
22. Shlipak MG, Simon JA, Vittinghoff E et al. Estrogen and progestin, lipoprotein(a), and the risk of recurrent coronary heart disease events after menopause. *JAMA* 2000; **283**: 1845–52.
23. Grady D, Wenger NK, Herrington D et al. Postmenopausal hormone therapy increases risk for venous thromboembolic disease. The Heart and Estrogen/Progestin Replacement Study. *Ann Intern Med* 2000; **132**: 689–96.
24. Miller J, Chan BK, Nelson HD. Postmenopausal estrogen replacement and risk for venous thromboembolism: a systematic review and meta-analysis for the US Preventive Services Task Force. *Ann Intern Med* 2002; **136**: 680–90.

16

Direct vascular actions of estrogens

AO Mueck and H Seeger

Background • **Introduction** • **Prospects – the significance of estradiol metabolites** • **References**

BACKGROUND

Numerous in vitro experiments and several clinical studies indicate that estrogens exert various positive effects on the vasculature. By modulating the synthesis of nitric oxide (NO), prostacyclin and endothelin, and blocking calcium channels, estrogens beneficially affect the vasotonus. Atherogenesis, which is considered an inflammatory, fibroproliferative process, may be delayed by estrogens via downregulation of inflammatory markers such as cell-adhesion molecules and chemokines. The delay is further based on inhibition of smooth muscle cell proliferation and downregulation of angiotensin receptor gene expression as well as by its antioxidative property. In addition, estrogens may stabilize the atherosclerotic plaque by reducing the expression of matrix metalloproteinases. The thrombogenic potency of the ruptured plaque may also be reduced by estrogens downregulating the synthesis of plasminogen activator inhibitor-1 (PAI-1). In addition, clinical studies suggest that other nonendothelial-derived vasoactive surrogate markers, such as serotonin and urodilatin, may be positively influenced by estrogens.

Differential effects of progestin addition were observed concerning the direct estrogenic effects on the vasculature. Antagonistic progestin effects have been observed for some markers and may depend on the type of progestin and on its administration mode. Thus, the role of progestin addition remains to be elucidated in further studies.

INTRODUCTION

Clinical studies and experimental in vitro investigations indicate that estrogens have beneficial direct effects on the vasculature (Fig. 16.1). These actions can mainly be divided into endothelium-dependent and endothelium-independent effects. By means of these direct effects estrogens elicit vasodilatory and anti-atherogenic actions. The mechanisms of these estrogen-induced actions may be genomic, mediated by both hitherto known estrogen receptors, i.e. α- and β-receptors, which have been detected in vascular cells, or nongenomically by direct action on membrane-associated G-proteins or as yet unknown membrane receptors. The role of additional progestin, however, has as yet not been fully explored. In this chapter the most important direct vascular actions of estrogens and the potential role of progestin addition are summarized. In vivo, direct vascular effects are measurable by means of blood flow methods and measurement of vasoactive

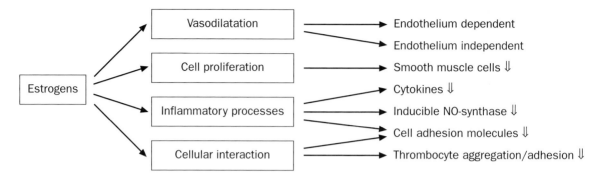

Figure 16.1 Direct vascular effects of estrogens.

markers. Here estrogenic-induced effects on biochemical mediators surrogating on vascular effects and/or as representatives of direct involvement in the vascular mechanism(s) of hormonal action are considered.

Direct effects on the vascular endothelium

Migration and proliferation of endothelial cells
Physiologic estrogen concentrations lead to an increase in the migration and proliferation of endothelial cells.[1] This effect was believed to contribute to an improved vessel repair under estrogens and perhaps to the formation of collaterals in the heart. However, new vessel formation or angiogenesis also plays an important role in the formation of tumors and in tumor spreading, i.e. metastasis. Recent work also indicates that angiogenesis is an important step in atherogenesis, and that neoangiogenesis may destabilize arteriosclerotic plaques.[2] Thus, the effect of estrogens on migration and proliferation of vascular endothelial cells might be beneficial regarding inhibition of atherosclerotic progression, but also harmful in terms of carcinogenesis. The effect of progestins on endothelial cell proliferation and migration has so far only been investigated for endothelial cells from human endometrium,[3] whereby progesterone was able to inhibit proliferation and migration.

NO
Estrogens are able to enhance the synthesis and activity of NO which is a potent vasodilatory,

anti-aggregatory and anti-atherosclerotic substance.[4] This effect seems to be mainly of genomic nature; however, endothelial NO-synthase can be activated by estrogens within 30 minutes, indicating an additional nongenomic mechanism.[5] Progesterone increased NO generation in rat aortas, which seems to be a rapid, nongenomic effect.[6] As yet, it remains unclear as to whether progesterone and synthetic progestins may attenuate the estrogen-induced beneficial effect on NO synthesis.

We performed a series of studies measuring vasoactive markers during hormonal replacement therapy whereby, among others, we evaluated the urinary excretion of cyclic guanosine monophosphate (cGMP), which can reflect NO production.[7,8] After 4 weeks of treatment in postmenopausal women with transdermal as well as oral estradiol replacement therapy a slight increase in cGMP was observed.[9,10] No deteriorating effect of oral or transdermal addition of the progestin norethisterone acetate sequentially added to oral or transdermal estradiol was found.[11] In a further prospective randomized study we also found no negative effect with the new progestin, dienogest on cGMP excretion continuously combined with oral estradiol valerate (Table 16.1).[12]

In several clinical studies the measurement of nitrate/nitrite as surrogate markers of NO production has revealed that estrogen replacement therapy (ERT) was associated with an increase of this marker in serum, whereas progestin addition had a divergent effect. Methoxyprogesterone

Table 16.1   Changes in urinary marker excretions of postmenopausal women after treatment with estradiol (2 mg/day) (n = 25) or estradiol (2 mg/day) + dienogest (2 mg/day) (n = 27) for 12 weeks compared to the pretreatment values

Marker	Difference (%)	P value
Estradiol group: within-group difference		
Week 6		
cGMP (NO)	+39.2	0.010
PGI_2-M/TxB_2-M	+55.6	0.005
5-HIAA	+65.1	0.002
Week 12		
cGMP (NO)	+49.6	0.0070
PGI_2-M/TxB_2-M	+99.9	0.0001
5-HIAA	+59.1	0.0100
Estradiol/dienogest versus estradiol: between-group difference		
Week 6		
cGMP (NO)	−9.8	0.56
PGI_2-M/TxB_2-M	−24.8	0.25
5-HIAA	−9.4	0.70
Week 12		
cGMP (NO)	+15.3	0.48
PGI_2-M/TxB_2-M	−37.1	0.08
5-HIAA	+6.9	0.80

cGMP, cyclic guanosine monophosphate, PGI_2-M, prostacyclins metabolite; TxB_2-M, thromboxane metabolite; 5-HIAA, 5-hydroxyindole acetic acid (serotonin metabolite).

acetate (MPA) attenuated the estradiol-induced increase of nitrate/nitrite, surrogate markers for the production of the vasodilating NO, in post-menopausal women.[13] Intermittent addition of MPA for 10 days every 3 months to 17β-estradiol, however, did not inhibit an increase in plasma NO levels after 6 months.[14] For norethisterone, however, published data are scarce, but norethisterone acetate (NETA) diminshed the estradiol-induced increase in nitrate/nitrite levels in postmenopausal women.[15] Long-term effects of oral and transdermal hormone replacement therapy (HRT) using NETA were investigated by Ylikorkala et al.[16] These authors found no changes in nitrate/nitrite levels after 1 year of treatment.

Thus, in clinical studies with post-menopausal women an estradiol-induced increase in NO can be observed. However, this effect alone cannot explain the strong vasodilatory estrogen action as seen, for example, in blood flow studies, suggesting that further mediators and various other mechanism(s) are involved. Progestin addition evidently can antagonize the estrogenic effect depending on the basal endothelial function, which might explain the different results in different study populations.

Prostacyclin
Several in vitro studies have demonstrated that estrogens increase the synthesis of prostacyclin, a potent vasodilatory and anti-aggregatory

Table 16.2 Ratio of prostacyclin ($PGF_{1\alpha}$) to thromboxane (TxB_2) metabolites in urine from postmenopausal women before and after oral or transdermal estradiol replacement therapy for 2 and 4 weeks. Means ± standard deviation

	6-keto-$PGF_{1\alpha}$/TxB_2	dinor-6-keto-$PGF_{1\alpha}$/dinor-TxB_2
Transdermal		
Before treatment	3.9±4.1	3.6±1.8
14 days treatment	4.6±3.5	4.9±3.8
28 days treatment	6.1±4.4*	7.5±5.4*
Oral		
Before treatment	4.9±7.0	5.8±4.5
14 days treatment	5.8±4.5*	8.2±8.8*
28 days treatment	5.8±4.1*	10.9±11.3*

* $P < 0.01$.

compound.[9,17,18] In in vitro experiments we showed that this estrogen-induced effect was not abrogated by the addition of MPA or NETA.[19] In clinical studies we have investigated stable urinary metabolites of prostacyclin and its counterpart thromboxane, as well as the ratio of these prostanoids. The results comparing oral versus transdermal estradiol replacement for 4 weeks in postmenopausal women are summarized in Table 16.2.[20] Following both oral and transdermal administration, estradiol treatment showed a significant increase in prostacyclin production, thus the ratio increased significantly after 4 weeks of treatment. The question arose as to whether time-dependent effects were in action and whether progestin addition could antagonize beneficial estrogen actions, such as leading to changes in the excretion of markers which surrogate on vasoconstrictory progestogenic effects. Therefore, we compared the effect of oral versus transdermal sequential estradiol/NETA replacement therapy in postmenopausal women.[11] As shown in Fig. 16.2, an increase of prostacyclins metabolite during the estrogen phase and an increase of thromboxane metabolite during combined phase were observed with both oral and transdermal administration, but

failed to show significance possibly due to high interindividual variations. Conceivably speculative, but the decrease in the quotient of prostacyclin to thromboxane, which is decisive for the resulting effects on vessels and which occurred following oral addition of NETA, can clearly be explained by a vasoconstrictory progestin effect, as progestins are thought to exert a vasoconstrictory effect on vessels.

Another research group has provided conflicting data on the effect of oral or transdermal HRT on urinary prostanoid excretion.[16,21,22] Oral estradiol/desogestrel for 6 months and oral and transdermal estradiol valerate (E2) NETA application for 12 months did not change prostanoid excretion significantly compared to the pretreatment values. However, in a third study an increase in thromboxane metabolites for oral E2/NETA but not for transdermal E2/MPA was found after treatment for 12 months.[21] In our study investigating the continuous addition of dienogest to estradiol no significant effect on the ratio of prostacyclin to thromboxane was observed after 3 months (Table 16.1).[12]

In a further study we compared two different oral contraceptives (OC) containing ethinylestradiol and levonorgestrel in the same ratio but with different absolute dosages.[23]

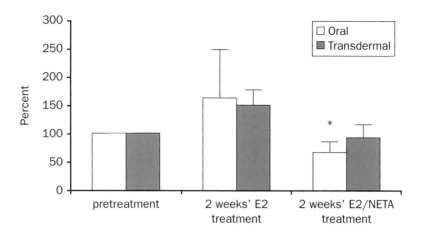

Figure 16.2 Ratio of prostacyclin metabolite to thromboxane metabolite (%) pretreatment value (100%) after oral hormonal treatment [2 weeks of estradiol valerate (E2) (2 mg/day) and 2 weeks of estradiol valerate + norethisterone acetate (NETA) (1 mg/day) (n = 20)] and transdermal hormonal treatment (2 weeks of estradiol patch (0.05 mg/day) and 2 weeks of combi-patch estradiol + norethisterone acetate (0.25 mg/day) (n = 17)]. Means ± standard error of the mean (SEM). *P < 0.05.

After 12 cycles of treatment the ratio of prosta-cyclin to thromboxane increased significantly for both preparations. We obtained comparable results testing other OC preparations contain-ing norethisterone and dienogest.[24] In OC the strong vasodilatory effect of ethinylestradiol might not be antagonized by the addition of progestins.

These data indicate that the ratio of prostacy-clin to thromboxane may be useful as a surro-gate marker for vasodilatory estrogenic effects reproducible in most studies but especially for possible vasoconstrictory actions of progestins. As with estrogen-induced NO stimulation, antagonizing progestin effects may be present or absent depending on the state of the arterial endothelium, which can also explain the differ-ent effects in blood flow studies.

Endothelin
Endothelin is a potent vasoconstrictory agent and appears to be upregulated in patients with cardiovascular diseases. In in vitro experiments estrogens were able to suppress serum and angiotensin-II-stimulated endothelial endothe-lin production.[17,19,25] Adding MPA or NETA we found no impact on the estradiol-induced downregulation of serum-stimulated endothe-

lin synthesis.[19] Progesterone was also able to inhibit the angiotensin-II-induced increase in endothelin production.[25] Several clinical studies on the effect of oral or transdermal HRT have demonstrated a beneficial reduction of endothe-lin blood levels.[26–28] One study failed to confirm these results for oral and transdermal HRT in nonsmoking women, but showed a reduction in smoking women for transdermal HRT.[16] In women with cardiovascular risk factors, con-flicting data have been presented. In hypercho-lesterolemic women oral and transdermal ERT reduced plasma endothelin values,[29] whereas in women with Type 2 diabetes mellitus and metabolic syndrome no effect of oral HRT or transdermal ERT was found.[30]

The beneficial effects of estrogens on the potent vasoconstrictor endothelin are considered an important mechanism of the vasodilatory and anti-atherogenic estrogenic effects.

PAI-1
PAI-1 is an important compound within the hemostatic system. Increased serum concentra-tions of PAI-1 may shift the fibrinolytic/coagu-latory balance towards an increased risk for arterial thrombosis. PAI-1 has been detected in high concentrations in atherosclerotic plaques

and therefore may accelerate arterial thrombosis following plaque rupturing.[31] Evidence is accumulating that PAI-1 may be an independent risk factor for cardiovascular diseases.[31] In recent investigations we found that estradiol reduces endothelial production of PAI-1 in human coronary endothelial,[19] which has already been shown in bovine aortic endothelial cells.[32] Progesterone also inhibited PAI-1 concentrations in bovine aortic endothelial cells.[32] We found that neither MPA nor NET seem to exert an antagonistic effect on the E2-induced decrease of PAI-1 synthesis in human coronary aortic endothelial cells.[19]

In a clinical study, only oral ERT but not transdermal ERT reduced PAI-1 serum levels after 3 months of treatment in healthy postmenopausal women.[33] The same also seems to be true for HRT using transdermal E2 gel and MPA or E2/progesterone where no decrease in PAI-1 levels were found,[34,35] whereas oral E2/P, CEE/P, CEE/MPA and E2/NETA reduced serum PAI-1 levels.[35–37] This effect was also observed for low-dose conjugated equine estrogen (CEE) combined with a progestin.[38,39] However, in postmenopausal women with established coronary artery disease (CAD), transdermal ERT and HRT lowered PAI-1 levels significantly.[40]

In summary, study results give conflicting data on the effect of ERT and HRT on PAI-1 serum levels.

Inflammatory markers

The inflammatory marker C-reactive protein (CRP) has gained more and more attention because of a series of clinical investigations indicating it to be an independent marker of upcoming coronary events.[41] It has been shown that oral estrogens increase serum levels of CRP.[42,43] However, this effect was not found for transdermal estrogens.[44] In a recent clinical study, administration of a statin reduced the estrogen-induced CRP increase.[45]

Adhesion molecules play a crucial role in the early stages of atherogenesis.[46] These molecules mediate the adhesion, rolling and tethering of leukocytes on endothelial cells. Thus, these molecules are expressed on the surface of endothelial cells. Recent investigations showed

that a soluble form of adhesion molecules can be measured in the serum.[47] Evidence is growing that they emerge from shedding of membrane-associated adhesion molecules and thus indirectly reflect the expression of adhesion molecules on endothelial cells. A possible pathophysiologic role of these soluble forms, however, remains to be determined. We have for the first time demonstrated effects of E2 on the soluble forms of E-selectin and intercellular adhesion molecule-1 (ICAM-1) in vitro and the influence of added progestins.[19] E2 is able to reduce the concentrations of both E-selectin and ICAM-1, and the addition of MPA and NET does not have a negative influence on this E2 effect. In fact, in the case of E-selectin the progestins may even have an enhancing action. Clinical studies with oral and transdermal ERT[33] and HRT[36,43] revealed a significant decrease in circulating blood levels of all three soluble cell adhesion molecules, E-selectin, ICAM-1 and vascular cell adhesion molecule-1 (VCAM-1). In postmenopausal women with established CAD the circulating levels of E-selectin, ICAM-1 and VCAM-1 were significantly decreased in women using HRT compared to nonusers.[49]

Evidence is growing that inflammatory markers are important in atherogenesis and may indicate high-risk patients. However, there are indications that these markers should not be measured in isolation but rather in context.

Monocyte chemoattracting protein-1 (MCP-1)

Chemokines such as MCP-1 are synthesized by vascular cells in the follow-up of inflammatory processes in order to recruit monocytes using their chemotacting properties.[50] Thus, the activity of this molecule is decisive in the early stages of atherosclerosis. Synthesis of MCP-1 can be triggered by cytokines or potent atherogenic substances such as oxidized low-density lipoprotein (LDL).[50] Physiologic estradiol concentrations inhibited the migration of monocytes exposed to MCP-1.[51] Progesterone had no effect on the migration of monocytes and abrogated the estradiol effect.[52] To our knowledge there have not been any investigations so far on the influence of sex hormones on cytokine-stimulated endothelial production of MCP-1. In recent investigations we were able to demonstrate that E2 can reduce tumor necrosis factor (TNF)-α-stimulated MCP-1 production.[19] This effect was not reinforced by the addition of MPA but interestingly by the addition of NET. Thus, with respect to the synthesis of this endothelial marker, differences in progestin action may exist. Clinical studies have shown that CEE combined with progesterone significantly lowered serum MCP-1 levels.[53] The same is true for 17β-estradiol combined with a progestin.[48]

Matrixmetalloproteinases (MMP)

Plaque stabilization has been shown to be important in preventing acute coronary syndromes such as myocardial infarct or stroke. Several factors contribute to plaque stabilization; these include collagenases such as MMP-1, which can be synthesized by macrophages and endothelial cells.[54] Since so far no studies have been performed on the effect of sex steroids on the production of MMP-1, we investigated the effect of E2 on the synthesis of the precursor of MMP-1, pro-MMP-1. The results revealed that E2 is able to reduce pro-MMP-1 concentrations, but only at high concentrations.[19] Interestingly, the addition of MPA as well as of NET elicited an enhanced reduction of MMP-1. However, another research group found a dose-dependent increase in MMP-2 levels in human coronary artery and umbilical artery smooth muscle cells.[55] In a clinical study, CEE alone or combined with MPA increased MMP-9 levels after 4 weeks in postmenopausal women with established CAD.[43]

Further investigations are necessary, since MMP are important markers not only in terms of plaque stability but also for angiogenesis and thus in the oncological research field.

Direct effects on vascular smooth muscle cells

Migration and proliferation

Proliferation of vascular smooth muscle cells, an early and critical event in the development and progression of atherosclerosis, appears to

be influenced by various growth factors and also directly or indirectly by sex steroids.[56,57] The mechanism by which sex steroids affect cell growth may be receptor dependent, since both estrogen and progesterone receptors were demonstrated in vascular smooth muscle cells.[56] 17β-Estradiol and progesterone are able to inhibit serum- and endothelin-1-stimlated growth of human umbilical vein smooth muscle cells.[58] We showed that 17β-estradiol significantly inhibited serum-stimulated growth of smooth muscle cells from human coronary artery (HCASMC).[59] The progestin MPA significantly enhances HCASMC growth. Furthermore, MPA antagonizes the estradiol-induced inhibition of HCASMC proliferation. In combination with estradiol the proliferative effect of MPA was dominant (Fig. 16.3). In contrast, for the progestin NET we were able to demonstrate a neutral effect of NET alone on cell growth and no impact of NET on the estradiol-induced inhibition of HCASMC proliferation.

The estrogen-induced inhibition of migration and proliferation of vascular smooth muscle cells is considered an important mechanism in inhibiting atherogenesis. This effect seems to be modulated by progestins in a positive or negative manner.

Calcium influx

Intracellular calcium availability is fundamental to the synthesis of endothelium-derived vasoactive substances like NO and prostacyclin, as well as to smooth muscle contraction.[60] For estradiol, a calcium-antagonistic effect was demonstrated in vascular animal smooth muscle cells.[61] In experiments at our laboratory we demonstrated for the first time an inhibition of calcium influx in human aortic cell cultures with estradiol, but not with estrone or estriol.[62] The magnitude of the calcium antagonistic effect of estradiol was about one-third of the effect of well-known antagonistic substances such as verapamil, nifedipine and diltiazem.[63] We also tested the calcium antagonistic effect of new 17α-estradiol derivatives, so-called scavenger estrogens, and found strong calcium antagonistic effects.[64] Since these substances are virtually devoid of estrogenic activity, they may

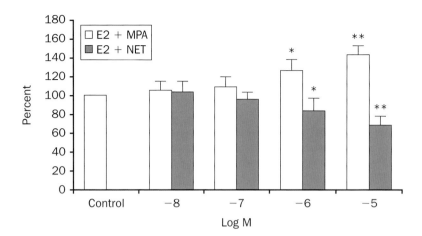

Figure 16.3 Difference between cell numbers of smooth muscle cells from human coronary artery after addition of estradiol (E2) + medroxyprogesterone acetate (MPA) and estradiol (E2) + norethisterone (NET) compared to control value (100%). Means ± standard deviation; duplicates from three different experiments. $*P < 0.05$; $**P < 0.01$.

offer advantages over 17β-estradiol in the prevention of cardiovascular diseases.

Furthermore, for the first time we tested the effect of various progestins alone and in addition to estrogens in human aortic cell cultures.[65] With progestins alone neither progesterone, nor chlormadinone acetate, dienogest or norethisterone, showed a significant effect on calcium influx. In combination with estradiol, progesterone, chlormadinone acetate and dienogest did not influence the effect of estradiol. In contrast, norethisterone dose dependently attenuated the effect of estradiol. Last but not least we also tested the effect of ethinylestradiol combined with levonorgestrel, 6-keto-desogestrel or gestodene and found that those progestins used in OC might not change the vasotonus interfering with calcium homeostasis.[59]

Thus, we were able to demonstrate in different experimental studies reproducible calcium antagonistic effects of estradiol, most of which were not antagonized by progestin addition, at least concerning healthy intact vasculature.

Angiotensin II receptor type 1 (AT1)
AT1 has been implicated in the pathogenesis of hypertension and atherosclerosis. Recent animal experiments demonstrated that 17β-estradiol induced a downregulation of AT1 receptors in ovarectomized rats and in cell cultures of smooth muscle cells.[66] In a further experiment the same group showed that prog-

esterone addition to smooth muscle cell cultures upregulated AT1 expression.[67]

LDL oxidation

Oxidized LDL is believed to contribute to risk factors of cardiovascular diseases such as hypertension as well as to the formation of atherosclerotic lesions.[68] Nutritive antioxidants like vitamin E and C are thought to inhibit the oxidation of LDL, and, therefore, are able to delay or even prevent atherosclerotic processes.[69]

17β-Estradiol has been shown to extend the onset of LDL oxidation in several in vitro investigations.[70–72] The progestins NETA and MPA did not inhibit the antioxidative activity of 17β-estradiol.[71,73,74] In a recent study, however, some progestins were shown to promote LDL oxidation and oppose the antioxidant effect of E2.[75] Most clinical studies on estrogens found a delay in the onset of LDL oxidation after treatment with HRT;[72,76,77] however, other studies failed to prove such an effect.[78–80] This discrepancy may be explained by different kinds of estrogen, duration and modes of administration.

Vasoactive markers of different origins

In addition to biochemical mediators originated from vascular cells, as summarized above, several other 'surrogate markers' may be of interest that are not synthesized in vascular cells but which are systemically stable and can act on the vasculature, and thereby modify vasotonus. For this reason, hormonal-induced changes in the concentrations of those systemic vasoactive mediators can only be measured in in vivo studies. We have performed clinical studies investigating the influence of ERT or HRT on the urinary excretion of serotonin, relaxin and urodilatin in postmenopausal women.

The indolamine *serotonin*, apart from its important functions in the brain, also has vasoactive properties, as demonstrated in several studies. For example, serotonin has been shown to have both vasodilative and vasoconstrictive effects on human coronary arteries.[81]

How this effect prevails depends mainly on the condition of the vascular endothelium, i.e. the vasodilative effect predominants if the endothelium is intact, whereas the vasoconstrictive one predominates if the endothelium is damaged.

Comparing oral and transdermal ERT we found a positive effect for both oral and transdermal estradiol after 2 and 4 weeks of treatment, which was more pronounced for transdermal ERT.[82] We observed different effects for sequentially combined oral and transdermal ERT using estradiol and norethisterone acetate.[11] The increase in urinary serotonin excretion after 2 weeks of estradiol was negatively influenced by the addition of oral NETA

Table 16.3   Delay of the transformation of low-density lipoprotein (LDL) to oxidized LDL after administration of the test substances

Compound	Concentration (μm)		
	0.25	**0.5**	**1.0**
Estradiol	< 5	30.5±6.1*	80.7±9.1†
A-Ring metabolites			
4-Hydroxyestradiol	149.2±14.1†	> 300†	> 300†
2-Hydroxyestradiol	146.5±16.2†	> 300†	> 300†
2-Hydroxyestrone	140.4±10.1†	> 300 †	> 300†
2-Hydroxyestriol	135.7±13.9†	> 300†	> 300†
4-Methoxyestradiol	130.4±14.3†	> 300†	> 300†
2-Methoxyestriol	127.1±11.9†	> 300†	> 300†
2-Methoxyestradiol	126.9±15.2†	> 300†	> 300†
2-Methoxyestrone	122.4±11.4†	> 300†	> 300†
D-Ring metabolites			
16α-Hydroxyestrone	< 5	28.1±4.3*	69.7±7.0†
Estrone	< 5	27.5±5.1*	65.3±7.9†
Estetrol	< 5	25.4±3.9*	62.4±6.8†
Estriol	< 5	23.7±4.7*	60.2±8.4†
Vitamin E	< 5	50.3±8.6*	108.4±9.8†

Figures represent minutes by which the time of the control values was exceeded, i.e. the time of uninfluenced LDL oxidation (96 minutes). Mean values ± standard deviation, $n = 9$. *$P < 0.05$, †$P < 0.01$.

but not by the addition of transdermal NETA. In a further study comparing oral estradiol with continuous combined administration of estradiol plus dienogest, we found serotonin excretion to be enhanced after 3 months of unopposed estradiol.[10] This effect was not negatively influenced by the addition of dienogest (Table 16.1).

The hormone *relaxin* is primarily synthesized in the ovaries and possesses a uterus-relaxing effect during pregnancy.[83] In recent studies it was shown that relaxin also has vasoactive properties: it can relax blood vessels and lower blood pressure.[84–86] Our investigations on the urinary excretion of relaxin showed that transdermal estradiol application postmenopause, i.e. using physiological estradiol concentrations, leads to a significant increase in relaxin production, whereas during oral application no distinct effect was observed.[87]

The structure of the peptide *urodilatin*, isolated from urine only in the 1990s, is similar to atrionatriuretic peptide (ANP).[88] It is presumably solely synthesized in the kidney, where it acts favorably on the balance of water and electrolytes.[88] Thus, measurement of urinary excretion of urodilatin mainly reflects renal effects.

In our studies, urodilatin excretion was stimulated by both oral and transdermal estradiol, being more pronounced for transdermal application.[89] Sequential addition of NETA to oral or transdermal ERT appears to reduce urodilatin production.[10] In contrast, continuous addition of dienogest to ERT caused a significant increase of urodilatin excretion after 3 months compared to ERT alone.[12]

In conclusion, surrogate markers for vasoactive action were beneficially influenced by estrogens in all of our studies. The effect of progestin addition seems to be different.

PROSPECTS – THE SIGNIFICANCE OF ESTRADIOL METABOLITES

Evidence is accumulating that, beyond the parent substance 17β-estradiol, estradiol metabolites, especially the A-ring metabolites, may be involved in the physiologic actions of estradiol on the cardiovascular system.[90] In a series of in vitro experiments we demonstrated that estradiol metabolites are able to increase prostacyclin synthesis[91] inhibit vascular smooth muscle cell proliferation[92] and delay LDL oxidation.[93, 94] In our investigations we were able to demonstrate that certain metabolities elicit a much higher antioxidative potency than their parent substance (Table 16.3).[94] These effects were especially pronounced for the A-ring metabolites, the so-called catechol estrogens. Our data indicate that estradiol metabolites may be involved in the physiologic inhibition of LDL oxidation. In addition, certain metabolites can stimulate cell proliferation of human osteoblasts[95] and may play a role in cancer development.[96] In the latter case, proliferative as well as antiproliferative and anti-angiogenic activities of estradiol metabolites have been shown.

Thus, future experimental studies investigating estrogenic effects should also include estradiol metabolites. Of special interest in this respect might be 2-methoxyestradiol, which has been shown to be a potent anticarcinogenic substance[96] but in addition elicits beneficial effects on the cardiovascular system.[97]

The positive influence of catechol estrogens on the vascular system additionally opens up new aspects for clinical pharmacology regarding the potential use of these substances for prevention and therapy of cardiovascular disease. As catechol estrogens are largely free of feminizing properties, it seems possible to use these substances independently of sex and of the endogenous hormone production.

REFERENCES

1. Morales DE, McGowan KA, Grant DS et al. Estrogen promotes angiogenic activity in human umbilical vein endothelial cells in vitro and in a murine model. *Circulation* 1995; **91**: 755–63.
2. Moulton KS, Heller E, Konerding MA et al. Angiogenesis inhibitors endostatin or TNP-470 reduce intimal neovascularization and plaque growth in apolipoprotein E-deficient mice. *Circulation* 1999; **99**: 1726–32.
3. Rodriguez-Mazaneque JC, Graubert M et al. Endothelial cell dysfunction following prolonged activation of progesterone receptor. *Hum Reprod* 2000; **15**: 39–47.

4. Anggard E. Nitric oxide: mediator, murderer, and medicine. *Lancet* 1994; **343:** 1199–206.

5. Caulin-Glaser TL, Sessa W, Sarrel P et al. The effect of 17β-estradiol on human endothelial cell nitric oxide production. *Circulation* 1994; **90:** 1–30 (abstract).

6. Selles J, Polini N, Alvarez C, Massheimer V. Progesterone and 17 beta-estradiol acutely stimulate nitric oxide synthase activity in rat aorta and inhbit platelet aggregation. *Life Sci* 2001; **69:** 815–27.

7. Broadus AE, Hardman JG, Kaminsky NI et al. Extracellular cyclic nucleotides. *Ann NY Acad Sci* 1971; **185:** 50–66.

8. Conrad KP, Vernier K. Plasma level, urinary excretion, and metabolic production of cGMP during gestation in rats. *Am J Physiol* 1989; **257:** R847–R853.

9. Mueck AO, Seeger H, Kaβpohl-Butz S et al. Urinary cGMP-excretion after hormone replacement therapy in postmenopausal women. *Exp Clin Endocr Diabetes* 1996; **104:** 392–6.

10. Mueck AO, Seeger H, Lippert C et al. Urinary excretion of vasoactive markers following estrogen replacement therapy in postmenopausal women. *Int J Clin Pharmacol Therap* 2000; **38:** 381–6.

11. Seeger H, Mueck AO, Teichmann AT et al. Effect of sequential estrogen/progestin treatment on biochemical markers in postmenopausal women comparing oral and transdermal application. *Clin Exp Obstet Gynecol* 2000; **27:** 17–20.

12. Mueck AO, Seeger H, Lüdtke R et al. Effect on biochemical vasoactive markers during postmenopausal HRT: estradiol vs estradiol/dienogest. *Maturitas* 2001; **38:** 305–13.

13. Imthurn B, Rosselli M, Jaeger AW et al. Differential effects of hormone-replacement therapy on endogenous nitric oxide (nitrite/nitrate) levels in postmenopausal women substituted with 17 beta-estradiol valerate and cyproterone acetate or medroxyprogesterone acetate. *J Clin Endocr Metab* 1997; **82:** 388–94.

14. Best PJ, Berger PB, Miller VM et al. The effect of estrogen replacement therapy on plasma nitric oxide and endothelin-1 levels in postmenopausal women. *Ann Intern Med* 1998; **128:** 285–8.

15. Rosselli M, Imthurn B, Keller PJ et al. Circulating nitric oxide (nitrite/nitrate) levels in postmenopausal women substituted with 17beta-estradiol and norethisterone acetate. A two-year follow-up study. *Hypertension* 1995; **25:** 848–53.

16. Ylikorkala O, Cacciatore B, Paakkari I et al. The long-term effects of oral and transdermal postmenopausal hormone replacement therapy on nitric oxide, endothelin-1, prostacyclin, and thromboxane. *Fertil Steril* 1998; **69:** 883–8.

17. Mikkola T, Turunen P, Avela K et al. 17-Beta estradiol stimulates prostacyclin, but not endothelin-1, production in human vascular endothelial cells. *J Clin Endocr Metab* 1995; **80:** 1832–6.

18. Mueck AO, Seeger H, Korte K et al. The effect of 17β-estradiol and endothelin 1 on prostacyclin and thromboxane production in human endothelial cell cultures. *Clin Exp Obstet Gynecol* 1993; **20:** 203–6.

19. Mueck AO, Seeger H, Wallwiener D. Medroxyprogesterone acetate versus norethisterone: effect on estradiol-induced changes of markers for endothelial function and atherosclerotic plaque characteristics in human female coronary endothelial cell cultures. *Menopause* 2002; **9:** 273–81.

20. Mueck AO, Seeger H, Wiesner J et al. Urinary prostanoids in postmenopausal women after transdermal and oral oestrogen. *J Obstet Gynaecol* 1994; **14:** 341–5.

21. Viinikka L, Orpana A, Puolakka J et al. Different effects of oral and transdermal hormonal replacement on prostacyclin and thromboxane A2. *Obstet Gynecol* 1997; **89:** 104–7.

22. Ylikorkala O, Hirvonen E, Saure A et al. Urinary excretion of prostacyclin and thromboxane metabolites in climacteric women: effect of estrogen–progestin replacement therapy. *Prostaglandins* 1990; **39:** 33–8.

23. Mueck AO, Seeger H, Petersen G et al. Effect of two low dose oral contraceptives containing levonorgestrel on biochemical markers surrogating on vasoactive action. *Contraception* 2001; **64:** 357–62.

24. Seeger H, Lüdtke R, Gräser T et al. Effect of oral contraceptives on the urinary excretion of biochemical markers indicating vasoactive action. *J Clin Pharmacol Therap* 2000; **25:** 221–6.

25. Morey AK, Razandi M, Pedram A et al. Oestrogen and progesterone inhibit the stimulated production of endothelin-1. *Biochem J* 1998; **330:** 1097–105.

26. Anwaar I, Rendell M, Gottsater A et al. Hormone replacement therapy in healthy postmenopausal women. Effects on intraplatelet cyclic guanosine monophosphate, plasma endothelin-1 and neopterin. *J Intern Med* 2000; **247:** 463–70.

27. Haenggi W, Bersinger NA, Mueller MD et al.

Decrease of serum endothelin levels with post-menopausal hormone replacement therapy or tibolone. *Gynecol Endocr* 1999; **13**: 202–5.

28. Ylikorkala O, Orpana A, Puolakka J et al. Postmenopausal hormone replacement decreases plasma levels of endothelin-1. *J Clin Endocr Metab* 1995; **80**: 3384–7.

29. Wilcox JG, Hatch IE, Gentzschein E et al. Endothelin levels decrease after oral and nonoral estrogen in postmenopausal women with increased cardiovascular risk factors. *Fertil Steril* 1997; **67**: 273–7.

30. Saltevo J, Puolakka J, Ylikorkala O. Plasma endothelin in postmenopausal women with type 2 diabetes mellitus and metabolic syndrome: a comparison of oral combined and transdermal oestrogen-only replacement therapy. *Diabetes Obes Metab* 2000; **2**: 293–8.

31. Kohler HP, Grant PJ. Plasminogen-activator inhibitor type 1 and coronary artery disease. *N Engl J Med* 2000; **342**: 1792–801.

32. Sobel MI, Winkel CA, Macy LB et al. The regulation of plasminogen activators and plasminogen activator inhibitor type 1 in endothelial cells by sex hormones. *Am J Obstet Gynecol* 1995; **173**: 801–8.

33. Vehkaavar S, Silveira A, Hakal AP et al. Effects of oral and transdermal estrogen replacement therapy on markers of coagulation, fibrinolysis, inflammation and serum lipids and lipoproteins in postmenopausal women. *Thromb Haemost* 2001; **85**: 619–25.

34. Kroon UB, Tengborn L, Rita H et al. The effect of transdermal oestradiol and oral progestogens on haemostasis variables. *Br J Obstet Gynaecol* 1997; **104**: 32–7.

35. Scarabin PY, Alhenc-Gelas M, Plu-Bureau G et al. Effects of oral and transdermal estrogen/progesterone regimens on blood coagulation and fibrinolysis in postmenopausal women. A randomized controlled trial. *Arterioscler Thromb Vasc Biol* 1997; **17**: 3071–8.

36. Koh KK, Jin DK, Yang SH et al. Vascular effects of synthetic or natural progestagen combined with conjugated equine estrogen in healthy postmenopausal women. *Circulation* 2001; **103**: 1961–6.

37. Teede HJ, McGrath BP, Smolich JJ et al. Postmenopausal hormone replacement therapy increases coagulation activity and fibrinolysis. *Arterioscler Thromb Vasc Biol* 2000; **20**: 1404–9.

38. Lobo RA, Bush T, Carr BR et al. Effects of lower doses of conjugated equine estrogens and medroxyprogesterone acetate on plasma lipids and lipoproteins, coagulation factors, and carbohydrate metabolism. *Fertil Steril* 2001; **76**: 13–24.

39. Schlegel W, Petersdorf LI, Junker R et al. The effects of six months treatment with a low-dose of conjugated oestrogens in menopausal women. *Clin Endocr* 1999; **51**: 643–51.

40. Falco C, Tormo G, Estelles A et al. Fibrinolysis and lipoprotein(a) in women with coronary artery disease. Influence of hormone replacement therapy. *Haematologica* 2001; **86**: 92–8.

41. Rifai N, Ridker PM. High-sensitivity C-reactive protein: a novel and promising marker of coronary heart disease. *Clin Chem* 2001; **47**: 403–11.

42a. Ridker PM, Hennekens CH, Rifai N et al. Hormone replacement therapy and increased plasma concentration of C-reactive protein. *Circulation* 1999; **100**: 713–16.

42b. Mueck AO, Seeger H, Armbruster FP et al. The influence of norethisterone acetate on urinary urodilatin excretion in postmenopausal women. *Clin Exp Obstet Gynecol* 1998; **25**: 76–8.

43. Zanger D, Yang BK, Ardans J et al. Divergent effects of hormone therapy on markers of inflammation in postmenopausal women with coronary artery disease on appropriate medical management. *J Am Coll Cardiol* 2000; **36**: 1797– 802.

44a Skouby SO, Gram J, Andersen LF et al. Hormone replacement therapy: estrogen and progestin effects on plasma C-reactive protein concentrations. *Am J Obstet Gynecol* 2002; **186**: 969–77.

44b. Mueck AO, Seeger H, Korte K et al. Natural and synthetic estrogens and prostacyclin production in human endothelial cells from umbilical cord and leg veins. *Prostaglandins* 1993; **45**: 517–25.

45. Koh KK, Schenke WH, Waclawiw MA et al. Statin attenuates increase in C-reactive protein during estrogen replacement therapy in postmenopausal women. *Circulation* 2002; **105**: 1531–3.

46. Chia MC. The role of adhesion molecules in atherosclerosis. *Crit Rev Clin Lab Sci* 1998; **35**: 573–602.

47. Ridker PM, Hennekens CH, Roitman-Johnson B et al. Plasma concentration of soluble intercellular adhesion molecule 1 and risk of future myocardial infarction in apparently healthy men. *Lancet* 1998; **351**: 88–92.

48. Stork S, Baumann K, von Schacky C et al. The effect of 17beta-estradiol on MCP-1 serum levels in postmenopausal women. *Cardiovasc Res* 2002; **53**: 642–9.

49. Caulin-Glaser T, Farrell WJ, Pfau SE et al. Modulation of circulating cellular adhesion mol-

ecules in postmenopausal women with coronary artery disease. *J Am Coll Cardiol* 1998; **31:** 1555–60.

50. Reape TJ, Groot TH. Chemokines and atherosclerosis. *Atherosclerosis* 1999; **147:** 213–25.

51. Yamada K, Hayashi T, Kuzuya M et al. Physiological concentration of 17beta-estradiol inhibits chemotaxis of human monocytes in response to monocyte chemotactic protein 1. *Artery* 1996; **22:** 24–35.

52. Okada M, Suzuki A, Mizuno K et al. Effects of 17beta-estradiol and progesterone on migration of human monocytic THP-1 cell stimulated by minimally oxidized low-density lipoprotein in vitro. *Cardiovasc Res* 1997; **34:** 529–35.

53. Koh KK, Son JW, Ahn JY et al. Effect of hormone replacement therapy on nitric oxide bioactivity and monocyte chemoattractant protein-1 levels. *Int J Cardiol* 2001; **81:** 43–50.

54. Galis ZS, Khatri JJ. Matrix metalloproteinases in vascular remodelling and atherogenesis. *Cric Res* 2002; **90:** 251–62.

55. Wingrove CS, Garr E, Godsland IF et al. 17beta-estradiol enhances release of matrix metalloproteinase-2 from human vascular smooth muscle cells. *Biochem Biophys Acta* 1998; **1406:** 169–74.

56. Chen Y-F, Oparil S. Effects of sex steroids in vascular injury. In: (Levin ER, Nadler JL, eds) *Endocrinology of Cardiovascular Function.* (Kluwer Academic Publishers: Dordrecht, 1998) 45–59.

57. Klagsbrun M. Vascular growth factors and the arterial wall. In: (Haber E, ed) *Molecular Cardiovascular Medicine.* (Scientific American: New York, 1995) 63–78.

58. Morey AK, Pedram A, Razandi M et al. Estrogen and progesterone inhibit vascular smooth muscle proliferation. *Endocrinology* 1997; **139:** 3330–9.

59. Seeger H, Wallwiener D, Mueck AO. Effect of medroxyprogesterone acetate and norethisterone acetate on serum-stimulated and estradiol-inhibited proliferation of human vascular smooth muscle cells. *Menopause* 2001; **8:** 5–9.

60. Lüscher TF, Vanhoutte PM (eds). *The Endothelium: Modulator of Cardiovascular Function.* (CRC Press: Boca Raton, 1991.)

61. Collins P, Rosano GMC, Jiang C et al. Cardiovascular protection by oestrogen – a calcium antagonist effect? *Lancet* 1993; **341:** 1264–5.

62. Mueck AO, Seeger H, Lippert TH. Calcium antagonistic effect of natural and synthetic extrogens – investigations on a nongenomic mechanism of direct vascular action. *Int J Clin Pharmacol Therap* 1996; **32:** 424–7.

63. Seeger H, Mueck AO, Lippert TH. Comparison of the effect of estradiol with calcium channel-blockers – in vitro investigations of calcium influx in human aortic smooth muscle cells. *Pharm Pharmacol Lett* 1995; **5:** 132–4.

64. Seeger H, Mueck AO, Oettel M et al. Calcium antagonistic effects of 17α-estradiol derivatives: in vitro examinations. *Gynecol Endocr* 1999; **13:** 246–8.

65. Lippert TH, Seeger H, Mueck AO et al. Effect of estradiol, progesterone, and progestogens on calcium influx in cell cultures af human vessels. *Menopause* 1996; **3:** 33–7.

66. Nickenig G, Baumer AT, Grohe C et al. Estrogen modulates AT1 receptor gene expression in vitro and in vivo. *Circulation* 1998; **97:** 2197–3001.

67. Nickenig G, Strehlow K, Wassmann S et al. Differential effects of estrogen and progesterone on AT1 receptor gene expression in vascular smooth muscle cells. *Circulation* 2000; **102:** 1828–33.

68. Steinberg D. Oxidative modification of LDL and atherogenesis. *Circulation* 1997; **95:** 1062–71.

69. Stephens NG, Parsons A, Schofield PM et al. Randomised controlled trial of vitamin E in patients with coronary artery disease: Cambridge Heart Antioxidant Study (CHAOS). *Lancet* 1996; **347:** 781–6.

70. Maziere C, Auclair M, Ronveaux M-F et al. Estrogens inhibit copper and cell-mediated modification of low density lipoprotein. *Atherosclerosis* 1991; **89:** 175–82.

71. McManus J, McEneny J, Young IS et al. The effect of various oestrogens and progestogens on the susceptibility of low density lipoproteins to oxidation in vitro. *Maturitas* 1996; **25:** 125–31.

72. Wakatsuki A, Ikenoue N, Sagara Y. Effects of estrogen on susceptibility to oxidation of low-density and high-density lipoprotein in postmenopausal women. *Maturitas* 1998; **28:** 229–34.

73. Mueck AO, Seeger H, Lippert TH. Estradiol inhibits LDL oxidation: do the progestins medroxyprogesterone acetate and norethisterone acetate influence this effect? *Clin Exp Obstet Gynecol* 1998; **25:** 26–8.

74. Seeger H, Mueck AO, Lippert TH. Effect of norethisterone acetate on the estradiol-induced inhibition of LDL-oxidation. *Pharm Pharmacol Lett* 1996; **3:** 105–6.

75. Zhu X, Bonet B, Knopp RH. Estradiol 17beta inhibition of LDL oxidation and endothelial cell cytotoxicity is opposed by progestins to different degrees. *Atherosclerosis* 2000; **148:** 31–41.

76a. Guetta V, Panza JA, Waclawiw MA et al. Effect of combined 17 beta-estradiol and vitamin E on low-density lipoprotein oxidation in post-menopausal women. *Am J Cardiol* 1995; **75:** 1274–6.

76b. Seeger H, Mueck AO, Lorkowski G et al. Effect of 17alpha-ethinylestradiol, levonorgestrel, 3-keto-desogestrel and gestodene on calcium influx via voltage-gated calcium channels in human aortic smooth muscle cells. *Contraception* 1996; **54:** 265–8.

77. Sack MN Rader DJ, Cannon 3rd RO, Oestrogen and inhibition of oxidation of low-density lipoproteins in postmenopausal women. *Lancet* 1994; **343:** 269–70.

78. McManus J, McEneny J, Thompson W et al. The effect of hormone replacement therapy on the oxidation of low-density lipoprotein in post-menopausal women. *Atherosclerosis* 1997; **135:** 73–81.

79. van der Mooren MJ, Demacker PN, Blom HJ et al. The effect of sequential three-monthly hor-mone replacement therapy on several cardiovas-cular risk estimators in postmenopausal women. *Fertil Steril* 1997; **67:** 67–73.

80. Wen Y, Doyle MC, Norris LA et al. Combined oestrogen–progestogen replacement therapy does not inhibit low-density lipoprotein oxida-tion in postmenopausal women. *Br J Clin Pharmacol* 1999; **47:** 315–21.

81. Golino P, Piscione F, Willerson JT et al. Divergent effects of serotonin on coronary-artery dimensions and blood flow in patients with coronary atherosclerosis and control patients. *N Engl J Med* 1991; **324:** 641–8.

82. Lippert TH, Filshie GM, Mueck AO et al. Serotonin metabolite excretion after post-menopausal estradiol therapy. *Maturitas* 1996; **24:** 37–41.

83. Lippert TH, Struck H, Voelter W. *Relaxin – Das wiederentdeckte Hormon.* (Springer-Verlag: Berlin, 1993.)

84. Han X, Habuchu Y, Giles WR. Relaxin increases heart rate by modulating calcium current in car-diac pacemaker cells. *Circ Res* 1993; **74:** 537–41.

85. St Louis J, Massiotte G. Chronic decrease of blood pressure by rat relaxin in spontaneously hypertensive rats. *Life Sci* 1985; **37:** 1351–7.

86. Ward DG, Thomas GR, Cronin MJ. Relaxin increases rat heart rate by a direct action on the cardiac atrium. *Biochem Biophys Res Commun* 1992; **186:** 999–1005.

87. Lippert TH, Seeger H, Armbruster FP et al. Urinary excretion of relaxin after estradiol treat-ment of postmenopausal women. *Clin Exp Obstet Gynecol* 1996; **23:** 65–9.

88. Meyer M. *Urodilatin – Von Entdeckung zu klinis-cher Anwendung. I.* (Holzapfel Verlag: München, 1997.)

89. Seeger H, Armbruster FP, Mueck AO et al. The effect of estradiol on urodilatin production in postmenopausal women. *Arch Gynecol Obstet* 1998; **262:** 65–8.

90. Lippert TH, Seeger H, Mueck AO. Estrogens and the cardiovascular system: role of estradiol metabolites in hormone replacement therapy. *Climacteric* 1999; **1:** 296–301.

91. Seeger H, Mueck AO, Lippert TH. Effect of estra-diol metabolites on prostacyclin synthesis in human endothelial cell cultures. *Life Sci* 1999; **65:** 167–70.

92. Seeger H, Mueck AO, Lippert TH. The antipro-liferative effect of 17β-estradiol metabolites on human coronary artery smooth muscle cells. *Med Sci Res* 1998; **26:** 481–2.

93. Seeger H, Mueck AO, Lippert TH. Effect of estra-diol metabolites on the susceptibility of low den-sity lipoprotein to oxidation. *Life Sci* 1997; **61:** 865–8.

94. Seeger H, Mueck AO, Lippert TH. The inhibitory effect of endogenous estrogen metabolites on copper-mediated oxidation of LDL. *Int J Clin Pharmacol Therap* 1998; **36:** 383–5.

95. Seeger H, Hadji P, Mueck AO. Endogenous estradiol metabolites stimulate the in vitro pro-liferation of human osteoblastic cells. *Int J Clin Pharmacol Ther* 2003; **41:** 148–52.

96. Lippert TH, Seeger H, Mueck AO. The impact of endogenous estradiol metabolites on carcinogen-esis. *Steroids* 2000; **65:** 357–69.

97. Dubey RK, Jackson EK. Cardiovascular protec-tive effects of 17β-estradiol metabolites. *J Appl Physiol* 2001; **91:** 1868–83.

17

Neurotropic and psychotropic action of estrogens: implications for Alzheimer's disease

P Schönknecht, J Pantel, J Schröder and K Beyreuther

Introduction • Estrogen replacement therapy (ERT) and Alzheimer's disease (AD) • Molecular biology of Alzheimer's disease (AD) and estrogen effects on the central nervous system (CNS) • Endogenous estrogen in Alzheimer's patients • Cerebrospinal fluid (CSF) estrogen and clinical characteristics of Alzheimer's disease (AD) • Modifying estrogen effects in Alzheimer's disease (AD) • 24S-Hydroxycholesterol in Alzheimer's disease (AD) • 17β-estradiol and cerebral glucose metabolism • Conclusions • References

INTRODUCTION

It is well known that estrogens exhibit several psychotropic effects in humans and that a relative lack of endogenous estrogens may even be involved in the pathogenesis of psychologic dysfunctions. Among those, depressive symptoms are the most common and accordingly estrogen replacement therapy (ERT) has been recommended as a mood-stabilizing intervention in postmenopausal women as well as for the treatment of the premenstrual syndrome.[1-3] In addition, recent studies have provided evidence of systematic activation effects of estrogens on cerebral activity and cognitive function.[4] In animal studies, a beneficial effect of estrogen on memory dysfunction and disturbances in cerebral energy metabolism,[5] as well as an estrogen-induced enhancement of glucose transporter expression in cerebral cortical neurons of primates,[6] have been shown. Consequently, the potential use of estrogens as a cognition enhancer in physiologic aging has

been previously considered. Apart from that, several epidemiologic studies have suggested that estrogen replacement might not only improve cognition in physiologic aging but may also exhibit beneficial effects on the onset and course of Alzheimer's dementia or Alzheimer's disease (AD), which is one of the most common and most devastating disorders of the elderly. The present chapter reviews current evidence in favor of beneficial neurotropic and psychotropic effects of estrogens in AD and also aims to address certain unresolved questions in the field.

ESTROGEN REPLACEMENT THERAPY (ERT) AND ALZHEIMER'S DISEASE (AD)

Among patients suffering from dementia, most cases (50–60%) could be characterized as AD. Clinically, mnestic and other cognitive dysfunction represent the core symptoms of AD. While symptoms are often subtle in the earliest stages of AD, their steady progression typically leaves the patient in an almost entirely helpless condition. Recent neuroimaging studies have demonstrated structural and functional cerebral changes in AD. These changes strike primarily the entorhinal cortex and medial temporal structures relevant for explicit memory functioning, but generally extend to almost the entire neocortex with progression of the disease. These findings do not only contribute to our understanding of the disease but can also facilitate clinical diagnosis (for reviews see Herholz et al,[7] and Pantel et al[8–10]). Further studies have identified increased tau and decreased β-amyloid levels as potential diagnostic markers.[11] In addition, the clinical diagnosis of AD requires exclusion of other forms of dementia such as vascular dementia or dementia due to cerebral neoplasm, infectious diseases or other pathologies.

Many epidemiological studies have investigated the potential of estrogens for modifying AD onset and progression. There was evidence for a beneficial effect of ERT on AD by an approximately 50% lower incidence of AD in women receiving ERT.[12,13] This finding was recently confirmed in prospective studies,[14,15] and led to the hypothesis of a therapeutic effect of estrogens on the course and severity of AD in postmenopausal women. Retrospective or uncontrolled studies investigating ERT for women with AD supported a facilitative effect of the hormone on memory function.[12] While these studies had methodologic limitations, such as open-label design, small sample size or short treatment duration, beneficial effects on memory and attention were also found in prospective, placebo-controlled, double-blind studies.[16,17] Recently, randomized, double-blind, placebo-controlled, parallel-group trials have been undertaken to define a therapeutic role for ERT in AD patients.[18–21] In the majority of these studies,[18–20] no differences in cognitive function between estrogen- and placebo-treated groups could be found. Those studies used conjugated estrogen, either 0.625 or 1.25 mg/day, for a treatment period ranging between 12 and 52 weeks. Sample sizes ranged from 42 to 120 AD patients and controls. Accordingly, the major

methodological limitations involved a small patient sample[19] and short treatment course.[20]

Asthana et al[21,22] indicated that conjugated equine estrogen administered orally may not be as effective in the central nervous system (CNS) as pure 17β-estradiol, the most potent endogenous human estrogen. Using a transdermal application of 17β-estradiol at doses of 0.05 and 0.10 mg/day for 8 weeks, Asthana et al[21] demonstrated a potential therapeutic role for this estrogen in a double-blind, placebo-controlled study of 20 postmenopausal AD patients. Significant effects of 17β-estradiol treatment were observed on attention, verbal memory and visual memory. However, evaluation of the importance of different estrogen compounds is rather difficult since oral estradiol treatment not only leads to elevated estradiol levels in serum but also to supraphysiologic levels of estrone.

MOLECULAR BIOLOGY OF ALZHEIMER'S DISEASE (AD) AND ESTROGEN EFFECTS ON THE CENTRAL NERVOUS SYSTEM (CNS)

Histopathologically, AD is associated with neurofibrillary tangle formation in the CNS. A microtubuli-associated protein, the tau protein, is assumed to be released into the cerebrospinal fluid (CSF) during neurofibrillary tangle formation, and has been found to be increased in patients with manifest AD[23] as well as in mild cognitive impairment or incipient AD.[11] The deposition of amyloid plaques in the brain, however, seems to be the major feature of AD pathology. Amyloid plaques are extracellular deposits of fibrillar aggregates mainly composed of a 4 kDa peptide, β-amyloid 1–42 (Aβ42), which is derived along with the peptide Aβ40 from the larger amyloid precursor protein (APP) by proteolytic cleavage.[24,25] Several studies have indicated that the deposition of Aβ42 constitutes an important process in the etiology of neuronal degeneration (for a review see Beyreuther et al[26]). Significantly, CSF Aβ42 concentrations have been shown to be a sensitive marker of AD pathology (for a review see Jensen et al[25]). Neuroimaging studies demonstrate that cerebral changes characteristic of AD primarily strike the temporal lobe with a particular focus on medial temporal substructures. These cerebral changes may be reliably assessed using quantitative magnetic resonance imaging (MRI).[8,27] Therefore, one might assume CSF Aβ42 levels to be associated with measures of temporal lobe rather than global cerebral atrophy. In line with this hypothesis, CSF Aβ42 levels in AD were found to be significantly correlated with the volume of the temporal lobes ($r = 0.46$ and 0.48, respectively) but not with other volumetric measures.[28] Similar findings obtained in a larger patient sample indicated that changes in cerebral Aβ42 levels are strongly associated with temporal lobe but not general brain atrophy, and thus emphasize the significance of Aβ in the etiology of AD.[29]

Several studies indicate that both genetically determined disturbances in APP metabolism with consecutive overexpression of the protein, and a pathologic enzymatic processing of APP to Aβ42 are essentially involved in amyloid plaque production. The Aβ42 release, however, has been supposed to be modified by several cofactors such as metallic elements (copper, zinc) or apolipoprotein E (ApoE). In addition, cholesterol and estrogens are supposed to play a major role in this process.

Estrogens can readily pass the blood–brain barrier and have several effects on the CNS (for a review see Henderson[30]). They enhance the outgrowth of neurites and promote the formation of dendrite spines and synapses.[31,32] In the brain, estrogens increase cerebral blood flow and glucose metabolism, and modulate acetylcholine metabolism.[33–35] Furthermore, the beneficial effect of estrogens on the CNS may be mediated by ApoE metabolism since estrogens have been found to decrease serum ApoE levels in postmenopausal women.[36]

In addition, estrogens have been characterized as having an important impact on Aβ42 formation in the CNS, a hallmark of AD. Experiments in cell cultures have indicated that physiologic concentrations of 17β-estradiol increase production of soluble APP at the expense of Aβ40 and Aβ42 production. Jaffe et al[37] demonstrated in vitro that physiologic concentrations of 17β-estradiol may modulate APP metabolism by increasing cellular release of the soluble, nonamyloidogenic components. Xu et al[38] investigated the effect of physiologic concentrations of 17β-estradiol on the APP metabolism of neurites and found not only an increase of soluble APP components but also significantly reduced Aβ42 and Aβ40 concentrations. Moreover, animal studies indicate that prolonged ovariectomy results in uterine atrophy with decreased serum 17β-estradiol levels and is associated with increased cerebral Aβ42 levels.[39] In the same study, 17β-estradiol treatment significantly reversed the ovariectomy-induced increase in brain Aβ42 levels.

The effect of estrogens on Aβ42 metabolism may be mediated by a morphological modification of the intracellular trans-Golgi compartments, where maturated APP is processed to Aβ42. Furthermore, estrogens support neuronal APP transport and act against the apparent dysregulation that leads to increased Aβ42 production.[38] The protective effects of estrogens may also be mediated by interactions not directly related to APP processing, such as modulation of neural functioning or prevention of oxidative toxicity due to glutamate, free radicals and Aβ40 or Aβ42.[40] Behl et al[41] showed that 17β-estradiol can prevent intracellular peroxide accumulation and, ultimately, the degeneration of hippocampal neurons.

Up to now, little has been known about potential differential effects of the various estrogens on the CNS. The majority of studies have focused on 17β-estradiol, which is generally considered to be the most potent estrogen, but others have considered estrone. The effects of other estrogens, such as estriol, or progestogens, such as progesterone, have not yet been investigated.

ENDOGENOUS ESTROGEN IN ALZHEIMER'S PATIENTS

Since a potential beneficial effect of ERT on the development and course of AD has been suggested in the studies discussed above, several investigators compared endogenous serum estrogen levels in demented and nondemented individuals (Table 17.1). At this point, an

Table 17.1 Serum estrogen levels in demented patients [Alzheimer's disease (AD)] and nondemented controls

Author (ref)	AD patients (g1)	Nondemented controls (g2)	Serum estrogen	Results
Honjo et al 1989[43]	$n = 7$	$n = 7$	Estrone-sulfate	g1 < g2 ($P < 0.05$)
Manly et al 2000[42]	$n = 50$	$n = 93$	Estrone	g1 < g2*
			Estradiol	g1 < g2 ($P < 0.05$)
Cunningham et al 2001[47]	$n = 52$	$n = 60$	Estrone	g1 > g2 ($P < 0.05$)
		Estradiol	g1 < g2*	
Senanarong et al 2002[44]	$n = 72$ demented	$n = 63$	Estradiol	g1 < g2*
		(AD $n = 37$)		
Hogervorst and Smith 2002[46]	$n = 66$	$n = 62$	Estrone	g1 > g2*
			Estradiol	g1 > g2 ($P < 0.05$)

* Not significant

important methodologic problem has to be addressed: in a considerable proportion of women, postmenopausal estrogen levels are below the detection limits of the assays available. Data from these subjects would be excluded from the sample if a simple comparison of estrogen level means across patients and controls was performed. This methodologic problem applies particularly to larger studies, which comprise a considerable proportion of women with subthreshold levels. One way to overcome this difficulty is to compare frequency differences among quartiles of hormone levels between patients and controls for significant differences of distribution.[42]

A pilot study conducted by Honjo et al[43] described lower estrone sulfate but not estradiol levels in seven female AD patients when compared to seven controls. In contrast, in a study of 50 patients compared to 93 nondemented controls, Manly et al[42] found postmenopausal AD patients to have lower serum estradiol levels. Although this difference failed to reach statistical significance, AD patients were much more likely to have estradiol levels < 20 pg/ml than estradiol levels > 20 pg/ml. Concerning estrone, no significant group differ-

ences arose. In a study by Senanarong et al,[44] elderly individuals with lower estradiol levels were found to have more impaired cognition as revealed by a modified version of the minimental status examination (MMSE).[45] In this study, the 72 patients with dementia (including 36 AD patients) were characterized by lower estradiol levels than the 63 nondemented controls.

These two studies were contrasted by recent findings of Hogervorst et al,[46] who reported AD patients to have significantly higher serum 17β-estradiol levels than controls. In this study, lower cognitive performance measured on the MMSE was associated with a high ratio of 17β-estradiol to total estrogen, and lower serum folate concentrations in the AD patients.

In a study of 52 postmenopausal women with AD and 60 nondepressed cognitively healthy controls, significantly higher serum levels for estrone but not estradiol were found in the AD group compared to the controls.[47] Based on the findings of Yaffe et al,[48] who reported an association between higher serum estrone levels and lower scores on digit symbol and Trail-Making B test in 532 women older than the age of 65, an antagonistic effect of estrone and estradiol has been hypothesized. In fact, estrone has a C2 hydroxylated subtype that acts as competitive inhibitor of estradiol.[49–51] Furthermore, these conflicting results can be explained by the metabolic exchange rate between estrone and estradiol. Under in vivo conditions, estrone can be rapidly converted to estradiol and acts as a reservoir for estradiol production.

CEREBROSPINAL FLUID (CSF) ESTROGEN AND CLINICAL CHARACTERISTICS OF ALZHEIMER'S DISEASE (AD)

Although several studies investigating serum estrogen and estrone levels among demented and nondemented individuals have revealed conflicting results, the endogenous CSF estrogen status in demented patients has not been investigated sufficiently well. Regarding CSF estrogen levels in pre- and postmenopausal healthy women, one study found no significant differences between these two groups.[52] Since the CSF–blood barrier has been supposed to protect the brain from the effects of peripheral estrogen deficiency, the impact of CSF estrogen status on Aβ42 metabolism needs to be further addressed.

Concerning this issue, we investigated 30 female patients with probable AD (NINCDS–ADRDA criteria[53]) and 11 female patients with nondementing diseases such as major depression (DSM-IV).[54] All patients were postmenopausal and had no history of ERT: severity of dementia was rated on the MMSE. CSF 17β-estradiol levels were determined using an electrochemiluminescence immunoassay on a Roche Elecsys 2010 immunoassay analyzer. For CSF Aβ40 and Aβ42 concentrations an enzyme-linked immunosorbent assay (ELISA), established previously by our group, was employed.[25,55] In addition, we measured tau protein concentrations using the innotest (Innogenetics) tau antigen kit.[23] In order to address the potential confounding effect of severity of dementia on the Aβ42 levels, MMSE scores were partialled out when the 17β-estradiol levels were correlated with Aβ40 and Aβ42 concentrations.

17β-Estradiol levels were significantly ($P < 0.05$) lower in the AD patients (16.0±3.0 pg/ml) compared to the patients with nondementing disease (19.1±5.2 pg/ml). While there were only minor, nonsignificant group differences with respect to age and body mass indices (BMI), MMSE scores were significantly lower in the AD patients compared to the controls (16.3±6.6 versus 26.7±1.8, respectively; $P < 0.005$). As expected, tau protein concentrations were significantly ($P < 0.005$) higher in the AD patients (591.8±282.3 pg/ml) compared to those with nondementing diseases (148.0±30.2 pg/ml).

Within the AD group, 17β-estradiol and Aβ42 levels were inversely correlated when severity of illness (MMSE scores) was partialled out ($r = -0.36$, $P = 0.05$) (Fig. 17.1). None of the other variables investigated, including tau protein concentration, were significantly correlated with 17β-estradiol levels. In summary, this study provides two major findings: firstly, evidence that female AD patients have lower CSF 17β-estradiol levels than nondemented female patients; and secondly, an indication that this deficit may have a mediating effect on Aβ42 metabolism. This finding is consistent with results from cell culture experiments demonstrating that 17β-estradiol can significantly decrease Aβ40 and Aβ42 release.[38] To our knowledge, this is the first clinical study which provides in vivo evidence supporting these experimental findings. We did not find any correlation between Aβ40 and 17β-estradiol levels. This, however, parallels the clinical finding of increased Aβ42 but not Aβ40 levels in patients with mild cognitive impairment and mild to moderate stages of AD.[25] Although significant correlation between BMI or severity of dementia and 17β-estradiol levels did not arise, differences in the respective measures have to be discussed as potential confounding variables.

MODIFYING ESTROGEN EFFECTS IN ALZHEIMER'S DISEASE (AD)

In a further study, we investigated CSF 17β-estradiol concentrations with respect to the clinical characteristics of the disease, as well as CSF

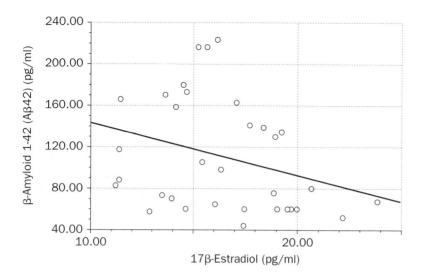

Figure 17.1 β-Amyloid 1–42 (Aβ42) versus cerebrospinal fluid (CSF) 17β-estradiol concentrations in female Alzheimer's patients.

tau protein concentration and potential medication effects in a larger sample of 59 postmenopausal patients with AD.[56] The study confirmed the previous findings that are summarized above; no significant correlations between CSF 17β-estradiol levels and severity of dementia, age, age at onset of disease or CSF tau protein levels were found. Subsequently, CSF 17β-estradiol levels were compared among those AD patients with and without neuroleptics. We found a trend towards slightly higher CSF 17β-estradiol levels in nine female AD patients on neuroleptics compared to 50 female AD patients without this medication. This difference, however, failed to reach statistical significance ($P = 0.08$). Based on the assumption that neuroleptic medication in AD might refer to subgroups of AD patients who require treatment because of behavioral or cognitive symptoms, we compared AD patients with and without neuroleptic medication with respect to other important clinical variables. However, neither age, age at onset of disease, severity of dementia, ApoE genotype nor CSF tau protein concentration differed significantly between groups.

24S-HYDROXYCHOLESTEROL IN ALZHEIMER'S DISEASE (AD)

There is growing evidence from cell culture experiments that cholesterol may influence estrogen metabolism. Results from recent studies indicate that accumulation of cholesterol in hippocampal neurons results in accelerated cleavage of APP into amyloidogenic components,[57] which leads to formation of amyloid plaques in susceptible brain regions of AD patients with consecutive neurodegeneration. Cholesterol is converted to 24S-hydroxycholesterol by cholesterol 24S-hydroxylase prior to being eliminated from the brain. This mechanism constitutes the major pathway of cholesterol homeostasis in the brain.[58,59]

Lütjohann et al[60] reported elevated plasma 24S-hydroxycholesterol concentrations in AD patients compared to controls. However, it can be hypothesized that CSF 24S-hydroxycholesterol may be a more appropriate indicator of cholesterol turnover in the brain than its plasma concentration because plasma 24S-hydroxycholesterol levels are strongly influenced by hepatic clearance.[61]

In order to confirm this hypothesis we investigated CSF 24S-hydroxycholesterol levels in 25 AD patients and 19 healthy controls. Fourteen samples from AD patients and 10 from controls with plasma cholesterol levels in the normal range of 150–230 mg/dl were preselected from the original sample. Plasma concentrations of cholesterol were determined by standard enzymatic procedures (Boehringer, Mannheim). CSF and plasma 24S-hydroxycholesterol and CSF cholesterol levels were measured using combined gas chromatography and mass spectrometry.[62]

In the AD patients, CSF 24S-hydroxycholesterol – but not plasma levels – were significantly increased compared to controls. Neither total CSF cholesterol nor total plasma cholesterol levels differed significantly between groups. Repeated analyses with BMI entered as a covariate revealed consistent results. Within the AD group, no significant correlation between 24S-hydroxycholesterol CSF levels and age, age of onset, severity of dementia, BMI nor plasma cholesterol arose. To address potential effects of the ApoE genotype, a two-way analysis of variance with diagnosis and ApoE genotype as independent factors was calculated. Again, a significant effect of diagnosis with significantly increased CSF 24S-hydroxycholesterol values in the AD patients emerged.

Based on this analysis it could be demonstrated that CSF 24S-hydroxycholesterol levels are significantly increased in AD patients compared to controls, and that this effect is not mediated by plasma cholesterol levels since, owing to the preselection of the samples, the latter did not significantly differ between the groups. However, we cannot exclude that high serum cholesterol levels may further enhance this effect. These results facilitate the hypothesis that 24S-hydroxycholesterol CSF concentrations reflect the disease process in AD since an increased brain cholesterol turnover or 24S-hydroxycholesterol metabolism could be associated with an acceleration of β-amyloid release.

17β-ESTRADIOL AND CEREBRAL GLUCOSE METABOLISM

Since neuroimaging studies provide evidence of hormone-related changes in brain areas such as the hippocampus, an area preferentially affected in AD,[8,63] one could hypothesize an association between regional cerebral activity and CSF 17β-estradiol concentrations in female patients with AD. We therefore investigated six female patients with probable AD with CSF 17β-estradiol measurements and positron emission tomography (PET). All patients were postmenopausal and had no history of ERT. Before injection of 225 MBq [^{18}F]2-fluoro-2-deoxy-D-glucose (^{18}F-FDG), blood glucose levels were determined and shown to be < 110 mg/dl in all patients. From 15 minutes before injection until 45 minutes after, patients rested in a quiet room with dimmed lighting. Emission scans over 20 minutes were acquired, followed by the transmission scans over 5 minutes using three [68]Ge line sources. Measurements were obtained with a whole-body body PET system, (ECAT EXACT HR+, CTI, Knoxville, TN, USA), covering 155 mm in the axial field of view (63 transversal slices, thickness of each slices 2.4 mm). Data were acquired in the more sensitive 3D mode without interslice tungsten septa, which was found to be equivalent to the 2D mode for quantification of radioactivities used in the clinical setting. The matrix size was 128 × 128 pixels. Basic image processing was done by MEDx 3.0 (Sensor Systems, Inc), using statistical parametric mapping (SPM).[64] All data were spatially normalized by affine 12-parameter transformation to standard stereotactic space based on the atlas of Talairach and Tournoux.[65] Normalized images were represented on a 78×76×85 matrix and smoothed by a Gaussian filter of 12 mm full width at half maximum (FWHM). Using a multisubject design, correlations were generated to assess the association of regional cerebral glucose metabolism and CSF 17β-estradiol concentration. The cerebral structures were identified by their coordinates according to the Talairach atlas.

The patients' mean age was 70.3 ($\pm$7.7), their mean MMSE score was 20.5 ($\pm$4.0) years and the mean CSF 17β-estradiol concentration was 12.86 pg/ml ($\pm$4.0). SPM analyses revealed a selective significant ($P < 0.001$) correlation between CSF 17β-estradiol concentration and cerebral glucose metabolism in the left hippocampus (Fig. 17.2).[66] This effect was not confounded by age or severity of dementia as

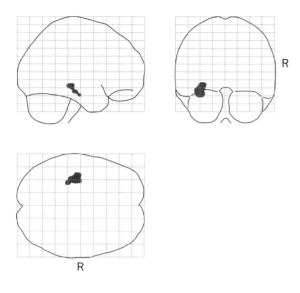

Figure 17.2 Spots indicating significant correlation of left hippocampal glucose metabolism and cerebrospinal fluid 17β-estradiol levels.

measured on MMSE. None of the other variables investigated, such as age, age at onset of disease and MMSE score, were significantly correlated with hippocampal glucose metabolism in the AD patients.

This represents the first clinical study indicating an association between CSF 17β-estradiol concentration and hippocampal glucose metabolism in postmenopausal women with AD. The findings confirm results from recent neuroimaging studies indicating a significant effect of estrogen on the hippocampus, an area physiologically involved in encoding and retrieval, and one affected even in early AD.[63,67] Recently, Maki et al[68] reported increased hippocampal blood flow over time in nondemented women receiving hormone therapy, which is consistent with our results.

Interestingly, we found an association of CSF 17β-estradiol concentration and hippocampal glucose metabolism in the left hemisphere only. This finding is in accordance with a recent study demonstrating unilateral left hemisphere defects of regional cerebral blood flow as measured by single photon emission computed tomography (SPECT) in female AD patients.[69] However, with respect to the small sample size

in our study, the respective findings need to be addressed in further studies. Similarly, in our study, the question remains unresolved as to whether the association between hippocampal glucose metabolism and CSF 17β-estradiol concentration represents a physiologic impact of estrogen on hippocampal activity in postmenopausal women per se or refers to specific estrogen effects on mechanisms which are directly involved in the pathology of the disorder such as Aβ42 release.

CONCLUSIONS

In conclusion, results from the studies discussed above suggest that estrogens may modify the onset and course of AD, at least in subgroups of patients. While the majority of the epidemiological studies indicate that ERT may delay the onset of the disease, results from treatment studies appear to be more controversial. One explanation for this discrepancy may be that optimal levels of 17β-estradiol are needed to maintain brain function but postmenopausal ERT may not restore estrogen homeostasis consistently in all women.

A modest, although significant, reduction of estrogen levels in serum and CSF of women with AD was described in several clinical studies. Again, this effect appeared particularly to strike subgroups of patients. Moreover, 17β-estradiol levels in the CSF were found to be moderately correlated with Aβ42 levels and hippocampal glucose uptake in AD patients.[66] These results have to be weighted against certain methodologic problems (such as the limited sensitivity of the assays available that prevents the exact determination of rather low postmenopausal estrogen levels) as well as against our limited knowledge on CNS effects of different subtypes of estrogen. Accordingly, the question remains unresolved as to whether the beneficial effect of estrogens in AD is mediated by a more global beneficial effect of estrogens on cerebral metabolism or refers to specific estrogen effects on the mechanisms involved in the pathogenesis of the disorder.

Since basic findings of the mechanisms of neurodegenerative disorders suggest at least two phases in their pathogenesis – initiation and propagation – it was hypothesized that estrogens may interact differentially in each phase.[70] Future studies should address the questions of whether the mode of application, required dose and specific type of estrogen may influence ERT effects on initiation and propagation of AD. In addition, the impact of age, early onset and severity of dementia, as well as of long-term treatment, on the potential beneficial effects of ERT need to be considered systematically.

Taken together, there is some evidence from the available studies that estrogens exhibit neurotropic and psychotropic effects in the brain which might enhance our preventive and therapeutic options in AD. However, it is premature to draw definite conclusions until further investigations have been performed.

REFERENCES

1. Halbreich U. Hormonal interventions with psychopharmacological potential: an overview. *Psychopharmacol Bull* 1997; **33**: 281–6.
2. Sherwin BB. Sex hormones and psychological functioning in postmenopausal women. *Exp Gerontol* 1994; **29**: 423–30.
3. Moline ML. Pharmacologic strategies for managing premenstrual syndrome. *Clin Pharm* 1993; **12**: 181–96.
4. Maki PM, Resnick SM. Effects of estrogen on patterns of brain activity at rest and during cognitive activity: a review of neuroimaging studies. *Neuroimage* 2001; **14**: 789–801.
5. Lannert H, Wirtz P, Schuhmann V, Galmbacher R. Effects of estradiol (-17β) on learning, memory and cerebral energy metabolism in male rats after intracerebroventricular administration of streptozotocin. *J Neuronal Transmem* 1998; **105**: 1045–63.
6. Cheng CM, Cohen M, Wang J, Bondy CA. Estrogen augments glucose transporter and IGF1 expression in primate cerebral cortex. FASEB 2001; **15**: 907–15.
7. Herholz K, Salmon E, Perani D et al. Discrimination between Alzheimer dementia and controls by automated analysis of multicenter FDG PET. *Neuroimage* 2002; **1**: 302–16.
8. Pantel J, Schröder J, Schad LR et al. Quantitative magnetic resonance imaging and neuropsychological functions in dementia of the Alzheimer type. *Psychol Med* 1997; **27**: 221–9.
9. Pantel J, Schönknecht P, Essig M et al. Progressive mental temporal lobe changes in Alzheimer's disease revealed by quantitative MRI: potential use for monitoring of drug-related changes. *Drug Development Res* 2002; **56**: 51–6.
10. Pantel J, Kratz B, Essig M et al. Parahippocampal volume deficits in subjects with aging-associated cognitive decline. *Am J Psychiatry* 2003; **160**: 379–82.
11. Schönknecht P, Pantel J, Volkmann M et al. Total and phosphorylated cerebrospinal fluid tau protein in Alzheimer's disease and vascular dementia. *Neurosci Lett* 2003; **339**: 172–4.
12. Henderson VW. The epidemiology of estrogen replacement therapy and Alzheimer's disease. *Neurology* 1997; **48**: 27–35.
13. Lamberts SWJ, van den Beld AW, van der Lely AJ. The endrocinology of aging. *Science* 1997; **278**: 419–24.
14. Tang M, Jacobs D, Stern Y et al. Effect of estrogen during menopause on risk and age at onset of Alzheimer's disease. *Lancet* 1996; **348**: 429–32.
15. Kawas C, Resnick S, Morrison A et al. A prospective study of estrogen replacement therapy and the risk of developing Alzheimer's disease: the Baltimore Longitudinal Study of Aging. *Neurology* 1997; **48**: 1517–21.
16. Honjo H, Ogino Y, Tanaka K et al. An effect of conjugated estrogen to cognitive impairment in women with senile dementia – Alzheimer's type: a placebo controlled, double-blind study. *J Jpn Menopause Soc* 1993; **1**: 167–71.
17. Fillit H. Estrogens in the pathogenesis and treatment of Alzheimer's disease in postmenopausal women. *Ann NY Acad Sci* 1994; **743**: 233–8.
18. Mulnard RA, Cotman CW, Kawas C et al. Estrogen replacement therapy for treatment of mild to moderate Alzheimer's disease: a randomized controlled trial. *JAMA* 2000; **283**: 1007–15.
19. Henderson VW, Paganini-Hill A, Miller BL et al. Estrogen for Alzheimer's disease in woman: randomized, double-blind, placebo-controlled trial. *Neurology* 1997; **54**: 295–301.
20. Wang P, Liao S, Liu R et al. Effects of estrogen on cognition, mood, and cerebral blood flow in AD. *Neurology* 2000; **54**: 2061–6.
21. Asthana A, Baker LD, Craft S et al. High-dose estradiol improves cognition for women with AD. *Neurology* 2001; **57**: 605–12.
22. Asthana S, Craft S, Baker LD et al. Cognitive

and neuroendocrine response to transdermal estrogen in postmenopausal woman with Alzheimer's disease: results of a placebo-controlled, double-blind, pilot study. *Psychoneuroendocrinology* 1999; **24:** 657–77.

23. Schönknecht P, Pantel J, Hartmann T et al. Cerebrospinal fluid tau levels in Alzheimer's disease are elevated when compared to vascular dementia but do not correlate with measures of cerebral atrophy. *Psychiatry Res* 2003; **120:** 231–8.

24. Haass C, Selkoe DJ. Cellular processing of β-amyloid precursor protein and genesis of the amyloid-β peptide. *Cell* 1993; **75:** 1039–42.

25. Jensen M, Schröder J, Blomberg M. et al. Cerebrospinal fluid A beta 42 is increased early in sporadic Alzheimer's disease and declines with disease progression. *Ann Neurol* 1999; **45:** 504–11.

26. Beyreuther K, Multhaupt G, Masters CL. Molecular neuropathology in the causation of Alzheimer's disease. In: (Stefanis C, Hippius H, eds) *Neuropsychiatry in Old Age: An Update.* (Hofgrefe and Huber Publishers: Seattle, Göttingen, 1996) 43–54.

27. Pantel J, Schröder J, Essig M et al. Quantitative magnetic resonance imaging in geriatric depression and primary degenerative dementia. *J Affect Disord* 1997; **42:** 69–83.

28. Schröder J, Pantel J, Ida N et al. Cerebral changes and cerebrospinal fluid-amyloid in Alzheimer's disease: a study with quantitative magnetic resonance imaging. *Molec Psychiatry* 1997; **2:** 505–7.

29. Schröder J, Pantel J. Morphologische und funktionelle Bildgebung. In: (Förstl H, ed) *Alzheimer Demenz.* (Springer: Berlin, 1999.)

30. Henderson V. Estrogen replacement therapy for the prevention and treatment of Alzheimer's disease. *CNS Drugs* 1997; **8:** 343–51.

31. Woolley CS, McEwen BS. Estradiol regulates hippocampal dendritic spine density via an N-methyl-D-aspartate receptor-dependent mechanism. *J Neurosci* 1994; **14:** 7680–7.

32. Lustig RH. Sex hormone modulation of neural development in vitro. *Hormone Behav* 1994; **28:** 383–95.

33. Ohkura T, Isse K, Akazawa K. et al. Long-term estrogen replacement therapy in female patients with dementia of the Alzheimer type: 7 case reports. *Dementia* 1995; **6:** 99–107.

34. Bishop J, Simpkins JW. Role of estrogens in peripheral and cerebral glucose utilization. *Rev Neurosci* 1992; **3:** 121–37.

35. Luine V. Estradiol increases choline acetyltransferase activity in specific basal forebrain nuclei and projection areas of female rats. *Exp Neurol* 1985; **89:** 484–90.

36. Urabe M, Yamamoto T, Kashiwagi T et al. Effect of estrogen replacement therapy on hepatic triglyceride lipase, lipoprotein lipase and lipids including apolipoprotein E in climacteric and elderly women. *Endocr J* 1996; **43:** 737–42.

37. Jaffe AB, Torna-Allerand CD, Greengard P, Gandy SE. Estrogen regulates metabolism of Alzheimer amyloid β precursor protein. *J Biol Chem* 1994; **269:** 13,065–8.

38. Xu H, Gouras GK, Greenfield JP et al. Estrogen reduces neuronal generation of Alzheimer β-amyloid peptides. *Nat Med* 1998; **4:** 447–51.

39. Petanceska S, Nagy V, Frail D, Gandy S. Ovariectomy and 17β-estradiol modulate the levels of Alzheimer's amyloid peptides in brain. *Neurology* 2000; **54:** 2212–17.

40. Mooradian AD. Antioxidant properties of steroids. *J Steroid Biochem Molec Biol* 1993; **45:** 509–11.

41. Behl C, Skutella T, Lezoualch F et al. Neuroprotection against oxidative stress by estrogens: structure-activity relationship. *Molec Pharmacol* 1997; **51:** 535–41.

42. Manly JJ, Merchant CA, Jacobs DM et al. Endogenous estrogen levels and Alzheimer's disease among postmenopausal women. *Neurology* 2000; **54:** 833–7.

43. Honjo H, Ogino Y, Naitoh K et al. In vivo effects by estrone sulfate on the central nervous system-senile dementia (Alzheimer's Type). *J Steroid Biochem* 1989; **34:** 521–5.

44. Senanarong V, Vannasaeng S, Poungvarin N et al. Endogenous estradiol in elderly individuals. *Arch Neurol* 2002; **59:** 385–9.

45. Folstein MF, Folstein SE, McHugh PR. Minimental state: a practical method for grading the cognitive state of patients for the clinician. *Psychiatry Res* 1975; **12:** 189–98.

46. Hogervorst E, Smith D. The interaction of serum folate and estradiol levels in Alzheimer's disease. *Neuroendocr Lett* 2002; **23:** 155–60.

47. Cunningham CJ, Sinnott M, Denihan A et al. Endogenous sex hormone levels in postmenopausal women with Alzheimer's disease. *J Clin Endocr Metab* 2001; **86:** 1099–103.

48. Yaffe K, Grady D, Pressman A, Cummings S. Serum estrone levels, cognitive performance, and risk of cognitive decline in older community women. *J Am Geriatr Soc* 1998; **46:** 816–21.

49. Lim SK, Won YJ, Lee JH et al. Altered hydroxylation of estrogen in patients with postmenopausal osteopenia. *J Clin Endoc Metab* 1997; **82:** 1001–6.

50. Vandewalle B, Lefebvre J. Opposite effects of estrogen and catecholestrogen on hormone-sensitive breast cancer cell growth and differentiation. *Molec Cell Endocr* 1989; **61:** 239–46.

51. Schneider J, Huh MM, Bradlow HL, Fishman J. Antiestrogen action of 2-hydroxyestrone on MCF-7 human breast cells. *J Biol Chem* 1984; **259:** 4840–5.

52. Molnár G, Kassai-Bazsa Z. Gonadotropin, ACTH, prolactin, sexual steroid and cortisol levels in postmenopausal women's cerebrospinal fluid (CSF). *Arch Gerontol Geriatr* 1997; **24:** 269–80.

53. McKhann G, Drachman D, Folstein M et al. Clinical diagnosis of Alzheimer's disease: report of the NINCDS–ADRDA work group under the auspices of Department of Health and Human Services Task Force on Alzheimer's disease. *Neurology* 1984; **34:** 939–44.

54. Schönknecht P, Pantel J, Klinga K et al. Reduced cerebrospinal fluid estradiol levels are associated with increased β-amyloid levels in female patients with Alzheimer's disease. *Neurosci Lett* 2001; **307:** 122–4.

55. Ida N, Hartmann T, Pantel J et al. Analysis of heterogeneous βA4 peptides in cerebrospinal fluid and blood by a newly developed sensitive Western blot assay. *J Biol Chem* 1996; **271:** 22,908–14.

56. Schönknecht P, Pantel J, Klinga K et al. Cerebrospinal fluid estradiol and β-amyloid levels in female patients with Alzheimer's disease. *Euro Psychiatry* 2002; **17:** 41s.

57. Fassbender K, Simons M, Bergmann C et al. Simvastatin strongly reduces levels of Alzheimer's disease beta-amyloid peptides Abeta 42 and Abeta 40 in vitro and in vivo *Proc Natl Acad Sci USA* 2001; **98:** 5371–3.

58. Lütjohann D, Breuer O, Ahlborg G et al. Cholesterol homeostasis in human brain: evidence for an age-dependent flux of 24S-hydroxycholesterol from the brain into the circulation. Proc Natl Acad Sci *USA* 1996; **93:** 9799–804.

59. Björkhem I, Lütjohann D, Breuer O et al. Importance of a novel oxidative mechanism for elimination of brain cholesterol. Turnover of cholesterol and 24(S)-hydroxycholesterol in rat brain as measured with 1802 techniques in vivo and in vitro. *J Biol Chem* 1997; **272:** 30,178–84.

60. Lütjohann D, Papassotiropoulos A, Björkhem I. et al. Plasma 24S-hydroxycholesterol (cerebrosterol) is increased in Alzheimer and vascular demented patients. *J Lipid Res* 2000; **41:** 195–8.

61. Bretillon L, Lütjohann D, Stahle L et al. Plasma levels of 24S-hydroxycholesterol reflect the balance between cerebral production and hepatic metabolism and are inversely related to body surface. *J Lipid Res* 2000; **41:** 840–5.

62. Dzeletovic S, Breuer O, Lund E, Diczfalusy U. Determination of cholesterol oxidation products in human plasma by isotope dilution mass spectrometry. *Annal Biochem* 1995; **225:** 73–80.

63. Schröder J, Buchsbaum MS, Shihabuddin L et al. Patterns of cortical activity and memory performance in Alzheimer's disease. *Biol Psychiatry* 2001; **49:** 426–36.

64. Friston KJ, Holmes AP, Worsley KJ et al. Statistical parametric maps in functional imaging: a general linear approach. *Hum Brain Mapp* 1995; **2:** 189–210.

65. Talairach JA, Tournoux P. *Co-planar Stereotaxic Atlas of the Human Brain.* (Thieme: Paris, 1988.)

66. Schönknecht P, Henze M, Hunt A et al. Cerebrospinal fluid estrogen levels are associated with hippocampal glucose metabolism. *Psychiatry Res: Neuroimaging* 2003; **124:** 125–7.

67. Schachter DL, Curran T, Reiman EM et al. Medial temporal lobe activation during episodic encoding and retrieval: a PET study. *Hippocampus* 1999; **9:** 575–81.

68. Maki PM, Resnick SM. Longitudinal effects of estrogen replacement therapy on PET cerebral blood flow and cognition. *Neurobiol Aging* 2000; **21:** 373–83.

69. Ott BR, Heindl WC, Tan Z, Noto RB. Lateralized cortical perfusion in woman with Alzheimer's disease. *J Gend Specif Med* 2000; **3:** 29–35.

70. Johnson JK, McCleary R, Oshita MH, Cotman CW. Initiation and propagation stages of beta-amyloid are associated with distinctive apolipoprotein E, age, and gender profiles. *Brain Res* 1998; **798:** 18–24.

18

Sexuality in postmenopause and senium

A Graziottin

Introduction • Classifications of female sexual dysfunctions (FSD) • Sexual desire disorders
• Sexual arousal disorders • Orgasmic disorders • Sexual pain disorders • New perspectives
• Conclusions • References

INTRODUCTION

'All passion spent.' The transition from the fertile age, the age of passion, to the passionless late senium, as Vita Sackville West gently describes it in her novel, can be abrupt or gradual. Biological, psychosexual and context-dependent factors may all modulate the emotional and sexual transition, and the perception that women and couples have. Of these three factors, the biological ones may cause the most abrupt decline of women's sexuality. This is particularly the case when the loss of hormones, typical of the menopause (especially when iatrogenic), is not addressed with appropriate and individually tailored hormonal replacement therapy (HRT), and/or when gynecologic or pelvic surgery further reduces the vaginal receptiveness both in anatomical and functional ways. Psychosexual and context-dependent factors, however, may have longer evolutions. Thus the challenge for the clinician is the appropriate diagnosis made by consideration of the most important interacting variables.

Female sexual dysfunction (FSD) is indeed a multicausal and multidimensional problem. It is age related, progressive and highly prevalent, affecting 20–45% of women.[1,2] For many women it is physically disconcerting, emotionally dis-

tressing and socially disruptive.[3] The media-genic emphasis on high-caliber sexual performances further increases the gap between an individual's reality and expectation of full sexual satisfaction. At the same time, the increasing discrepancy between the biological age and the age one feels psychologically and emotionally increases the expectations about a high quality of life, inclusive of sexuality, until the late decades of life. The physician is therefore increasingly requested to be competent in giving appropriate therapeutic answers when FSD is complained of: unfortunately, the general lack of a formal training makes this task particularly difficult.

The purpose of this chapter, therefore, is to offer a clinical approach to FSD for physicians working with peri- and postmenopausal women. The aim is threefold: (1) to help them to feel more comfortable in addressing the patient's request for a rigorous diagnosis and treatment of her sexual complaint, when biologically based; (2) to correctly refer her to a competent specialist – e.g. psychosexologist, couple therapist, psychotherapist, psychiatrist – when the FSD seems to depend more on psychodynamic and/or interpersonal factors, and/or referral of the partner to the uroandrologist if there is a specific male sexual disorder (MSD), secondarily inducing FSD; (3) to effectively improve doctor–patient communication. By asking about sexuality, the health care provider informs the patient that it is appropriate to openly discuss these issues in the medical setting and validates an older woman's self-perception as a sexual being. Otherwise, it is hard to provide an effective intervention if there is no mention of a problem!

CLASSIFICATIONS OF FEMALE SEXUAL DYSFUNCTIONS (FSD)

Classifications of FSD have varied among different diagnostic systems.[4,5] According to the World Health Organization (WHO) International Classifications of Diseases–10 (ICD–10), the definition of sexual dysfunction includes 'the various ways in which an individual is unable to participate in a sexual relationship as he or she would wish'.[4] The Diagnostic and Statistical Manual of Mental Disorders (DSM-IV) of the American Psychiatric Association defines sexual dysfunctions as 'disturbances in sexual desire and in the psychophysiological changes that characterize the sexual response cycle and cause marked distress and interpersonal difficulty'.[5] Unfortunately, this persistent focus on the mental, nonorganic side of FSD contributed to a substantial lack of attention to the potential biological basis of these disorders for many years.

The recently convened International Consensus Development Conference on Female Sexual Dysfunction[3] expanded nosographic criteria, with contributions from an interdisciplinary consensus conference panel consisting of 19 world experts in FSD. Leading disorders were classified as:

(1) sexual desire disorders:
   (a) hypoactive sexual desire disorder;
   (b) sexual aversion disorders;
(2) sexual arousal disorders;
(3) orgasmic disorders;
(4) sexual pain disorders:
   (a) dyspareunia;
   (b) vaginismus;
   (c) other sexual pain disorders.

Further subtyping differentiates the diagnosis of FSD according to: (1) the *temporal onset*: lifelong versus acquired; (2) the *context-dependent dynamic*: generalized versus situational; (3) the *etiology*: classified as organic, psychogenic, mixed, unknown. In comparison to previous classifications, the latter is the principal change, as it enables an exploration of the biological side of FSD for a full diagnosis mandatory. This acknowledges that, for women as well as for men, a healthy, functional body is a necessity, although not a sufficient condition, for a satisfying sexual response, particularly around and after the menopause, when a number of biological factors – endocrine, vascular, metabolic, muscular, neurological, connective and immunitary – may affect the general health and combine to worsen the physical potential of a full sexual response.[6] This certainly does not refute the importance of intimacy and love issues, and of psychodynamic and interpersonal factors, that seem to be more critical in contributing to sexual satisfaction in women,[2,6–8] but puts them in perspective in relation to the biological scenario.[6]

Definition of different FSD and paying attention to the subtyping may help the clinician in correctly approaching the complaint(s). In this diagnostic path, special attention should be paid to medical etiologies that are more relevant in the postmenopausal years, whilst psychodynamic and/or relational issues will be only mentioned briefly.

SEXUAL DESIRE DISORDERS

Definition

(1) 'Hypoactive sexual desire disorder is the persistent or recurrent deficiency (or absence) of sexual fantasies/thoughts, and/or desire for or receptivity to sexual activity, which causes personal distress.'[3]
(2) 'Sexual aversion disorder is the persistent or recurrent phobic aversion to and avoidance of sexual contact with a sexual partner, which causes personal distress.'[3]

'. . . Sexual fantasies/thoughts, and/or desire . . .' stresses the importance of mental activity dedicated to anticipating, dreaming about and/or fantasizing about sexual encounters. In women, this is more typical of the first months or years of a relationship. In stable, long-lasting relationships between couples many women report that the leading motivation to sex is the intimacy need, which may then trigger the sexual response leading to increased willingness to be receptive to the partner's initiative.[7,8] Receptivity specifically addresses the issue of female willingness to have intercourse. However, this attitude may be biologically crippled, among others, by postmenopausal exacerbation of vaginal dryness, unless the woman is on HRT.[6,9] The dryness may cause discomfort until dyspareunia arises, that may secondarily cause a loss of libido. This simple example addresses three points: the frequent overlapping, or comorbidity, of different FSD; the usefulness of a circular model where different moments of the physiologic response are interconnected and may explain positive or negative feedbacks (Fig. 18.1);[6] the need for the clinical history to differentiate which disorder appeared first and which appeared subsequently.

'Sexual aversion ...', with the key word 'phobic', indicates that the FSD has a strong unconscious basis. It is usually accompanied by neurovegetative symptoms of various intensities, e.g. tachypnea, tachycardia, sweating and/or increased muscular tension, with a subjective feeling of fear and anguish, that sometimes may be also evoked by gynecologic examination. The phobic reaction induces the '... avoidance of sexual contact' to avoid the unpleasant feeling of anguish.

The 'personal distress' criterion strongly suggests that the woman herself has to be sufficiently motivated to seek treatment because she is personally disturbed by the FSD in order to classify the disorder as a true FSD and to commence with clinical treatment.

Prevalence

Hypoactive sexual desire disorder is the most frequently complained of FSD. Population data indicate a prevalence of 33% in women between the ages of 18 and 59,[1] which may reach 45% in

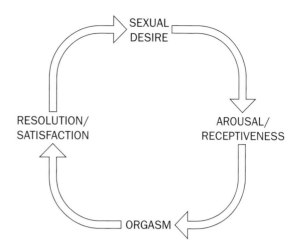

Figure 18.1 This model, formulated by the presenting author, contributes to the understanding of: 1) frequent overlapping of sexual symptoms reported in clinical practice, as different dimensions of sexual response are correlated from a physiopathologic point of view; 2) potential negative or positive feedback mechanisms operating in sexual function.

The model also addresses two critical aspects: a) the 'specificity' of receptiveness, as the female characteristic of sex drive and arousal, when coitus is involved. In this sense, dyspareunia could be considered not only a pain symptom but a specific receptiveness disorder; b) the importance of the human dimension of 'satisfaction', that goes beyond the physiologic phase of resolution and encompasses both physical and emotional correlates of the erotic experience.

The clinician should therefore be alerted to potential problems in any critical component of sexual function, particularly from the medical point of view, to make appropriate differential diagnosis and suggest best medical, psychosexual and/or couple therapy.

This model may be more typical in the early phase of a new relationship, when physical and emotional components of sex drive concur to enhance the sexual function; after physical or emotional distancing; in the few days postovulation for women premenopausally, who are sensitive to the increase in testosterone that occurs at ovulation; in the immediate postmenopause of women with previous polycystic ovary syndrome, who may have an increased androgen production in response to the increased level of LH; in case of androgen replacement therapy (ART), more so when supraphysiologic doses are given. The model of R. Basson (Fig. 18.2) is more fitting the arousal dynamic in a stable couple, when need for intimacy may be the leading force. (Modified from Graziottin[6] with permission.)

clinical samples, particularly after the menopause,[2,9] although figures vary greatly among studies due to methodological biases.[2,10] Unbiased prevalence estimates from population samples are rare and incidence estimates are nonexistent.[3]

Physiologic scenario

Sexual desire indicates sexual appetite, which then motivates a person to sexual activity and focuses his/her attention on that goal.[6,11-13] The basic drive is biologically rooted in the instinctual rhinecephalic and limbic brain, which is strongly hormone dependent,[6,11-14] and represents the core of sexual behavior. Androgens are the leading hormones that trigger sex drive

in women and men.[6,13-23] In humans the biological drive is progressively enriched by emotional and affective meanings,[7,8,15-18] the need for intimacy first seems to be particularly relevant to women.[2,7,8] The subjective experience of being 'turned on' is accompanied by, and partly consists of, various physiologic changes, many of which are in preparation for sexual behavior.[6,11] This sexually activated mental state may be countered and influenced by the mood of the moment,[6-8,11,15,16] more so in the perimenopausal transition when mood disorders may rebound on and cripple libido,[6,7,13,15] despite the availability of a willing partner. Factor analysis helps to put into perspective the many factors that co-occur and thus modulate sexual activity during the menopausal transition (Table 18.1).[2]

Table 18.1 Sexual activity outcomes identified by factor analysis (*n* = 200 women)

Outcome	Mean (standard deviation) or percentage	No.	Range
Satisfaction with sexual relationship	23.2 (4.7)	6	6–30
Sexual desire	10.0 (4.1)	3	0–20
Frequency of sexual intercourse	58.2 (50.9)	1	0–364
Arousal compared to when in the 40s			
Less now	39.0%		
Same now	52.0%		
More now	9.0%		
Difficulty reaching orgasm			
Never	25.0%		
Seldom	37.8%		
Sometimes	22.2%		
Usually/always	15.0%		
Pain during intercourse			
Never	77.5%		
Seldom/always	22.5%		

Women reported a quite high average satisfaction with their sexual relationship (mean of 23.2 on a scale ranging from 6 to 30), a mean frequency of intercourse of once a week, an average reduction of desire by 50% (mean of 10 on a scale ranging from 0 to 20), reduction in arousal of 39%, difficulties in orgasm by 37.2 of them (although no comparison is reported for that parameter with respect to premenopause), whilst pain is complained of by 22.5%. A trend towards a reduction in all aspects of sexual function is reported. Menopause is significantly associated to lower sexual desire and decreased arousal. In multiple regression analysis, other factors such as health, marital status (or new partner), mental health and smoking had a greater impact on women's sexual functioning than menopause status. (Adapted from Avis et al,[2] with permission.)

Menopause may represent a critical turning point of sexual desire, as biological,[6,9,13,17–23] motivational-affective and cognitive factors[7,8,15,16] may all undergo significant changes. With menopause comes the loss of the primary biological goal, i.e. reproduction; therefore, the motivation for intercourse may well remain the pursuit of pleasure, recreational sex[13] as well as instrumental sex, when intercourse is performed as a means to obtain advantages and express motivations different from pleasure and/or procreation.[6–8,18,24] In stable and aging couples, intimacy needs are increasingly reported to be the leading motivation for intercourse (Fig. 18.2),[2,7,8] particularly after the menopause, when many women report that the coital experience gradually loses its central character whilst more tender behavior, like holding, caressing and hugging, become more and more gratifying.

When the etiology of the hypoactive sex drive appears to be mainly biological and related to the menopause, HRT may well improve sex drive, through direct and indirect mechanisms.[17–31] Directly, it may restore central and peripheral neuroendocrine sexual pathways leading to a better physical response.[17–22,25–27,29,30] Indirectly, well-adjusted HRT may also improve insomnia, mood disorders, anxiety and thus the general perception of wellbeing in some women. Poor health and psychologic disturbances may contribute further to a loss in sexual drive,[2,6] and to the inability to respond to former sexual cues.[7,8] HRT may be the treatment of choice when the main complaint is female androgen deficiency syndrome,[25] secondary to bilateral ovariectomy and characterized by loss of libido, loss of assertiveness, loss of vital energy (that may mimic, but which is not, depression), loss of pubic hair, reduced muscle mass, plus changes in body image due to the increase in centripetal fat.

Diagnostic work-up

When a woman complains of FSD in the perimenopause and late postmenopause, the very first step for the clinician is to define the complaint with a number of appropriate

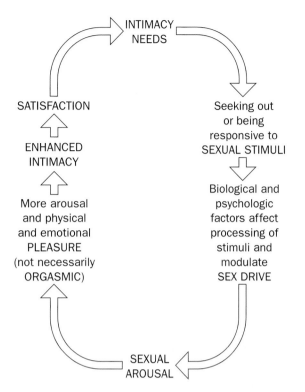

Figure 18.2 Alternative model of the female sex response cycle. This model focuses on the priority of intimacy needs, as the motivational leading force of female receptivity. The entities of intimacy (as a driving force) and sexual stimuli do not feature in the traditional cycle of Masters and Johnson[24] revisited in Fig. 18.1. According to Rosemary Basson's model,[7,8] that seems to be predominant in long lasting relationships and after the menopause, the woman senses an opportunity to be sexual, starting from a state of sexual neutrality. She may be motivated to respond to her partner's initiative, primarily because her intimacy with the partner will be thereby enhanced. This motivation may also be aided by the expectation that although she has no sexual hunger currently, the experience is likely to become physically as well as emotionally pleasurable, provided that no major biological factors are preventing or crippling it. If the physical and emotional outcome is positive, the couple intimacy is enhanced, with increasing satisfaction of sense of commitment, bonding, tolerance of each other's imperfections, caring and affection.[8] This model also stresses the dependence of female sexuality on male initiative in the majority of long lasting stable couples: marital status, satisfaction with the current relationship, partner's general and sexual health are reported to be among the strongest predictors of postmenopausal female sexual activity.[2,41] (Adapted from Basson[8] with permission.)

Box 18.1   Short form of a sexual history

How do you feel?

Are you currently sexually active?

If no, is that fine for you?

If yes, how's your sex life? Do you have a stable relationship?

If your sex life is dissatisfying, what's the main complaint you have?

Is it a desire disorder (are you still interested in sex)?

Do you feel an arousal/lubrication disorder with vaginal dryness?

Do you have increasing difficulties in getting orgasm?

Do you feel pain during or after intercourse? Or do you suffer from cystitis 24–72 hours after intercourse?

If you have one or more of these disorders, have they been lifelong or did they appear or worsen after the menopause?

How's your couple relationship, and your partner's general and sexual health?

Do you feel that your sexual problem is more dependent on physical or couple problems?

Are you personally interested in improving your sex life?

---

questions[15,17] and proper examination. A short form of sexual history is reported in Box 18.1. In the paper an extended version is discussed, to offer the reader the opportunity to build up a diagnostic detailed and meaningful clinical reasoning. Since loss of sex drive is the most frequently reported complaint, it will be discussed in greater detail as an example of wording on FSD and sexual wellbeing. A useful set of questions follows.

(1) *When did you notice this change in your sex drive? Have you always suffered from a low libido* [lifelong] *or has your libido fallen recently* [acquired] *? If acquired, was this loss coincidental with, or did it appear after the menopause?* These questions help to differentiate between long-lasting hypoactive sexual desire, which may well have more psychodynamic and interpersonal etiologies, from the disorder acquired around the menopause, which may be more related to hormonal changes,[17–26] particularly if the woman associates the change with the immediate period after ovariectomy (with or without hysterectomy).[18,19,25] *Is it the only disorder you feel, or do you also feel vaginal dryness,*[6,13,17] *have difficulties in lubrication*[32,33] *and/or orgasm?*[30] *Do you feel pain during and/or after intercourse?*[27,28,34] These questions help to diag-

nose comorbidity (Fig. 18.1), to establish the triggering and leading disorder (i.e. dyspareunia may cause secondary loss of libido), and to address treatment multidimensionally.

(2) *Is the loss of your sex drive generalized, that is, do you not feel any sexual interest in any situation or towards anybody, or is it limited to your current partner or to a specific situation* [situational]? The generalized loss addresses more biological and/or personal factors (hormonal menopausal loss, problems of hypoandrogenism,[18,19,20–23,25] depression,[2,12,13,18] phobic attitude towards sexual contacts, not feeling attractive any more). The situational loss immediately focuses the attention on interpersonal etiologies (marital crisis,[2] loss of love and intimacy,[7,8,15,16,18] and/or partner's problems, either physical or sexual[2,18,35,36]). It indicates more likely context-dependent etiologies. The referral of the male partner to the uroandrologist may be essential when the female problem (the symptom carrier) is induced by a persistent male problem, mostly erection disorder (ED) (the symptom inducer), not yet referred to the clinician.[35,36] From the initial occurrence of ED, usually there is a lag time of months or years before a man seeks medical help. In this long interval, full of reactive depression, frustration, anger, shame, heavy

silences and loss of emotional and physical intimacy, up to 62% of female partners report a dysfunctional sexuality, namely loss of libido and arousal difficulties, that may interact with biological factors, thus contributing to worsening the sexual drive and the sexual response.[35,36]

(3) *What has been the average frequency of intercourse in the last 6 months, and who usually initiates the intercourse?* Average reported frequency is once per week[2,18,24] in the perimenopausal sexually active group: the real frequency roughly indicates how deeply the female loss of sex drive may have affected the sexual relationship.

(4) *Are you satisfied with your current relationship? Do you feel that this loss of libido might be more dependent on psychological or couple problems?* According to Avis et al,[2] in multiple regression analysis, personal health, marital status (or new partner), mental health and smoking all have a greater impact on sexual functioning than menopause per se when perimenopausal women are studied (Table 1). Bachman and Leiblum[18] reported similar findings in women in their 60s. Both studies describe a gradual decline both in sexual interest and arousal after the menopause in half of the subjects on average, in spite of marital satisfaction, probably due to the loss of sexual hormones and age-related changes. However, the maintenance of all sexual parameters is definitely better in sexually active postmenopausal women when compared to the abstinent ones: the former report higher levels of sexual desire ($P < 0.03$), greater sexual satisfaction ($P < 0.007$), more comfort in expressing sexual preferences ($P < 0.009$), greater premenopausal sexual satisfaction ($P < 0.01$) and less genital atrophy ($P < 0.0005$).[18] The availability of a secure and loving relationship with a functional partner may counter and attenuate the biological trend towards a decrease in sexual response, both from the physical point of view and motivationally, i.e. maintaining receptiveness.[2,18,32,33] Trophic factors and neuromediators released in response to arousal may co-occur to partially maintain the genital trophism and functionality

in spite of the loss of ovarian hormones.[32] Single women, a cohort that increases dramatically with increasing age,[17] report suffering more from loneliness and frustration due to lack of intimacy (holding, hugging, tenderness) than from the loss of eroticism per se. However, physicians should be warned not to involuntarily provoke an iatrogenic increase in sexual drive, which would further frustrate these women, with inappropriate hormonal treatment with androgens and androgen-derived drugs.

(5) *Focusing on your libido, do you have erotic dreams, sexual day dreams and/or voluntary sexual fantasies?* If yes, this indicates a good hormonal profile (if the woman is on HRT, this indicates optimal androgenic balance,[18–25,29] as well a substantial integrity of the mental sexual processes). However, only half of postmenopausal women report maintenance of[2,18] or even an increase (9%) in sexual desire and erotic dreams.[2,18] Some studies correlate this increase to higher free testosterone levels,[18–22] although this is not confirmed by others.[2]

(6) *Do you prefer sexual contacts to be noncoitus oriented, or only tender and loving, with physical intimacy without overt sexual meanings?* This question, useful when the woman reports aversion to sexual contact, may suggest a phobic attitude towards intercourse, and/or sexual pain-related disorders (dyspareunia, vaginismus, postcoital cystitis, clitoralgia, either spontaneous or after arousal and congestion) and genital inflammations that should be looked for (vestibulitis, vaginitis, vulvitis,),[27,28] as they all may cause a secondary loss of libido due to pain. In many other cases, particularly in elderly patients, awareness of intimacy needs and progressive lack of motivation to coitus may shift the intercourse to tenderness. This adjustment may be perfect for the woman (not causing personal distress, indeed) and causing disappointment and frustration in the partner. A couple therapist may help the partners to address the different expectations, i.e. the need for intimacy for her and the need for arousal for him, in a constructive and loving way.

(7) *Is there any autoerotic activity, with orgasm?* If yes, this indicates sufficient hormonal levels, good libido, good perception of one's body and lack of inhibition (but when compulsive it may indicate psychosexual and/or psychiatric problems). However, particularly in single women, negative guilty feelings, which an understanding doctor can address and relieve, may be an issue.[17]

The clinician should be comfortable with these quite intimate questions, choosing the ones he/she feels most at ease with. If the clinical history suggests a possible *biological etiology*, the gynecologist should undertake the following.

(1) *Assess the patient's hormonal equilibrium.* The most common situations are as follows.

(a) *The woman is naturally menopausal and is not taking HRT.* Well-tailored HRT usually restores premenopausal sexuality[18–23,29,37–41] if other negative biological, personal or relational factors are not involved.

(b) *The woman has undergone surgical menopause.* Her loss of libido typically has a sudden onset, within the first months after bilateral oophorectomy, that on average deprives the woman of 50% of her androgen production.[18–23,25] Androgen replacement therapy (ART) increases libido in women who are androgen deficient (e.g. after surgical menopause)[18–23,25] but it does not seem to affect sexual arousal and behavior in naturally menopausal women.[21] That is, physiologic replacement of deficient plasmatic levels may restore libido, whilst supplementation to supraphysiologic levels does not (but it may increase side effects which are likely to be dose dependent). Androgens could have a threefold action: (i) increase susceptibility to psychosexual stimulation, contributing to the sexually activated mental state, typical of a good libido;[11,12,14,23–25,29,39,40] (ii) increase sensitivity of the external genitalia, facilitating the nitric oxide pathways that leads to clitoral congestion;[30,38] (iii) increase the intensity of sexual gratification.[22,25,29] In the study of Shifren et al[40] it was shown that transdermal testosterone treatment in women with impaired sexual function after oophorectomy significantly improved sexual function – desire, arousal, frequency of sexual activity and pleasure, and psychologic wellbeing – with better scores with the higher dose (300 μg/day of testosterone transdermally) in comparison to the smaller one (150 μg/day testosterone transdermally) and placebo. Topical testosterone cream is an approved treatment for vulvar lichen sclerosus.[19,30] It has been claimed to improve clitoral sensitivity, heighten arousal and ease clitoral orgasm, thus leading to a higher sexual satisfaction that might enhance libido, but controlled studies are still lacking to the present author's knowledge.

(c) *The woman is on HRT, reports a reasonably good couple adjustment with no changes after the menopause and yet she complains of loss of libido.* Prolactin assessment is advised, as a persistent prolactin increase has an inhibiting effect on libido, and on the sexual cascade of neurovegetative and vascular responses via the dopaminergic system.[14] A precise inquiry about antidepressant use, particularly the selective serotonin reuptake inhibitors (SSRI), is mandatory as they may have a specific inhibitory effect on sex drive.[26] Sex hormone-binding globulin (SHBG) levels should be checked, together with free testosterone levels, as oral HRT may increase it, causing a lowering of free testosterone.[11,19] In women with conserved ovaries, another recent study by Kokçu et al[29] suggested that tibolone, thanks to its androgenic properties, offers a better impact on female sexual performance [sexual desire ($P < 0.001$) and coital frequency, ($P = 0.014$)] in comparison to conjugated estrogen–medroxyprogesterone acetate therapy (which improves subjective wellbeing, vasomotor symptoms and vaginal dryness, but not sex drive and coital frequency).

In summary, evidence suggests that *hormones, in their complex interplay, seem to control the intensity of libido and sexual behavior, rather than its direction,*[15] which is more dependent on motivational-affective and cognitive factors.[7,8,15,16] Estrogens contribute to the maintenance of secondary sex characters, to the central and peripheral scenario of femininity, that can be enhanced by appropriate levels of androgens,[18–23,25,29,39,40] while prolactin may inhibit the physiologic cascade of events involved in the sexual response.[14] However, consensus on the prominent role of sexual hormones has not been reached so far,[2,18,33,41] as other factors, e.g. health, quality of premenopausal sex life and marital status, seem to be the leading ones for other researchers.

(2) Assess the trophism of the pelvic floor structures
Negative feedback from the genitals, because of poor arousal secondary to vulvovaginal dystrophia, dyspareunia[27] and/or vulvodynia,[30] orgasmic difficulties either as a result of clitoral involution and/or hypotonic pelvic floor,[17,34] may secondarily cause or contribute to a further loss of sex drive.

(3) Assess potential drug-dependent FSD
Addiction (alcohol and smoking primarily) may contribute to FSD and their potential roles should be investigated.[2,6] Particularly in the elderly, the probability of chronic multidrug treatment for ongoing multiple pathologies is increasingly likely. The possibility of a specific negative effect of different diseases and drugs on the human sexual response is currently being intensively investigated and should be considered carefully in each individual patient complaining of acquired FSD.[6,11,14,17,26]

(4) Assess relationship factors
Relationship factors, implications about the quality of a couple's relationship,[7,8] the partner's attitudes and problems, e.g. erectile deficit[35,36] and his real desirability,[6] may further modulate the intensity and direction of sexual desire and contribute to the contradictory findings in the variability of libido in the perimenopausal years.[10,41] Male sexual disorders, that increase dramatically with age, may cause dysfunctional FSD in up to 62% of partners according to Renshaw.[35] This long-lasting dissatisfaction may further contribute to female loss of desire[36] until complete sexual inactivity, at least with that partner, is reached.

SEXUAL AROUSAL DISORDERS

Definition

Sexual arousal disorder is the persistent or recurrent inability to attain or maintain sufficient sexual excitement, causing personal distress, which may be expressed as a lack of subjective excitement, or genital (lubrication/swelling) or other somatic responses.[3]

The definition indicates that in women their *subjective* perception of inadequate excitement may be the leading complaint, if it causes personal distress. At the same time, and differently from men who are more focused on the genital reaction leading to erection, women may suffer from inadequate central arousal, nongenitals peripheral arousal and/or genital arousal.[32]

Prevalence

Arousal disorders were reported in 19–20% of women in an epidemiologic survey.[1] This figure can rise to 39–50% in postmenopausal sexually active patients.[2,9,18] Vaginal dryness is reported as a specific complaint with increasing years after the menopause, particularly in thin women who do not have the endocrine contribution from the androgenic conversion to estrogens in the adipose tissue, and in those with a very low frequency of intercourse. No data are reported for prevalence of specific subtypes of arousal disorders. Decrease of salivary secretion during arousal and oral intimacy may only be inferred by studies reporting that up to 45% of women after the menopause complain of some degree of mouth dryness, this figure rises to 65% in women on medication other than HRT.[42,43]

Physiologic scenario

Mental arousal may be triggered through different pathways: biologically by androgen, most likely with the participation of apomorphine,[26] credited to participate to the cascade of physiologic events; psychologically by motivational forces like intimacy needs, where the wording indicates all the affective needs of love, tenderness, attention, bonding and commitment (Fig. 18.2).[7,8] Mental arousal may activate both nongenital peripheral and genital arousal. It is also likely that physical stimulation, with nongenital and genital foreplay, and response to sexual cues, may further increase both mental and genital arousal.[7,8] With successful sexual arousal most women produce increased quantities of the vaginal transudate.[24] This neurogenic transudate production arises because the blood vessels supplying the capillary bed become vasodilated due to the release of the neurotransmitter vasoactive intestinal peptide (VIP) at the parasympathetic nerve endings of the sacral nerves S2, S3 and S4.[32,37] Estrogens are credited to be powerful permitting factors for VIP.[32,37] The enhanced transudate produced passes through the intercellular channels of the epithelium and reaches the surface of the vagina with a high Na^+ concentration.[32,37] It may be variably enriched by the cervical secretion, with its content in sialoproteins and the secretion of the Bartholin glands. The reduction in vaginal lubrication is one of the commonest complaints of postmenopausal women. Sarrel[44] noted that when the plasma estradiol concentration was < 50 pg/ml (fertile normal range being 100–200 pg/ml) vaginal dryness is reported. A decreased blood flow is the most likely cause of the reduction, as it has been shown that VIP does not increase vaginal blood flow when injected into menopausal women. Whether this is due to lack of VIP receptors that are under estrogen control or whether the action of VIP is mediated by an estrogen-sensitive mechanism further downstream from the VIP receptor is not known.[37] Laan and Everaerd[33] and Laan and Lunsen,[45] however, interpreted their results of measuring vaginal blood flow by photophletismography in sexually aroused postmenopausal women in terms of inadequate erotic stimulation (and pre-existing arousal disorder) rather than a post-menopausal vasculogenic dysfunction.

After the menopause, physiologic studies indicate: that there is an increase in vaginal pH from 3.5–4.5 to 5.0–5.4, due to decreased glycogen production and metabolism to lactic acid;[37,46–48] an average reduction of 50% of vaginal secretions; an average reduction by half of

transvaginal potential difference. Changes in quantity of secretions leading to the feeling of dryness become subjectively perceived 4–5 years after the menopause. After 1 month of conjugated estrogens (either 0.625 or 1.25 mg/day orally) there is a rapid increase in blood flow, with a reduction in pH, and increases in vaginal secretion and transvaginal potential differences.[46] Topical treatment with small vaginal tablets containing only 25 mg of 17β-estradiol have recently been shown to be as effective and better tolerated than 1.25 mg conjugated equine estrogen vaginal cream to relieve symptoms of atrophic vaginitis, including dryness and arousal difficulties.[48]

Diagnostic work-up

Due to the frequent comorbidity, and the many common etiologies between different FSDs, many questions may overlap with the ones previously presented for hypoactive sexual desire. The questions listed below focus specifically on arousal disorder around the menopause.

(1) *When did you notice you had more difficulty in becoming aroused? Have you had this difficulty previously, since the beginning of your sex life* [lifelong], *or is it a new experience, worsening in the postmenopause* [acquired]*?*

(2) *Is it generalized or do you have this problem only with your current partner or in certain situations* [situational]*?* As mentioned, the generalized issue addresses more personal (biological and/or psychodynamic) factors, whilst the situational one indicates a more likely interpersonal etiology. In the latter case, couple dynamics and/or partner's problems should be addressed.

(3) *Do you feel easily mentally excited, or do you feel 'neutral' and need your partner to take the initiative to start to be 'turned on'? When you start feeling excited, do you feel that all your body responds, or that somehow something is 'blocked' in your genitals?* A selective genital poor response may suggest vascular factors (heavy smoking, hypercholesterolemia, atherosclerosis)[31] and/or

severe atrophic genital involution due to long-lasting loss of sexual hormones.[17,39] It may be reported more clearly in women resuming sexual activity after years of abstinence (as it may be in new relationships in single, widowed, separated or divorced women). *Do you suffer from a dry mouth? If yes, have you noticed that it does not change when you kiss your partner?* This may indicate a nongenital peripheral arousal disorder, superimposed to the salivary glands involution,[6,32,42,43] secondary to long-lasting hypoestrogenism. *Are you normally lubricated during foreplay and does the lubrication suddenly disappear when intercourse begins?* This may suggest not only a *phobic reaction* to coitus (in common with vaginismus) but also the appearance of *pain of different etiologies* (see dyspareunia).[27,28] Pain is the strongest reflex inhibitor of arousal in nonmasochistic women.

In cases of complaint about arousal disorders, the clinician should assess the following.

(1) *The patient's hormonal profile.*[6,9,11,17–25,32,37,40,42,43,46]

(2) *The patient's general and pelvic health*, focusing on pelvic floor trophism: vaginal, clitoral, vulvar, connective and muscular, looking for both hypertonic and hypotonic pelvic floor conditions.[6,30,34]

(3) *Biological factors* causing introital and/or pelvic pain (see dyspareunia).[27,28]

(4) *Vascular factors* that may impair the genital arousal response (smoking, hypercholesterolemia, atherosclerosis).[31]

(5) *The patient's marital status and partner-related problems* (general and sexual health).[17,35,36,41]

(6) *Psychodynamic factors*, either personal or interpersonal.[7,8,33,41,45]

If the arousal problem appears to be acquired and generalized and worsening after the menopause, then HRT may be the treatment of choice. Estrogen, for vaginal lubrication and congestion, and androgen, for clitoral and

vestibular response, may offer the best improvement, as they act in different parts of the sexual circuit, improving sex drive and arousal (central, nongenitals peripheral and genital), thus favoring the orgasmic response. Sometimes, systemic treatment requires the addition of a topical dose[30,48] to optimize the genital response.[19] Topical estrogenic treatment alone may be sufficient to restore normal vaginal lubrication, provided that other interpersonal inhibiting factors are not in play.[9,17,27,32,37,46] Topical androgen treatment may improve the clitoral arousal (congestion and engorgement),[30] although no prospective studies have been reported so far to the present author's knowledge. Rehabilitation of the pelvic floor is necessary to ease the reflex contraction in response to dryness that causes further pain and inhibition of lubrication when coitus is initiated.[27,34] It may also be useful to improve the tone of the elevator ani, thus increasing vaginal sensitivity and pleasure, provided that lubrication and trophism have been hormonally restored.[27] Nonhormonal drugs, such as sildenafil,[26] may be considered in women complaining of arousal disorders who cannot use hormones (e.g. because of hormone-dependent cancer) or because they do not want to. Preliminary results are encouraging when the diagnosis of pure (or dominant) female arousal disorders is made.[47] Studies on apomorphine on female desire and arousal are also ongoing.

ORGASMIC DISORDERS

Definition

Orgasmic disorder is the persistent or recurrent difficulty, delay in or absence of attaining orgasm following sufficient sexual stimulation and arousal, which causes personal distress.

Prevalence

Orgasmic disorder has been reported in an average of 25% of women during their fertile years in an epidemiologic study.[1] After the menopause, 20% of women consulting a menopausal clinic quote that 'their clitoris is dead' according to Sarrel and Whitehead,[9] and even more (if properly listened to) report increasing difficulty and delay in achieving orgasm. In the most recent population-based sample of postmenopausal women,[2] difficulty reaching orgasm was reported as 'always' by 15.0%, 'sometimes' by 22.2% and 'seldom' by 37.8%: only 25% said they never had orgasmic difficulties (Table 18.1).

Physiologic scenario

Orgasm is a sensory motor reflex that may be triggered by a number of different stimuli, physical and mental,[24,32] not even requiring direct genital stimulation.[32] Mental orgasm, that has been demonstrated under laboratory conditions (for the increase of the pain threshold when the orgasm was referred to being mentally perceived),[32] requires an optimal sex drive and intense mental arousal, both biological and motivational. Genital orgasm requires the integrity of the cavernosal structures that, engorged and adequately stimulated, convey sensory pleasant stimuli to the medullary center and the brain.[24,32] Short medullary reflexes may trigger the muscular response, characterized by the involuntary contraction (three to eight times, in single or repetitive sequences) of the levator ani. The medullary reflex may be eased or blocked, respectively, by corticomedullary fibers that may convey both excitatory stimuli, when central arousal is maximal, or inhibitory ones, when arousal is poor or when performance anxiety prevents abandonment and activates adrenergic input that disrupts the arousal response. Inhibitory fibers are mostly serotoninergic: this explains the inhibitory effects of SSRI on orgasm, both in men and women.[26] A biological correlate has recently been suggested for the complaint of worsening clitoral responsiveness with age, particularly after the menopause. The clitoral cavernosal erectile tissue consists of smooth muscle and connective tissue. Tarcan et al[38] utilized computer-assisted histomorphometric image analysis to determine the age-associated changes in the content of smooth muscle and connective tissue, in the clitoral cavernosa

bodies, using clitoris obtained from fresh cadavers (age 11–90) and from patients undergoing clitoral surgery (age 6 months to 15 years). Smooth muscle in the clitoral cavernosa in the 6 months to 15 years group was 65±1.5%, in the 44–54 years group it was 50±1.2% and in 55–90 years group it was 37±1.3% (ANOVA $P = 0.0001$). This study revealed a strong link between an increase in age and a decrease in clitoral cavernosal smooth muscle fibers, which may play an as yet undetermined pathophysiology in age-associated clitoral sexual dysfunction. It also indicates that vulvar aging is a full-thickness process,[30] involving all genital structures, cutaneous and mucosal, submucosal, cavernosal, vascular, muscular and neurologic, thus impairing the complex biological background of the sexual response. The cavernosal involution also involves the female equivalent of the male corpus spongiosum, previously thought to be distributed under the labia minora, in the form of the two, symmetric vestibular bodies, and more recently proven to also be distributed around the distal urethra.[49] This may explain the periurethral engorgement during arousal, reinforcing urethral continence and competence during intercourse and orgasm; the reduction or loss of it after the menopause, because of the cavernosal involution, may facilitate the unpleasant leakage at orgasm which some women complain of. Incontinence may be so disruptive to cause a secondary block of the orgasmic reflex, increasingly reported in women suffering from urge, stress or mixed incontinence.[50]

Diagnostic work-up

(1) *When did you notice having orgasmic difficulty? Did you always have persistent or recurrent orgasmic difficulty* [lifelong], *or did you notice its appearance or worsening after the menopause* [acquired]? Tarcan et al's[38] study suggested an age-dependent deterioration of the cavernosal, vascular tissue. Postmenopausal full-thickness vulvar involution may further worsen the congestive phase of the orgasmic response, more so in women suffering from lichen sclerosus.[30] Topical androgen treatment, approved for

lichen sclerosus, (2% testosterone propionate powder in vaseline jelly, applied topically once a day) is anecdotally reported to improve physical sensation and clitoral pleasure within 3–6 months of initiating treatment. No controlled studies focusing on the effect of topical androgen treatment on sexuality have so far been reported to the author's knowledge.

(2) *Is it generalized (in every situation and independent of the partner) or is it situational?* If generalized, it suggests a biological component, particularly if sex drive is maintained. Antidepressant use (SSRI and clomipramine in particular[51]) should be investigated, as their use is one of the most frequent and overlooked causes of acquired, generalized, biologically based (and reversible) orgasmic difficulties in women (as well as in men).

(3) *What, in your opinion, is causing your orgasmic difficulty?* This question is useful in diagnosing other interfering factors. For example, worsening incontinence;[50,52,53] pain;[27] depression;[2] too rapid foreplay;[2,7,8] loss of sex drive and arousal (Fig. 18.1); alcohol abuse;[2,6] dissatisfaction with the current relationship.[2,7,8] *Do you feel a selective loss in your clitoral sensitivity and pleasure ability and/or a reduction in your coital pleasure?* If the complaint is focused on the clitoris, and involution or dystrophia is present, then topical androgen treatment may be useful. If it is coital, two further points of attention should be raised. (a) *Do you have a decreased coital sensation?* This may suggest a worsening hypotonia of the perivaginal muscles.[50,52,53,56] Menopausal loss of estrogens may cause not only a gradual loss of pelvic connective tissue up to 10 years after the menopause[54] but also a loss of the muscular component,[25,55] thus affecting the tone of the muscle itself. As vaginal pleasure and sensitivity are physically dependent on the tone of perivaginal muscles, this decrease may selectively damage the coital component of the orgasmic experience. HRT, contributing to maintaining better connective, muscular and vascular trophism, may indirectly concur to maintenance of a better orgasmic response.[25,31,54,55,57] (b) *Do you feel pain during*

intercourse? Pain of whatever origin[50,53,57–62] may cause a reflex block of the arousal and of the orgasmic response.[27,28]

The physician working with the perimenopausal woman, according to the scenario emerging from the clinical history, should assess the following.

(1) *The patient's hormonal balance.*[6,18–22]

(2) *Signs and symptoms and vulvar dystrophia,*[30,38] specifically of clitoral and vaginal involution; worsening consequences of ritual genital mutilations should be evaluated.

(3) *Signs and symptoms of incontinence,*[50,53] of hypotonic[34] or hypertonic pelvic floor conditions.[27]

(4) *Iatrogenic orgasmic disorders*, when potentially orgasm-inhibiting drugs are prescribed.[26,51]

(5) *Marital problems.*[35,36,41]

(6) *Psychological disturbances*, depression, anxiety[7,8,51] and neurological diseases.[58]

SEXUAL PAIN DISORDERS

Definition

(1) Dyspareunia is the recurrent or persistent genital pain associated with sexual intercourse.
(2) Vaginismus is the recurrent or persistent involuntary spasm of the musculature of the outer third of the vagina that interferes with vaginal penetration, which causes personal distress.
(3) Noncoital sexual pain disorders are recurrent or persistent genital pain induced by noncoital sexual stimulation.

Dyspareunia is a comprehensive definition that indicates the situation(s) where intercourse is characterized by pain of different etiologies (Box 18.2). Vaginismus focuses on the muscular

Box 18.2 Etiology of introital dyspareunia
Psychosexual
Hormonal/dystrophic
Inflammatory
Muscular
Iatrogenic
Traumatic
Neurologic
Vascular
Connective and immunity

component of the disorder, which is usually psychogenically triggered by fear of penetration, of conscious or unconscious etiology. Noncoital sexual pain disorder addresses the possibility of pain in sexual behaviors other than intercourse, i.e. during foreplay, evoking or worsening clitoralgia or vestibular pain, and/or in lesbian couples.

Prevalence

Fifteen per cent of coitally active women[1] and up to 22.5–33%[2,3] of postmenopausal women complain of various degrees of dyspareunia. Vaginismus is reported in an average of 1% of fertile women.[24] No prevalence figures specific for vaginismus are available for the post-menopause period. The category of noncoital sexual pain disorders is new and prevalence data have not yet been produced.

Physiologic scenario

Vaginal receptiveness is a prerequisite for inter-course. This ability requires *anatomical and functional integrity* of the many tissue components, both in resting and aroused states. Normal trophism,[30] mucosal and cutaneous, adequate hormonal impregnation,[32,37,47] lack of inflammation, particularly at the introitus,[56] normal tonicity of the perivaginal muscles,[27] and vascular,[31,57] connective[54] and neurological[58] integrity, and normal immunity[62] responses are all credited to be necessary conditions to guarantee the

vaginal habitability. However, some contradictory findings are reported.[33,45,59] Vaginal receptiveness may be further modulated by psychosexual, mental and interpersonal, factors, with poor arousal the consequent sign.[7,8] *Fear of penetration* may cause a defensive contraction of perivaginal muscles – leading to *vaginismus* – that can be controlled both consciously and unconsciously. This contraction may also be secondary to *genital pain*, of whatever cause.[27,30,50,58,60–61] It may be triggered by nongenital, nonsexual causes, such as urological factors (urge incontinence, when tightening the pelvic floor may be secondary to the aim of reinforcing the ability to control the bladder through a hypercontracted pelvic floor) or anorectal problems (anismus, hemorrhoids, rhagades).[60]

Medical ('organic') factors – too often under-evaluated in the clinical setting – may cause pain and/or combine with psychogenic (psychosexual) factors contributing to further pain during intercourse.[6,7,8,27,28,33,45] They include hormonal/dystrophic,[6,9,13,17–22,27] inflammatory,[56] muscular,[27,34,61] iatrogenic,[27,60] neurologic and/or post-traumatic,[58] vascular,[32,57] connective and immune causes.[62] Other FSD – loss of libido,[2,3,6,15,16] arousal disorders,[7,8,32,37,47] orgasmic difficulties[2,30] and/or sexual pain-related disorders[3,30] may frequently partially overlap with dyspareunia.

Diagnostic work-up

(1) *Is it a lifelong or acquired disorder? If lifelong, were you afraid of feeling pain before your first intercourse?* If lifelong, dyspareunia is often caused by vaginismus and/or coexisting, lifelong low libido and arousal disorders.[18,27,41] If fear of pain and a phobic attitude towards intercourse prevented penetration, lifelong severe vaginismus is probably revealed. Not infrequently, primary vaginismus is occasionally diagnosed around the menopause when the woman is induced to seek medical help, and have her first gynecologic visit, because of a severe menopausal syndrome. *If acquired, do you remember the situation or what happened when it started? Is it improving or worsening over time*

and/or around periods? If it appeared after the menopause, how did you try to relieve it? This cluster of questions may highlight the most frequent medical condition that leads to dyspareunia in the fertile age: vestibulitis.[56] Other triggering physical factors may be iatrogenic as well:[27] colporrhaphy and posterior perineorrhaphy, mostly in the peri- and postmenopausal years, are the surgical procedures resulting in the complication of dyspareunia. Physical genital trauma and/or sexual abuse[28] may also cause an acquired dyspareunia and should be investigated. Pudendal nerve entrapment syndrome, leading to dyspareunia, may appear up to 15 years after coccygeal sacral physical trauma or pelvic surgery.[58]

(2) *Is it generalized or situational?* Pain may emerge from a combination of factors: psychogenic poor arousal, secondary to the frustration of intimacy needs,[7,8] worsened by the poor vascular response secondary to hypoestrogenism,[32,37,47] thus increasing the vulnerability to mechanical coital microlesions of the introital mucosa, worsening pain and maintaining it for hours or up to 2–3 days after intercourse.

(3) *Where does it hurt? At the beginning of the vagina, in the mid-vagina or deep in the vagina? Location of the pain* and *its onset* within an episode of intercourse are the strongest predictors of presence and type of organicity.[28] *Introital dyspareunia* may be more frequently caused by poor arousal,[7,8,27] vestibulitis,[56] vulvar dystrophia,[30] painful outcome of vulvar physical therapies,[27,60] perineal surgery (episiorrhaphy, colporrhaphy, posterior perineorrhaphy),[27] pudendal nerve entrapment syndrome and/or pudendal neuralgia,[58] or Sjögren's syndrome.[62] *Mid-vaginal pain*, acutely evoked during physical examination by a gentle pressure on the sacrospinous insertion of the elevator ani muscle, is more frequently due to levator ani myalgia,[27,34,61] the most frequently overlooked biological cause of dyspareunia. If *deep*, pain suggests other organic factors: e.g. endometriosis (which may be reactivated by cyclic HRT: continuous combined treatment is preferred when endometriosis is present); pelvic inflammatory disease (PID) (nonprotected intercourse outside the normal relationship is increasing in perimenopausal women and their partners, bringing with it an increased risk of sexually transmitted diseases); adhesions, referred abdominal pain, outcomes of radiotherapy and abdominal cutaneous nerve entrapment syndrome.[27]

(4) *When do you feel pain? Before, during or after intercourse?*[28] Pain *before* intercourse suggests a phobic attitude towards penetration, usually associated with vaginismus and/or the presence of vestibulitis if previous attempts at intercourse have caused a mechanical microtrauma of the introital mucosa. Pain *during* intercourse is more frequently reported. This information, combined with the previous. 'Where does it hurt?' question, proves to be the most predictive of the organicity of pain.[28] Pain *after* intercourse indicates that mucosal damage was provoked during intercourse, possibly because of poor arousal, concurring to vestibulitis, pain and defensive contraction of the pelvic floor.

(5) *Do you feel other accompanying symptoms, vaginal dryness, pain or paresthesias in the genitals and pelvic areas? Or do you suffer from cystitis 24–72 hours after intercourse?* Vaginal dryness, either secondary to loss of estrogen and/or to poor genital arousal, may coincide with dyspareunia. Clitoralgia and/or vulvodynia, spontaneous and/or worsening during sexual arousal may be associated with dyspareunia and hypertonic pelvic floor muscles.[34,57,61] Postcoital cystitis[27] should suggest a hypoestrogenic condition and/or the presence of hypertonic pelvic floor muscles: it should specifically be investigated in the postmenopause and senium as it may benefit from HRT and a specific rehabilitation of the pelvic floor aimed at relaxing the myalgic perivaginal muscles. Accompanying symptoms such as vulvar pruritus, vulvar dryness and/or feeling of a burning vulva should be investigated, as they may suggest the presence of vulvar lichen sclerosus,[30,62] which may worsen the introital dyspareunia. Vestibulitis[56] may concur to noncoital sexual pain disorder during foreplay. Neurogenic pain may cause not only

dyspareunia but also clitoralgia. Eye and mouth dryness, when accompanying dyspareunia and vaginal dryness, should suggest Sjögren's syndrome, a connective and immune disease.[63]

(6) *How intense is the pain you feel?* Focusing on the intensity and characteristics of pain[27,28] is a relatively new approach in addressing dyspareunia issues. A shift from nociceptic to neuropathic pain is typical of chronic dyspareunia; treatment may require a systemic and local analgesic approach.

Diagnostic work-up

In cases of complaint about sexual pain disorders the physician should assess the following.

(1) *The patient's hormonal profile.*[6,17,19–22,27]

(2) *A physically accurate examination to define the 'pain map',*[27] inclusive of pelvic floor trophism,[27,30] muscular tone,[34,52,61] signs of inflammation,[56] poor outcomes of pelvic surgery,[27] associated urogenital and rectal pain syndromes,[60] myogenic[34,61] or neurogenic pain,[57] and vascular problems.[31,57]

(3) *Psychosexual factors* – poor arousal first[7,8,33] – that may contribute to poor lubrication and consequent mechanical trauma during intercourse.

(4) *Marital issues.*[2,35,36,41]

Pain is rarely purely psychogenic and dyspareunia is no exception. Like all pain syndromes, it usually has one or multiple biological etiologic factors. Psychosexual factors, mostly low libido, lifelong or acquired, because of the persisting pain, and arousal disorders, lifelong or acquired, due to the inhibitory effect of pain, should be addressed in parallel, in order to give a comprehensive, integrated and more effective treatment.

NEW PERSPECTIVES

The recent outburst of interest in FSD is finally leading to the testing of new drugs and devices to treat the biological basis of FSD, although with >20 years' delay in comparison to men. At present the following studies are of interest.

- Studies on testosterone patches are very promising.[40]
- Studies on dehydroepiandrosterone (DHEA) suggest that its complex beneficial effects on many biological parameters and their psychophysiologic correlates[64,65] might also have a beneficial effect on sexual function, male and female, by improving vital energy, a general sense of wellbeing, libido and motivation for a more intense life, inclusive of sex. More studies are needed to confirm the preliminary reports.
- Studies on sildenafil[47] and apomorphine[26] are ongoing: preliminary results seem less promising than in the male counterpart, thus stressing the importance of relational and psychosexual factors in women, the need for a careful diagnosis and of a clear personal motivation of the woman in improving her own sexuality. When these conditions are met, positive results are obtained in pre- and postmenopausal women with sildenafil.[47]
- Studies on the so-called Eros clitoral therapy device (EROS-CTD), a small device designed to specifically improve clitoral arousal through the induction of mechanical engorgement, have shown positive results in increasing genital sensations and arousal, vaginal lubrication, enhanced ability to orgasm and overall satisfaction.[66] These significant improvements, reported in different studies, were acknowledged by the Food and Drug Administration (FDA) on April 28, 2000: this device is therefore the first approved treatment of arousal disorders in women.

CONCLUSIONS

FSD is a multifactorial disorder increasingly reported during gynecologic consultation, particularly during and after the menopause. With an appropriate *clinical history*, the physician should be able to: (1) diagnose the leading and accompanying disorder(s) – hypoactive sexual desire, arousal disorders, orgasmic difficulties, sexual pain disorders – paying equal attention to both biological and psychodynamic and/or interpersonal factors; (2) put the problem in a lifespan perspective, with adequate subtyping: lifelong versus acquired, focusing on the potential etiologic role of menopause and loss of sexual hormones and/or coexisting health problems; generalized versus situational, paying attention to marital status and the partner's related problems; (3) focus on a preliminary definition of potential etiology (organic, psychogenic, mixed or unknown). The clinical history, clinical examination and tests will all help to recognize the most important factors contributing to the present complaint.

During the *diagnostic work-up*, the physician should: (1) assess the potential role of hormonal factors, loss of estrogens and, specifically, of androgens, that trigger both libido and arousal, central and peripheral; and/or potential increase of prolactin that may further inhibit libido; (2) diagnose pelvic floor dysfunctions and genital anatomic factors, including poor outcome of surgery, that may lead to a disappointing physical response; (3) recognize psychobiologic factors that may interfere with the motivational-affective basis of sexual response, namely depression, anxiety, chronic stress and insomnia, all of which may worsen after the menopause; (4) diagnose concurrent diseases and iatrogenic factors that may increasingly interfere with the biology of sexual response, particularly in elderly patients, both per se and for treatment-related side effects; (5) inquire about relational conflicts and/or marital delusions and partner-specific problems, primarily erectile deficit. All these aspects should be at least briefly evaluated to effectively address the patient's, indeed the couple's, complaint in the most effective way.

With a well-tailored *etiologic treatment* the physician may greatly contribute to the reduction of the biological causes of FSD. The psychosexologist or couple's therapist will be able to address motivational and relational factors more effectively once the physical equilibrium has been restored. The uroandrologist is the referral doctor if MSD is complained of as well. A multidisciplinary team approach will ultimately give the best-tailored response. Apart from addressing the FSD complaint in a competent way when the issue is openly raised, a physician who is prepared to listen can contribute towards improving the quality of (sexual) life of his/her aging patients by simply asking them 'How's your sex life?'.

REFERENCES

1. Laumann EO, Paik A, Rosen RC. Sexual dysfunction in the United States. Prevalence and predictors. *JAMA* 1999; **281**: 537–44.
2. Avis NE, Stellato R, Crawford S et al. Is there an association between menopause status and sexual functioning? *Menopause* 2000; **7**: 297–309.
3. Basson R, Bertian J, Burnett A et al. Report of the International Consensus Development Conference on Female Sexual Dysfunction: Definitions and Classifications. *J Urol* 2000; **163**: 888–93.
4. World Health Organization: ICD–10. *International Statistical Classification of Diseases and Related Health Problems*, 10th edn. (World Health Organization: Geneva, 1992.)
5. American Psychiatric Association. *DSM-IV. Diagnostic and Statistical Manual of Mental Disorders*, 4th edn. (American Psychiatric Press Inc: Washington DC, 1994.)
6. Graziottin A. Libido: the biologic scenario. *Maturitas* 2000; **43** (Suppl 1): S9–S16.
7. Basson R. The female sexual response: a different model. *J Sex Marital Ther* 2000; **26**: 51–65.
8. Basson R. The female sexual response revisited. *J Soc Obstet Gynecol Can* 2000; **22**: 383–7.
9. Sarrel PM, Whitehead MI. Sex and menopause: defining the issue. *Maturitas* 1985; **7**: 217–24.
10. Myers LS. Methodological review and meta-analysis of sexuality and menopause research. *Neurosci Behav Rev* 1995; **19**: 331–341.
11. Bachman G (ed). Menopause and female sexuality *J Women's Health & Gender-based Med* 2000; **9** (S1): S25–S32.
12. Levin RJ. Human male sexuality: appetite and arousal, desire and drive. In: (Legg C, Boott D, eds) *Human Appetite: Neural and Behavioural Bases*. (Oxford University Press: Oxford, 1994 127–64.
13. Graziottin A. The biological basis of female sexuality. *Int Clin Psychopharmacol* 1998; **13**: S15–S22.
14. Pfaus JG, Everitt BJ. The psychopharmacology of

sexual behaviour. In: (Bloom FE, Kupfer D, eds) *Psychopharmacology*. (Raven Press: New York, 1995) 743–58.

15. Levine SB. An essay on the nature of sexual desire. *J Sex Mar Ther* 1984; **10**: 83–96.

16. Kaplan HS. *Disorders of sexual desire*. (Simon and Schuster: New York, 1979.)

17. Graziottin A. Sexuality and the menopause. In: (Studd J, ed) *The Management of the Menopause – Annual Review*. (Parthenon Publishing: London, 1998) 49–57.

18. Bachmann GA, Leiblum SR. Sexuality in sexagenarian women. *Maturitas* 1991; **13**: 43–50.

19. Notelovitz M. *A Practical Approach to Postmenopausal Hormone Therapy*. Ob/gyn, Special edition, (Mac Mahon: New York, 2002.)

20. Sherwin BB, Gelfand MM, Brender W. Androgens enhance sexual motivation in females: a prospective, crossover study of sex steroid administration in surgical menopause. *Psychosom Med* 1987; **47**: 339–51.

21. Myers LS, Dixen J, Morrissette D et al. Effects of estrogen, androgen and progestin on sexual psychophysiology and behaviour in postmenopausal women. *J Clin Endocr Metab* 1990; **70**: 1124–31.

22. Davis SR, McCloud P, Strauss BJG, Burger H. Testosterone enhances estradiol's effects on postmenopausal bone density and sexuality. *Maturitas* 1995; **21**: 227–36.

23. Miller KK. Androgen deficiency in women *J Clin Endocr Metab* 2001; **86**: 2395–401.

24. Masters WH, Johnson VE. *Human Sexual Response*. (Little, Brown: Boston, 1966) 5–131.

25. Sands R, Studd J. Exogenous androgens in postmenopausal women. *Am J Med* 1995; **98**: 76–9.

26. Graziottin A, Maraschiello T. *Farmaci e sessualità*. (Airon Ed: Milano, 2002.)

27. Graziottin A, Castoldi E. Dyspareunia: what should we look for? In: (Graziottin A, ed) *Menopause and Sexuality*. Menopause Rev 1999; **IV**: 33–42.

28. Meana M, Binik YM, Khalifé S, Cohen D. Dyspareunia: sexual dysfunction or pain syndrome? *J Neural Mental Dis* 1997; **185**: 561–9.

29. Kokçu MB, Çetinkaya F, Alper T, Malatyaliogly E. The comparison of effects of tibolone and conjugated estrogen–medroxyprogesterone acetate therapy on sexual performances in postmenopausal women. *Maturitas* 2000; **36**: 75–80.

30. Graziottin A. Organic and psychologic factors in vulval pain: implications for management. *Sex Mar Ther* 1998; **13**: 329–38.

31. Goldstein I, Berman J. Vasculogenic female sexual dysfunction: vaginal engorgement and clitoral erectile insufficiency syndrome. *Int J Imp Res* 1998; **10**: S84–S90.

32. Levin RJ. The mechanisms of human female sexual arousal. *Ann Rev Sex Res* 1992; **3**: 1–48.

33. Laan E, Everaerd W. Determinants of female sexual arousal: psychophysiological theory and data. *Ann Rev Sex Res* 1995; **6**: 32–76.

34. Travell JG, Simons DG. *Myofascial Pain and Dysfunction, The Trigger Points Manual – The Lower Extremities*. (Williams & Wilkins: Baltimore, 1992.

35. Renshaw DC. Coping with an impotent husband. *Illinois Med J* 1981; **159**: 29–33.

36. Barnes T. The female partner in the treatment of erectile dysfunction: what is her position? *Sex Mar Ther* 1998; **13**: 233–8.

37. Levin RJ. The impact of the menopause on the physiology of genital function. In: (Graziottin A, (ed). *Menopause and Sexuality*. Menopause Rev 1999; **IV**: 23–32.

38. Tarcan T, Park K, Goldstein I et al. Histomorphometric analysis of age related structural changes in human clitoral cavernosal tissue. *J Urol* 1999; **161**: 940–4.

39. Madelska K, Cummings S. Tibolone for postmenopausal women: systematic review of randomized trials. *J Clin Endocr Metab* 2002; **87**: 16–23.

40. Shifren JL, Glenn D, Brauntsein MD. et al. Transdermal testosterone treatment in women with impaired sexual function after oophorectomy. *N Engl J Med* 2000; **343**: 682–8.

41. Dennerstein L, Lehert P, Burger H et al. In: (Studd J, ed) *The Management of the Menopause. The Millennium Review: Menopause and Sexual Functioning*. (Parthenon Publishing: London, 2000) 203–10.

42. Streckfus CF, Baur U, Brown LJ et al. Effects of estrogen status and aging on salivary flow rates in healthy caucasian women. *Gerontology* 1998; **44**: 32–9.

43. Ben Aryeth H, Gottlieb I, Ish Shalom S, David A. Oral complaints related to menopause. *Maturitas* 1996; **24**: 185–90.

44. Sarrel PM. Ovarian hormones and vaginal blood flow using laser Doppler velocimetry to measure effects in aclinical trial of post-menopausal women. *Int J Imp Res* 1998; **18**: S91–S93.

45. Laan E, Lunsen RHW. Hormones and sexuality in postmenopausal women: a psychophysiologic study. *J Psychosoc Obstet Gynecol* 1997; **18**: 126–33.

46. Levin RJ. Measuring the menopause genital changes – a critical account of laboratory procedures past and for the future. In: (Graziottin A, ed) *Menopause and Sexuality*. Menopause Rev 1999; **IV:** 49–57.

47. Berman JR, Berman LA, Lin H et al. Effect of sildenafil on subjective and physiologic parameters of the female sexual response in women with sexual arousal disorders *J Sex Marital Ther* 2001; **27:** 411–20.

48. Rioux JE, Devlin MC, Gelfand MM. et al. 17 beta estradiol vaginal tablet versus conjugated equine estrogen vaginal cream to relieve menopausal atrophic vaginitis. *Menopause* 2000; **7:** 156–61.

49. O'Connell HE, Hutson JM, Anderson CR, Plenter RJ. Anatomical relationship betweeen urethra and clitoris. *J Urol* 1998; **159:** 1892–7.

50. Barlow DH, Cardozo L, Francis RM et al. Urogenital ageing and its effect on sexual health in older British women. *Br J Obstet Gynecol* 1997; **104:** 87–91.

51. Rosen RC, Lane R, Menza M. Effects of SSRIs on sexual function: a critical review. *J Clin Pharmacol* 1999; **19:** 67–85.

52. Kegel A. Sexual function of the pubococcygeus muscle. *West J Surg* 1952; **60:** 521–4.

53. Cardozo L, Bachmann G, McClish D et al. Meta-analysis of estrogen therapy in the management of urogenital atrophy in postmenopausal women: second report of the hormones and urogenital therapy committee. *Obstet Gynecol* 1998; **92:** 722–7.

54. Brincat M (ed). *Hormone Replacement Therapy and the Skin*. (Parthenon Publishing: New York, 2002) 8–20.

55. Meeuwsen IB, Samson MM, DuursmaVerhaar HJ. Muscle strength and tibolone: a randomized, double-blind, placebo-controlled trial. *Br J Obstet Gynaecol* 2002; **109:** 77–84.

56. Bergeron S, Binik YM, Khalife S, Pagidas K. Vulvar vestibulitis syndrome: a critical review. *Clin J Pain* 1997; **13:** 27–42.

57. Berman JR, Berman LA, Werbin TJ et al. Clinical evaluation of female sexual function: effects of age and estrogen status on subjective and physiologic sexual responses. *Int J Imp Res* 1999; **11:** S31–S38.

58. Shafik A. Pudendal canal syndrome as a cause of vulvodynia and its treatment by pudendal nerve decompression. *Eur J Obstet Gynecol Reprod Biol* 1998; **80:** 215–20.

59. Weber AM, Walters MD, Schover LR, Mitchinson A. Vaginal anatomy and sexual function. *Obstet Gynecol* 1995; **86:** 946–9.

60. Wesselmann U, Burnett AL, Heinberg LJ. The urogenital and rectal pain syndromes. *Pain* 1997; **73:** 269–94.

61. De Lancey JO, Sampselle CM, Punch MR. Kegel dyspareunia: levator ani myalgia caused by overexertion. *Obstet Gynecol* 1993; **82:** 658–9.

62. Hagedorn M, Buxmeyer B, Schmitt Y, Buknecht T. Survey of genital lichen sclerosus in women and men. *Arch Gynecol Obstet* 2002; **266:** 86–91.

63. Mulherin DM, Sheeran TP, Kumararatne DS et al. Sjögren's syndrome in women presenting with chronic dyspareunia. *Br J Obstet Gynaecol* 1997; **104:** 1019–23.

64. Labrie F, Luu-The V, Labrie C. Simard J. DHEA and its transformation into androgens and estrogens in peripheral target tissues: intracrinology. *Front Neuroendocrinol* 2001; **22:** 185–212.

65. Stomati M, Monteleone P, Casarosa E, et al. Six-month oral dehydroepiandrosterone supplementation in early and late postmenopause. *Gynecol Endocr* 2000; **14:** 342–63.

66. Wilson SK, Delk JR, Billups KL. Treating symptoms of female sexual arousal disorder with the Eros-Clitoral Therapy Device. *J Gend Specif Med* 2001; **4:** 54–8.

19

Estrogens and urogenital atrophy

D Robinson and L Cardozo

Introduction • Epidemiology • Urogenital atrophy • Urinary incontinence • Economic considerations • Estrogen receptors and hormonal factors • Progesterone and androgen receptors • Lower urinary tract function • Bladder function • Neurologic control • Urethra • Collagen • Urogenital atrophy • Lower urinary tract symptoms • Estrogens in the management of incontinence • Estrogens in the management of stress incontinence • Estrogens in the management of urge incontinence • Estrogens in the management of recurrent urinary tract infection • Estrogens in the management of urogenital atrophy • Selective estrogen receptor modulators (SERM) • Conclusions • References

INTRODUCTION

Urogenital atrophy is a manifestation of estrogen withdrawal following the menopause and symptoms may appear for the first time > 10 years after the last menstrual period.[1] The female genital and lower urinary tract share a common embryologic origin from the urogenital sinus and both are sensitive to the effects of female sex steroid hormones. Estrogen is known to have an important role in the function of the lower urinary tract throughout adult life, and estrogen and progesterone receptors have been demonstrated in the vagina, urethra, bladder and pelvic floor musculature.[2–5] Estrogen deficiency occurring following the menopause is known to cause atrophic changes within the urogenital tract,[6] and is associated with urinary symptoms such as frequency, urgency, nocturia, incontinence and recurrent infection. These may co-exist with symptoms of vaginal atrophy such as dyspareunia, itching, burning and dryness.

The role of estrogen replacement in the treatment of these symptoms of urogenital atrophy has still not been clearly defined despite several randomized trials and widespread clinical use. This chapter presents an overview of the pathogenesis and management of urogenital symptoms, and the role of estrogen replacement therapy (ERT).

EPIDEMIOLOGY

Increasing life expectancy has led to an increasingly elderly population and it is now common for women to spend a third of their lives in the estrogen-deficient postmenopausal state.[7] The average age of the menopause is 50 years although there is some cultural and geographical variation.[8] Worldwide, in 1990 there were approximately 467 million women ≥ 50 years of age and this is expected to increase to 1200 million over the next 30 years.[9] Furthermore, postmenopausal women comprise 15% of the population in industrialized countries, with a predicted growth rate of 1.5% over the next 20 years. Overall, in the developed world 8% of the total population have been estimated to have urogenital symptoms,[10] representing 200 million women in the US alone.

UROGENITAL ATROPHY

The prevalence of symptomatic urogenital atrophy is difficult to estimate since many women accept the changes as being an inevitable consequence of the aging process and thus do not seek help. It has been estimated that 10–40% of all postmenopausal women are symptomatic,[11] although only 25% are thought to seek medical help. In addition, vaginal symptoms associated with urogenital atrophy are reported by two out of three women by the age of 75.[12]

More recently a study assessing the prevalence of urogenital symptoms in 2157 Dutch women has been reported.[13] Overall 27% of women complained of vaginal dryness, soreness and dyspareunia, whilst the prevalence of urinary symptoms such as leakage and recurrent infections was 36%. When considering severity, almost 50% reported moderate to severe discomfort although only a third had received medical intervention. Interestingly women who had previously had a hysterectomy reported moderate to severe complaints more often than those who had not.

The prevalence of urogenital atrophy and urogenital prolapse has also been examined in a population of 285 women attending a menopause clinic.[14] Overall 51% of women were found to have anterior vaginal wall prolapse, 27% posterior vaginal prolapse and 20% apical prolapse. In addition, 34% of women were noted to have urogenital atrophy, 40% complaining of dyspareunia. Whilst urogenital atrophy and symptoms of dyspareunia were related to menopausal age the prevalence of prolapse showed no association.

Whilst urogenital atrophy is an inevitable consequence of the menopause women may not always be symptomatic. A recent study of 69 women attending a gynecology clinic were asked to fill out a symptom questionnaire prior to examination and undergoing vaginal cytology.[15] Urogenital symptoms were found to be relatively low and were poorly correlated with age and physical examination findings, although not with the vaginal cytologic maturation index. Women who were taking ERT had higher symptom scores and physical examination scores. It would appear that urogenital atrophy is a universal consequence of the menopause, although often women may be minimally symptomatic and hence treatment should not be the only indication for replacement therapy.

URINARY INCONTINENCE

The prevalence of urinary incontinence is known to increase with age, affecting 15–35% of community-dwelling women > 60 years of age,[16] with other studies reporting a prevalence of 49% in women > 65 years of age.[17] In addition, rates of 50% have been reported in elderly nursing-home residents.[18] A recent cross-sectional population prevalence survey of 146 women aged 15–97 found that 46% experienced symptoms of pelvic floor dysfunction defined as stress or urge incontinence, flatus or fecal incontinence, symptomatic prolapse or previous pelvic floor surgery.[19]

Little work has been done to examine the incidence of urinary incontinence although a study in New Zealand of women > 65 years of age found 10% of the originally continent developed urinary incontinence in the 3-year study period.[20]

ECONOMIC CONSIDERATIONS

The economic cost of urogenital atrophy is difficult to estimate due to under-reporting and also since some of the cost is borne by the patients themselves without involving the health services. The price of incontinence is slightly easier to estimate although is still affected by under-reporting. It is comprised of direct – supplies and provision of medical staff – and indirect – loss of earnings and productivity – costs. A study performed in 1994 in Scotland estimated that the cost of pad supplies alone in the UK may be in the region of £57.3 million year whilst the cost of incontinence has been estimated at $16 billion year in the US. More recent data from the UK have shown the annual expenditure on incontinence to be £163 million, with appliances and containment accounting for £59 million and £69 million, respectively, and the cost of drugs and surgery being £23 million and £12 million, respectively.[21]

ESTROGEN RECEPTORS AND HORMONAL FACTORS

The effects of the steroid hormone 17β-estradiol are mediated by ligand-activated transcription factors known as estrogen receptors, which are glycoproteins sharing common features with androgen and progesterone receptors. The classic estrogen receptor (ERα) was first discovered by Elwood Jensen in 1958 and cloned from uterine tissue in 1986,[22] although it was not until 1996 that the second estrogen receptor (ERβ) was identified.[23]

Estrogen receptors have been demonstrated throughout the lower urinary tract and are expressed in the squamous epithelium of the proximal and distal urethra, vagina and trigone of the bladder,[24] although not in the dome of the bladder, reflecting its different embryological origin. Pubococcygeous and the musculature of the pelvic floor have also been shown to be estrogen sensitive,[25,26] although estrogen receptors have not yet been identified in the levator ani muscles.[27]

More recently the distribution of estrogen receptors throughout the urogenital tract has been studied with both α and β receptors being found in the vaginal walls and uterosacral ligaments of premenopausal women, although the latter was absent in the vaginal walls of postmenopausal women.[28] In addition, α receptors are localized in the urethral sphincter and when sensitized by estrogens are thought to help maintain muscular tone.[29] Interestingly estrogen receptors have also been identified in mast cells in women with interstitial cystitis[30] and in the male lower urinary tract.

PROGESTERONE AND ANDROGEN RECEPTORS

In addition to estrogen receptors both androgen and progesterone receptors are expressed in the lower urinary tract, although their role is less clear. Progesterone receptors are expressed inconsistently, having been reported in the bladder, trigone and vagina. Their presence may be dependent on estrogen status. In addition, whilst androgen receptors are present in both the bladder and urethra their role has not yet been defined.[31]

More recently the incidence of both estrogen and progesterone expression has been examined throughout the lower urinary tract in 90 women undergoing gynecologic surgery; 33 were premenopausal, 26 postmenopausal without hormone replacement therapy (HRT) and 31 postmenopausal and taking HRT.[32] Biopsies were taken from the bladder dome, trigone, proximal urethra, distal urethra, vagina and vesicovaginal fascia adjacent to the bladder neck. Estrogen receptors were found to be consistently expressed in the squamous epithelia although were absent in the urothelial tissues of the lower urinary tract of all women, irrespective of estrogen status. Progesterone receptor expression, however, showed more variability, being mostly subepithelial, and was significantly lower in postmenopausal women not taking ERT.

LOWER URINARY TRACT FUNCTION

In order to maintain continence, urethral pressure must remain higher than intravesical pressure at all times except during micturition.[33] Estrogens play an important role in the continence mechanism, with bladder and urethral function becoming less efficient with age.[34] Elderly women have been found to have a reduced flow rate, increased urinary residuals, higher filling pressures, reduced bladder capacity and lower maximum voiding pressures.[35] Estrogens may affect continence by increasing urethral resistance, raising the sensory threshold of the bladder or by increasing α-adrenoreceptor sensitivity in the urethral smooth muscle.[36,37] In addition exogenous estrogens have been shown to increase the number of intermediate and superficial cells in the vagina of postmenopausal women,[38] and these changes have also been demonstrated in the bladder and urethra.[39]

More recently a prospective observational

study has been performed to assess cell proliferation rates throughout the tissues of the lower urinary tract.[40] Fifty-nine women were studied of whom 23 were premenopausal, 20 were postmenopausal and not taking HRT, and 20 were postmenopausal and taking HRT. Biopsies were taken from the bladder dome, trigone, proximal urethra, distal urethra, vagina and vesicovaginal fascia adjacent to the bladder neck. The squamous epithelium of estrogen-replete women was shown to exhibit greater levels of cellular proliferation than in those women who were estrogen deficient.

BLADDER FUNCTION

Estrogen receptors, although absent in the transitional epithelium of the bladder, are present in the areas of the trigone which have undergone squamous metaplasia.[24] Estrogen is known to have a direct effect on detrusor function through modifications in muscarinic receptors[41,42] and by inhibition of movement of extracellular calcium ions into muscle cells.[43] Consequently estradiol has been shown to reduce the amplitude and frequency of spontaneous rhythmic detrusor contractions,[44] and there is also evidence that it may increase the sensory threshold of the bladder in some women.[45]

NEUROLOGIC CONTROL

Sex hormones are known to influence the central neurologic control of micturition although their exact role in the micturition pathway has yet to be elucidated. Estrogen receptors have been demonstrated in the cerebral cortex, limbic system, hippocampus and cerebellum,[46,47] whilst androgen receptors have been demonstrated in the pontine micturition center and the pre-optic area of the hypothalamus.[48]

URETHRA

Estrogen receptors have been demonstrated in the squamous epithelium of both the proximal and distal urethra,[24] and estrogen has been shown to improve the maturation index of urethral squamous epithelium.[49] It has been suggested that estrogen increases urethral closure pressure and improves pressure transmission to the proximal urethra, both promoting continence.[50-53] Estrogens have been shown to cause vasodilatation in the systemic and cerebral circulation, and these changes are also seen in the urethra.[54-56] The vascular pulsations seen on urethral pressure profilometry secondary to blood flow in the urethral submucosa and urethral sphincter have been shown to increase in size following estrogen administration,[57] whilst the effect is lost following estrogen withdrawal at the menopause.

COLLAGEN

Estrogens are known to have an effect on collagen synthesis and they have been shown to have a direct effect on collagen metabolism in the lower genital tract.[58] Changes found in women with urogenital atrophy may represent an alteration in systemic collagenase activity,[59] and urodynamic stress incontinence and urogenital prolapse has been associated with a reduction in both vaginal and periurethral collagen.[60-62] There is a reduction in skin collagen content following the menopause[63] and rectus muscle fascia has been shown to become less elastic with increasing age resulting in a lower energy requirement to cause irreversible damage.[64] Changes in collagen content have also been identified, the hydroxyproline content in connective tissue from women with stress incontinence being 40% lower than in continent controls.[65]

UROGENITAL ATROPHY

Withdrawal of endogenous estrogen at the menopause results in well-documented climacteric symptoms such as hot flushes and night sweats in addition to the less commonly reported symptoms of urogenital atrophy. Symptoms do not usually develop until several years following the menopause when levels of endogenous estrogens fall below the level required to promote endometrial growth.[66] This temporal relationship would suggest estrogen withdrawal as the cause.

Vaginal dryness is commonly the first reported symptom and is caused by a reduction in mucus production within the vaginal glands. Atrophy within the vaginal epithelium leads to thinning and an increased susceptibility to infection and mechanical trauma. Glycogen depletion within the vaginal mucosa following the menopause leads to a decrease in lactic acid formation by Döderlein's lactobacillus and a consequent rise in vaginal pH from around 4 to between 6 and 7. This allows bacterial overgrowth and colonization with Gram-negative bacilli, compounding the effects of vaginal atrophy and leading to symptoms of vaginitis such as pruritis, dyspareunia and discharge.

LOWER URINARY TRACT SYMPTOMS

Epidemiologic studies have implicated estrogen deficiency in the etiology of lower urinary tract symptoms with 70% of women relating the onset of urinary incontinence to their final menstrual period.[6] Lower urinary tract symptoms have been shown to be common in postmenopausal women attending a menopause clinic, with 20% complaining of severe urgency and almost 50% complaining of stress incontinence.[67] Urge incontinence in particular is more prevalent following the menopause and the prevalence would appear to rise with increasing years of estrogen deficiency.[68] There is, however, conflicting evidence regarding the role of estrogen withdrawal at the time of the menopause. Some studies have shown a peak incidence in perimenopausal women[69,70] whilst other evidence suggests that many women develop incontinence at least 10 years prior to the cessation of menstruation with significantly more premenopausal women than postmenopausal women being affected.[66,71]

Cyclical variations in the levels of both estrogen and progesterone during the menstrual cycle have also been shown to lead to changes in urodynamic variables and lower urinary tract symptoms, with 37% of women noticing a deterioration in symptoms prior to menstruation.[72] Measurement of the urethral pressure profile in nulliparous premenopausal women shows that there is an increase in functional urethral length midcycle and early in the luteal phase corresponding to an increase in plasma estradiol.[73] Furthermore, progestogens have been associated with an increase in irritative bladder symptoms[74,75] and urinary incontinence in those women taking combined HRT.[76] The incidence of detrusor overactivity in the luteal phase of the menstrual cycle may be associated with raised plasma progesterone following ovulation, and progesterone has been shown to antagonize the inhibitory effect of estradiol on rat detrusor contractions.[77] This may help to explain the increased prevalence of detrusor overactivity found in pregnancy.[78]

Urinary tract infection is also a common cause of urinary symptoms in women of all ages. This is a particular problem in the elderly with a reported incidence of 20% in the community and > 50% in institutionalized patients.[79,80] Pathophysiologic changes such as impairment of bladder emptying, poor perineal hygiene and both fecal and urinary incontinence may partly account for the high prevalence observed. In addition, as previously described, changes in the vaginal flora due to estrogen depletion lead to colonization with Gram-negative bacilli which, in addition to causing local irritative symptoms, also act as uropathogens. These microbiologic changes may be reversed with ERT following the menopause, which offers a rationale for treatment and prophylaxis.

ESTROGENS IN THE MANAGEMENT OF INCONTINENCE

Estrogen preparations have been used for many years in the treatment of urinary incontinence[81,82] although their precise role remains controversial. Many of the studies performed have been uncontrolled observational series examining the use of a wide range of different preparations, doses and routes of administration. The inconsistent use of progestogens to provide endometrial protection is a further confounding factor making interpretation of the results difficult.

In order to clarify the situation a meta-analysis from the Hormones and Urogenital Therapy

(HUT) Committee has been reported.[83] Of 166 articles identified which were published in English between 1969 and 1992 only six were controlled trials and 17 were uncontrolled series. Meta-analysis found an overall significant effect of estrogen therapy on subjective improvement in all subjects and for subjects with urodynamic stress incontinence alone. Subjective improvement rates with estrogen therapy in randomized controlled trials ranged from 64 to 75%, although placebo groups also reported an improvement of 10–56%. In uncontrolled series, subjective improvement rates were 8–89%, with subjects with urodynamic stress incontinence showing improvements of 34–73%. However, when assessing objective fluid loss there was no significant effect. Maximum urethral closure pressure was found to increase significantly with estrogen therapy, although this outcome was influenced by a single study showing a large effect.[84]

A further meta-analysis performed in Italy has analyzed the results of randomized controlled clinical trials on the efficacy of estrogen treatment in postmenopausal women with urinary incontinence.[85] A search of the literature (1965–1996) revealed 72 articles, of which only four were considered to meet the meta-analysis criteria. There was a statistically significant difference in subjective outcome between estrogen and placebo although there was no such difference in objective or urodynamic outcome. The authors concluded that this difference could be relevant, although the studies may have lacked objective sensitivity to detect this.

The role of ERT in the prevention of ischemic heart disease has recently been assessed in a 4-year randomized trial, the Heart and Estrogen/progestin Replacement Study (HERS),[86] involving 2763 postmenopausal women < 80 years of age with intact uteri and ischemic heart disease. In the study 55% of women reported at least one episode of urinary incontinence each week, and were randomly assigned to oral conjugated estrogen plus medroxyprogesterone acetate or placebo daily. Incontinence improved in 26% of women assigned to placebo as compared to 21% receiving HRT, while 27% of the placebo group complained of worsening symptoms

compared with 39% in the HRT group ($P = 0.001$). The incidence of incontinent episodes per week increased by an average of 0.7 in the HRT group and decreased by 0.1 in the placebo group ($P < 0.001$). Overall, combined HRT was associated with worsening stress and urge urinary incontinence, although there was no significant difference in daytime frequency, nocturia or number of urinary tract infections.

More recently the effects of oral estrogens and progestogens on the lower urinary tract have been assessed in 32 female nursing home residents[87] with an average age of 88. Subjects were randomized to oral estrogen and progesterone or placebo for 6 months. At follow-up there was no difference between severity of incontinence, prevalence of bacteriuria or the results of vaginal cultures, although there was an improvement in atrophic vaginitis in the placebo group.

ESTROGENS IN THE MANAGEMENT OF STRESS INCONTINENCE

In addition to the studies included in the HUT meta-analysis, several authors have also investigated the role of estrogen therapy in the management of urodynamic stress incontinence only. Oral estrogens have been reported to increase the maximum urethral pressures and lead to symptomatic improvement in 65–70% of women,[88,89] although other work has not confirmed this.[90,91] More recently two placebo-controlled studies have been performed examining the use of oral estrogens in the treatment of urodynamic stress incontinence in postmenopausal women. Neither conjugated equine estrogens and medroxyprogesterone[92] or unopposed estradiol valerate[93] showed a significant difference in either subjective or objective outcomes. Furthermore, a review of eight controlled and 14 uncontrolled prospective trials concluded that estrogen therapy was not an efficacious treatment for stress incontinence but may be useful for symptoms of urgency and frequency.[94]

From the available evidence, estrogen does not appear to be an effective treatment for stress incontinence although it may have a synergistic role in combination therapy. Two placebo-controlled studies have examined the use of oral and vaginal estrogens with the α-adrenergic agonist phenylpropanolamine used separately and in combination. Both studies found that combination therapy was superior to either drug given alone, and whilst there was subjective improvement in all groups[95] there was only objective improvement in the combination therapy group.[96] This may offer an alternative conservative treatment for women who have mild urodynamic stress incontinence.

ESTROGENS IN THE MANAGEMENT OF URGE INCONTINENCE

Estrogens have been used in the treatment of urinary urgency and urge incontinence for many years but there have been few controlled trials to confirm their efficacy. A double-blind placebo-controlled crossover study using oral estriol in 34 postmenopausal women produced subjective improvement in eight women with mixed incontinence and 12 with urge incontinence,[97] However, a double-blind multicenter study of the use of estriol (3 mg/day) in postmenopausal women complaining of urgency has failed to confirm these findings,[98] showing both subjective and objective improvement but not significantly better than placebo. Estriol is a naturally occurring weak estrogen which has little effect on the endometrium and does not prevent osteoporosis, although has been used in the treatment of urogenital atrophy. Consequently it is possible that the dosage or route of administration in this study was not appropriate in the treatment of urinary symptoms and higher systemic levels may be required.

The use of sustained release 17β-estradiol vaginal tablets (Vagifem, Novo Nordisk) has also been examined in postmenopausal women with urgency and urge incontinence or a urodynamic diagnosis of sensory urgency or detrusor overactivity. These vaginal tablets have been shown to be well absorbed from the vagina and to induce maturation of the vaginal epithelium within 14 days.[99] However, following a 6-month course of treatment the only significant dif-

ference between active and placebo groups was an improvement in the symptom of urgency in those women with a urodynamic diagnosis of sensory urgency.[100] A further double-blind, randomized, placebo-controlled trial of vaginal 17β-estradiol vaginal tablets has shown lower urinary tract symptoms of frequency, urgency, urge and stress incontinence to be significantly improved, but no objective urodynamic assessment was performed.[101] In both of these studies the subjective improvement in symptoms may simply represent local estrogenic effects reversing urogenital atrophy rather than a direct effect on bladder function.

To try to clarify the role of estrogen therapy in the management of women with urge incontinence a meta-analysis of the use of estrogen in women with symptoms of an overactive bladder has been reported by the HUT Committee in 2001 (unpublished work). In a review of 10 randomized placebo controlled trials estrogen was found to be superior to placebo when considering symptoms of urge incontinence, frequency and nocturia, although vaginal estrogen administration was found to be superior for symptoms of urgency. In those taking estrogens there was also a significant increase in first sensation and bladder capacity as compared to placebo

ESTROGENS IN THE MANAGEMENT OF RECURRENT URINARY TRACT INFECTION

Estrogen therapy has been shown to increase vaginal pH and reverse the microbiologic changes that occur in the vagina following the menopause.[102] Initial small uncontrolled studies using oral or vaginal estrogens in the treatment of recurrent urinary tract infection appeared to give promising results,[103,104] although unfortunately this has not been supported by larger randomized trials. Several studies have been performed examining the use of oral and vaginal estrogens but these have given mixed results.

Kjaergaard et al[105] compared vaginal estriol tablets with placebo in 21 postmenopausal women over a 5-month period and found no significant difference between the two groups.

However, a subsequent randomized, double-blind placebo-controlled study assessing the use of estriol vaginal cream in 93 postmenopausal women during an 8-month period did reveal a significant effect.[106]

Kirkengen et al[107] randomized 40 postmenopausal women to receive either placebo or oral estriol and found that although initially both groups had a significantly decreased incidence of recurrent infections, after 12 weeks estriol was shown to be significantly more effective. These findings, however, were not confirmed subsequently in a trial of 72 postmenopausal women with recurrent urinary tract infections randomized to oral estriol or placebo. Following a 6-month treatment period and a further 6-month follow-up, estriol was found to be no more effective than placebo.[108]

More recently a randomized, open, parallel-group study assessing the use of an estradiol-releasing silicone vaginal ring (Estring; Pharmacia & Upjohn, Sweden) in postmenopausal women with recurrent infections has been performed, which showed the cumulative likelihood of remaining infection free was 45% in the active group and 20% in the placebo group.[109] Estring was also shown to decrease the number of recurrences per year and to prolong the interval between infection episodes.

ESTROGENS IN THE MANAGEMENT OF UROGENITAL ATROPHY

Symptoms of urogenital atrophy do not occur until the levels of endogenous estrogen are lower than that required to promote endometrial proliferation.[66] Consequently it is possible to use a low dose of ERT in order to alleviate urogenital symptoms whilst avoiding the risk of endometrial proliferation and removing the necessity of providing endometrial protection with progestogens.[110] The dose of estradiol commonly used in systemic estrogen replacement is 25–100 µg/day, although studies investigating the use of estrogens in the management of urogenital symptoms have shown that 8–10 µg/day of vaginal estradiol is effective.[111] Thus only 10–30% of the dose used to treat

vasomotor symptoms may be effective in the management of urogenital symptoms. Since 10–25% of women receiving systemic HRT still experience the symptoms of urogenital atrophy,[112] low-dose local preparations may have an additional beneficial effect.

A recent review of estrogen therapy in the management of urogenital atrophy has been performed by the HUT Committee.[113] Ten randomized trials and 54 uncontrolled series were examined from 1969 to 1995, assessing 24 different treatment regimens. Meta-analysis of 10 placebo-controlled trials confirmed the significant effect of estrogens in the management of urogenital atrophy.

The route of administration was assessed, and oral, vaginal and parental (transcutaneous patches and subcutaneous implants) were compared. Overall the vaginal route of administration was found to correlate with better symptom relief, greater improvement in cytologic findings and higher serum estradiol levels.

With regard to the type of estrogen preparation, estradiol was found to be most effective in reducing patient symptoms but conjugated estrogens produced the greatest cytologic change and the greatest increase in serum levels of estradiol and estrone.

Finally the effect of different dosages was examined. Low-dose vaginal estradiol was found to be the most efficacious according to symptom relief, although oral estriol was also effective. Estriol had no effect on the serum levels of estradiol or estrone, whilst vaginal estriol had a minimal effect. Vaginal estradiol was found to have a small effect on serum estrogen but not as great as systemic preparations. In conclusion it would appear that estrogen is efficacious in the treatment of urogenital atrophy and low-dose vaginal preparations are as effective as systemic therapy.

More recently the use of a continuous low-dose estradiol-releasing silicone vaginal ring (Estring), releasing estradiol 5–10µg/day, has been investigated in postmenopausal women with symptomatic urogenital atrophy.[109] There was a significant effect on symptoms of vaginal dryness, pruritis vulvae, dyspareunia and urinary urgency, with improvement being reported in > 90% of women in an uncontrolled study. Patient acceptability was high and whilst the maturation of vaginal epithelium was significantly improved there was no effect on endometrial proliferation.

These findings were supported by a 1-year multicenter study of Estring in postmenopausal women with urogenital atrophy which found subjective and objective improvement in 90% of patients for up to 1 year. However, there was a 20% withdrawal rate with 7% of women reporting vaginal irritation, two having vaginal ulceration and three complaining of vaginal bleeding although there were no cases of endometrial proliferation.[114] Long-term safety has been confirmed by a 10-year review of the use of the estradiol ring delivery system which has found its safety, efficacy and acceptability to be comparable to other forms of vaginal administration.[115] A comparative study of safety and efficacy of Estring with conjugated equine estrogen vaginal cream in 194 postmenopausal women complaining of urogenital atrophy found no significant difference in vaginal dryness, dyspareunia and resolution of atrophic signs between the two treatment groups. Furthermore, there was a similar improvement in the vaginal mucosal maturation index and a reduction in pH in both groups, with the vaginal ring being found to be preferable to the cream.[116]

SELECTIVE ESTROGEN RECEPTOR MODULATORS (SERM)

A recent development in hormonal therapy has been the development of SERM. These drugs have estrogen-like actions in maintaining bone density and in lowering serum cholesterol but have anti-estrogenic effects on the breast[117] and do not cause endometrial stimulation.[118] In theory, partial estrogen antagonists may lead to a downregulation of estrogen receptors in the urogenital tract, and consequently cause an increase in lower urinary tract symptoms and symptomatic urogenital atrophy. Early work would suggest that some SERM in development (levormeloxifene and idoxifene) may

increase the risk of urogenital prolapse,[119] although there were some methodologic problems noted in the study. However, in an analysis of three randomized, double-blind, placebo-controlled trials investigating raloxifene in 6926 postmenopausal women there appeared to be a protective effect, with fewer treated women having surgery for urogenital prolapse – 1.5 versus 0.75% ($P < 0.005$).[120] At present the long-term effect of SERM on the urogenital tract remains to be determined and there are little data regarding effects on urinary incontinence and urogenital atrophy

CONCLUSIONS

Estrogens are known to have an important physiologic effect on the female lower genital tract throughout adult life, leading to symptomatic, histologic and functional changes. Urogenital atrophy is the manifestation of estrogen withdrawal following the menopause, presenting with vaginal and/or urinary symptoms. The use of ERT in the management of lower urinary tract symptoms has been examined, as well as in the treatment of urogenital atrophy, although only recently has it been subjected to randomized placebo-controlled trials and meta-analysis.

Estrogen therapy alone has been shown to have little effect in the management of urodynamic stress incontinence but when used in combination with an α-adrenergic agonist to an improvement in urinary leakage may be seen. When considering the irritative symptoms of urinary urgency, frequency and urge incontinence, estrogen therapy may be of benefit, although this may simply represent reversal of urogenital atrophy rather than a direct effect on the lower urinary tract. The role of ERT in the management of women with recurrent lower urinary tract infection remains to be determined but there is now some evidence that vaginal administration may be efficacious. Finally, low-dose vaginal estrogens have been shown to have a role in the treatment of urogenital atrophy in postmenopausal women, appearing to be as effective as systemic preparations.

REFERENCES

1. Iosif CS. Effects of protracted administration of oestriol on the lower genitourinary tract in postmenopausal women. *Acta Obstet Gynecol Scand* 1992; **251:** 115–20.
2. Cardozo LD. Role of oestrogens in the treatment of female urinary incontinence. *J Am Geriatr Soc* 1990; **38:** 326–8.
3. Iosif S, Batra S, Ek A, Astedt B. Oestrogens receptors in the human female lower urinary tract. *Am J Obstet Gynecol* 1981; **141:** 817–20.
4. Batra SC, Fossil CS. Female urethra, a target for oestrogen action. *J Urol* 1983; **129:** 418–20.
5. Batra SC, Iosif LS. Progesterone receptors in the female urinary tract. *J Urol* 1987; **138:** 130–4.
6. Iosif C, Bekassy Z. Prevalence of genitourinary symptoms in the late menopause. *Acta Obstet Gynecol Scand* 1984; **63:** 257–60.
7. American National Institute of Health Population Figures. US Treasury Department. NIH. 1991.
8. Research on the menopause in the 1990's. Report of a WHO Scientific Group. WHO Technical Report Series 866, Geneva, Switzerland. 1994.
9. Hill K. The demography of the menopause. *Maturitas* 1996; **23:** 113–27.
10. Barlow D, Samsioe G, van Geelan H. Prevalence of urinary problems in European countries. *Maturitas* 1997; **27:** 239–48.
11. Greendale GA, Judd JL. The menopause: health implications and clinical management. *J Am Geriatr Soc* 1993; **41:** 426–36.
12. Samsioe G, Jansson I, Mellstrom D, Svanborg A. The occurrence, nature and treatment of urinary incontinence in a 70 year old population. *Maturitas* 1985; **7:** 335–43.
13. Van Geelen JM, Van de Weijer PH, Arnolds HT. Urogenital symptoms and resulting discomfort in non-institutionalised Dutch women aged 50–75 years. *Int Urogynecol J Pelvic Floor Dysfunct* 2000; **11:** 9–14.
14. Versi E, Harvey MA, Cardozo L et al. Urogenital prolapse and atrophy at menopause: a prevalence study. *Int Urogynaecol J Pelvic Dysfunct* 2001; **12:** 107–10.
15. Davila GW, Karapanagiotou I, Woodhouse S et al. Are women with urogenital atrophy symptomatic? *Obstet Gynecol* 2001; **97** (Suppl 1): S48.
16. Diokno AC, Brook BM, Brown MB. Prevalence of urinary incontinence and other urological symptoms in the non-institutionalised elderly. *J Urol* 1986; **136:** 1022.
17. Yarnell J, Voyle G, Richards C, Stephenson T. The prevalence and severity of urinary incontinence in women. *J Epidemiol Commun Health* 1981; **35:** 71–4.
18. Ouslander JG. Urinary incontinence in nursing homes. *J Am Geriatr Soc* 1990; **38:** 289–91.
19. MacLennan AH, Taylor AW, Wilson AW, Wilson D. The prevalence of pelvic floor disorders and their relationship to gender, age, parity, and mode of delivery. *Br J Obstet Gynaecol* 2000; **107:** 1460–70.
20. Kok AL, Voorhorst FJ, Burger CW et al. Urinary and faecal incontinence in community residing elderly women. *Age Ageing* 1992; **21:** 211.
21. Department of Health, 2001.
22. Green S, Walter P, Kumar V et al. Human oestrogen receptor cDNA: sequence, expression and homology to v-erbA. *Nature* 1986; **320:** 134–9.
23. Kuiper G, Enmark E, Pelto-Huikko M et al. Cloning of a novel oestrogen receptor expressed in rat prostate and ovary. *Proc Natl Acad Sci USA* 1996; **93:** 5925–30.
24. Blakeman PJ, Hilton P, Bulmer JN. Mapping oestrogen and progesterone receptors throughout the female lower urinary tract. *Neurourol Urodyn* 1996; **15:** 324–5.
25. Ingelman-Sundberg A, Rosen J, Gustafsson SA. Cytosol oestrogen receptors in urogenital tissues in stress incontinent women. *Acta Obstet Gynecol Scand* 1981; **60:** 585–6.
25. Smith P. Oestrogens and the urogenital tract. *Acta Obstet Gynecol Scand* 1993; **72:** 1–26.
26. Bernstein IT. The pelvic floor muscles: muscle thickness in healthy and urinary-incontinent women measured by perineal ultasonography with reference to the effect of pelvic floor training. Oestrogen receptor studies. *Neurourol Urodyn* 1997; **16:** 237–75.
28. Chen GD, Oliver RH, Leung BS et al. Oestrogen receptor α and β expression in the vaginal walls and uterosacral ligaments of premenopausal and postmenopausal women. *Fertil Steril* 1999; **71:** 1099–102.
29. Screiter F, Fuchs P, Stockamp K. Oestrogenic sensitivity of α receptors in the urethral musculature. *Urol Int* 1976; **31:** 13–19.
30. Pang X, Cotreau-Bibbo MM, Sant GR, Theoharides TC. Bladder mast cell expression of high affinity oestrogen receptors in receptors in patients with interstitial cystitis. *Br J Urol* 1995; **75:** 154–61.

31. Blakeman PJ, Hilton P, Bulmer JN. Androgen receptors in the female lower urinary tract. *Int Urogynecol J* 1997; **8**: S54.

32. Blakeman PJ, Hilton P, Bulmer JN. Oestrogen and progesterone receptor expression in the female lower urinary tract, with reference to oestrogen status. *BJU Int* 2000; **86**: 32–8.

33. Abrams P, Blaivas JG, Stanton SL et al. The standardisation of terminology of lower urinary tract dysfunction. *Br J Obstet Gynaecol* 1990; **97**: 1–16.

34. Rud T, Anderson KE, Asmussen M et al. Factors maintaining the urethral pressure in women. *Invest Urol* 1980; **17**: 343–7.

35. Malone-Lee J. Urodynamic measurement and urinary incontinence in the elderly. In: (Brocklehurst JC, ed) *Managing and Measuring Incontinence*. Proceedings of the Geriatric Workshop on Incontinence, July 1988.

36. Versi E, Cardozo LD. Oestrogens and lower urinary tract function. In: (Studd JWW, Whitehead MI, eds) *The Menopause*. (Blackwell Scientific Publications: Oxford, 1988) 76–84.

37. Kinn AC, Lindskog M. Oestrogens and phenylpropanolamine in combination for stress incontinence. *Urology* 1988; **32**: 273–80.

38. Smith PJB. The effect of oestrogens on bladder function in the female. In: (Campbell S, ed) *The Management of the Menopause and Postmenopausal Years*. (MTP: Carnforth, 1976) 291–8.

39. Samsioe G, Jansson I, Mellstrom, D, Svandborg A. Occurrence, nature and treatment of urinary incontinence in a 70 year old female population. *Maturitas* 1985; **7**: 335–42.

40. Blakeman PJ, Hilton P, Bulmer JN. Cellular proliferation in the female lower urinary tract with reference to oestrogen status. *Br J Obstet Gynaecol* 2001; **8**: 813–16.

41. Shapiro E. Effect of oestrogens on the weight and muscarinic receptor density of the rabbit bladder and urethra. *J Urol* 1986; **135**: 1084–7.

42. Batra S, Anderson KE. Oestrogen induced changes in muscarinic receptor density and contractile responses in the female rat urinary bladder. *Acta Physiol Scand* 1989; **137**: 135–41.

43. Elliott RA, Castleden CM, Miodrag A, Kirwan P. The direct effects of diethylstilboestrol and nifedipine on the contractile responses of isolated human and rat detrusor muscles. *Eur J Clin Pharmacol* 1992; **43**: 149–55.

44. Shenfield OZ, Blackmore PF, Morgan CW et al. Rapid effects of oestriol and progesterone on tone and spontaneous rhythmic contractions of the rabbit bladder. *Neurourol Urodyn* 1998; **17**: 408–9.

45. Fantl JA, Wyman JF, Anderson RL et al. Post menopausal urinary incontinence: comparison between non-oestrogen and oestrogen supplemented women. *Obstet Gynecol* 1988; **71**: 823–8.

46. Maggi A, Perez J. Role of female gonadal hormones in the CNS. *Life Sci* 1985; **37**: 893–906.

47. Smith SS, Berg G, Hammar M (eds). *The modern management of the menopause. Hormones, mood and neurobiology – a summary*. (Parthenon Publishing: Carnforth, UK, 1993) 204.

48. Blok EFM, Holstege G. Androgen receptor immunoreactive neurones in the hypothalamic preoptic area project to the pontine micturition centre in the male cat. *Neurourol Urodyn* 1998; **17**: 404–5.

49. Bergman A, Karram MM, Bhatia NN. Changes in urethral cytology following oestrogen administration. *Gynecol Obstet Invest* 1990; **29**: 211–13.

50. Rud T. The effects of oestrogens and gestogens on the urethral pressure profile in urinary continent and stress incontinent women. *Acta Obstet Gynecol Scand* 1980; **59**: 365–70.

51. Hilton P, Stanton SL. The use of intravaginal oestrogen cream in genuine stress incontinence. *Br J Obstet Gynaecol* 1983; **90**: 940–4.

52. Bhatia NN, Bergman A, Karram MM et al. Effects of oestrogen on urethral function in women with urinary incontinence. *Am J Obstet Gynecol* 1989; **160**: 176–80.

53. Karram MM, Yeko TR, Sauer MV et al. Urodynamic changes following hormone replacement therapy in women with premature ovarian failure. *Obstet Gynecol* 1989; **74**: 208–11.

54. Ganger KF, Vyas S, Whitehead RW et al. Pulsatility index in the internal carotid artery in relation to transdermal oestradiol and time since the menopause. *Lancet* 1991; **338**: 839–42.

55. Jackson S, Vyas S. A double blind, placebo controlled study of postmenopausal oestrogen replacement therapy and carotid artery pulsatility index. *Br J Obstet Gynaecol* 1998; **105**: 408–12.

56. Penotti M, Farina M, Sironi L et al. Long term effects of postmenopausal hormone replacement therapy on pulsatility index of the internal carotid and middle cerebral arteries. *Menopause J N Am Menopause Soc* 1997; **4**: 101–4.

57. Versi E, Cardozo LD. Urethral instability: diagnosis based on variations in the maximum

urethral pressure in normal climateric women. *Neurourol Urodyn* 1986; **5**: 535–41.

58. Falconer C, Ekman-Ordeberg G, Ulmsten U et al. Changes in paraurethral connective tissue at menopause are counteracted by oestrogen. *Maturitas* 1996; **24**: 197–204.

59. Kushner L, Chen Y, Desautel M et al. Collagenase activity is elevated in conditioned media from fibroblasts of women with pelvic floor weakening. *Int Urogynecol* 1999; **10**: 34.

60. Jackson S, Avery N, Shepherd A et al. The effect of oestradiol on vaginal collagen in post-menopausal women with stress urinary incontinence. *Neurourol Urodyn* 1996; **15**: 327–8.

61. James M, Avery N, Jackson S et al. The patho-physiological changes of vaginal skin tissue in women with stress urinary incontinence: A controlled trial. *Int Urogynecol* 1999; **10**: 35.

62. James M, Avery N, Jackson S et al. The bio-chemical profile of vaginal tissue in women with genitourinary prolapse: a controlled trial. *Neurourol Urodyn* 1999; **18**: 284–5.

63. Brincat M, Moniz CF, Studd JWW. Long term effects of the menopause and sex hormones on skin thickness. *Br J Obstet Gynaecol* 1985; **92**: 256–9.

64. Landon CR, Smith ARB, Crofts CE, Trowbridge EA. Biochemical properties of connective tissue in women with stress incontinence of urine. *Neurourol Urodyn* 1989; **8**: 369–70.

65. Ulmsten U, Ekman G, Giertz G. Different bio-chemical composition of connective tissue in continent and stress incontinent women. *Acta Obstet Gynecol Scand* 1987; **66**: 455.

66. Samicoe G. Urogenital ageing – a hidden prob-lem. *Am J Obstet Gynecol* 1998; **178**: S245–S249.

67. Cardozo LD, Tapp A, Versi E et al (eds). The lower urinary tract in peri- and post-menopausal women. In: *The Urogenital Deficiency Syndrome.* (Novo Industri AS: Bagsverd, Denmark, 1987) 10–17.

68. Kondo A, Kato K, Saito M et al. Prevalence of hand washing incontinence in females in com-parison with stress and urge incontinence. *Neurourol Urodyn* 1990; **9**: 330–1.

69. Thomas TM, Plymat KR, Blannin J et al. Prevalence of urinary incontinence. *BMJ* 1980; **281**: 1243–5.

70. Jolleys JV. Reported prevalence of urinary incontinence in a general practice. *BMJ* 1988; **296**: 1300–2.

71. Burgio KL, Matthews KA, Engel B. Prevalence, incidence and correlates of urinary inconti-nence in healthy, middle aged women. *J Urol* 1991; **146**: 1255–9.

72. Hextall A, Bidmead J, Cardozo L, Hooper R. Hormonal influences on the human female lower urinary tract: a prospective evaluation of the effects of the menstrual cycle on symptoma-tology and the results of urodynamic investiga-tion. *Neurourol Urodyn* 1999; **18**: 282–3.

73. Van Geelen JM, Doesburg WH, Thomas CMG. Urodynamic studies in the normal menstrual cycle: the relationship between hormonal changes during the menstrual cycle and the urethral pressure profile. *Am J Obstet Gynecol* 1981; **141**: 384–92.

74. Burton G, Cardozo LD, Abdalla H et al. The hormonal effects on the lower urinary tract in 282 women with premature ovarian failure. *Neurourol Urodyn* 1992; **10**: 318–19.

75. Cutner A, Burton G, Cardozo LD et al. Does progesterone cause an irritable bladder? *Int Urogynecol J* 1993; **4**: 259–61.

76. Benness C, Gangar K, Cardozo LD, Cutner A. Do progestogens exacerbate urinary inconti-nence in women on HRT? *Neurourol Urodyn* 1991; **10**: 316–18.

77. Elliot RA, Castleden CM. Effect of progesta-gens and oestrogens on the contractile response of rat detrusor muscle to electrical field stimu-lation. *Clin Sci* 1994; **87**: 342.

78. Cutner A. *The urinary tract in pregnancy.* MD thesis, University of London, 1993.

79. Sandford JP. Urinary tract symptoms and infec-tion. *Ann Rev Med* 1975; **26**: 485–505.

80. Boscia JA, Kaye D. Assymptomatic bacteria in the elderly. *Infect Dis Clin N Am* 1987; **1**: 893–903.

81. Salmon UL, Walter RI, Gast SH. The use of oestrogen in the treatment of dysuria and incontinence in postmenopausal women. *Am J Obstet Gynecol* 1941; **14**: 23–31.

82. Youngblood VH, Tomlin EM, Davis JB. Senile urethritis in women. *J Urol* 1957; **78**: 150–2.

83. Fantl JA, Cardozo LD, McClish DK, and the Hormones and Urogenital Therapy Committee. Oestrogen therapy in the management of incontinence in postmenopausal women: a meta-analysis. First report of the Hormones and Urogenital Therapy Committee. *Obstet Gynecol* 1994; **83**: 12–18.

84. Henalla SM, Hutchins CJ, Robinson P, Macivar J. Non-operative methods in the treatment of female genuine stress incontinence of urine. *Br J Obstet Gynecol* 1989; **9**: 222–5.

85. Zullo MA, Oliva C, Falconi G et al. Efficacy of oestrogen therapy in urinary incontinence. A meta-analytic study. *Minerva Gynecol* 1998; **50:** 199–205.

86. Grady D, Brown JS, Vittinghoff E et al. Postmenopausal hormones and incontinence: the Heart and Estrogen/progestin Replacement Study. *Obstet Gynecol* 2001; **97:** 116–20.

87. Ouslander JG, Greendale GA, Uman G et al. Effects of oral oestrogen and progestin on the lower urinary tract among female nursing home residents. *Am Geriatr Soc* 2001; **49:** 803–7.

88. Caine M, Raz S. The role of female hormones in stress incontinence. Proceedings of the 16th Congress of the International Society of Urology, Amsterdam, The Netherlands.

89. Rud T. The effects of oestrogens and gestagens on the urethral pressure profile in urinary continent and stress incontinent women. *Acta Obstet Gynecol Scand* 1980; **59:** 265–70.

90. Wilson PD, Faragher B, Butler B et al. Treatment with oral piperazine oestrone sulphate for genuine stress incontinence in postmenopausal women. *Br J Obstet Gynecol* 1987; **94:** 568–74.

91. Walter S, Wolf H, Barlebo H, Jansen H. Urinary incontinence in postmenopausal women treated with oestrogens: a double-blind clinical trial. *Urol Int* 1978; **33:** 135–43.

92. Fantl JA, Bump RC, Robinson D et al. Efficacy of oestrogen supplementation in the treatment of urinary incontinence. *Obstet Gynecol* 1996; **88:** 745–9.

93. Jackson S, Shepherd A, Brookes S, Abrams P. The effect of oestrogen supplementation on post-menopausal urinary stress incontinence: a double-blind, placebo controlled trial. *Br J Obstet Gynecol*. 1999; **106:** 711–18.

94. Sultana CJ, Walters MD. Oestrogen and urinary incontinence in women. *Maturitas* 1995; **20:** 129–38.

95. Beisland HO, Fossberg E, Moer A et al. Urethral insufficiency in post-menopausal females: treatment with phenylpropanolamine and oestriol separately and in combination. *Urol Int* 1984; **39:** 211–16.

96. Hilton P, Tweddel AL, Mayne C. Oral and intravaginal oestrogens alone and in combination with alpha adrenergic stimulation in genuine stress incontinence. *Int Urogynecol J* 1990; **12:** 80–6.

97. Samsicoe G, Jansson I, Mellstrom D, Svanberg A. Urinary incontinence in 75 year old women.

Effects of oestriol. *Acta Obstet Gynecol Scand* 1985; **93:** 57.

98. Cardozo LD, Rekers H, Tapp A et al. Oestriol in the treatment of postmenopausal urgency: a multicentre study. *Maturitas* 1993; **18:** 47–53.

99. Nilsson K, Heimer G. Low dose oestradiol in the treatment of urogenital oestrogen deficiency – a pharmacokinetic and pharmacodynamic study. *Maturitas* 1992; **15:** 121–7.

100. Benness C, Wise BG, Cutner A, Cardozo LD. Does low dose vaginal oestradiol improve frequency and urgency in postmenopausal women. *Int Urogynecol J* 1992; **3:** 281.

101. Eriksen PS, Rasmussen H. Low dose 17β-oestradiol vaginal tablets in the treatment of atrophic vaginitis: a double-blind placebo controlled study. *Eur J Obstet Gynecol Reprod Biol* 1992; **44:** 137–44.

102. Brandberg A, Mellstrom D, Samsioe G. Low dose oral oestriol treatment in elderly women with urogenital infections. *Acta Obstet Gynecol Scand* 1987; **140:** 33–8.

103. Parsons CL, Schmidt JD. Control of recurrent urinary tract infections in postmenopausal women. *J Urol* 1982; **128:** 1224–6.

104. Privette M, Cade R, Peterson J et al. Prevention of recurrent urinary tract infections in postmenopausal women. *Nephron* 1988; **50:** 24–7.

105. Kjaergaard B, Walter S, Knudsen A et al. Treatment with low dose vaginal oestradiol in postmenopausal women. A double blind controlled trial. *Ugeskr Laeger* 1990; **152:** 658–9.

106. Raz R, Stamm WE. A controlled trial of intravaginal oestriol in postmenopausal women with recurrent urinary tract infections. *N Engl J Med* 1993; **329:** 753–6.

107. Kirkengen AL, Anderson P, Gjersoe E et al. Oestriol in the prophylactic treatment of recurrent urinary tract infections in postmenopausal women. *Scand J Prim Health Care* 1992; **10:** 142.

108. Cardozo LD, Benness C, Abbott D. Low dose oestrogen prophylaxis for recurrent urinary tract infections in elderly women. *Br J Obstet Gynaecol* 1998; **105:** 403–7.

109. Eriksen B. A randomised, open, parallel-group study on the preventative effect of an oestradiol-releasing vaginal ring (Estring) on recurrent urinary tract infections in postmenopausal women. *Am J Obstet Gynecol* 1999; **180:** 1072–9.

110. Mettler L, Olsen PG. Long term treatment of atrophic vaginitis with low dose oestradiol vaginal tablets. *Maturitas* 1991; **14:** 23–31.

111. Smith P, Heimer G, Lindskog M, Ulmsten U.

Oestradiol releasing vaginal ring for treatment of postmenopausal urogenital atrophy. *Maturitas* 1993; **16:** 145–54.

112. Smith RJN, Studd JWW. Recent advances in hormone replacement therapy. *Br J Hosp Med* 1993; **49:** 799–809.

113. Cardozo LD, Bachmann G, McClish D et al. Meta-analysis of oestrogen therapy in the management of urogenital atrophy in postmenopausal women: second report of the Hormones and Urogenital Therapy Committee. *Obstet Gynecol* 1998; **92:** 722–7.

114. Henriksson L, Stjernquist M, Boquist L et al. A one-year multicentre study of efficacy and safety of a continuous, low dose, oestradiol-releasing vaginal ring (Estring) in postmenopausal women with symptoms and signs of urogenital aging. *Am J Obstet Gynecol* 1996; **174:** 85–92.

115. Bachmann G. Oestradiol-releasing vaginal ring delivery system for urogenital atrophy. Experience over the last decade. *J Reprod Med* 1998; **43:** 991–8.

116. Ayton RA, Darling GM, Murkies AL et al. A comparative study of safety and efficacy of low dose oestradiol released from a vaginal ring compared with conjugated equine oestrogen vaginal cream in the treatment of postmenopausal vaginal atrophy. *Br J Obstet Gynaecol* 1996; **103:** 351–8.

117. Park WC, Jordan VC. Selective oestrogen receptor modulators (SERMs) and their roles in cancer prevention. *Trends Molec Med* 2002; **8:** 82–8.

118. Silfen SL, Ciaccia AV, Bryant HU. Selective oestrogen receptor modulators: tissue selectivity and differential uterine effects. *Climacteric* 1999; **2:** 268–83.

119. Hendrix SL, McNeeley SG. Effect of selective oestrogen receptor modulators on reproductive tissues other than endometrium. *Ann NY Acad Sci* 2001; **949:** 243–50.

120. Goldstein SR, Neven P, Zhou L et al. Raloxifene effect on frequency of surgery for pelvic floor relaxation. *Obstet Gynecol* 2001; **98:** 91–6.

20

Estrogens in the treatment of premenstrual, postnatal and perimenopausal depression

J Studd

Introduction • **Premenstrual syndrome (PMS)** • **Postnatal depression** • **Climacteric depression** • **Conclusions** • **References**

INTRODUCTION

There is increasing awareness amongst psychiatrists and gynecologists that depression is more common in women than in men and that much of this depression is improved with estrogens and becomes worse with progestogens.

On Boxing Day 1851, Charles Dickens attended the patients' Christmas dance at St Luke's Hospital for the insane. On describing his visit in an article for *Household Words* he commented that the experience of the asylum proved that insanity was more prevalent amongst women than men. Of the 18,759 inmates over the century, 11,162 had been women. He adds, 'It is well known that female servants are more frequently affected by lunacy than any other class of persons.'

Charles Dickens was as great an observer as any Nobel prize winner and indeed this passage is one of the very few references in Victorian literature that makes the point between gender and depression, but there are none to my knowledge relating reproductive function to depression. Jane Eyre's red room and Berthe Mason's monthly madness may be coded examples of this from Charlotte Brontë's pen.

Modern epidemiology confirms that depression is more common in women than men whether we look at hospital admissions, population studies, suicide attempts or the prescription of antidepressants.[1] The challenge remains to determine whether this increase in depression is environmental, reflecting women's perceived role in contemporary society, or whether it is due to hormonal changes.

It is clear that this excess of depression in women starts at puberty and is no longer present in the sixth and seventh decades. The peaks of depression occur at times of hormonal fluctuation in: (1) the premenstrual phase; (2) the postpartum phase; and (3) the climacteric perimenopausal phase, particularly in the 1–2 years before periods cease. This triad of hormone-responsive mood disorders often occur in the same vulnerable woman. The depression of these patients can usually be treated effectively by estrogens, preferably by the transdermal route and in a moderately high dose. Transdermal estrogen patches of 200 µg has been the dose used in published placebo-controlled studies but the 100 µg dose is frequently effective.

The 45-year-old depressed perimenopausal woman who is still menstruating will often give a history of previous postnatal depression and depression before periods. They will often be in a very good mood during pregnancy and also have systemic manifestations of hormonal fluctuation in the form of menstrual headaches or menstrual migraine. Such a woman will often say that she *last felt well during her last pregnancy*. She then developed postnatal depression for several months. When her periods returned the depression became cyclical and as she approached the menopause the depression became more constant. Reproductive events also affect the course of bipolar disorder in women: 67% of such women had a history of postpartum depression. Of these, all had episodes of depression after subsequent pregnancies. Subsequently women who were not using hormone replacement therapy (HRT) were significantly more likely than those who were using HRT to report worsening of the depression symptoms during the perimenopause or menopause.

The problem with this clear clinical history of a woman who will probably respond to estrogens is that psychiatrists believe that such patients are also ideal for the use of antidepressants. This is because they would recognize that they would have had a pre-morbid history of depression and therefore they would have chronic relapsing depressive illness. The fact that this depression is postnatal or premenstrual in timing usually escapes them. It is sad that both gynecologists and psychiatrists are products of their own training with too little overlap in knowledge. The patients thus become victims of this professional schism.

The clue to the use of estrogens came with the important and somewhat eccentric paper by Klaiber et al,[2] who performed a placebo-controlled study of very high-dose estrogens in patients with chronic relapsing depression. They had various diagnoses and were both premenopausal and postmenopausal. They were given Premarin 5 mg/day with an increase in dose of 5 mg each week until a maximum of 30 mg/day was used. There was a huge improvement in depression on these high doses *compared to placebo* and the only patients who had a substantial improvement in their Hamilton depression score ≥ 15 were on the active treatment. But this important work has not been repeated because of anxiety over high-dose estrogens.

PREMENSTRUAL SYNDROME (PMS)

This condition is mentioned in the fourth century BC by Hippocrates but became a medical epidemic in the nineteenth century. Victorian physicians were aware of menstrual madness, hysteria, chlorosis, ovarian mania, as well as the more commonplace neurasthenia. In the 1870s Maudsley,[3] the most distinguished psychiatrist of the time, wrote 'The monthly activity of the ovaries which marks the advent of puberty in women has a notable effect upon the mind and body; wherefore it may become an important cause of mental and physical derangement . . .' This and other female maladies were recognized, rightly or wrongly, to be due to the ovaries. As a consequence, bilateral oophorectomy – Battey's operation[4] or Lawson Tait's operation – became fashionable, being performed in approximately 150,000 women in North America and Northern Europe in the 30 years from 1870. (Although Battey of Georgia, USA, and Tait of Birmingham, UK, insisted that their names were used to describe the operation of normal ovariotomy, it was first performed by Alfred Hegar of Germany in 1872.)

Longo,[5] in his brilliant historical essay on the decline of Battey's operation, posed the question of whether it worked or not. Of course they had no knowledge of osteoporosis and the devastation of long-term estrogen deficiency; therefore, on balance, the operation was not helpful as a long-term solution but it probably did, as was claimed, cure the 'menstrual/ovarian madness', which would be a quaint Victorian way of labeling severe PMS. The essential logic of this operation was to remove cyclical ovarian function but happily this can now effectively be achieved by simpler medical therapy. Only in 1931 was the term *premenstrual tension* introduced by Frank,[6] who described 15 women with the typical symptoms of PMS as we know it. Greene and Dalton[7] extended the definition to premenstrual syndrome in 1953, recognizing the wider range of symptoms.

Severe PMS is a poorly understood collection

of cyclical symptoms which cause considerable psychologic and physical distress. The psychologic symptoms of depression, loss of energy, irritability, loss of libido and abnormal behavior, as well as the physical symptoms of headaches, breast discomfort and abdominal bloating may occur for up to 14 days each month. There may also be associated menstrual problems, pelvic pain, menstrual headaches and the woman may only enjoy as few as seven good days per month. It is obvious that the symptoms mentioned can have a significant impact on the day-to-day functioning of women. It is estimated that up to 95% of women have some form of PMS but in about 5% of women of reproductive age they will be affected severely with disruption of their daily activities. Considering these figures it is disturbing that many of the consultations at our specialist PMS clinics start with women saying that for many years they have been told that there are no treatments available and that they should simply 'live with it'. In addition, many commonly used treatments for PMS, particularly progesterone or progestogens, have been shown by many placebo-controlled trials not to be not only ineffective but they commonly make the symptoms worse as these women are progesterone or progestogen intolerant.

The exact cause is uncertain but fundamentally it is due to the hormonal or biochemical changes (whatever they are) that occur with ovulation, and the resulting complex interaction between ovarian steroids, the gamma-aminobutyric acid (GABA) system and the seratonin and other neuroendocrine factors that occur with ovulation. These neural endocrine changes produce the varied symptoms in women who are somehow vulnerable to changes in their normal reproductive hormone levels. These cyclical chemical changes, probably due to progesterone or one of its metabolites such as allopregnanalone, produce the cyclical symptoms of PMS.

Estrogens

PMS does not occur if there is no ovarian function.[8] Obviously, it does not occur before puberty or after the menopause or after oophorectomy. It also does not occur during pregnancy. However, it is important to realize that hysterectomy with conservation of the ovaries does not often cure PMS,[9] as patients are left with the usual cyclical symptoms and cyclical headaches without the periods. This condition, best-called the *ovarian cycle syndrome*,[10] is usually not recognized to be hormonal in etiology as there is no reference point of menstruation. The failure to make this diagnosis is regrettable because these monthly symptoms of depression, irritability, mood change, bloating and headaches, which might affect the woman most days with only a good week each month, can easily be treated with transdermal estrogens which suppress ovarian function and thus remove the symptoms.

A medical Battey's operation can be achieved by the use of gonadotropin-releasing hormone (GnRH) analogues, and Leather et al[11] have demonstrated that 3 months of Zoladex therapy cures all the symptom groups of PMS. The women do, of course, have hot flushes and sweats but these are usually far preferable to the cyclical depression, irritability and headaches. The long-term risk of Zoladex therapy is bone demineralization but the same group showed that add-back with a product containing 2 mg of estradiol valerate and cyclical levonorgestrel (Nuvelle, Schering Health) maintains the bone density at both the spine and the hip.[12] Most of the PMS symptoms remain improved with this add-back but bloating, tension and irritability recur, probably due to the cyclical progestogen. Livial may be a better add-back preparation.

In a Scandinavian study, Sundstrom et al[13] used low-dose GnRH analogues (100 µg buserelin) with good results on the symptoms of PMS, but the treatment still caused anovulation in as many as 56% of patients. Danazol is another method to treat PMS by inhibiting pituitary gonadotropins, but it has side effects including androgenic and virilizing effects. When used in the luteal phase only it only relieved mastalgia but not the general symptoms of PMS, even though side effects were minimal.[14]

Greenblatt et al[15] showed the effects of

anovulatory doses of estrogen implants for the use of contraception. The first study for its use in PMS was by Magos et al,[16] using 100 mg estradiol implants, the dose that had been shown to inhibit ovulation by using ultrasound and day 21 progesterone measurements in earlier studies by the same group. This showed a huge 84% improvement with placebo implants but the improvements of every symptom cluster was greater in the active estradiol group. In addition, the placebo effect usually waned after a few months compared with a continued response to estradiol. These patients, of course, were also given 12 days of oral progestogen per month to prevent endometrial hyperplasia and irregular bleeding.[17] It was clear that the addition of progestogen attenuated the beneficial effect of estrogen. Subsequently a placebo-controlled trial of cyclical norethisterone in well-estrogenized hysterectomized women reproduced the typical symptoms of PMS.[18] This study of cyclical oral progestogen in the estrogen-primed woman is the model for PMS. It is also significant that progestogen intolerance is one of the principal reasons why older, postmenopausal women stop taking HRT,[19] particularly if they have a past history of PMS or progesterone intolerance. It is common for progestogens to cause PMS-like symptoms in these women in the same way endogenous cyclical progesterone secretion is the probable fundamental cause of PMS.

Our group still uses estradiol implants, often with the addition of testosterone for loss of energy and loss of libido, in our PMS clinics but we have reduced the estradiol dose, never starting with 100 mg. We will now insert pellets of estradiol 50 or 75 mg with 100 mg of testosterone. These women must have endometrial protection by either oral progestogen or a Mirena (Schering Healthcare) levonorgestrel-releasing intrauterine system (LNG IUS).[20] As women with PMS respond well to estrogens but are often intolerant to progestogens, it is commonplace for us to reduce the orthodox 13-day course of progestogen to 10 or 7 days starting, for convenience, on the first day of every calendar month. Thus, the menstrual cycle is reset.

The Mirena IUS also plays a vital role in preventing PMS-like symptoms as it performs its role of protecting the endometrium without systemic absorption. A recent study has shown a 50% decrease in hysterectomies in our practice since the introduction of the Mirena IUS in 1995.[17] With its profound effect on menorrhagia and the possibility of fewer progestogenic side effects, Mirena looks a very promising component of PMS treatment in the future.

Hormone implants are not licensed in all countries and are unsuitable for women who may wish to easily discontinue treatment in order to become pregnant. Estradiol patches are an alternative and our original double-blind crossover study used 200 μg estradiol patches twice weekly.[21] This produced plasma estradiol levels of 800 pmol/l and suppressed luteal phase progesterone and ovulation. Once again this was better than placebo in every symptom cluster of PMS and is now our treatment of choice in severe PMS.

Subsequently a randomized but uncontrolled observational study from our PMS clinic indicated that PMS sufferers could have the same beneficial response to 100 μg patches as they do with the 200 μg dose. They also have fewer symptoms of breast discomfort, bloating and there is less anxiety from the patient or general practitioner about high-dose estrogen therapy.[22] Twenty-one-day progesterone assays in the patients receiving 100 μg showed low anovulatory levels, prompting the intriguing question that even this moderate dose might reliably suppress ovulation and be contraceptive. Clearly, a great deal of work must be done before we can suggest that this treatment is effective birth control but it is of great importance because many young women on this therapy for PMS will be pleased if it is also an effective contraceptive. This is a study which needs to be conducted.

The original studies outlined in this chapter are all scientifically valid placebo-controlled trials showing a considerable improvement in PMS symptoms with estrogens. Although this treatment is used by most gynecologists in the United Kingdom, its value has not been exploited by psychiatrists anywhere in the world. We believe that the benefit of this therapy in severe PMS is due to the inhibition of ovulation but there is probably also a central mental tonic effect. Klaiber et al,[2] in their study of high-dose Premarin, showed this, and other psychoendocrine studies of climacteric depression[23] and postnatal depression[24] have shown the benefit of high-dose transdermal estrogens for these conditions which is not related to or dependent upon suppression of ovulation.

Ultimately there are some women who, after treatment with estrogens and Mirena coils, will prefer to have a hysterectomy in order to remove all cycles with a virtual guarantee of improvement of symptoms. This should not be seen as a failure or even treatment of last resort as it does have many other advantages.[25] It is important that women who have had a hysterectomy and bilateral salpingo-oophorectomy have effective replacement therapy, ideally with replacement of the ovarian androgens. Implants of estradiol 50 mg and testosterone 100 mg are an ideal route and combination of hormones for this long-term therapy posthysterectomy, with a continuation rate of 90% at 10 years.[17] We have an unpublished study of 47 such patients who have had a hysterectomy, bilateral salpingo-oophorectomy and implants of estradiol and testosterone for severe PMS who have gone through many years of treatment with transdermal estrogens and cycle progestogens or Mirena coils. The symptoms are improved in all patients and all but one was 'very satisfied' with the outcome.

POSTNATAL DEPRESSION

Postnatal depression is another example of depression being caused by fluctuations of sex hormones, therefore having the potential to be effectively treated by hormones. It is a common condition which affects 10–15% of women following childbirth and may persist for > 1 year in 40% of those affected. There does seem to be a lack of any overall influence of psychosocial background factors in determining vulnerability to this postpartum disorder although it can be recurrent.

Although common, the disease is often not reported to the health care professional, particularly the general practitioner or the visiting midwife, as exhaustion and depression is regarded as normal. Indeed, the symptoms of postnatal depression may be confused with the normal sequelae of childbirth. The symptoms can consist of depressed mood with lack of pleasure with the baby or any interest in her surroundings. There may be sleep disturbance, either insomnia or hypersomnia. There may be loss of weight, loss of energy and certainly loss of libido together with agitation, retardation and feelings of worthlessness or guilt. Frequent thoughts of death and suicide are common.

Postnatal depression is not more common after a long labor, difficult labor, Cesarean section or separation from the baby after birth, nor is it determined by education or socioeconomic group. The only environmental factor which seems to be important is the perceived amount of support given by the partner. There is no doubt that the first 6 months or so after delivery can be an exhausting time, full of anxiety and insecurity in mothers with the new responsibility of the baby. Even allowing for that, there does seem to be a clear hormonal aspect to this condition.

Postnatal depression is severe and more prolonged in women who are lactating and lower estradiol levels are found in depressed women following delivery than with controls. It is probable that the low estradiol levels with breastfeeding and the higher incidence of depression are related in a causative way.

We studied the effect of high-dose transdermal estrogens in this condition in an attempt to close the circle of studies treating this triad of hormone responsive depressions – premenstrual depression, climacteric depression and postnatal depression. This was a double-blind placebo-controlled trial of 60 women with major depression which began within 3 months of childbirth and persisted for up to 18 months postnatally.[24] They had all been resistant to antidepressants and the diagnosis of postnatal depression was made by two psychiatrists who were expert in the field. We excluded breastfeeding women from the study. They were given either placebo patches or transdermal estradiol patches 200 µg/day for 3 months without any added progestogen. After 3 months, cyclical Duphaston 10 mg/day was added for 12 days each month. The women were assessed monthly by self-rating their depressive symptoms on the Edinburgh postnatal depression score (EPDS) and by clinical psychiatric interview. Both groups were severely depressed with a mean EPDS score of 21.8 before treatment. During the first month of therapy the women who received estrogen improved rapidly and to a greater extent than controls. None of the other factors – age, psychiatric, obstetric or gynecologic history, severity and duration of current episode of depression, and concurrent antidepressant medication – influenced the response to treatment.

The study showed that the mean EPDS score was less with the active group at 1 month and then maintained for 8 months, and that the percentage with EPDS scores > 14 (diagnostic of postnatal depression) was reduced by 50% at 1 month and by 90% at 5 months. This was much better than the placebo response. Not only did this study show that transdermal estrogens were effective for the treatment of postnatal depression but a subsequent study by Lawrie et al[26] showed that depot progestogen was worse than placebo, causing deterioration in the severity of postnatal depression. Thus we again have the picture of the mood-elevating effect of estrogens and the depressing effect of progestogen.

An uncontrolled study showed similar improvements using sublingual estradiol in 23 women with major postnatal depression.[26] These women had plasma levels of 79.0 pmol/l before the treatment with sublingual estradiol. The estradiol levels were 342 pmol/l at 1 week and 480 pmol/l at 8 weeks. There was improvement in 12 out of the 23 patients at 1 week and after 2 weeks there was recovery in 19 of the 23 patients. The mean Montgomery Asberg depression rating scale (MADRS) was 40.7 before treatment, 11 at 1 week and 2 at 8 weeks. At the end of the second week of treatment the MADRS scores were compatible with clinical recovery in 19 out of the 23 patients. This study

stressed the rapidity of response to the estradiol therapy and this was our observation also. However, it must be stressed that this is an uncontrolled study in women with a very low, almost postmenopausal, levels of estradiol. Another placebo-controlled study is required together with information about bleeding patterns to support or refute our original paper.[24]

It would support the hormonal pathogenesis of this condition if we could mimic postnatal depression by hormonal manipulation. This was done in a study by Bloch et al[28], who studied 16 women, eight with a history of postnatal depression. They induced hypogonadism with leuprolide acetate, and stimulated pregnancy by add-back supraphysiologic doses of estradiol and progesterone for 8 weeks and then withdrew both steroids. Five of the eight women, 62.5% with a history of postnatal depression and none of the women without a prior history, developed significant mood symptoms during the withdrawal period.

This study supported the view that there was an involvement of the reproductive hormones, estradiol and progesterone, in the development of postpartum depression in a set group of women. Furthermore, the study showed that women with a history of postpartum depression are differentially sensitive to the mood-destabilizing effects of gonadal steroids.

CLIMACTERIC DEPRESSION

Like many aspects of depression in women, the diagnosis of climacteric depression and its treatment remains controversial. Whereas gynecologists who deal with the menopause have no difficulty in accepting the role of estrogens in the causation and the treatment of this common disorder, psychiatrists seem to be implacably opposed to it. This may be because there is no real evidence of an excess of depression occurring *after* the menopause nor any evidence that estrogens help *post*menopausal depression, or what used to be called involutional melancholia. This is quite true and indeed many women with long-standing depression improve considerably when their periods stop. This is because the depression created by PMS – heavy painful periods, menstrual headaches and the exhaustion that attend excess blood loss – disappears. Therefore, the longitudinal studies of depression carried out by many psychologists, particularly those as notable as Hunter,[29] have shown no peak of depression in a large population of menopausal women. The depression that occurs in women around the time of the menopause is at its worst in the 2–3 years before the periods stop. This, of course, is perimenopausal depression and is, no doubt, related to premenstrual depression as it becomes worse with age and with falling estrogen levels.

The earliest placebo-controlled study which defined the precise menopausal syndrome showed that estrogens helped hot flushes, night sweats and vaginal dryness. They also had a mood-elevating effect.[30] This work was further supported by the work of Campbell and Whitehead[31] who used Premarin and by the study of Montgomery et al[23] using higher dose estradiol implants. This study of 90 peri- and postmenopausal women with depression showed considerable improvement in the treatment group compared with placebo but only in the perimenopausal women. There was no improvement in the depression in the postmenopausal women with this treatment when compared with placebo. This effect is not transient and we have shown that the improvement in depression is maintained even at 23 months.

At last, after 15 years, psychiatrists, particularly in the USA, are coming round to the view that transdermal estrogens are effective in the treatment of depressed perimenopausal women. In 2001, Soares et al[32] studied 50 such women, 26 with major depressive disorder, 11 with dysthymic depression and 30 with minor depressive illness. They treated them with 100 µg estradiol patches in a 12-week placebo-controlled study. There was a remission of depression in 17 out of 25 of the treatment patients (68%) and in only five out of the 25 placebo patients (20%). This improvement occurred regardless of the Diagnostic and Statistical Manual of Mental Disorders (DSM-IV) diagnosis.

Rasgon et al[33] studied 16 perimenopausal women with unipolar major depressive disorder for an 8-week open-protocol trial comparing low-dose (0.3 mg) Premarin plus fluoxetine daily. There was a greater response with estrogen alone. All but two of the total patients responded but the response was greater in the estrogen replacement therapy (ERT) patients and it was significant that the reduction of depression scores began rapidly after the first week of treatment.

More recently, Harlow et al[34] studied a large number (976) of perimenopausal women with a history of major depression and those without. The patients with a history of depression had higher follicle-stimulating hormone (FSH) levels and lower estradiol levels at enrolment to the study, and those women with a history of antidepressant medication had three times the rate of early menopause. A similar excess rate was found in perimenopausal women who had had a history of severe depression.

It is reassuring for those 'menopausologists' who have been trying to persuade the world of psychiatry that estrogens have a place in the treatment of depressed women and pleasing to read at last the view that 'Periods of intense hormonal fluctuations have been associated with the heightened prevalence and exacerbation of underlying psychiatric illness, particularly the occurrence of premenstrual dysphoria, puerperal depression and depressive treatment during the perimenopause. It is speculated that sex steroids such as estrogens, progestogens, testosterone and dehydroepiandrosterone (DHEA) exert a significant modulation of brain functioning. There are preliminary, although promising data on the use of estradiol (particularly transdermal estradiol) to alleviate depression during the menopause.'[34] At last we are getting through!

Progestogen intolerance

Women having moderately high-dose estrogen therapy must of course have cyclical progestogen if they still have a uterus in order to prevent irregular bleeding and endometrial hyperplasia. The problem is that women with hormone-responsive depression enjoy a mood-elevating effect with estrogens but this is attenuated by the necessary progestogen.[35] This hormone can produce depression, tiredness, loss of libido, irritability, breast discomfort and, in fact, all of the symptoms of PMS, particularly in women with a history or previous history of PMS. A randomized trial of norethisterone versus placebo in estrogenized hysterectomized women (see above) clearly showed this and in fact the paper was subtitled a *A model for the causation of PMS*.[16]

If women become depressed with 10–12 days of progestogen then it may be necessary to halve the dose, decrease the duration or change the progestogen used.[36] It is our policy to routinely shorten the duration of progestogen in women with hormone-responsive depression because adverse side effects with any gestogen are almost invariable. We would therefore use transdermal estrogens either 100 or 200 μg of an estradiol patch or a 50 mg estradiol implant and then we would reset the menstrual bleeding by prescribing norethisterone 5 mg for the first 7 days of each calendar month. This will produce a regular bleed on about day 10 or 11 of each calendar month.

If heavy periods occur (and they usually do not), the duration of progestogen is extended to the more orthodox 12 days. At this stage many women would prefer to have a Mirena coil inserted so there will be no bleeding, no cycles nor any need to take oral progestogen with its side effects. It is not unusual for those women who at this stage understand the benefits of estrogens and the problems of their menstrual cycles, to request hysterectomy and bilateral salpingo-oophorectomy with HRT with estradiol and testosterone.[37] This is a fact of medical life and patient choice but it will be at least another 15 years before psychiatrists attempt to leap over that hurdle.

CONCLUSIONS

- Estrogen therapy is effective for the treatment of postnatal depression, premenstrual depression and perimenopausal depression: the triad of hormone-responsive mood disorders.
- Transdermal estradiol 100 or 200 μg patches producing plasma levels of approximately 500 and 800 pmol/l, respectively, should be used as patients often require plasma levels > 600 pmol/l for efficacy.
- Consider adding testosterone for depression libido and energy.
- Patients require a cyclical progestogen or a Mirena coil if they still have a uterus.
- The most effective long-term medical therapy is estradiol patches or an implant of estradiol and testosterone with a Mirena coil in situ.
- Ultimately, a hysterectomy plus bilateral salpingo-oophorectomy and implants with estradiol and testosterone may be requested.

REFERENCES

1. Paney N, Studd JWW. The psychotherapeutic effects of oestrogens *Gynecol Endocr* 1998; **12**: 353–65.
2. Klaiber EL, Broverman DM, Vogel W, Kobayashi Y. Estrogen therapy for severe persistent depressions in women. *Arch Gen Psychiatry* 1979; **36**: 550–9.
3. Maudsley H. Sex in mind and education. *Fortnightly Rev* 1874.
4. Battey R. Battey's operation – its matured results. *Trans Georgia Med Ass* 1873.
5. Longo LD. The rise and fall of Battey's operation: a fashion in surgery. *Bull Hist Med* 1979; **53**: 244–67.
6. Frank RT. The hormonal basis of premenstrual tension. *Arch Neurol Psychiatry* 1931; **26**: 1053–7.
7. Greene R, Dalton K. The premenstrual syndrome. *BMJ* 1953; **I**: 1007–14.
8. Studd JWW. Premenstrual tension syndrome. *BMJ* 1979; **I**: 410.
9. Backstrom T, Boyle H, Baird DT. Persistence of symptoms of premenstrual tension in hysterectomized women. *Br J Obstet Gynaecol* 1981; **88**: 530–6.
10. Studd JWW. Prophylactic oophorectomy at hysterectomy. *Br J Obstet Gynaecol* 1989; **96**: 506–9.
11. Leather AT, Studd JWW, Watson NR, Holland EFN. The treatment of severe premenstrual syndrome with goserelin with and without 'add-back' estrogen therapy: a placebo-controlled study. *Gynecol Endocr* 1999; **13**: 48–55.
12. Leather AT, Studd JWW, Watson NR, Holland EFN. The prevention of bone loss in young women treated with GNRH analogues with 'add back' oestrogen therapy. *Obstet Gynecol* 1993; **81**: 104–7.

13. Sundstrom I, Myberg S, Bixo M et al. Treatment of premenstrual syndrome with gonadotropin-releasing hormone agonist in a low dose regimen. *Acta Obstet Gynecol Scand* 1999; **78:** 891–9.

14. O'Brien PM, Abukhalil IE. Randomized controlled trial of the management of premenstrual syndrome and premenstrual mastalgia using luteal phase-only danazol. *Am J Obstet Gynecol* 1999; **180:** 18–23.

15. Greenblatt RB, Asch RH, Mahesh VB, Bryner JR. Implantation of pure crystalline pellets of estradiol for conception control. *Am J Obstet Gynecol* 1977; **127:** 520–7.

16. Magos AL, Brewster E, Singh R et al. The effects of norethisterone in postmenopausal women on oestrogen replacement therapy: a model for the premenstrual syndrome. *Br J Obstet Gynaecol* 1986; **93:** 1290–6.

17. Studd JWW, Domoney C, Khastgir G. The place of hysterectomy in the treatment of menstrual disorders. In: O'Brien S, Cameron I, MacLean A (eds) *Disorders of the Menstrual Cycle.* (London: RCOG Press: 2000) **29:** 313–32.

18. Magos AL, Brewster E, Singh R et al. The effects of norethisterone in postmenopausal women on oestrogen replacement therapy: a model for the premenstrual syndrome. *Br J Obstet Gynaecol* 1986; **93:** 1290–6.

19. Bjorn I, Backstrom T. Drug related negative side-effects is a common reason for poor compliance in hormone replacement therapy. *Maturitas* 1999; **32:** 77–86.

20. Panay N, Studd JWW. Progestogen intolerance and compliance with hormone replacement therapy in menopausal women. *Hum Reprod* 1997; **3:** 159–71 (update).

21. Watson NR, Studd JWW, Savvas M et al. Treatment of severe premenstrual syndrome with oestradiol patches and cyclical oral norethisterone. *Lancet* 1989; **23:** 730–2.

22. Smith RNH, Studd JWW, Zambleera D, Holland EFN. A randomised comparison over 8 months of 100 mcg and 200 mcg twice weekly doses in the treatment of severe premenstrual syndrome. *Br J Obstet Gynaecol* 1995; **102:** 6475–84.

23. Montgomery JC, Brincat M, Tapp A et al. Effect of oestrogen and testosterone implants on psychological disorders in the climacteric. *Lancet* 1987; **I:** 297–9.

24. Gregoire AJP, Kumar R, Everitt B et al. Transdermal oestrogen for treatment of severe postnatal depression. *Lancet* 1996; **3347:** 930–3.

25. Khastgir G, Studd JWW. Patients outlook, experience and satisfaction with hysterectomy, bilateral oophorectomy and subsequent continuation of hormone replacement therapy. *Am J Obstet Gynecol* 2000; **183:** 1427–33.

26. Lawrie TA, Hofmeyr GJ, De Jager M et al. A double blind randomised placebo controlled study of postnatal norethisterone enanthate: the effect on postnatal depression and hormones. *Br J Obstet Gynaecol* 1998; **105:** 1082–90.

27. Ahokas A, Kaukoranta J, Wahlbeck K, Aito M. Oestrogen deficiency in severe postpartum depression. Successful treatment with sublingual physiologic 17 beta oestradiol a preliminary study. *J Clin Psychiatry* 2001; **62:** 332–6.

28. Bloch M, Schmidt PJ, Danaceau M et al. Effects of denerbal steroids in women with a history of postpartum depression. *Am J Psychiatry* 2000; **57:** 924–30.

29. Hunter MS. Depression and the menopause. *BMJ* 1996; **313:** 1217–8.

30. Utian WH. The true clinical features of postmenopause and oophorectomy and their response to oestrogen therapy. *S Afr Med J* 1972; **46:** 732–7.

31. Campbell S, Whitehead M. Oestrogen therapy and the menopausal syndrome. *Clin Obstet Gynecol* 1977; **4:** 31–47.

32. Soares CN, al Maida OP, Joffe E, Cohen LS. Efficacy of oestradiol for the treatment of depressive disorders in perimenopausal women: a double blind randomised placebo controlled trial. *Arch Gen Psychiatry* 2001; **58:** 529–34.

33. Rasgon NL, Altshuler LL, Fairbanks LA et al. Estrogen replacement therapy in the treatment of major depressive disorder in perimenopausal women. *J Clin Psychiatry* 2002; **63:** 545–8.

34. Harlow BL, Wise LA, Otto MW et al. Depression and its influence on reproductive endocrine and menstrual cycle markers associated with perimenopause: the Harvard Study of Moods and Cycles. *Arch Gen Psychiatry* 2003; **60:** 29–36.

35. Smith RN, Holland ES, Studd JWW. The symptomatology of progestogen intolerance. *Maturitas* 1994; **18:** 87–91.

36. Panay N, Studd JWW. Progestogen intolerance and compliance with hormone replacement therapy in menopausal women. *Hum Reprod Update* 1997; **3:** 159–71.

37. Watson NR, Studd JWW, Savvas M, Bayber R. The longterm effects of oestrogen implant therapy for the treatment of premenstrual syndrome. *Gynecol Endocr* 1990; **2:** 99–107.

21

Anti-aging and esthetic endocrinology

CJ Gruber and JC Huber

Introduction • Molecular basis of aging • Aging of the skin • Aging of subcutaneous tissue • Aging of the sensorium • Conclusions • References

INTRODUCTION

Besides differential effects on bone mass and the cardiovascular system, sexual steroids are also involved in other extragenital systems due to the different expression of estrogen receptors in various tissues. The clinical success achieved with hormone replacement therapy (HRT) in the treatment of urogenital problems,[1] arthropathia climacterica[2] and psychovegetative symptoms[3] is beyond doubt. These extragenital effects of ovarian steroids also include those related to the metabolism of skin and hair, changes in body composition and subcutaneous fat distribution, and are relevant to the esthetic wellbeing of women.

Sexual steroids are small molecules which, when properly formulated and applied topically to the skin, may also be transported into and through the skin. That is why they are suitable for transdermal application in these respects. Another benefit in this field is that these steroids may be applied to tissue specifically in order to achieve a topical esthetic effect but to avoid systemic reactions. Therefore new indications for HRT are found and a new field in endocrine research, known as *esthetic endocrinology*, is gaining more and more interest.

MOLECULAR BASIS OF AGING

For a long time the process of aging has been regarded as a mechanistic development comparable to the material fatigue of a machine. Summation of mechanical and genetic defects would yield the end of maintainance of life. The successful cloning of higher animals through somatic cell nucleus transfer contradicts some of the theories supported earlier and proves a marked rejuvenation capacity of the adult genome. At least two main functions of human life are related to aging: reproductive function and metabolism. One major principle of evolution – the maintainance of one's own species – obliges individual members to reproduce. Energetic processes are committed to sustain youth. Once the reproductive capacity is lost an exacerbation of aging symptoms is recognizable. With respect to metabolism, it is indispensable for the maintainance of life but yields higher mitotic activity of cells and therefore accelerates aging of these components. In yeast, a well-known model of aging, the lifespan of the organism is directly correlated with the intensity of mitotic activity. On the genetic level, it is known that certain areas of DNA can temporarily be forced into a resting state through the so-called process of *gene silencing*. Gene silencing is subject to control by a protein named the *silent information regulator* (SIR). A complex of SIR subtypes, SIR-2, SIR-3, SIR-4, rich in SIR-2, tethered to the respective coding part of DNA, yields an increased lifespan. Deletion on SIR-2, in contrast, shortens the lifespan. SIR-2 functions as a nicotinamide adenine dinucleotide (NAD)-dependent deacetylase of histone, acting on specific lysine residues. This enzymatic reaction compacts the structure of chromatine and slows transcription of the respective genes. The SIR system can easily be influenced through nutritional habits. High levels of glucose inactivate SIR-2 through a cascade involving the ras system. When the intake of calories is reduced, most effectively during the nocturnal hours of rest, and the level of blood glucose is low, this pathway is obstructed and the activity of SIR-2 is enhanced. In contrast, SNF-1, a kinase, is increasingly expressed during feasting and aging. It activates genes that metabolize carbon hydrogens and is therefore associated with aging. In accordance with these observations two principal strategies of anti-aging seem feasible from current knowledge: hypothermia and restriction of caloric intake. Maintainance of a low-calorie diet for long periods of time has led to an increase in total lifespan in a variety of organisms, including higher animals such as rodents, by up to 30%. Taking the widespread health hazards linked to obesity in Western societies, counseling patients to restrict their caloric intake on a permanent basis seem justified for various reasons. More difficult to achieve in humans is a hypothermic state. From current estimations, lowering the core body temperature by 1°C would result in a dramatic increase in life expectancy. High temperature is associated with high activity. In the lack of more precise methods it therefore seems reasonable to recommend periodical phases of rest to patients seeking anti-aging strategies. However, when nocturnal blood glucose levels are low in humans the body temperature also decreases for an 8–10 hour period. To restrict food prior to sleep might therefore constitute valuable advice for these patients.

AGING OF THE SKIN

Hormonal influences on the skin

In the epidermis, keratinocytes are important targets for various steroids, including calcitriol. During their cell cycle, keratinocytes express their own vitamin D receptors for calcitriol-mediated reactions.[4] Besides, other sexual steroid receptor-related proteins are also consistently observed in the epidermis, the sebaceous glands, hair follicles and sweat ducts, thus confirming the influence of sexual steroids on the upper skin.[5] Expression of estrogen receptors in the epidermis seems to be constitutive. The activated estrogen receptor complex is able to enhance the expression of growth factors such as insulin-like growth factor (IGF)-1, a mitosis-enhancing protein for keratinocytes.[6,7] Langerhans cells are also under the influence of ovarian steroids. Homing effects of this cell type, for instance, is controlled by progesterone, and the number of dendritic cells increases during the luteal phase as shown in the vaginal epithelia.[8] The melanocytes, the third target cell in the epidermal layer, are also stimulated by 17β-estradiol. The subsequent effects are known to patients suffering from chloasma, either solely or in connection with pregnancy.[9] Pigmentation in susceptible women can be aggravated by sun exposure and oral contraceptives and deposition of melanin can be found in the epidermis, dermis or both.[10] Although the exact mechanism of action still remains to be elucidated, a hormonal etiology is strongly suggested, including increased production of melanocyte-stimulating hormone.

Changes in the lipid composition of the stratum corneum, as a result of either altered synthesis or processing, can be responsible for scaling disorders. Steroid sulfatase activity is important for stratum corneum synthesis and is influenced by steroids or steroid sulfates.[11]

The dermis consists of an extracellular matrix and a cell compartment constituted of fibroblasts, macrophages and mast cells. The extracelullar matrix is composed of two classes of macromolecules – the collagens and the polysaccharide glucosamine glycans. Fibroblasts were shown to express estrogen receptors and there is increasing evidence that sexual steroids are involved in both the main biological functions of dermal fibroblasts, in collagen synthesis and in the production of glucosamine glycans.

In the different parts of the body, different types of collagen exist. The expression of collagen subfamilies depends on the distinct activation of various promoters in the genes encoding for collagen synthesis, but age is also recognized as a regulating factor. In addition, ovarian hormones are involved in the subtle expression of the different collagen subtypes. Aging and the inherent changes in the steroid hormone balance are therefore accompanied by major changes in collagen biosynthesis and metabolism. In 1973 Grosman[12] demonstrated that the ratio of type III: type I collagen is greater in younger skin than in the skin of older people. Additionally, the balance of collagen synthesis and degradation is important for skin integrity and also underlies steroid hormonal influence. Skin degradation depends on the activity of proteinases such as the matrix metalloproteinases and cathepsin secreted from connective tissue cells. Matrix metalloproteinases are are stored in lysosomes in the form of procollagenases and are continuously secreted into the extracellular matrix. Through their enzymatic activity they are the major degrading agents of the helico-collagen under physiologic conditions. They are activated by endogenous pro-collagenase activators such as stromelysin. Several metalloproteinase inhibitors, referred to as tissue inhibitors of metalloproteinases (TIMP), control the activity of metalloproteinases.[13] The action of progesterone on TIMP production suggests that ovarian steroids are able to affect the translation and/or the stability of TIMP mRNA.[14] When plasma progesterone levels are high, collagen breakdown and turnover are low. This is due to the fact that progesterone inhibits collagenase synthesis and also to its action on TIMP. Progesterone also suppresses the transcription factor nuclear factor kappa B (NFκB), which is not only involved in inflammatory diseases but also in menstruation, parturition and ovulation. In suppressing this transcription factor, progesterone develops anti-inflammatory and antiproteinase proper-

ties. The progesterone receptor attached to its ligand prevents NFκB-mediated transcriptional activity via the formation of a transcriptionally inactive complex with NFκB. Secondly, progesterone was shown to enhance the production of NFκB inhibitor (NFκB-I, thereby suppressing the activity of inflammatory enzymes, prostaglandins and proteinases.[15] Another important mechanism for skin aging is exposure to ultraviolet (UV) light (extrinsic skin aging). UV irradiation leads to sustained elevations of matrix metalloproteinases that degrade skin collagen. Treatment with topical tretinoin inhibits irradiation-induced matrix metalloproteinases but not their endogenous inhibitors.[16] Theoretically, progesterone is superior to tretinoin in the prevention of extrinsic skin aging.

Hormone therapy of skin aging symptoms

As outlined above, collagen production in dermal fibroblasts is directly enhanced by 17β-estradiol. Brincat et al[17,18] investigated the skin collagen content in menopausal woman with and without HRT some years ago. The HRT group had a significantly higher collagen content than the untreated group. They also investigated the effect of estrogen and testosterone application in women. It was demonstrated that skin collagen also decreased proportionally after menopause. This decrease could be prevented by HRT but also, more interestingly with respect to the new discipline of esthetic endocrinology, by topical administration of estrogens.[19] A body of evidence supports these observations but a few reports do not. A study published recently, for example, showed that a 1-year treatment with systemic estrogen alone or combined with progestin did not change the amount of collagen or the rate of collagen synthesis in postmenopausal women.[20] The contradictory outcome of this study might be due to the fact that skin samples were taken from the lower abdomen. Abdominal, gluteo/femoral cutis and subcutis as well as facial skin all display different steroid hormone concentrations and aromatase activity, and might also differ in their steroid hormone receptor density. These are relative comparisons between these different regions. In addition, the duration and dosage of 17β-estradiol seems to be of critical importance as far as the topical application of estrogen is concerned and in this context more data are needed. The effects of topical estradiol on skin collagen and elastin were also investigated by measuring skin hydroxyprolin, the levels of carboxyterminal pro-peptide of human type I pro-collagen and the amino, terminal pro-peptide of human type III pro-collagen.[21] The increase in type I and type III pro-collagen indicated that topical estradiol treatment stimulates collagen synthesis.

Another useful estrogenic effect in the prevention of intrinsic skin aging is the fact that 17β-estradiol increases the production of glucosamine glycans by enhancing N-acetyl galactose transferase and oligosaccharide transferase.[22] In the stratum germinativum, the mitotic rate is enhanced during HRT. In accordance, skin quality is usually improved by orally ingested estradiol as well as after topical application of estrogens. Schmidt et al[23] investigated skin aging symptoms in perimenopausal females with estradiol and estriol. They used either 0.3% estriol or 0.01% estradiol topically applied as a cream to the facial skin and investigated the different parameters of skin aging. Both treatment groups showed an improvement of skin quality at the end of treatment. The therapeutic effect in the group treated with topical estriol was far superior with regard to the extent of skin aging parameters such as wrinkle depth and skin moisture. In a placebo-controlled study, Creidi et al[24] investigated the effect of topically applied conjugated estrogen on aging facial skin. Premarin cream was significantly more effective than placebo on epidermal thickness and in reducing fine wrinkles. Skin thickness not only depends on the collagen fibers in the subcutis but is also influenced by the thickness of the epidermis.

Table 21.1 refers to the above observations and proposes an example of a topical formula as it is used in our center. It contains 0.06% 17β-estradiol for the prevention of intrinsic skin aging and vitamin C for its antioxidant capacity in order to counteract extrinsic skin aging. Oleum jojobae is beneficial to dryness of skin, a

Table 21.1   Example of a topical formulation for the prevention of skin aging

Component	Amount
17β-Estradiol	0.06%
Sojabase	0.5%
Oleum jojobae	2–8%
Complex acid ascorbate	2.0%
Bellaternity	50.0 g

symptom often noticed in the peri- and post-menopausal period. 'Sojabase' is a solution of soy bean lecithin in propylene glycol useful for the production of liposomal dispersions. As a basis we use a soybean-based formulation called Bellaternity, rich in phospholipids with both saturated and unsaturated fatty acids, ceramides, hyaluronic acid and other components. According to the individual needs, other components can be added to such formulae. Green tea extracts, for instance, contain phytosteroids, with partially estrogenic and anti-oxidant properties, and have been mentioned in the chemoprevention of skin tumors. Coenzyme Q_{10} has also been shown to be useful in the prevention of skin aging. Clinical trials using laktokine and hydrochinone, a tyrosinase inhibitor, are currently underway for use in the reduction of chloasma.

Although the importance of progesterone for collagen synthesis and degradation has theoretically been established, it has not been studied to the same extent as estradiol. Similarly, the homing effect of progesterone on Langerhans cells has not undergone the same clinical evaluation in the cutis as it has in the vaginal epithelium. Still, in the light of the above results, it seems reasonable to introduce progesterone as a hormone to be applied topically to the aging skin. Such a topical lotion is given in Table 21.2. Retinol has been used in dermatological routines for a long time. Given the impact of sexual steroids on melanocytes and melanin production, it is at present merely recommended to avoid excessive exposure to sunlight immediately after application of such formulae to the

Table 21.2 Example of a topical lotion for the prevention of skin aging

Component	Amount
Progesterone	2.0%
Sojabase	0.5%
Oleum jojobae	2–8%
Retinol	0.06%
Bellaternity	50.0 g

skin or to postpone their application to the evening. The same recommendation is reasonable for the oral intake of hormones.

Hormone therapy of hair loss

Male pattern baldness in women is induced by androgens.[25] Testosterone and estradiol, together with the thyroid hormones, influence the hair cycle. Whereas androgens stimulate vellus hair to turn into terminal hair all over the body, the situation is reversed on the scalp. Androgens convert terminal hair into vellus hair thereby causing male pattern baldness and hair loss.[26] In the scalp hair follicle, androgens shorten the anagen phase of the hair follicle cycle, causing the hair follicle to regress. However, hair follicles in other regions of the body, such as the chin or genital skin, have a different response to androgens. Here, androgens cause stimulation and a lengthening of the hair. The biologically active androgen metabolite to the hair follicle is dihydrotestosterone,[27] the testosterone derivative reduced by the 5α-reductase enzyme. There are two isoforms of 5α-reductase – type 1 and type 2 – which regulate the tissue-specific dihydrotestosterone production. Young women and men with alopecia androgenetica have higher levels of 5α-reductase, more androgen receptors and lower levels of aromatase in hair follicles of the frontal scalp compared to the occipital region.[28] Estrogens, in a similar way to keratinocytes, exert mitotic effects on the hair follicles and arrest hair growth in the anagen phase. Most women

notice an enhancement of hair growth during pregnancy. This is partly due to an increase in the proportion of anagen hair and also to an increase in hair thickness. Postpartal hair loss is due to the synchronous transition of anagen-phase hair into the telogen phase. Menopausal hair loss is likewise often triggered by estrogen deficiency, although a relative excess of androgens may also have a causal effect.

Female pattern hair loss, which is more diffuse with all regions of the scalp being affected, is often triggered by estrogen deficiency. Besides hypoestrogenemia and hyperandrogenemia, other endocrine disorders such as hypothyroidism, chronic illness, intoxication, infections, physical and chemical agents, congenital and developmental defects, and inflammatory dermatosis can also cause hair loss.[29] Likewise, iron deficiency should also be ruled out.

For the treatment of isolated male pattern hair loss in women, extensive evaluation of serum hormone levels including androgens are worthless in most cases, unless severe endocrine disease is suspected. Once again, this indicates a local hormonal unbalance rather than systemic alteration in the matters of esthetic endocrinology. Although various treatments, including the use of topical and systemic 5α-reductase inhibitors, have been suggested, the only proven treatment for promoting hair growth in women with alopecia androgenetica is a topical minoxidil lotion (Table 21.3).[30]

The 2 or 5% minoxidil solution must be applied twice daily. Concerning the respective clinical trials, a treatment period of at least 32 weeks seems necessary. As reported recently, a

Table 21.3 Minoxidil lotion components

Component	Amount
Minoxidil	2.5 or 5.0%
Milk protein complex (MPC)	3.0%
Propylenglycol	3.0%
Misc cum aeth dil qsf sol	100.0 g

Table 21.4 Topical scalp preparation	
Component	**Amount**
17α-Estradiol	0.01%
Progesterone	2.0%
Propylenglycol	15.0%
Sojabase	5.0%
Milk protein complex (MPC)	3.0%
Misc cum aeth dil qs f sol	100.0 g

type 1 steroid 5α-reductase inhibitor might be a promising compound for the treatment of androgen-dependent hair loss, as type 1 isoenzyme is expressed in the human scalp.[31]

Estrogen replacement therapy (ERT) can prevent female pattern hair loss, especially when it begins during the menopause. As estradiol induces the production of the sex hormone-binding globulin (SHBG), it also reduces androgen activity. Although no controlled clinical trials have been conducted, estrogens can be applied topically onto the scalp (Table 21.4).

Promising candidates for topical application do not only include 17β-estradiol but also 17α-estradiol. The latter compound exerts estrogenic as well as anti-androgenic effects. In the case of vitamin deficiencies, above all vitamin H and biotin are able to support endocrinological treatments to stop hair loss.

Hormone therapy of acne and hirsutism

Endocrinologic treatment strategies in patients with hyperandrogenic symptoms are widely accepted for esthetic reasons. Hyperandrogenic appearance in women poses a psychosocial problem and women who are embarrassed by these conditions are among the most grateful of patients. Acne and hirsutism are common features of hyperandrogenemia and can be successfully treated by suppressing ovarian activity with anti-androgens and 5α-reductase inhibitors.[32,33] In many patients affected by hyperandrogenic symptoms the serum levels of testosterone, androstendion and sulfate ester of

dehydroepiondrosterone (DHEAS) are within the normal limits. This suggests a paracrine and local disorder[34] rather than a systemic alteration. An enhanced activity of skin 5α-reductase appears to explain much of the abnormality and specific markers of this activity in the blood have been suggested as useful.[35] Nevertheless, serious underlying endocrine disorders must be ruled out in patients with clinical signs of hyperandrogenism before focusing attention on esthetic endocrinology. Furthermore, the use of anti-androgens is contraindicated in women of reproductive age unless adequate measures of contraception guarantee their safety.

Acne vulgaris is the result of an obstruction of sebaceous follicles by excessive amounts of sebum produced by sebaceous glands in the follicles combined with numerous desquamated epithelial cells from the follicle walls. The obstruction causes the formation of a microcomedo, which hosts an anaerobic microorganism *Propionibacterium acnes*. Many patients with acne probably have sebaceous glands that are hypersensitive to androgens rather than an overproduction of androgens. The clinical expression of these pathophysiologic events ranges from inflammatory to non-inflammatory forms of acne.[36] Therapeutic strategies aim at reducing sebum production and epithelial desquamation and antagonizing androgen action. Additionally, the proliferation of *P. acnes* can be suppressed by antibiotics such as erythromycin, clindamycin and tetracycline. Tretinoin, a natural metabolite of vitamin A, when given in pharmacologic dosages profoundly reduces sebum production.[37] Three topical agents that affect the desquamation of follicular epithelial cells are currently available: tretinoin, isotretinoin and salicylic acid.[38,39] They slow down the desquamation process, act against comedogenesis and reduce the number of comedones. On the hormonal sector, systemic drugs that influence sebum production further include estrogens,[40] spironolactone[41] and the anti-androgen cyproterone acetate.[42] A combined estrogen–antiandrogen/progestin oral contraceptive is most apparent in having beneficial effects. Some encouraging attempts

Table 21.5 Composition of a liposomal vehicle for the treatment of acne	
Component	**Amount**
Sojabase	4.0%
Cyproterone acetate (CPA)	0.75%
Bellaternity	61.6%
Aqua destillata	33.65%
Misc fiat lotion	50.0 g

have recently been made to avoid systemic cyproterone acetate effects by using this drug topically for treating acne. As a steroidal progestogen, cyproterone acetate can be applied percutaneously via a liposomal vehicle (Table 21.5) and can thus approach the target cells topically, bypassing the enterohepatic circulation. Results of new clinical trials indicate a sufficient resorption and an esthetic effect of topical cyproterone acetate preparations.[43]

Endocrine treatment of acne can be combined in a simultaneous or sequential fashion with antibiotics or retin-A derivatives. In contrast to cyproterone acetate, 5α-reductase inhibitors are not likely to be promising candidates for acne therapy as the major marker of 5α-reductase activity is decreased in women with acne.[44]

Hirsutism is the presence of excessive hair growth in androgen-sensitive skin in women. The condition may indicate an underlying disorder of androgen production but in most cases hirsutism results from a combination of mildly increased androgen production and an increase in skin sensitivity to androgens. A strong genetic impact of local hyperandrogenemia can often be observed. The quality of hair that grows in any area of the body is determined by both hormones and innate characteristics of the hair follicle. Before puberty, most of the body is covered by fine unpigmented hair called vellus hair. On most areas, androgens promote the conversion of vellus hair to pigmented, terminal hair. The extent to which this conversion occurs depends not only on the rate of androgen production but

also on the duration of exposure to androgens and the intrinsic potential of the hair follicle. Therefore, the therapeutic success of hormonal treatment is small when compared to patients with acne or androgenetic hair loss. The altered conversion of testosterone into dihydrotestosterone by the action of 5α-reductase is seen as one cause of a tissue-specific hyperandrogenemia.[45] 5α-Reductase can be stimulated by elevated androgen levels in the circulation as well as by genetic factors.[46] Numerous studies have in fact documented that 5α-reductase increases in the skin of hirsute women with or without hyperandrogenism.[47] Besides the well-known therapeutic modalities such as ovulation suppression, the application of progestogens is described. Spironolactone was investigated intensively in patients with hirsutism and proved to be efficacious.[48,49] The 5α-reductase inhibitor finasteride is an agent undergoing clinical trials for the treatment of benign prostatic hyperplasia which is the compound that has been found to be successful in patients with hirsutism[50] and PCO patients.[51,52] Flutamide, another antiandrogen used to treat hirsutism, is similar in efficacy to that of spironolactone and cyproterone acetate. It is a nonsteroidal selective anti-androgen which can act on androgen binding at the receptor. This drug is used efficaciously in the treatment of advanced prostatic carcinoma and was recently evaluated in hirsute women.[53] However, flutamide is expensive, has caused fatal hepatitis and should therefore be used with caution. Although finasteride-containing creams can be administered topically (Table 21.6), their efficacy so far lacks clinical confirmation.[54]

Table 21.6 Composition of a finasteride-containing cream for treatment of hirsutism	
Component	**Amount**
Finasteride	0.15%
Sojabase	2.0%
Propylenglycol	q.s.
Bellaternity	50.0 g

Mechanical forms of hair removal such as shaving, plucking, and the application of depilatory creams can control hirsutism, but they will not change the underlying disorder. A combination of mechanical removal and medical therapy offers a reasonable prospect for improvement.

AGING OF SUBCUTANEOUS TISSUE

Hormonal influences on subcutaneous tissues

Abdominal obesity frequently occurs in post-menopausal women. Steroid hormones have a profound impact on the subcutaneous layer, and sexual steroids exert a strong influence on the fat and muscle distribution.[55–57] Clinically, it is observed that body composition is subject to change throughout life. The selective accumulation of body fat in different regions depends on the balance of inflow and outflow of free fatty acids from adipocytes. As demonstrated, progesterone and estradiol enhance lipoprotein lipase activity in the gluteo-femoral area of the female body.[58,59] Progesterone and estradiol administration is followed by an increase in lipoprotein lipase activity and an enlargement of fat cells, most apparent in the lower region. Although other factors enrich the complexity of this process, young women have a high level of lipoprotein lipase activity and enlarged fat cells in the gluteo-femoral region. Accumulation of fat in this area probably fulfills reproductive functions in the course of evolution. These schematics disappear upon entry into the menopausal stage but can be restored by the administration of ERT and progesterone replacement therapy.[60] This observation has an implication for HRT in general. Women on estrogen substitution occasionally suffer from body composition changes, especially in the gluteo-femoral region. This side-effect can be ameliorated by reducing the dosage of estrogen and progesterone. Cortisol in contrast clearly centralizes fat deposition, as seen clinically after corticosteroid therapy and in morbus Cushing.[61,62] Because progesterone occupies glucocorticoid receptors it can be assumed that progesterone counteracts the effects of cortisol on the accumulation of the visceral fat. Androgens have a strong influence on body composition and their anabolic effect has obviously been overemphasized in the past. Recent studies demonstrate that regional lipolysis is enhanced by testosterone. Androgens stimulate the expression of β_3-adrenergic receptors on the surface of the adipocytes, which is an important step towards lipolysis and free fatty acid mobilization.[63,64] Testosterone therefore counteracts lipid accumulation by increasing the rate of lipid mobilization via the β_3-adrenergic receptors.

In the thighs, subcutaneous tissue is composed of three layers of fat with two planes of connective tissue between them. On the thighs of women, especially where the 'pinch test' for the 'mattress phenomenon' is performed, the uppermost subcutaneous layer consists of what are termed large 'standing fat-cell chambers', the average size of which, as seen in cross section, is 0.5×1.5 cm. They are separated from each other by septa of connective tissue (retinacula cutis). These retinacula cutis (binders of the skin) run in a radial, arched way and anchor into the overlying corium. The architecture of the subcutaneous tissue is gender specific. In males, connective tissue between the fat cells is widely crossed, with the anatomic consequence of the fat-cell chambers remaining small. However, in females, and also in states of androgen deficiency, the lower fat is divided by the connective fibers into large fat units, the papillae adiposae.[65] Moreover, the corium is thicker in the skin of male thighs than in women. In women, the 'pinch test' – tangentially applied pressure or pull – can indeed fold or furrow the surface of the skin, whereas in normal men, status protrusus cutis does not appear, unlike the condition found in men with a deficiency of androgens. These gender-specific phenomena are probably under the control of androgens. Unlike in men with normal androgen levels, so-called cellulite is observed in primary or secondary hypogonadal men and the 'mattress phenomenon' becomes positive in this group. Additionally, these men display a female fat distribution in the thigh–hip region, gynecomastia and a female pattern of public hair growth. Histologically, most hypogonadal men are found to have the skin structure, subcutaneous tissue and standing fat-cell chambers characteristic of women. Particularly interesting findings were observed in patients with Klinefelter's syndrome. Those with normal serum androgen levels had a skin structure that was typically masculine. Those with definite androgen deficiency had a feminine skin structure and a positive 'mattress' sign. As all patients with Klinefelter's syndrome have XXY chromosomal patterns, this indicates that sex-typical skin structure of the thighs and hips is hormonally, but not genetically, determined.[66]

Hormone therapy of cellulite

Cellulite is a frequent esthetic problem in women. Androgens have an important clinical impact on a woman's sexual desire, wellbeing and energy, lipid metabolism, and subcutaneous fat layers. In view of these clinical aspects, androgen replacement therapy is of interest in postmenopausal women. After menopause ovarian production of androgens continues for several years and serves as an aromatizable steroid reserve. As a side-effect, hyperandrogenemic stigmata can occur in these women. However, androgens also play a positive role in esthetic endocrinology. As depicted above, androgen deficiency exerts negative effects on the consistency of the subcutaneous fat tissue, on its architecture and, above all, favors the progression of cellulite. A small number of isolated studies indicate that topical androstanolone may ameliorate the 'mattress phenomenon' and may at least bring about a marked esthetic improvement with respect to cellulite. In this context, it must be noted that only androgen compounds which are not aromatized in the body shall be used in the topical treatment of cellulite (Table 21.7). Large, placebo-controlled and prospective studies are still needed to confirm the clinical efficacy of this treatment. However, difficulties in finding methods to objectively evaluate cellulite have rendered these efforts unsuccessful so far.

Table 21.7 Composition for an androgen-containing compound for the treatment of cellulite

Component	Amount
Sojabase	2.5%
Androstanolone	2.0%
Retinol	0.06%
Ethanol	15.0%
Carbomer	q.s.
Misc f. Lipo-Gel	80.0 g

Hormone therapy of abdominal obesity

Weight gain is one of the major problems in menopause. Special care should be given to evaluating estradiol, progesterone and androgen levels in peri- and postmenopausal women. As described above, these hormones are mainly involved in lipogenesis and lipolysis. HRT is widely accepted but is often accompanied by weight problems. If weight problems occur in the gluteo-femoral region in women on estrogen–progesterone substitution, a reduction of estrogen and progesterone dosage is recommended. Because cortisol competes with progesterone at the receptor site in the greater omentum, progesterone possibly antagonizes the cortisol-induced storage of triglycerides in this area. However, androgens are the most promising candidates to treat weight gain in the abdominal region.

A proper androgen balance is necessary for successful weight control in women. While orally applied high-dose androgens increase insulin resistance, androgens administered via the percutaneous route have no impact on insulin resistance. Table 21.8 gives an example of an androgen gel to be applied to the abdominal region with DHEAS as androgen. Under a similar medication using androstanolone (see Table 21.7) a marked reduction of subcutaneous fat in the abdominal region without any concomitant changes in lipid parameters was observed.[67] Notably, the accompanying

Table 21.8 Composition of an androgen-containing gel for application to the abdomen	
Component	Amount
Dehydroepiandrosterone	4.4 or 8.8%
Propylene glycol	q.s.
Bellaternity	50.0 g

changes in body composition were partly restored in the premenopausal state.

AGING OF THE SENSORIUM

Hormone therapy of eye aging diseases

The incidence of primary open-angle glaucoma is much higher in men than in women < 50 years of age. This difference between the sexes becomes less pronounced after this age, which leads to a relationship between intraocular pressure and a reduction of estrogens and progestins in postmenopausal women. Increased intraocular pressure is a significant risk factor for visual impairment in glaucoma patients. Intraocular pressure is maintained as a result of a balance between secretion of aqueous humor by the ciliary processes and reabsorption or outflow of the aqueous humor through the trabecular meshwork, into Schlemm's canal, and the veins. Nitric oxide systemically regulates the resistance in blood vessels and has important regulatory roles in the vascular endothelium and smooth muscle cells throughout the body. The ciliary muscle and outflow pathway of aqueous humor in the eye are sites enriched with nitric oxide synthase. It is known that estrogens cause acute vasodilation by increasing the formation and release of nitric oxide and prostacyclin in endothelial cells.[68] They also reduce the vascular smooth muscle tone by opening specific calcium channels through a cyclic guanosine–monophosphate-dependent mechanism.[69] Consistently, systemic HRT has been shown to reduce the intraocular pressure of postmenopausal women suffering from glaucoma.[70] The reduction reached statistical significance and ranged at about 2 mmHg. Postmenopausal women suffering from glaucoma may therefore constitute a new target group for estrogen substitution.

A second disease of the eye related to age is keratoconjunctivitis sicca. This disorder manifests itself mainly through a sensation of dryness and foreign bodies in the conjunctival region. Since these complaints are among the most frequent in postmenopausal women, the reduction of endogenous sex steroids in aging women has been proposed as a causal factor. The previously demonstrated importance of sex steroids for the integrity of the conjunctiva has prompted our group to undertake prospective randomized trials to compare the effectiveness of 17β-estradiol eye drops to commercial tear substitutes.[71] After 4 months of local ERT a significant beneficial change in the quantity of tear fluid as assessed by the Schirmer's test was seen. In terms of visual analog scale scores, a similar effect was observed. This indicates that 17β-estradiol eye drops are successful, in the treatment of keratoconjunctivitis sicca and are, after all, superior to commercial tear substitutes. 17β-Estradiol eye drops are constituted of an oily solution whereas estriol is soluble in aqueous solution (Table 21.9).

Hormone therapy of age-related hearing loss

In a prospective, randomized, double-blind, placebo-controlled trial, tibolone, a synthetic steroid, has been shown to modify the auditory brainstem response in postmenopausal women.[72] After 12 weeks, auditory brainstem responses and hormone levels were measured.

Table 21.9 Composition of estriol-containing eye drops	
Component	Amount
Estriolsuccinat-Natrium	0.025%
Sol NaCl 0.9%	5.0%
Natrium-Hyaluronat RK 0.5%s	(ad) 10.0 g

Comparisons of the auditory brainstem response latency data from the two treatment groups showed a significant decrease in wave II, III and V peak latencies in women receiving tibolone. No significant differences in pre- and post-treatment circulating hormone concentrations were observed between the tibolone and placebo groups. Furthermore, there was no significant increase in hormone levels in either of the groups at 12 weeks. These findings show an improvement in auditory function via brainstem auditory neural pathways sensitive to tibolone in postmenopausal women. Tibolone may therefore offer new therapeutic strategies in otologic disorders related to aging and hormone deficiency.

CONCLUSIONS

It is beyond doubt that the cessation of sex hormone production in postmenopausal women is linked to an accelerated aging process. In evolutionary terms, entering the postreproductive period of life brings with it some unfavorable consequences. Aging symptoms of the cardiovascular system, brain or other organs can impose serious, sometimes life-threatening problems. On the other hand, age-related symptoms of the skin, the hair or the body composition pose only cosmetic problems, but have gained importance in today's society. Systemic as well as local hormone replacement has to be weighed up against its risks such as breast cancer or risk of deep venous thrombosis. However, if administered correctly and tailored to the individual patient it promotes wellbeing and slows some of the symptoms of aging, including those of an esthetic nature.

REFERENCES

1. Fantl JA, Cardozo L, McClish D, and the Hormones and Urogenital Therapy Committee. Estrogen therapy in the management of urinary incontinence in postmenopausal women: a meta-analysis. First report of the hormones and urogenital therapy committee. *Obstet Gynecol* 1994; **83**: 12–18.

2. Metka M, Heytmanek G, Enzelsberger H et al. Der Gelenkschmerz in der Prä- und Postmeno-pause: Arthropathia climacterica. *Geburtsh u Frauenheilk* 1988; **48**: 232–4.

3. Fillit H, Luine V. The neurobiology of gonadal hormones and cognitive decline in late life. *Maturitas* 1997; **26**: 159–64.

4. Stumpf WE, Koike N, Hayakawa K et al. Distribution of 1,25-dihydroxyvitamin D3(22-ox), in vivo receptor binding in adult and developing skin. *Arch Dermatol Res* 1995; **278**: 294–303.

5. Hasselquist MB, Goldberg N, Schroeter A, Spelsberg TC. Isolation and characterisation of the estrogen receptor in human skin. *J Clin Endocr Metab* 1980; **50**: 76–82.

6. Misra PB, Nickoloff BJ, Morhenn VB et al. Characterisation of insulin-like growth factor-1/somatomedin-C receptors on human keratinocyte monolayers. *J Invest Dermatol* 1986; **87**: 265–73.

7. Nickoloff BJ, Misra PB, Morhenn VB et al. Further characterisation of keratinocyte somatomedin C/insulin-like growth factor (SM-C/IGF-1) receptor and the biological responsiveness of culture keratinocytes to SM-C/IGF-1. *Dermatologica* 1988; **117**: 265–73.

8. Marx Preston A, Spira Alexandra I, Gettie A et al. Progesterone implants enhance SIV vaginal transmission and early virus load. *Nature Med* 1996; **10**: 1084–9.

9. Murray JC. Pregnancy and the skin. *Dermatol Clin* 1990; **8**: 327–34.

10. Smith AG, Shuster S, Thody AF et al. Chloasma, oral contraceptives, and plasma immune reactive beta-melanocytic-stimulating hormone. *J Invest Dermatol* 1977; **68**: 169–70.

11. Roop D. Defects in the barrier. *Science* 1995; **267**: 474–5.

12. Grosman N. Studies on the hyaluronic acid protein complex, the molecular size of hyaluronic acide and the exchangeability of chloride in skin of mice before and after oestrogen treatment. *Acta Pharmacol Toxicol* 1973; **33**: 201–8.

13. Simon C, Gimeno MJ, Mercader A et al. Cytokines–adhesion molecules–invasive proteinases. The missing paracrine/autocrine link in embryonic implantation. *Molec Hum Reprod* 1996; **2**: 405–24.

14. Sato T, Ito A, Mori Y et al. Hormonal regulation of collagenolysis in uterine cervical fibroblasts. Modulation of synthesis of procollagenase, prostromelysin and tissue inhibitor of metalloproteinases by progesterone and oestradiol-17β. *Biochem J* 1991; **275**: 645–50.

15. van der Burg B, van der Saag PT. Nuclear factor-kappa-B/steroid hormone receptor interactions

as a functional basis of anti-inflammatory action of steroids in reproductive organs. *Molec Hum Reprod* 1996; **2**: 433–8.

16. Fisher GJ, Wang ZQ, Datta SD et al. Pathophysiology of premature skin aging induced by ultraviolet light. *N Engl J Med* 1997; **337**: 1419–28.

17. Brincat M, Moniz CJ, Studd JWW et al. Long-term effects of the menopause and sex hormones on skin thickness. *Br J Obstet Gynaecol* 1985; **92**: 256–9.

18. Brincat M, Versi E, Moniz CF et al. Skin collagen changes in postmenopausal women receiving two different regimen oestrogen therapy. *Obstet Gynecol* 1987; **70**: 123–7.

19. Bincat M, Moniz CF, Studd JWW et al. Sex hormones and skin collagen content in postmenopausal women. *BMJ* 1983; **187**: 1337–8.

20. Haapasaari KM, Raudaskoski T, Kallioinen M et al. Systemic therapy with estrogen or estrogen with progestin has no effect on skin collagen in postmenopausal women. *Maturitas* 1997; **27**: 153–62.

21. Formosa M, Brincat MP, Cardozo LD, Studd JWW. Collagen. The significance in skin, bones, and bladder. In: (Lobo RA, ed) *Treatment of the Postmenopausal Woman: Basic and Clinical Aspects*. (Raven Press: New York, 1994) 143–51.

22. Grosman N, Hirdberg E, Schon J. The effect of oestrogenic treatment of the acid mucopolysacharide pattern in skin of mice. *Acta Pharmacol Toxicol* 1971; **30**: 359–64.

23. Schmidt JB, Binder M, Macheiner W et al. Treatment of skin ageing symptoms in perimenopausal females with estrogen components. A pilot study. *Maturitas* 1994; **20**: 25–30.

24. Creidi P, Faivre B, Agache P et al. Effect of conjugated oestrogen (Premarin®) cream on ageing facial skin. A comparative study with a placebo cream. *Maturitas* 1994; **19**: 211–23.

25. Bergfeld WF. Etiology and diagnosis of androgenetic alopecia. *Clin Dermatol* 1988; **6**: 102–7.

26. Lynfield YL. Effort of pregnancy on the human hair cycle. *J Invest Dermatol* 1960; **55**: 323–7.

27. Paulson RJ, Serafini PC, Catalino JA, Lobo RA. Measurements of $3\alpha,17\beta$-androstenediol glucuronide in serum and urine and the correlation with skin 5α-reductase activity. *Fertil Steril* 1986; **46**: 222–6.

28. Sawaya ME, Price VH. Different levels of 5 alpha-reductase type I and type II, aromatase, and androgen receptors in hair follicles of women and men with androgenetic alopecia. *J Invest Dermatol* 1997; **109**: 296–300.

29. Nielsen TA, Reichel M. Alopecia: diagnosis and management. *Am Family Physician* 1995; **51**: 1513–22.

30. DeVillez RL, Jacobs JB, Szpunar CA, Warner ML. Androgenetic alopecia in the female. Treatment with 2% topical minoxidil solution. *Arch Dermatol* 1994; **130**: 303–7.

31. Neubauer BL, Gray HM, Hanke CW et al. LY191704 inhibits type I steroid 5α-reductase in human scalp. *Clin Endocr Metab* 1996; **81**: 2055–60.

32. Burke BM, Cunliffe WJ. Oral spironolactone therapy for female patients with acne, hirsutism or androgenetic alopecia. *Br J Dermatol* 1985; **112**: 124–5.

33. Kuhnz W, Staks T, Jütting G. Pharmacokinetics of cyproterone acetate and ethinylestradiol. *Contraception* 1993; **48**: 557–75.

34. Bardin CW, Lipsett MB. Testosterone and androstenedione blood production rates in normal women and women with idiopathic hirsutism or polycystic ovaries. *J Clin Invest* 1967; **46**: 891–7.

35. Carmina E, Lobo RA. Evidence for increased androsterone metabolism in some normoandrogenic women with acne. *J Clin Endocr Metab* 1993; **76**: 1111–14.

36. Strauss JS, Klingman AM. The pathologic dynamics of acne vulgaris. *Arch Dermatol* 1969; **82**: 779–90.

37. Strauss JS, Rapini RP, Shalita AR et al. Isotretinoin therapy for acne: results of a multicenter dose–response study. *J Am Acad Dermatol* 1984; **10**: 490–6.

38. Chalker DK, Lesher Jr JL, Smith Jr JG et al. Efficacy of topical isotretinoin 0.05% gel in acne vulgaris: results of a multicenter, double-blind investigation. *J Am Acad Dermatol* 1987; **17**: 251–4.

39. Leyden JJ, Marples RR, Mills OH, Klingman AM. Tretinoin and antibiotic therapy in acne vulgaris. *South Med J* 1974; **67**: 20–5.

40. Strauss JS, Pochi PE. The effect of cyclic progestagen–estrogen therapy on sebum and acne in women. *JAMA* 1964; **190**: 815–19.

41. Muhlemann MF, Carter GD, Cream JJ et al. Oral spironolactone: an effective treatment of acne vulgaris in women. *Br J Dermatol* 1986; **115**: 227–32.

42. Hammerstein J, Meckies J, Leo-Rossberg I, Moltz L, Zielske F. Use of cyproterone acetate (CPA) in the treatment of acne, hirsutism, and virilism. *J Steroid Biochem* 1975; **6**: 827–36.

43. Gruber DM, Sator MO, Joura EA et al. Topical cyproterone acetate treatment in women with acne: a placebo-controlled trial. *Arch Dermatol* 1998; **134**: 459–63.

44. Joura EA, Geusau A, Schneider B et al. Serum 3α-androstanediol-glucuronide is decreased in nonhirsute women with acne vulgaris. *Fertil Steril* 1996; **66**: 1033–5.

45. Russell DW, Wilson JD. Steroid 5α-reductase: two genes/two enzymes. *Ann Rev Biochem* 1994; **63**: 25–61.

46. Mauvais-Jarvis P. Regulation of androgen receptor and 5α-reductase in the skin of normal and hirsute women. *Clin Endocr Metab* 1986; **15**: 307–17.

47. Serafini P, Lobo RA. Increased 5alpha-reductase activity in idiopatic hirsutism. *Fertil Steril* 1985; **43**: 74–78.

48. Lobo RA, Shoupe D, Serafini P et al. The effects of two doses of spironolactone of serum androgens and anagen hair in hirsute women. *Fertil Steril* 1985; **43**: 200–5.

49. Barth JH, Cherry CA, Wojnarowska F, Dawber RPR. Spironolactone is an effective and well tolerated systemic antiandrogen therapy for hirsute women. *J Clin Endocr Metab* 1989; **68**: 966–70.

50. Venturoli S, Marescalchi O, Colombo FM et al. A prospective randomized trial comparing flutamide, finasteride, ketokonazole, and cyproterone acetate–estrogen regimens in the treatment of hirsutism. *J Clin Endocr Metab* 1999; **84**: 1304–10.

51. Tolino A, Petrone A, Sarnacchiaro F et al. Finasteride in the treatment of hirsutism: new therapeutic perspectives. *Fertil Steril* 1996; **66**: 61–5.

52. Ciotta L, Cianci A, Calogero A, Palumbo LA. Clinical and endocrine effects of finasteride, a 5α-reductase inhibitor, in women with idiopathic hirsutism. *Fertil Steril* 1995; **64**: 299–306.

53. Falsetti L, De Fusco D, Eleftheriou G, Rosina B. Treatment of hirsutism by finasteride and flutamide in women with polycystic ovary syndrome. *Gynecol Endocr* 1997; **11**: 251–7.

54. Price DM, Allen S, Pegram GV. Lack of effect of topical finasteride suggests an endocrine role for dihydrotestosterone. *Fertil Steril* 2000; **74**: 414–5.

55. Borkan GA, Hults DE, Gerzof SG, et al. Age changes in body composition revealed by computer tomography. *J Gerontol* 1983; **38**: 673–7.

56. Ley CJ, Lee B, Stevenson JC. Sex and menopause

– associated changes in body fat distribution. *Am J Clin Nutr* 1992; **55**: 950–4.

57. Longcope C. Androgen and estrogen conversion ratios in aging women. *Maturitas* 1979; **2**: 13–17.

58. Rebuffé-Scrive M, Basdevant A, Guy-Grand B. Effect of local application of progesterone on human adipose tissue lipoprotein lipase. *Horm Metab Res* 1983; **15**: 566–71.

59. Eckel RH. Lipoprotein lipase – a multifunctional enzyme relevant to common metabolic diseases. *N Engl J Med* 1989; **320**: 1060–8.

60. Haarbo J, Marslew U, Gotfredsen A, Christiansen C. Postmenopausal hormone replacement therapy prevents central distribution of body fat after menopause. *Metabolism* 1991; **40**: 1323–6.

61. Yen SS. The polycystic ovarian syndrome. *Clin Endocr* 1980; **12**: 177–207.

62. Marin P, Darin N, Amemeiya T et al. Cortisol secretion in relation to body fat distribution in obese premenopausal women. *Metabolism* 1992; **41**: 882–6.

63. Marin P, Holmang S, Jonsson L et al. The effects of testosterone treatment on body composition and metabolism in middle-aged obese men. *Int J Obesity* 1992; **16**: 991–7.

64. Lovejoy JC, Bray GA, Bourgeois MO et al. Exogenous androgens influence body composition and regional body fat distribution in obese postmenopausal women – a clinical research center study. *J Clin Endocr Metab* 1996; **81**: 2198–203.

65. Nürnberger F, Müller G. So-called cellulite: an invented disease. *J Dermatol Surg Oncol* 1978; **4**: 221–9.

66. Nürnberger F, Riedel-Pauls W, Gräf KJ et al. Status protrusus cutis und Sexualhormone beim Klinefelter-Syndrom. *Z Hautkr* 1979; **54**: 47–57.

67. Gruber DM, Sator MO, Kirchengast S et al. Effect of percutaneous androgen replacement therapy on body composition and body weight in postmenopausal women. *Maturitas* 1998; **29**: 253–9.

68. Kim HP, Lee JY, Jeong JK et al. Nongenomic stimulation of nitric oxide release by estrogen is mediated by estrogen receptor α localized in caveolae. *Biochem Biophys Res Commun* 1999; **263**: 257–62.

69. White RE, Darkow DJ, Lang JL. Estrogen relaxes coronary arteries by opening BKCa channels through a cGMP-dependent mechanism. *Circ Res* 1995; **77**: 936–42.

70. Sator MO, Joura EA, Frigo P et al. Hormone

replacement therapy and intraocular pressure. *Maturitas* 1997; **28:** 55–8.

71. Sator MO, Joura EA, Golaszewski T et al. Treatment of menopausal keratoconjunctivitis sicca with topical oestradiol. *Br J Obstet Gynaecol* 1998; **105:** 100–2.

72. Sator MO, Franz P, Egarter C et al. Effects of tibolone on auditory brainstem responses in postmenopausal women – a randomized, double-blind, placebo-controlled trial. *Fertil Steril* 1999; **72:** 885–8.

22

Skin and connective tissue

MP Brincat, Y Muscat Baron and R Galea

The skin • The connective tissue • The menopause and the skin • Aging and the skin • Skin esthetics and menopause• Acne, wound healing and estrogen • Conclusions • References

THE SKIN

The skin is one of the largest organs in the body containing a sizeable proportion of total body collagen. This organ is composed of a population of cells of diverse embryonic origin which under normal conditions exist side by side in complete harmony, forming a complex mosaic. Skin is composed of two main layers, namely the epidermis and, internal to this layer, the dermis.

The thin outer layer, the epidermis, is composed of keratinocytes (keratin-producing cells) of ectodermal origin intermingled with melanin-producing cells, the melanocytes, which arise from a specialized embryonic ectodermal tissue, the neural crest. The other layer is the dermis, a stroma that forms the main bulk of the skin and is intimately bound with the overlaying epidermis; finger-like processes or dermal papillae project upwards into corresponding recesses in the epidermis. In contrast to the epidermis, the dermis is predominantly fibrous and contains blood vessels. It is of mesodermal origin like all connective tissue (including bone and the circulatory system). It also contains several structures derived from the embryonic ectoderm, e.g. sweat glands and hair follicles. The fibers present in the dermis consist of two main types of fibrous protein,

collagen (97.5%) and elastin (2.5%).[1] Collagen constitutes approximately one-third of the total mass of the body and 20% of total protein. It is a major constituent of all connective tissues, some 88% of which is found in the dermis and in bones, the amount of collagen being almost equally shared. Collagen fibers are responsible for the main mass and resilience of the dermis. This collagen is mainly disposed in an arrangement parallel to the skin surface. The elastin fibers on the other hand form a subepidermal network and are only thinly distributed. Collagen is produced by fibroblasts. These cells contain abundant endoplasmic reticulum where secreted proteins such as collagen are synthesized out of the main types of collagen found in connective tissues, types I–III, V and XI. The connective tissue of the adult body in the main is composed of type I. Collagen type I represents 90% of all the adult connective tissue component and is responsible for one-third of the adult dried body mass.[2]

THE CONNECTIVE TISSUE

Each component of the connective tissue is responsible for the specific properties and function of the body organs. Collagen type I, through its toughness and moderate elasticity, imparts stability, maintaining the physical integrity of the organ, concomitantly allowing the organ to function adequately. A delicate balance exists in the total amount of collagen present. A reduction in collagen content in bone and skin leads to osteoporosis and dermatological conditions, respectively both related to the aging process. Inappropriate deposits of collagen are responsible for end-stage atheroma formation in the arterial circulation.

The elastic property of connective tissue in the case of skin dermis is important as the skin is constantly undergoing topological changes. The tough characteristics of collagen type I prevents excessive distortion when the skin is stretched. Simultaneously, the more elastic collagen type III is responsible for greater extensibility of the skin. The rod-like collagen molecule is 1.4 nm in diameter and is composed of three polypeptide units called alpha chains. The three polypeptide units form a triple helix with a left-hand twist. By preventing the premature formation of collagen fibers, collagen propeptides are responsible for the transport and correct deposition of collagen.

Each type of collagen has a distinct amino acid sequence. The main amino acids in collagen are proline and hydroxyproline, which together comprise about 25% of the 1050 amino acid residues in each polypeptide chain. The collagen protein is composed of two basic peptide chains called alpha 1 and alpha 2. The various combinations of these two alpha chains forming a triple-helix structure determined the type of collagen protein produced. Accordingly, the various combinations of alpha chains produced correlate with the characteristic attributes of the collagen type required by the structure and function of the organ concerned. The stability of the triple helix is also maintained by the presence of a large number of hydroxyl groups. Additional strength is provided to the collagen fibrils by interfibrillar crosslinks present at the ends of the alpha chains. These crosslinks are composed of aldehyde radicals produced extracellularly from lysil and hydroxylysil residues by the action of the enzyme lysil oxidase.

Type I collagen is composed of two alpha I chains and one alpha 2 chain. This combination of alpha chains gives type I collagen the toughness required by supporting organs such as the skin and bone. Type III collagen, also found in skin, is composed of three alpha 1 chains, allowing for the elastic and expansive properties of the skin dermis.

The distribution of the different collagen types throughout the human body varies with growth and development. The rate of change of the collagen types varies most rapidly during fetal life but also occurs later during adulthood.

At 5 weeks' gestation the collagen bundles are made of fine fibrils of collagens draped in mesenchymal cells derived from the mesoderm. The amount of collagen slowly increases to surround the mesenchymal cells, with the collagen bundles increasing in number and diameter throughout the embryonic stage. Collagen type I and collagen type III are evenly distributed and collagen type V is found on dermal surfaces.[3]

With increasing gestation, collagen type I becomes the predominant collagen. During fetal life collagen type I constitutes 70% of all collagen protein, collagen type III 20% and collagen type II 7%. With increasing age collagen type I comprises 90% of collagen, collagen type III 7% and collagen type II decreases to < 2%.[4] This ratio of collagen type is demonstrated in the skin dermis.

Changes in skin vasculature during the menopause

The dermis and the epidermis are nourished by blood vessels that pass upwards from the subcutaneous layer. In the dermis they form relatively small channels (arterioles) that pass towards the undersurface of the epidermis forming a rich capillary network in the dermal papillae. It is these vessels that are responsible for the menopausal flush, the most characteristic symptom of the menopause affecting some 75% of all women in their first menopausal year[5] and still affecting 25% 5 years later.[6] Alberts et al[7] have shown a vascular response to estrogen applied to the ears of oophorectomized rabbits. In animal studies, estrogens appear to alter the vascularization of the skin.[8] Vascular dilatation has also been noted to occur in humans within seconds of estrogen administration, mainly due to the increase in endothelial formation of the vasodilatory nitric oxide and prostacyclin.[9]

Changes in the dermis during the menopause

Connective tissue consists of an extracellular matrix and cellular elements. The extracellular matrix is composed of two classes of macromolecules, the collagens and the polysaccharide glycosaminoglycans (GAG). GAG chains allow rapid diffusion of water molecules and are responsible for the turgor in the compressive forces. Collagen fibrils, on the other hand, resist stretching of the tissues. By weight, GAG amount to < 5% of the fibrous protein, the rest are composed largely of collagen with some elastin.[10] Although the bulk of the body collagen is remarkably stable, a fraction of the collagen in all tissues is continuously degraded and even replaced in old age. Such changes in overall collagen metabolism can be approximately followed by assaying excretion of peptide-bound hydroxyproline in urine,[11] since excretion of these substances is largely caused by collagen degradation.[12] Changes in collagen metabolism can also be assayed by urinary assay of collagen pyridinium crosslinks. Collagen changes with age, both in quality, type and amount.[3] Growth of connective tissue involves collagen biosynthesis and this is reflected in an increased level of intracellular post-translational enzymes. Both the rates of translation and the levels of these enzymes decrease with age.[12,13] In one study, collagen markers indicated that, after the menopause, the rate of collagen breakdown (osteoclastic activity) increased dramatically when compared to a faster rate of collagen production (osteoblastic activity). With hormone replacement therapy (HRT) this situation was reversed, i.e. osteoblastic activity and evidence of collagen formation were reduced. This however was greatly affected by the greater decrease in collagen breakdown which would

lead to an overall positive balance, thereby explaining the increase in bone mass and possibly also the increase in dermal skin thickness in women on estrogen replacement therapy (ERT).[14]

THE MENOPAUSE AND THE SKIN

The menopause is a major event in the life of a woman. This hypoestrogenic state gives rise to profound effects on all organs containing connective tissue. Albright et al,[15] as early as 1940, speculated that postmenopausal osteoporosis was part of a generalized connective tissue disorder, having observed that the skin of women with this disorder was noticeably thin. McConkey et al[16] showed that transparent skin on the back of the hand was most common in women > 60 years of age and the prevalence of osteoporosis in women with transparent skin was 83 versus 12.5% in women with opaque skin. In fact, postmenopausally, there is a decline in skin thickness and skin collagen, causing skin deterioration as evidenced by dry, wrinkled, flaky and easily bruised skin. There is also a decline in bone mass. These two organs in the body, containing some 80% of all the connective tissues in the body, show a deterioration which can be prevented and even reversed with appropriate and adequate estrogen replacement.[17–20]

Atrophy of the dermis after the menopause is due to a decrease in the dermal skin collagen content of the dermis. The amounts of hydroxyproline and glycosylated hydroxylysine[21,22] in type I collagen, and of immature and reducible crosslinks, decrease with age.[23] To what extent these changes are fundamental to the aging process is still unknown. This decrease is not only arrested but is reversed by HRT.[20] There is nonsignificant evidence from the National Health and Nutrition Examination Survey that estrogen prevents dry skin and skin wrinkling.[18] Skin aging that has been treated by topical estrogen shows positive influences on skin turgor and collagen content.[19]

Most of the studies have measured the thickness of dermis, since this is the layer which is mainly connective tissue. Subcutaneous tissue is an added variable and studies using

Harpenden's callipers, which also includes subcutaneous fat, have been conflicting.[24] Ultrasound can nowadays be used to measure skin thickness. Ultrasound examination has been used by dermatologists when assessing dermal malignancies. Good reproducibility has been obtained using high frequency (22.5 mHz) ultrasound to determine the thickness of the skin excluding the subcutaneous tissue. The dermal skin thickness itself – composed as it is of connective tissue including the predominant protein collagen as well as elastin (small amounts) and glycoaminoglycans – has more than one variable that is affected by ERT and the menopause. In rat work for example,[25] castrated rats that were given estrogens had a 70% increase in their glycosaminoglycans content in 2 weeks. Similar increases in women would lead to skin thickness increases that far outstrip those which would be expected from collagen content increases alone.

A change in the connective tissue of the dermis occurs, as is reflected by increased mucopolysaccharide incorporation, hydroxyproline turnover and alterations in ground substance. In addition to increased dermal turnover of hyaluronic acid, the dermal water content is enhanced with estradiol therapy.[26] Rauramo and Punnonen[27] observed that oral estrogen therapy in oophorectomized women caused thickening of the epidermis for 3 months, which persisted for 6 months.

The epidermis and the menopause

Punnonen,[28] using two different strengths of estrogens in castrated women, showed a statistically significant thickening of the epidermis after 3 months with both strengths, but this thickness persisted only with the lower dose. A third of patients on the higher dose started getting significant thinning of the epidermis possibly because the dosage and treatment was too strong and therefore was exerting a corticosteroid-like effect.

Dermal collagen and the menopause

Comparing a group of patients who had been on estradiol and testosterone implants for 2–10 years to a group of untreated postmenopausal women, it was shown that the treated group had a highly significant greater skin collagen content than the untreated group. Optimum skin collagen was obtained after 2 years of an optimum (calculated) estrogen regimen. Too high or too low levels of estradiol gave lower levels of collagen.[29] The same conclusions were also reported in relation to the epidermis.[30]

Skin, corticosteroids and hormone replacement

Connective tissue disorders and endocrine diseases have been shown to have a significant effect on skin. Shuster and Bottoms[31] noted correlations between collagen content and skin thickness in patients with systemic sclerosis and hirsutism. Increased collagen content was noted in hirsute women. Women treated with androgens also had an elevated collagen content.[31] Thin skin with telagectasiae are known to occur with corticosteroid therapy. Skin thickness appears to increase when estrogen treatment is given to postmenopausal women on long-term corticosteroids.[32,33]

AGING AND THE SKIN

The findings of skin changes with aging are conflicting. Shuster et al[34] showed that the best way of expressing skin collagen content was by measuring the collagen content of a skin biopsy of 1 mm of skin surface. This method appears to take into consideration the change of the total dermal mass. This study revealed a reduction of total skin collagen with age. However, this was not confirmed by Hall et al,[35] who confirmed high skin collagen contents in males compared to females but could not demonstrate any relationship between skin collagen control and aging.

The decline in skin collagen content after the menopause occurs at a much more rapid rate in the initial postmenopausal years than in the later ones. Some 30% of skin collagen is lost in the first 5 years after the menopause,[36] with an average decline of 2.1% per postmenopausal year over a period of 20 years. The increase in skin collagen content after 6 months of sex hormone therapy depends on the collagen content at the start of treatment.[36] In women with a low skin collagen, estrogens are initially of therapeutic and later of prophylactic value, while in those with mild loss of collagen content in the early postmenopausal years estrogens are of prophylactic value. Thus, a deficiency in skin collagen can be corrected but not overcorrected.

Skin collagen and skin thickness responses

Skin collagen content has been shown to have a strong correlation with dermal skin thickness.[36] Using 100 mg subcutaneous estradiol implants, significant increases in skin thickness and the metacarpal index occurred over a 1-year period. Most of the increase occurred in the first 6 months. Optimal skin collagen was obtained after 2 years of implant treatment. Elevated skin hydroxyproline, indicating increasing skin collagen content, was noted following topical estrogen. Skin blisters were assayed, and an increase in both PICP and PINP was noted following estrogen gel applications.[36] Brincat et al[37] and Castelo Barcia et al[38] have shown that following the menopause skin collagen content and skin thickness are increased in women on HRT compared to age-matched women on no treatment. Prospective studies have shown that skin thickness, skin collagen and bone mass increase in postmenopausal women who start ERT. The mechanical properties of the skin have been shown to be improved with HRT and to reach premenopausal levels.[39] In this study, the mechanical properties of this were defined by extensibility and elasticity measurements using a computerized device. Computerized measurements of skin deformability and viscoelasticity revealed differences between women on ERT, postmenopausal women on no treatment and nonmenopausal controls. This parallels the changes noted elsewhere with skin collagen. A sharp increase in skin extensibility was shown during the perimenopause in untreated women. ERT appeared to limit the age-related increase in cutaneous extensibililty, thereby exerting a preventive effect on skin slackness. No effect of HRT was found on other parameters of skin viscoelasticity. HRT has a beneficial effect on some mechanical properties of skin and this may slow the progress of intrinsic cutaneous aging.[39]

Brincat et al[40–42] found significant correlations between skin (dermal) collagen, skin thickness (measured radiologically) and the metacarpal index, both in postmenopausal women who had been on HRT and in untreated postmenopausal women. The common factor is the connective tissue present in all three sites. These findings were irrespective of the woman's age, number of years since the menopause, original skin thickness or metacarpal index.

Skin thickness changes has many potential implications regarding other tissues. One study that is currently underway has indicated that ERT indicated in postmenopausal women on long-term corticosteroids led to an increase in skin thickness over a period of 6 months up to 4 years.[32,33]

Attempts to identify the correct value of skin thickness measurement in an effort to screen for postmenopausal osteoporosis have been underway for some time.[40] Skin thickness does seem to have a role in screening for osteoporosis. Of course, the whole field of adequate prediction of fractures, whether by skin thickness, bone density or any other method, is fraught with huge difficulties due to the fact that there are so many variable contributions to when and where an individual will fracture. Even relatively expensive tests such as bone density measurements seem to be not much better than skin thickness measures in predicting fractures, so as a screening test the faster and considerably cheaper skin thickness assessment by high frequency ultrasound or radiological methods is still an attractive proposition. Bone densitometry assessments would then be utilized as a second tier of screening, or possibly even relegated to a purely diagnostic role and in assessing response to therapy.

SKIN ESTHETICS AND MENOPAUSE

Older skin is predominantly affected by three main factors: chronological aging, estrogen deficiency and photoaging. HRT is known to reverse the effects of estrogen deficiency but has no effect on the changes due to photoaging, such as solar lentigines or telangiectasia.[41]

With advance age, an increase is evident in intracellular concentrations of protocollagen lysylhydroxyproline transferase (the enzyme responsible for collagen breakdown), while a decrease is observed in both the collagen content and the production of glycosaminoglycans in the connective tissue.[42] The loss of the connective tissue component and the glycosaminoglycans of the skin dermis leads to increased rigidity and diminished elasticity. The resultant skin aging, of the face in particular, is characterized by a progressive increase in extensibility associated with a loss of elasticity.[43] The resultant effect is wrinkling, dryness, atrophy and a progressive deepening of facial creases. The First National Health and Nutrition Examination Survey indicated that estrogen may partially reverse these skin characteristics, particularly atrophy and dryness, in postmenopausal women.[44] Computerized measurements of skin deformability and viscoelasticity have revealed a marked increase in skin extensibility in untreated perimenopausal women, which can be limited by estrogen replacement therapy, therefore, helping to prevent skin slackness.[45] Optical profilometry and computerized image analysis has shown that HRT exerts a beneficial effect on facial skin by reducing the age-related rheological changes without limiting the number and depth of wrinkles.[46] Also, the water holding capacity of the skin has been shown to increase with HRT.[47] The maximal effect at preventing skin aging appears to occur if estrogens are started early. Interestingly, smokers are known to develop a high wrinkle score, which has not been shown to respond to estrogen replacement therapy.[48]

ACNE, WOUND HEALING AND ESTROGEN

Whilst aging is associated with a slower rate of cutaneous wound healing, it may be paradoxically associated with an improvment in the quality of scarring.[49–51] Ashcroft et al[52] demonstrated a significant delay in acute wound healing in young ovariectomized rodents, which was reversed by estrogen replacement. These effects appeared to involve an estrogen-induced increase in the secretion of latent transforming growth factor-β1 by the dermal fibroblasts.

Sex steroids have also been used for the treatment of atrophic acne scars. Estril iontophoresis was associated with photographic and clinical improvement of acne scars in 100% of patients in one study.[53] This method requires further assessment but may replace the more invasive treatments currently offered, such as bovine collagen implantation, chemical peeling and dermabrasion.

CONCLUSIONS

It is an old adage that skin is a manifestation of inner health but its own health is also important in the self-esteem of the individual with its quality, elasticity, translucence and hydration having important cosmetic implications.

The hypoestrogenemic state prevailing in the menopause has a profound effect on the skin that is not simply age related but, as with bone loss, leads to rapid deterioration which can be prevented and even reversed with appropriate and adequate ERT. These effects have been demonstrated in the epidermis, dermis, collagen content of the dermis, glycosaminoglycan content of the dermis and skin thickness. The mechanical properties of the skin after menopause have been shown to benefit from HRT. Skin and bone each contain some 40% of the total body collagen. Collagen marker studies have shown that the bone changes associated with the menopause are connective tissue changes. This connective tissue deficiency, in bone, is mirrored in the individual's skin changes, although the correlation is not exact. The deleterious effects of the menopause on connective tissue in skin, like those in bone, can be reversed by HRT in part or totally in most women.

REFERENCES

1. Bailey AJ, Etherington DJ. Metabolism of collagen and elastin. In: (Florkin M, Neuberger A, Van Dienen LLM, eds) *Comprehensive Biochemistry* (New York: Elsevier: 1980) 408–31.

2. Hall D. Gerontology and collagen diseases. *Clin Endocr Metab* 1974; **2**: 23.

3. Smith L, Holbrook WJ. Collagen changes during embryological development. *Am J Anat* 1986; **4**: 507–10.

4. Dumas M, Chaudagne C, Bonet F. In vitro biosynthesis of type I and III collagen by human fibroblasts from donors of increasing age. *Med Ageing Dev* 1994; **73**: 179–87.

5. McKinlay SM, Jeffreys M. The menopausal syndrome. *Br J Prev Med Soc Med* 1974; **28**: 108–15.

6. Thompson B, Hart SA, Durno D. Menopausal age and symptomatology in a general practice. *J Biosoc Sci* 1973; **5**: 71–2.

7. Reynolds S, Foster F. Peripheral vascularisation of oestrogen observed in ears of rabbit. *J Pharmacol Exp Ther* 1940; **68**: 173–7.

8. Goodrich SM, Wood JE. The effect of oestradiol 17B on peripheral venous distensibility and velocity of venous blood flow. *Am J Obstet Gynecol* 1966; **96**: 407–12.

9. Chen Z, Yuhanne I, Galcheva-Gargova Z et al. Estrogen receptor alpha mediates the nongenomic activation of endothelial nitric oxide. Synthesis by oestrogen. *J Clin Invest* 1999; **103**: 401–6.

10. Alberts B, Bray D, Laws J et al. Cell – cell adhesion and the extracellular matrix. In: (Alberts B et al, eds) *Molecular Biology of the Cell, Volume 12.* (Garland Publishing: New York, 1983) 673–718.

11. Kivirikko KI. Urinary excretion of hydroxyproline in health and disease. *Int Rev Connect Tiss Res* 1973; **5**: 93–163.

12. Krane SM, Kontrwitz FG, Byrne M et al. Urinary excretion of hydroxylysine and its glycosides as an index of collagen degradation. *J Clin Invest* 1977; **59**: 819–27.

13. Amen H, Crara J, Ryhanent L et al. Assay of proto collagen lysyl hydroxylase activity in the skin of human subjects and changes in the activities with age. *Clin Chim Acta* 1973; **47**: 289–94.

14. Muscat Baron Y, Brincat M, Galea R. Changes in collagen markers in hormone treated and untreated postmenopausal women. *Maturitas* 1997; **27**: 171–7.

15. Albright F, Bloomberg E, Smith PH. Postmenopausal osteoporosis. *Tran Ass Am Phys* 1940; **55**: 298–305.

16. McConkey B, Fraser GR, Bligh AS, Whitely M. Transparent skin and osteoporosis. *Lancet* 1963; **1**: 693–5.

17. Punnonen R, Vilska S, Rauramo L. Skinfold thickness and long-term post-menopausal hormone replacement therapy. *Maturitas* 1987; **5**: 259–62.

18. Dunn LB Damesyn M, Moore AA et al. Does estrogen prevent skin aging? Results from the First National Health and Nutrition Examination Survey (NHANES I). *Arch Dermatol* 1997; **133**: 339–42.

19. Schmidt JB, Binder M, Demschik G et al. Treatment of skin aging with topical estrogens. *Int J Dermatol* 1996; **35**: 669–74.

20. Maheux R, Naud F, Rioux M et al. A randomized, double-blind, placebo-controlled study on the effect of conjugated estrogens on the skin thickness. *Am J Obstet Gynecol* 1994; **170**: 642–9.

21. Barnes MJ, Constable BJ, Morton LF et al. Age-related variations in hydoxylation of lysine and proline on collagen. *Biochem J* 1974; **139**: 461–8.

22. Murai A, Miyahara T, Shiozawa S. Age related variations in glycosylation of hydroxyproline in human and rat skin collagens. *Biochem Biophys Acta* 1975; **404**: 345–8.

23. Risteli J, Kivirikko KI. Intracellular enzymes of collagen biosynthesis in rat liver as a function of age and in hepatic injury induced by dimethylnitrosamine: changes in prolyl hydroxylase, lysyl hydroxylase, collagen galactosyltransferase and collagen glucosyltransferase activities. *Biochem J* 1976; **158**: 361–7.

24. Tan CY, Stratham B, Marks R, Payne PA. Skin thickness measurements by pulsed ultrasound: its reproductibility, validation and variability. *Br J Dermatol* 1994; **96**: 1392–4.

25. Grosman N, Hindberg E, Schen J. The effect of oestrogenic treatment on the acid mucopolysaccharide pattern in the skin of mice. *Acta Pharmacol Toxicol* 1971; **30**: 458–64.

26. Varila E, Rantala I, Ikarinem A et al. The effect of topical oestriol on skin collagen of postmenopausal women. *Br J Obstet Gyndecol* 1995; **102**: 985–9.

27. Rauramo L, Punnonen R. Wirking einer oralen estrogentherapie mit oestriolsuccinat auf die haut hastiertre. *Frauen Haut Gerchluts Kr* 1969; **44**: 463–70.

28. Punnonen R. Effect of castration and peroral therapy on skin. *Acta Obstet Gynecol Scand* 1973; **21**: 1–4.

29. Brincat M, Moniz CF, Studd JWW et al. Sex hormones and skin collagen content in postmenopausal women. *BMJ* 1983; **287**: 1337.

30. Shahrad P, Marks RA. Pharmacological effect of oestrone on human epidermis. *Br J Dermatol* 1977; **97**: 383–6.

31. Shuster S, Bottoms E. Senile degeneration of skin collagen. *Clim Sci* 1963; **25**: 487–91.

32. Muscat Baron Y, Brincat M, Galea R. Bone density and skin thickness changes in postmenopausal women on long term steroid therapy. In: (Wren BG, ed) *Progress in the Management of the Menopause*. Proceedings of the 8th International Congress on the Menopause, Sydney, Australia, 3–7 November 1996, 179–82.

33. Muscat Baron Y, Brincat M, Galea R. Increased reduction in bone density and skin thickness changes in postmenopausal women on long term corticosteroid therapy. *Climacteric* 1999; **27**: 174–7.

34. Schuster J, Black M, McVitor E. The influence of age and sex on skin thickness, skin collagen and density. *Br J Dermatol* 1975; **93**: 639.

35. Hall DA, Reed FB, Noki G, Vince JD. The relative effects of age and corticosteroid therapy on the collagen profile of dermis from subjects with rheumatoid arthritis. *Age Ageing* 1974; **3**: 15–22.

36. Brincat M, Moniz CJ, Studd JWW et al. Long term effects of the menopause and sex hormones on the skin thickness. *Br J Obstet Gynaecol* 1985; **92**: 256–9.

37. Brincat M, Moniz CJ, Studd JWW et al. Sex hormones and skin collagen content in postmenopausal women. *BMJ* 1983; **287**: 1337–8.

38. Castelo-Barcia C, Pons F, Gratacos E et al. Gonzales Merlo J. Relationship between skin collagen and bone changes during ageing. *Maturitas* 1994; **18**: 199–206.

39. Pierard G E, Letawe L, Dowlati A, Pierard-Franchimant L. Effect of hormone replacement therapy for menopause on the mechanical properties of skin. *J Am Soc* 1995; **43**: 662–4.

40. Brincat M, Studd JWW, Moniz CF et al. Skin thickness and skin collagen mimic an index of osteoporosis in the postmenopausal woman. In: (Christiansen C, Riis B, Eds) *Osteoporosis 1*. Proceedings of the Copenhagen International Symposium on Osteoporosis, 1993, 353–5.

41. Schmidt JB, Binder M, Macheiner W et al. Treatment of skin ageing symptoms in perimenopausal females with estrogen compounds. A pilot study. *Maturitas* 1994; **20**: 25–30.

42. Anttinen H, Orava S, Ryhanen L et al. Assay of protocollagen lysyl hydroxylase activity in the skin of human subjects and changes in the activity with age. *Clin Chim Acta* 1973; **47**: 289–94.

43. Henry F, Pierard-Franchimont C, Cauwenbergh G et al. Age-related changes in facial skin contours and rheology. *J Am Geriatr Soc* 1995; **45**: 220–2.

44. Dunn LB, Damesyn M, Moore AA et al. Does estrogen prevent skin ageing? Results from the First National Health and Nutrition Examination Survey (NHANES I). *Arch Dermatol* 1997; **33**: 339–42.

45. Pierard GE, Letawe C, Dowlati A et al. Effect of hormone replacement therapy for menopause on the mechanical properties of the skin. *J Am Geriatr Soc* 1995; **43**: 662–5.

46. Henry F, Pierard-Franchimont C, Cauwenbergh G et al. Age-related changes in facial skin contours and rhetology. *J Am Geriatr Soc* 1995; **45**: 220–2.

47. Sator PG, Schmidt JB, Sator MO et al. The influence of hormone replacement therapy on skin ageing: a pilot study. *Maturitas* 2001; **39**: 43–55.

48. Castelo-Branco C, Figueras F, Matinez de Osaba MJ et al. Facial wrinkling in postmenopausal women: effects of smoking status and hormone replacement therapy. *Maturitas* 1998; **29**: 75–86.

49. Ramamurthy NS, McClain SA, Pirila E et al. Wound healing in aged normal and ovariectomised rats: effects of chemically modified doxycycline (CMT – 8) on MMP expression and collagen synthesis. *Ann N Y Acad Sci* 1999; **878**: 720–3.

50. Pirila E, Ramamurthy NS, Maisi P et al. Wound healing in ovariectomised rats: effects of chemically modified tetracycline (VMT-*) and estrogen on matrix metalloproteinases – 8, -13 and type I collagen expression. *Curr Med Chem* 2001; **8**: 281–94.

51. Ashcroft GS, Greenwelk-Wild T, Horan MA et al. Topical estrogen accelerates cutaneous wound healing in aged humans associated with an altered inflammatory response. *Am J Pathol* 1999; **115**: 1137–46.

52. Ashcroft GS, Dodsworth J, Van Boxtel E et al. Estrogen accelerates cutaneous wound healing associated with an increase in TGF-beta1 levels. *Nat Med* 1997; **3**: 1209–15,

53. Schmidt JB, Binder M, Macheiner W et al. New treatment of atrophic acne scars by iontophoresis with estriol and tretinoin. *Int J Dermatol* 1995; **34**: 53–7.

23

Lifestyle counseling

AS Wolf

Introduction • Nutrition (eating and drinking habits) • Physical activity, exercise and sports • Alcohol, tobacco smoking and caffeine • How can lifestyle counseling be promoted? • References

INTRODUCTION

Although life expectancies for women and men have increased considerably in the industrial nations during the last 100 years, thanks to social change, medical progress and improved hygienic standards, certain illnesses such as cardiovascular diseases (CVD), stroke, malign tumors, dementia and osteoporosis have increased dramatically. The questionable advantages of better life circumstances for people in the industrialized nations, providing a surplus of food and therefore the consumption of too much fat, sugar and a high calorie intake, as well as increasing ecological damage, have lead to a 4.5 times higher incidence of malign diseases in those nations compared to unindustrialized, underdeveloped countries. Women and men from Southeast Asia have a comparatively significantly lower risk of cancer of the breast, colon, endometrium, and prostate than the populations of Europe and the United States (US).

Also, an extreme discrepancy exists in the incidence and mortality rate of breast cancer cases in Western industrial countries compared to Southeast Asia. The number of breast cancer cases per 100,000 women per year in Japan and China is 21.2, compared to an incidence of 83.2 in the US. The mortality rate for Japanese women is 5.8%, compared with 23.9% in the US. Comparable discrepancies also exist in CVD and osteoporosis.

Besides ethnogenetic characteristics, different social and cultural practices in the eastern Asian population, religious beliefs and attitudes towards life, and especially differences in nutrition – small amounts of saturated fats but plenty of fiber, green tea and the use of soy as a base nutrition – are of significance.

The significance of nutrition and lifestyle has been elucidated in several migration studies of Japanese migrants in Hawaii and Australia, as well as Chinese immigrants in the US, by protocoled nutritional analyses. The findings were that Japanese immigrants developed the risk of developing colon cancer after one generation and the risk of developing breast cancer after two generations in their new environment. However, Scotch could lower this increased risk of developing colon cancer, shown in migrants to Australia.

Even if there is no direct scientifically proven correlation between nutrition and the initiation of cancer, the Western lifestyle is considered to be the main promoter for the higher incidence of malign diseases in industrialized countries. Today there is little doubt that daily lifestyle habits exert a profound impact on short- and long-term health and the quality of life.

'Lifestyle' describes routine habits of everyday life concerning:

- nutrition (eating and drinking habits);
- physical activity and sports;
- the use of alcohol and nicotine, as well as drug abuse;
- exposure to environmental toxins;
- stress and coping with it;
- individual social interaction and psychologic, emotional burdens.

In this chapter the problems of lifestyle counseling of elderly women is discussed.

NUTRITION (EATING AND DRINKING HABITS)

Nutrition in old age

When compared to those of younger people, eating habits of the elderly are considered to be smaller in quantity, lower in frequency and less balanced, and unfortunately often providing below the recommended levels of macro- and micronutrients. Their vulnerability to diseases, mainly infectious ones, lack of drive and general functional decrease seems to be attributable to malnutrition rather than aging.[1]

Another frequent problem of the eating habits of elderly people is weight gain, which is mostly a consequence of incorrect nutrition, combined with other factors such as a decrease in lean body mass, an increase in body fat, interactions of nutrition with medication and reduced physical activity.

Another problem of older women and men is the increasing demand for micronutrients and vitamins (e.g. vitamins K and E) due to increasing metabolism. An additional demand of micronutrients occurs in cases of tobacco consumption and in pathologic situations such as during and after diseases, homocystemia and metabolic disorders.

Intrinsic functional and organic aging processes, a handicap for the elderly

Older people tend to exhibit a decrease in lean body mass and proteins from 45% in younger

years to 27% in the 70s, with increasing body fat. The intracellular water content decreases from 42 to 33%, leading to a reduction in the whole body water content from 50 to 45% of body weight. The general vital body functions decrease from the ages of 15–22 in women and 18–25 in men, in an almost linear fashion. This leads to a lower requirement of macronutrients, changes of sensory perception and feelings of thirst.

Parallel to these involuntary processes on the sensory organs (eyes and ears), the perception of smell and taste also decreases. While the liking for sweet food remains intact into old age, the taste for salty and hot food (which requires more intense stimulation) decreases. About 60% of 65 to 80-year-old people have disorders of smell, partially potentiated by the lack of zinc. Additionally, the subjective feeling of thirst regresses, with a consequent decrease of plasma volume and cellular dehydration without equivalent feelings of thirst.

Changes of digestive organs and their function

One cause for the altered nutrition of older people is the involuntary process of bone loss, which encourages peroidontitis, disorders of chewing and loss of teeth, followed by replacement with dentures. Decreased secretion from the buccal glands, and loss of mucine and antibacterial substances, is associated with dryness of the mouth, burning sensations, pain of the tongue, pain during swallowing and inflammation of the gums. Other changes occur within the distal part of the esophagus with disorders of peristalsis and swallowing, heartburn and inflammation. The secretion of gastric, pancreatic, intestinal and gallbladder liquids are slowed down. An excretory pancreatic insufficiency leads to decreased resorption of fatty acids and fat-soluble vitamins, as well as to a decrease of vitamin B12. The presence of *Helicobacter pylori*, as well as H2-blockers and proton-pump inhibitors, decrease the resorption of vitamin B12.

Glands and muscles of the colon decrease,

Table 23.1   Causes of insufficient and ineffective nutrition during aging

Cause of poor nutrition	Effect of poor nutrition
Preference of nutrients or food	Avoidance of certain foods (e.g. vegetables, wholegrain products, milk) because of ignorance, lack of interest in cooking, laziness, possible intolerance, difficulty with chewing and swallowing. Loss of micronutrients during preparation of meal, improper conservation of food and inadequate preparation in private household or kitchen, overcooking of meals due to problems of chewing and swallowing (thermal destruction of vitamins, decreasing micronutrients)
Diseases of the gastrointestinal tract	Disorder of resorption (gastritis, exocrine pancreatic insufficiency, intestinal infections, colitis, cancer, resections), food intolerance (against lactose and gluten)
Daily habits	Alcohol abuse, use of tobacco
Increased demand for calories and nutrients	Diseases such as cancer, post-surgery, severe infections, convalescence
Increased demand for calories and nutrients due to aging	Higher demand for vitamins D and B12, folic acid and antioxidant vitamins
Medications	Altered metabolism, decrease of resorption, higher loss of macro- and micronutrients due to use of antibiotics, diuretics, laxatives, antineoplastic medication, H2-blocking, antirheumatics and antiepileptics After radiation and chemotherapy
Psychosocial factors	Isolation and loneliness, depression, immobility, beginning or existing dementia

leading to reduced peristalsis and a tendency for constipation and the development of diverticulosis, exacerbated by a lack of potassium.

Up to the 70s the kidneys decrease in size and weight up to one-third of their original measurements, and the number of glomeruli decrease by about 50%, leading to a decreased hydration rate of about 50%.

Changes of the immune system (immunosenescence)

During the aging process the immunologic response to antigens (microbes, malign cells, vaccination) is decreased, leading to a higher incidence of severe infections and malignant diseases. These changes are caused by a loss of replication of CD4 T cells, as well as a lack of antioxidative vitamins.

What is a healthy diet for the elderly?

For the nutrition of the elderly, scientifically proven standards and recommendations are less useful because the elderly cannot transfer them into their daily nutrition. Most elderly people want to continue with what they are used to eating. It seems very difficult to change dietary habits according to a cognitive process. Food counseling should be directed at an affordable diet and realized in small but effective steps.

Basic recommendations are:[2-4]

- wholegrain products;
- fruits and vegetables;
- milk and dairy products;
- high-quality protein;
- enough liquid (water).

Less recommended are:

- all sweets, including chocolate;
- high-fat food – red meat, sausages and full-fat cheese;
- alcoholic beverages.

More specific recommendations are:

- carbohydrates: use of non-glycemic polysaccharides in vegetables, fruit, legumes, wild rice, wholegrain products;
- protein: lean meat, preference for fish (especially cold-water fish), lean milk products and/or skimmed milk, eggs;
- fat: instead of saturated fat in meat, plant oils such as olive oil and/or any other plant oil, very little butter or margarine is preferred.
- as sources for diverse vitamins, trace elements and minerals:

  vitamin A: vegetables, low-fat milk resp. dairy products;
  B vitamins: meat, fish, wholegrain bread, fruits, vegetables;
  folic acid: milk, foliated vegetables (spinach, lettuce);
  vitamin C: citrus fruits, vegetables (bell peppers);
  iron: meat, wholegrain bread, vegetables;
  calcium: skimmed milk, lean milk products, vegetables;
  potassium: fruits, vegetables.

The decreasing demand for energy but constant need for micronutrients should favor any food with high densities of micronutrients and those low in calories with super-proportional contents of essential nutrients. These demands are realized in all wholegrain products, vegetables (including frozen), sour products, salad vegetables, potatoes and fruit, which should form the basis of daily nutrition. Recommended daily quantities are:

150–300 g vegetables and salad;
150–200 g fruit (unpeeled) and rice;
200–250 g of bread products, especially wholegrain ones.

This guarantees a sufficient supply of vitamin C, folic acid and betacarotene. Vitamin C in particular is necessary for the resorption of iron, especially in elderly with sub- and antacidity of gastric liquids or under medication with antacids. Plant foods are rich in vitamins such as B1, B6, biotine and pantothenic acid, minerals such as potassium, magnesium and trace elements (zinc and iodine), vitamins (C, folic acid) and fiber.

Vegetables and fruit contain additional secondary plant substances such as carotenoids, flavonoids, and phytoestrogens with antioxidative, antimicrobial and cancer-protective effects. Plant products should be supplemented by a daily consumption of milk (skimmed milk is highly recommended) and/or dairy products and cheese up to 100–200 g/day. To limit calorie and fat intakes, products low in fat should be used, such as fat-reduced or skimmed milk, and low-fat cheese and yoghurt. Additional sources of calcium are spinach, broccoli (calabrese), cabbage and fennel.

Lactose from milk and fresh cheese, as well as lactic acids from dairy products, enhance bowel movement and digestion, and increase the amount of lactobacillus whilst decreasing the content of *Escherichia coli* and candida. For an increment of vitamin D, fat, cold-water fish and eggs, as well as white meat (poultry or veal), are necessary. Cold-water fish (cod, red barb, flat fish, salmon, mackerel and herring) are rich in iodine and long-chain polyunsaturated fatty acids (PUFA) such as the docosahexaen acids and the eicosapentaen acids. These omega-3 unsaturated fatty acids are metabolized to prostaglandin I2 and I3 with vasodilatatory and aggregation inhibitory effects, replacing the pro-inflammatory eicosanoids (prostaglandin E, F, thromboxane, etc.).

Lean meat supplies high-quality proteins, iron, zinc, and vitamins B1, B6 and B12. Eggs are a good source of proteins, and vitamins A and B12, so are useful in a well-balanced diet. Today, in many countries meat has developed to become a food relatively low in fat, by means of altered methods of breeding. Additionally, ham, corned beef and sausages from poultry are recommended low-fat options. The daily consumption of fat should not exceed 60–75 g, mostly from plant oils and very little butter or fat-reduced margarine. Plant oils are free of cholesterol and rich in vitamin E as well as PUFA such as linolete and alphalinolenic acid (especially olive and rapeseed oils).

Drinking sufficiently, a very frequent problem

The reduced feeling, forgetting and the refusal of adequate drinks, often associated with loss of liquid through exsiccation (by diarrhea, fever, and dementia), are the main reasons for dryness of the elderly. The recommended daily drinking volume is > 1.5 l/day under normal climatic conditions and normally heated rooms. Higher daily amounts are recommended in cases of protein-rich food, fever, diarrhea and hypocaloric nourishment. As thirst is not an equivalent indicator for regulation of liquid or water deficits in the older person, a daily fixed plan for drinking should be established. The best supplement is water, rich in calcium and magnesium, vegetables or fruit juices, teas (fruit teas or green tea) and decaffeinated coffee. The use of alcohol is discussed later.

Food supplements in elderly persons

It is possible for the elderly to obtain the necessary micro- and macronutrients by eating a balanced diet. However, the content of micronutrients can be limited or restricted in many plant foods due to frequent harvests (fewer micronutrients), by industrial processing, conservation, radiation, transport methods and storage due to an alteration by gene technology, and use of fertilizers and pesticides leading to a higher levels of contamination with environmental toxins. Another situation for the necessity of additional supplementation is due to diseases which may demand up to a three-fold elevation of micronutrients, especially in cases of resorptive disorders like gastritis, exocrine pancreatic insufficiency, colitis, during nutritional therapy (because of osteoporosis, rheumatic diseases and homocystinemia) as well as severe deficiency diseases (in tumor patients). In cases of poor appetite and in patients who are underweight additional supplementation with soups and broths rich in calories and essential micronutrients are needed. In severe cases, parenteral nutrition is indicated.

Can an anti-aging diet prevent the aging process?

In the medical literature caloric restriction and special dieting are recommended for the prevention of aging. The aim of caloric restriction is to decrease nutritionally induced diseases like CVD, stroke, Type 2 diabetes [noninsulin-dependent diabetes mellitus (NIDDM)], osteoporosis and malignant diseases (e.g. breast, prostate and colon cancers), with the reduction of radical oxygen species (ROS), absorption of scavengers and enhancing hormone secretion.

Caloric restriction can be achieved by:

- restriction of calories (generally);
- dieting: selective decrease of macronutrients, according to the underlying diseases;
- dinner canceling.

Caloric restriction

In rodents and primates, reduction of calories (in rodents 50%, in primates 70% used for unrestrained feeding) led to an increase in lifespan of between 15 and 35%. The main effect was achieved by silencing the genes necessary for oxidative phosphorylation[5] and energy metabolism with a decrease of their mRNA activity.[6]

The biological effects of calorie restriction are:

- sustained cellular glucose–insulin regulation;
- increase of reparative processes of DNA damages;
- enhancement of immune functions, lean mass and protein synthesis;
- decrease of ROS, oxidative tissue damage and production of age products (advanced glucosylation end-products);
- reduction of gene activity;
- decrease of retardation of aging diseases such as autoimmune diseases, malign diseases, hypertonia, renal insufficiency and cataract.

Increased life expectancy was only achieved by a reduction of total calories, not after a partial restriction of carbohydrates. The effects were even noted when the experiments were started in the middle ages of the animals, leading to an increase of lifespan of 10–20%.[7] The clinical advantage of caloric restriction are:

- a decrease in fat depots;
- a reduction in glucose, insulin, triglycerides, cholesterol, ROS and age products
- increased neurotransmitter receptors, immunity, kidney function;
- increased human growth hormone, as well as melatonin.

Comparable prolongation of lifespan after caloric restriction could be achieved by elimination of the fat-specific insulin-receptor in knockout mice.[8] These data indicate that leanness and not food restriction is the key contributor to extended longevity, an effect which requires further analysis and confirmation.

Humans restricted for a 2-year period in a 'biosphere' model developed a comparable physiologic, hormonal and biochemical pattern resembling those of rodents and primates. The final conclusion of these experiments was that selective restriction of caloric intake is associated with a marked weight loss, but remaining subjects were in excellent health and sustained a high level of physical and mental activity throughout the 2-year experimental period.[9] In view of a general recommendation, calorie restriction should not be recommended before the twentieth year of age, starting slowly and reducing calories until the subject reaches 10–20% below the fixed body weight, which is defined as the weight during normal diet habits. In these cases, complex carbohydrates with additional micronutrients of vitamins and trace elements are recommended, with a further increase of micronutrients during stress, injuries and infections.[7]

Diet for the prevention and treatment of age-associated diseases

CVD

For primary prevention, saturated fat (especially in red meat, eggs, dairy products) should be avoided, with a preference for white meat, cold-water fish (due to PUFA) and skimmed-milk products. In general, a Mediterranean-type diet reduces cardiovascular risk in up to 37% of people (risk of cardiovascular death, nonfatal acute myocardial infarction, unstable angina, stroke, heart failure, embolism, stable angina, postangioplasty restenois and phlebitis). It is likely that certain nutrients characteristic of the Mediterranean diet, such as omega-3 fatty acids, oleic acid and antioxidative vitamins, possess specific and proven cardioprotective effects.[10,11]

Malignant diseases

A fundamental observation in cancer epidemiology is that the incidence and mortality of different cancers vary dramatically across the globe. In addition, the rates of cancer among populations migrating from low- to high-incidence countries change remarkably. In many cases migrating people adapted this risk within their new environment within one to three generations.[4,10] This stresses the fact that the primary cause of cancer development is not genetic but rather environmental factors and lifestyle. Factors involved in the increasing incidence of cancers are tobacco, dietary fat, lack of fiber and plant antioxidants, as well as lack of other protective substances (polyphenols, carotinoids, phytoestrogens).[6] Although there is a comprehensive desire to define monocausal relations between cancer incidence and aspects of lifestyle, the reduction to one mechanism is not adequate. In cohort studies the development of breast cancer in relation to the ingested amount of dietary fat as a cause of cancer was not confirmed or excluded.[11,12] However, one should consider that countries with a low breast cancer risk are primarily developing countries and traditional Eastern societies where lifestyle is notably different to that in Western countries.[12] This includes differences in reproductive behavior, physical activity, body composition and diet other than fat consumption. One problem in finding a direct correlation between diet and cancer is the impossibility of an individual to remember their exact diet in detail and to follow a strict protocol. It seems that current dietary assessment combined with consideration of dietary habits during childhood and adulthood may be useful, but this link is not completely understood.[4] In a meta-analysis of pooled data from nearly 5000 cases of breast cancer, there was no significant relationship between fat intake and breast cancer. However, in a small number of women who were reported to have < 15% energy from fat, a significant twofold increase of breast cancer was observed. This shows that a major fat reduction is not to be recommended.[13] Hyperinsulinemia however, which is the consequence of a high-carbohydrate/low-fat diet and most commonly associated with being overweight, appears to be of greater importance, as insulin acts as a remarkable growth factor binding to any receptor of the tyrosine-kinase family [like insulin-like growth factor (IGF)-1]. For this reason obesity and sedentary lifestyle carry higher risks for increased breast cancer.[14,15] A similar suspicion was expressed between dietary fat uptake and the incidence of colon cancer. Case control studies adjusting fat intake after adequately adjusting for the total energy intake showed no positive association.[16] In addition there was no association between cancer and red meat consumption in prospective studies.[17]

Role of diet in the prevention of coronary heart disease (CHD)

Metabolic studies with determinations of low- and high-density lipoprotein (LDL and HDL, respectively) cholesterol, and total cholesterol showed that women with a high intake of trans-fat and low intake of polyunsaturated fat (compared with women eating low trans-fat and high polyunsaturated fat) had a three times higher risk for CHD.[18] Therefore, a diet with reduced saturated fat may reduce CVD.

Role of filling substances and dietary fiber

Through observation and animal experiments, a view was reached that a high-fiber diet reduces the risk of colon cancer. However, prospective studies in men and women found no relationship between dietary fiber (from cereals) neither for risk of colon cancer nor for colon adenomas. But fiber does seem to reduce the risk for CHD by up to 30%, as well as the risk for Type 2 diabetes and diverticulosis.[19–21]

Is the 'five-a-day' campaign still justified?

From the World Cancer Research Fund,[22] the 'five-a-day' campaign recommended eating five portions of fruit and/or vegetables per day to protect against cancers of the colon, rectum, stomach, lung, esophagus, thorax and mouth. While case control studies found that fruit and vegetables can protect against stomach cancer, prospective studies could not confirm this in almost 1000 incidences of stomach cancer analyzed.[23] The cancer-reducing possibility was apparently overestimated, at least concerning stomach diseases. There are problems in comparing observational studies and case control studies with cohort and prospective studies, several of which are biased. Also, the category of fruit and vegetables is very unspecific and the daily amount is not stated accurately. The biological effects of fruit and vegetables are related to the amount of protective substances contained in them and there is still a considerable lack of knowledge of how the relationship between fruit, vegetables and cancer protection works.[4] Folic acid, which provides a methyl group used for DNA methylation and gene regulation, could be one of the substances beneficial in protecting against cancer. Folic acid consumption seems to protect against cancer during the early stages of colon carcinogenesis, especially in cases of a methylenetetrahydrofolatereductase-gene (MTHF) polymorphism. For the development of colon cancer, several risk factors have been defined from cohort studies in men.[12,19] A lower risk was described as:

- a body mass index (BMI) $< 25 \text{ kg/m}^2$;
- > 30 minutes of vigorous to moderate physical activity per day;
- alcohol consumption $< 15/\text{g/day}$ or $15\text{–}30 \text{ g/}$ day with a folic acid supplement;
- a folic acid supplement of 100 µg/day;
- less than three package years of lifetime smoking;
- less than two servings of red meat per week.

In big cohorts only 3.1% of the population fell into the low-risk group.

Conclusions
Dietary changes can help reduce cancer development. From today's evidence-based data the following recommendations concerning nutrition and food can be made:[12,24]

- Weight control and regular physical activity have highest priority for the prevention of cancer and CVD.
- Replacement of saturated and trans-fat with unsaturated fat and oil (plant oils and PUFA) will reduce CVD but not cancer.
- Replacement of fat with carbohydrates is counter productive.
- Consumption of fruits and vegetables as well as wholegrain products, all high in fiber, is recommended, but benefits are higher for CVD than cancer.
- Adequate folic acid intake, $> 100 \text{ µg/day}$, especially if alcohol is consumed (in which case supplements are advised), lowers the risk of disease.

Vitamins, trace elements, minerals and fatty acids

Free radicals
Free radicals are incomplete molecules with a missing electron and high biochemical reactivity with any neighboring structure such as proteins, DNA, RNA, lipids and carbohydrates. The majority of radicals are generated during energy generation within mitochondria during the process of oxidative phosphorylation, producing adenosine 3-phosphate and free radicals. These are ROS, a term for the group of activated oxygen molecules, hydroxyl radicals, hydrogen peroxide and nitric oxide radicals. Per day in each cell, $> 10,000$ radicals are produced. For their inactivation a system of antioxidative enzymes normally balances radical activity, e.g. gluthathion-peroxidase, catalase-stransferase, superoxide dismutase (SOD), cystine, gluthathion, coenzyme Q_{10}, and vitamins A, C and E, as well as betacarotene.

In 1956, Harman[25] first described the impact between free radicals and aging as well as aging-dependent diseases. As a consequence, radicals react aggressively, leading to autodestruction of mitochondria, their enzymes, mitochondrial DNA, and the lamina and crista apparatus, to point mutations of the DNA and lipid oxidation of the cell membrane. Conditions producing high concentrations of radicals are:

- increased calorie intake;
- environmental toxins: soluble/aerogenic toxins, chronic insolation, herbicides, pesticides, food additives;
- chronic inflammation caused by tobacco smoking, radiation, stress, competitive enduring sports, overdemanding lifestyle and lack of sleep.

For the prevention of radical production and biochemical radical influences the following recommendations are given:

- restriction of calories, with eventual normalization of BMI;
- intake of antioxidative vitamins, especially in terms of an 'antioxidative network', using vitamins C and E, betacarotene, coenzyme

Q_{10}, alpha-lipoic acid, lycopin, *Ginkgo biloba*, flavonoids, estradiol, phytoestrogens, selenium and zinc;

- removal of chronic inflammatory processes (e.g. paradontitis, dental inflammation, arthritis, rheumatoid inflammation);
- avoiding any direct insolation.

Potential of vitamin supplementation[26,27]

Vitamin E (alpha or gamma-tocopherol)

Vitamin E is a lipophilic substance and only absorbed in the presence of cholesterol lipids. It is connected to LDL cholesterol and transported via the lymphatic system into the blood. Vitamin E aggregates to lipids and is mostly placed in the extracellular space close to the lipid cell membranes. Its properties are: that it is an antioxidative substance, therefore protecting against arteriosclerosis (by blocking LDL oxidation); protection against malign diseases; dermoprotection by means of reduction of local inflammatory processes. The daily necessary application is 10–15 mg alpha-tocopherol per day, as a scavenger 400 mg (2 × 200 mg)/day.

Normally, only 30% of alpha-tocopherol is absorbed. The preventive potency of vitamin E alone is weak in primary prevention, as several studies showed a little lower incidence of cardiovascular events. In cases of pre-existing arteriosclerosis (secondary prevention), the preventive effect was not detectable concerning the valuable endpoints: neither the overall mortality nor the incidences of cardiovascular death were decreased after tocopherol in concentrations of 300–800 mg/day.[28–31]

Vitamin C (ascorbic acid)

The water-soluble ascorbic acid migrates into the cytoplasm and exerts an intracellular scavenger activity. Its biological properties are not only reduced on radical scavenging but it also develops synergistic effects to vitamin E. In addition it stimulates the metabolism of cholesterol by induction of cholesterol-reducing enzymes and stimulates the synthesis of adrenal hormones, testosterone, carnithin, collagen and neurotransmitters like norepinephrin and serotonin. The recommended daily dosage as a vitamin is 50–75 mg/day and as an antioxidant 250–500 mg/day.

Besides these properties, epidemiologic studies show only weak effects of vitamin C. Vitamin C reduces the intensity and length of common cold infections. Several studies show an increase in bone density, especially in the hip. A risk reduction of any cancer has only been described in the NHANES II study,[32] while others have not found any significant effects. Cardiovascular mortality is reduced about 20% and the risk for the development of stroke is reduced by about 24% when > 93 mg/day of vitamin C is taken.[33]

Vitamin C supplementation is needed in

Table 23.2 Meta-analysis of the efficiency of vitamin E compared to placebo for the secondary prevention of heart attack, stroke and cardiovascular mortality

Study	Dosage/day (mg)	Study's length (years)	Number of patients	RR (95% CI)	Vitamin E (%)	Placebo (%)
CHAOS	50	5.3	904	0.90 (0.67–1.22)	20.2	21.5
GISSI	300	3.5	11,334	0.98 (0.34–0.83)	4.0	6.6
HOPE	400	4.5	9541	1.05 (0.95–1.16)	16.2	15.5
MRC/BHF	600	5.0	20,536	1.00 (0.94–1.06)	10.2	10.4

RR, Relative risk; CI, confidence interval.

cases of malnutrition or when food is poorly prepared and vitamin C is destroyed, e.g. by storing or cooking. In cases of reduced resorption (intestinal disease), and increased demand during pregnancy, lactation or stress, as well as other diseases (especially infections), tobacco smoking or when food is vitamin C reduced (in particular in the elderly) supplements are recommended.[32]

Alpha-lipoic acid
This is a physiologic substance with vitamin cofactor activity. Its biological properties are antioxidative, regenerating vitamins C and E, complex binding of heavy metals, regulation of glucose utilization, and prevention of diabetic neuropathy and lens cataract, and increasing fatty acid metabolism.[5]

The daily dosage for an antioxidant is 50–100 mg/day and for therapeutic reasons 200–1000 mg/day. Alpha-lipoic acid should be combined with biotin.

Coenzyme Q_{10} (ubiquinone)
Coenzyme Q_{10} is the central enzyme in the mitochondrial respiratory chain. It stabilizes the insulin level and enhances energy production in bones and heart. It is a lipophilic substance and works in cooperation with vitamin E as a lipid protector. In patients undergoing statin treatment the concentrations of coenzyme Q_{10} are tremendously reduced, so supplementation is necessary in these cases. It is present in soy, nuts, almonds, mackerel, sardines, legumes, spinach and garlic.[2]

Folic acid
High concentrations of folates are available in leafy green plants, e.g. spinach, salad leaves, and asparagus, grains and liver. Folates are resorbed and activated into tetrahydrofolic acids. The daily demand for folate is about 400 µg/day.

Folic acid's main property is to metabolize homocysteine into methionine (with reduction of pathologically elevated homocysteine concentrations in the blood) and to reduce the risk of colon cancer, which has been observed in newer epidemiologic studies. There is an inter-relation between folate and vitamin B12 metabolism, as vitamin B12 blocks as a cofactor the homocysteine–methyltransferase reaction with generation of active tetrahydrofolate. For this reason an equivalent dosage of folic acid should be combined with vitamin B12 for the activation of folate metabolites.[2]

Vitamin B12 (cobalamin)
Vitamin B12 exists with a similar group of molecules with a cobalt atom in its center. The most important forms of vitamin B12 are methylcobalamide and 5-desoxyadenosyl-cobalamin which is stored in the liver. Its physiologic activity is to metabolize homocysteine to methionine by activating folic acid. In addition, it is necessary for the synthesis of myelin and DNA.

Vitamin B3 (niacin)
Another important B vitamin is B3, which exists in two physiologic forms as nicotinamide and niacinamide. Normally, niacin is generated through the metabolism of tryptophan to niacin. Working as an antioxidant, it coregulates glucose consumption and cell metabolism, and decreases lipoprotein (a).

Vitamin B6 (pyridoxine)
Vitamin B6 forms the coenzyme pyridoxal phosphate, a necessary enhancer of niacin, glucose regulation, and neurotransmitter synthesis, and a coactivator of vitamin B12 for the activation of folic acid (homocysteine to methionine).

Minerals and trace elements

The most essential minerals are calcium, magnesium, zinc, copper, manganese and molybdenum.

Calcium
As the most important mineral, calcium is the basic substance of the skeletal system and teeth together with phosphorus and magnesium. Only 1% of calcium ions circulate in the body fluid, with the greater part enclosed in the bone substance. Calcium homeostasis is regulated by

an interplay of parathormone and 1–25-dihydroxycholecalciferol (calcitonin). Lack of calcium is originated by defective calcium turnover, which is the leading cause of osteoporosis. For osteoporosis, an oral prophylaxis of 1000–1500 mg calcium is needed together with 400–800 international units (IU) of vitamin D/day.

Magnesium

High amounts of magnesium are found in the heart and skeletal muscles, brain, liver, kidney and bones (> 50%). Only 10% are free ions, mostly bound to ATP. Magnesium catalyzes > 300 enzymatic systems, especially ATP-dependent ones, and regulates the sodium/potassium ion pump and therefore sensoric transmissions in nerves and muscle cells, and serves as a physiologic calcium antagonist. A daily amount of 300–400 mg is required, available in major amounts in wheat, germs, oats, corn and rice.

Zinc

Zinc is the second most important trace element. About 2–3 g of zinc are contained in hair, testicles, bones, muscles, ovaries and pancreas. Zinc catalyzes many important enzyme systems: folic acid deconjugase (metabolizes absorbed folic acid and polyglutamate to resorbable monoglutamate), delta-6-desaturase (metabolizes omega-6 fatty acids, e.g. linolic acids into gamma-linolenic acid); alcohol dehydrogenase; retinol dehydrogenase; and is part of all antioxidant enzymes (glutathion-s-transferase, SOD, catalase) and ceratogenesis.

Zinc stimulates immunity by increasing the gamma-interferon production and enhances antibody production by B cells. A high content of zinc is available in oysters, pig liver, oats, veal, fat and cheese. The daily demand is 7–10 mg and 10–11 mg during pregnancy. A lack of zinc leads to defective wound healing, erythematous alterations of the skin, alopecia, white spots on finger nails, depression, hyperacitivity, phobia and susceptibility to infections.[2] Optimal pharmacologic preparations of zinc are those bound to aspartate, orothate, histidinate and piccolinate. Inorganic

sulfates and chlorides have only a low resorption of about 10–30%.

It should be noted that zinc, iron, copper and calcium disturb one another during intestinal resorption. For optimal resorption any zinc preparation should be given before meals, higher dosages can reduce the copper absorption and lead to hyperchromic anemia, and the absorption of selenium can be decreased by high amounts of zinc. The daily demand for chrome, copper, manganese and molybdenum is normally met by a balanced diet.

Essential fatty acids [PUFA, and omega-3 and -6 unsaturated fatty acids (FA)]

Unsaturated fatty acids are essential and have distinct functions in the body. They are part of the cell membrane, especially linoleic and linolenic acids (omega-6 FA), and are metabolized to eicosanoids (prostaglandins). Eicosanoids are regulatory substances for essential cell functions like cell growth and regeneration, regulation of vessel dilatation, blood pressure, aggregation of platelets, skin trophic, inflammatory processes and autoimmunology. Appropriate fatty acids are omega-linoleic and -linolenic acids, metabolized to eicosopentain acid (EPA) and decosahexain acid (DHA). Omega-3 unsaturated FA are rich in EPA and DHA and are metabolized into prostaglandins PG-I 2 and PG-I 3. A large randomized study showed that PUFA and not vitamin E significantly lower the risk of primary endpoints (common death, cardiovascular death and other fatal events in high-risk patients after primary heart infarction) by 10–30%.[28]

Carotenoids, flavonoids, phytoestrogens

Epidemiologic studies comparing individuals from Southeast Asian countries to Western industrialized countries show a lower risk of breast, colon and prostate cancers, as well as osteoporosis and CVD. Even within Europe there is a remarkable difference in incidence between Northern/Western and Southern European countries (Italy, France, Portugal). Several studies showed the Mediterranean diet[10] – rich in fiber, low in saturated fat – and

Asian diets – enriched with soy products – to be protective.[34,35] Nutrition in Northern/Western countries is highly concentrated in macronutrients and rich in fat, composed of > 40% saturated fat, with supplementary additives such as nitrosamine, and lipophilic environmental toxins in fast food, perhaps responsible for increased rates of cancer. In contrast, a diet with large amounts of fruit and vegetables, as well as wholegrain products, contains the antioxidant vitamins A, E and C, is rich in fiber and fermented nutrients, and high in secondary plant substances. Most of these secondary plant derivatives belong to one of three groups: (1) carotenoids; (2) glucosinolates; (3) polyphenols (flavonoids, phytoestrogens, sulfates).

Carotenoids

The most important substances are beta-carotene, lycopene, xanthophyll and lutein (xeaxanthin). Lycopene is the red substance in tomatoes which works as a potent antioxidant. It is only active when the cells are broken down, as after cooking, in tomato sauce, tomato juice and ketchup. However, commercially available tomato juices have only weak antioxidative activities of 34 mg vitamin C equivalent per 250 ml, which is comparably low. Xanthophylls, lutein and xeaxanthin also work as antioxidants, and block mono-oxigenases. Most of them are in higher concentrations in spinach and lettuce.

Glucosinolates

The most important metabolite is indole-III-carbinol, which is found in high concentrations in broccoli and cabbage. Indoles inhibit cytochrome P-450 mono-oxigenases, which activate carcinogens and stimulate glutathion-s-transferase, an antioxidant enzyme. Its major importance is the inhibition of epigallo-catechin-gallinat, a carcinogenic agent within the gallbladder liquid which enhances colon cancer initiation.

Polyphenols

Flavonoids More than 500 different forms of flavonoids exist, representing the color of any fruit and vegetable. Flavonoids are located in the peel of fruit and vegetables. The major important flavonoids are quercetin (especially in green tea, which suppresses mamma carcinoma cell lines, inhibits proliferative enzymes and works as a scavenger) and resveratrol, the color substance in red wine and red grape juice, which is a highly active antioxidant and inhibits cyclogenase activity by the inhibition of platelet clotting.

Phytoestrogens This large group is biochemically divided into isoflavones (genistein, daidzein, glycetin) and lignans (enterodiol, enterolacton). Isoflavones are high in concentration in soy, red clover, green tea, lignans in fruits, berries, wholegrain products, vegetables and linseeds. Their biochemical activity is based on their isosteric similarity to 17β-estradiol with a relatively high binding affinity to the estradiol receptor ERα and especially ERβ. Phytoestrogens work at different levels, mainly as modulators of ER:[34]

- they bind to ER in high numbers, replacing 17β-estradiol competitively;
- they inhibit tyrosinekinase, which is the main signal transducer of growth factors, e.g. insulin, IGF-1, epidermal growth factor (EGF);
- they stimulate SHBG;
- they inhibit the enzymes necessary for tumor proliferation such as 17β-hydroxysteroid dehydrogenase, angiogenetic enzymes, aromatase.

The clinical properties of phytoestrogens are:

- they decrease climacteric complaints;
- they help prevent osteoporosis;
- they help prevent arteriosclerosis and CVD;
- they help prevent breast, prostate, colon and endometrial cancer.

Clinical effects of isoflavones (genistein, daidzein, glycetin) in protecting against breast cancer are based on a few epidemiologic studies.[36,37] But the hope to inhibit breast cancer development by additional intake of soy phytoestrogens was not significantly effective for non-Asians.[38] For effective protection against breast cancer (and eventually colon cancer), an Asian lifestyle including food based on soy must be started in early childhood and maintained through adulthood.[37] Phytoestrogens in general are only weakly effective in reduction of menopausal complaints and work by their additional properties within their naturally textured soy products rich in fiber, lowering LDL cholesterol, increasing HDL cholesterol and stimulating osteoblast capacity.

PHYSICAL ACTIVITY, EXERCISE AND SPORTS

For the elderly person aerobic exercise and sport of a moderate to vigorous intensity is recommended. Overwhelming literature supports the concept that regular physical activity reduces the risk of coronary disease and its endpoints (sudden cardiovascular death, heart infarction) in primary and secondary prevention, with an additional protective effect against malign diseases. The basic and precise recommendation for the elderly is described as being 'at least 30 minutes of moderate intensive physical activity on most days of the week'.[39] Moderate intense physical activity is defined as any sport or physical activity consuming 4–7 kilocalories/minute, which is 3–6 met (1 met is the energy equivalent to the approximate rate of oxygen consumption of a seated adult at rest). One met is approximately 1 kilocalorie/kg/hour.[39]

Moderate physical activities are:[39,40]

- walking briskly (3–4 miles/hour);
- cycling (10 miles/hour);
- swimming with moderate effort;
- conditioning exercises;
- racket sports;
- table tennis;
- golf (including pulling cart or carrying clubs);
- canoeing leisurely (2–4 miles/hour);
- general housework (cleaning, mowing the lawn, home repairs, painting).

Before beginning any sport of a moderate intensity (e.g. brisk walking, slow jogging, cycling, etc.) after the age of 45, a graded exercise tolerance test should be performed. All recommendations should be prescribed with respect to an individual's personal risk for CVD and/or specific symptoms. Counseling and prescription should be as specific as possible, based on an individual's needs and opportunities. Any recommendation should include an exact program with time for warming up (normally 5 minutes) and duration of the exercise (in minutes), with an indication of the approximate velocity and suggested mileage if applicable. It should also include time to cool down and the frequency/week (normally 4–7 times/week). Pulse monitoring throughout the exercise is useful, which should normally not exceed 100–130/beats/minute. The normal training pulse should be within 65–75% of the maximal pulse frequency after exhaustion.

Major benefits from physical activity, exercise and sports

Reduced risk for CVD

The protective effect of physical activity has been confirmed in several cohort studies. Overall mortality rate was reduced by > 20% when exercise exeeded 30 minutes/day for 1 year of moderate intensity, confirmed by cardiorespiratory fitness mearurements. The health-promoting effect of physical activity appears in a dose-dependent response fashion for 50–2000 kilocalories/week.[41,42] The basic effects of physical activity are the decrease of total cholesterol, increase of HDL cholesterol and decrease of hypertension in a dose-dependent manner.[43] In diabetic patients the peripheral glucose consumption with decreasing insulin and increasing insulin sensitivity is of further importance.[40]

Reduction of breast cancer

Several epidemiologic studies have demonstrated a reduction in the risk of breast cancer among physically active women. Possible explanations for the observed decrease of breast cancer are multiple in origin. The reduction of estrogen production, the reduction of body weight with lowering cholesterol and increasing glucose consumption and enhanced immunity, with insulin possibly playing the key role.[15] In case-controled studies, moderate exercise decreased the relative risk for developing breast cancer by up to 0.53.[44–48] Further benefits of exercise are a reduction in the BMI, optimizing circulation, and reduction of depression and stress.

Reduction of osteoporosis

The benefit of exercise on bone density depends on the specific force, and therefore the activity, which then provides stimulus for the osteoblast. The exercise needed to enhance bone mass depends on the frequency, type of activity and intensity of physical effort. Weight training stresses skeletal areas most at risk for osteoporotic fractures (femoral neck, spine) and resistance or weight can be increased as muscles become stronger. Also muscle training in fitness studios is able to reinforce bone strength. For more active women, backpacking, cross-country skiing and rowing are good choices. In addition, exercise that enhances muscular equilibrium, to avoid falling and the risk of hip fractures, is also needed.[49,50]

ALCOHOL, TOBACCO SMOKING AND CAFFEINE

Alcohol

There are many publications reflecting the impact of alcohol on health status. Alcohol is reported to have beneficial effects concerning reduction of CVD and cancers.

As a drug, alcohol's use is widespread and well accepted by many societies. It is readily available and is advertised and promoted as being desirable, smart and sophisticated. One-third of the population are nondrinkers, one-third drinks moderately, another third drinks more than average. Used at low concentrations, i.e. moderate alcohol consumption, only a few health problems exist, depending on gender and individual alcohol tolerance, as alcohol tolerance depends on the amount of alcohol dehydrogenase, from which women have about half to one-third that of men.

There are mixed messages about alcohol use, considered below.

Alcohol decreases cardiovascular risk

In both sexes, low to moderate alcohol consumption decreases cardiovascular risk but increases the risks of breast and colon cancers and disturbs liver function. Moderate daily alcohol consumption is defined as 1–2 measures of distilled liquor, 1–2 glasses of wine or 1–2 beers. Heavy alcohol consumption is considered more than this and is strongly associated with the development of hypertension, and may therefore increase the risk of CVD. Low to moderate alcohol consumption is 10–25 g/day (equivalent to 125–250 ml of wine or 300–600 ml of beer) and is cardioprotective by increasing HDL cholesterol, decreasing thrombophilia, reducing subjective stress sensitivity and enhancing stress control.[51] Additional protection comes from polyphenols and flavonoids, especially from resveratol in red wine. Therefore the consumption of wine seems to protect better than liquor or beer, as demonstrated by meta-analysis of cardiovascular mortality and moderate wine consumption in different populations.[52] In general, 10–20 g of alcohol increases HDL cholesterol by about 12–15%;[52] furthermore, red wine enhances nitric oxide-associated vasodilation (Fig. 23.1).[53,54] In women, coronary risk can be reduced by moderate alcohol consumption of 10–12 g/day, but it should be noted that women in general have a very low coronary risk before the menopause, so the additional protection against CVD is little when compared to the increased risk of breast cancer. Light to moderate alcohol consumption of 15 g/day for women and 30 g/day for men has only negligible disease risks. The alcohol-specific risk is often potentiated by additional risks such as tobacco smoking, actual liver disease of another etiology, hypertension, chronic pancreatitis, other metabolic disorders, familial breast cancer or alcohol addiction (chronic drinkers). It has been pointed out that alcohol should not be used as a coronary therapeutic method, not even in small doses. In a meta-analysis surveying 51 different studies between 1966 and 1998, 28 cohort studies were pooled for dose–response functions of alcohol (Fig. 23.2). The risk of CHD decreased from 0 to 20 g alcohol/day up to 72 g/day; over 89 g/day

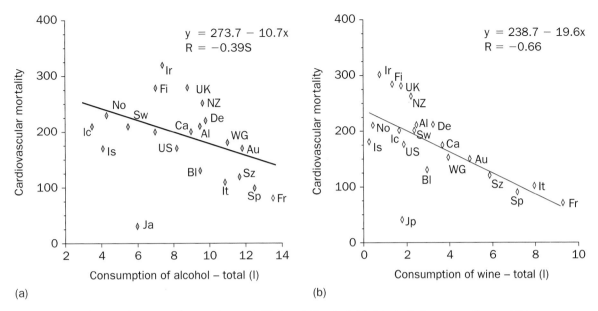

Figure 23.1 Distribution of cardiovascular mortality in relation to (a) total alcohol consumption and (b) consumption of wine. A greater reduction in cardiovascular mortality is seen to be achieved by wine in comparison to other alcoholic beverages within 21 industrial countries. (From Groenbaek et al,[54] with permission.)

the risk increased, showing less protection and harmful effects in women and in men living in countries outside the Mediterranean area.[51]

Alcohol increases the risk of breast cancer
Almost all studies show a positive correlation

and a linear increase in breast cancer incidence with the amount of daily alcohol consumption. In a pooled analysis of cohort studies evaluating 322,647 women for up to 11 years, including 4335 patients with invasive breast cancer, the relative risk (RR) for 10 g alcohol/day was 1.09, for

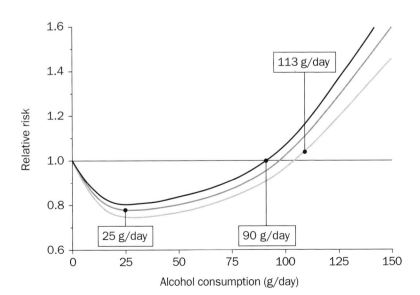

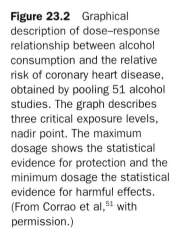

Figure 23.2 Graphical description of dose–response relationship between alcohol consumption and the relative risk of coronary heart disease, obtained by pooling 51 alcohol studies. The graph describes three critical exposure levels, nadir point. The maximum dosage shows the statistical evidence for protection and the minimum dosage the statistical evidence for harmful effects. (From Corrao et al,[51] with permission.)

30–60 g alcohol/day it was 1.41 with no further increase > 60 g alcohol/day. The type of alcoholic beverage did not influence the estimated risk.[35] In a meta-analysis of alcohol consumption and all-cause mortality, in 20 studies a total of 60,225 male deaths and 74,824 female deaths were registered. All studies showed a U-shaped curve with a nadir (lowest point at which mortality was least). Nadirs differed from country to country: United Kingdom (UK) was 17 g alcohol/week, United States (US) was 70 g alcohol/week, whereas in Italy the nadir was sevenfold of the US at 500 g alcohol/week.[52] The nadir in women was at a much lower level (27 g/week for the UK, depending on the different content of alcohol dehydrogenase in women and men). The data suggest that women and men in Italy, Australia and Denmark have lower nadirs than those in the US and UK. Furthermore, the nadir for women is considerably lower than for men in a proportion of 77 to 29.[52] Finally, it can be stated that alcohol is not healthy for everyone and it poses considerable health risks in many individuals.

Tobacco smoking

Cigarette smoking is one of the leading preventable causes for CHD and cancer, accounting for 18% of all newly diagnosed cancers of lung, oral cavity, larynx, esophagus, bladder, kidney, pancreas, stomach, cervix and colon, and 20% of all heart diseases. Prospective studies from different countries state that smokers have a 2–4 times greater risk of developing CVD and for sudden death than nonsmokers. Smoking also increases the risk of stroke, which interacts synergistically with other risk factors (hypertension, diabetes). About 3 million people die each year from smoking-related diseases, which will rise to over 10 million deaths up to the year 2025. The distribution of smoking-relating deaths is as follows:[55]

- heart diseases   40%
- lung cancer   90%
- other cancers   33%
- stroke   6%
- other diseases   2%.

Worldwide, there are an estimated 1.1 million smokers. There are almost twice as many smokers of lower educational levels, a phenomenon observed worldwide, so that by 2025 only 15% of the world smokers will live in rich countries. Men still smoke in significantly greater numbers than women (27 versus 22.6%), with an ethnic prevalence. The major public health concern is cigarette smoking among younger individuals and especially young girls. All smoking initiation occurs before high school graduation.[56] The main reasons for smoking are social factors, psychologic factors (fear of weight gain), economic factors (smoking is more frequent among lower socioeconomic groups) and the addictive aspects of nicotine. For smoking cessation many strategies have been developed including behavioral treatments, nicotine fading, stress-coping strategies and pharmacologic interventions, as well as an increase in physical activity.[56]

Any smoking cessation program must be intense and should be based on different individualized guidelines. An intervention program should include at least four to seven sessions and should be extended over at least 2 weeks. The program should include coping skills training and problem-solving strategies, as well as putting strong emphasis on support for quitting. However, it must be noted that only certain strategies will be effective for a given subset of smokers. The older the woman and the more excessive the smoking habit, the more problematic is any effort to finally quit smoking.

Caffeine

Caffeine is a mild stimulant that occurs naturally in more than 60 plants. The main component is methylxanthine which directly stimulates certain neurotransmitters and affects the whole body. One beneficial effect is the boost of athletic performance, especially for delaying exhaustion. Adverse effects are: trembling, nervousness, insomnia, muscle tension, irritability, headaches and disorientation. These effects usually occur in people not adapted to caffeine consumption. The effects of caffeine vary considerably from person to person, especially when comparing 'coffeeholics' and non-coffee drinkers. A dose of 250 mg administered to a regular coffee drinker usually has no significant effect on blood pressure, heart rate, respiration, blood cholesterol or anxiety; however, noncoffee drinkers might develop inappropriate symptoms. In general there is no evidence-based study on the considerable side-effects of caffeine on CVD, blood cholesterol and cancer. Even for benign breast diseases (caffeine increases the estradiol concentration) no relationship was found between caffeine consumption and fibrocystic diseases.

HOW CAN LIFESTYLE COUNSELING BE PROMOTED?

Physicians and medical doctors (MD) play key roles in spreading the beneficiary message for a healthy lifestyle. For this reason they must be educated and trained in the disciplines concerning lifestyle counseling. Since health is not a lack of disease but covers the whole physical, emotional and psychosocial capability of a human being, physicians must change their role along with changing historic paradigms.

Nearly all physicians have been educated in diagnosis and treatment of diseases but very little about health and its promotion – the aims of 'salutogenesis' must be internalized first. As the second step, MD must learn how to coach their patients in health-related problems, which is different to the adopted traditional doctor's setting. Many physicians will have to rethink their entire role, since many of them are complaining about burnout as a sign of poor health. After an intense education of physicians in health promotion and disease prevention, the motivation of the public can start. Any possibility for distribution of health promotion and motivation must be used in paper and electronic media. Any health activity must start in the early years (preschool, with health as a discipline during school education, etc.) and be continued in health-related videos and radio and TV transmissions.

Health promotion and prevention should be introduced nationwide and should reach all age groups. Health authorities should focus more than ever on health-related topics, and a nationwide fund to promote health, disease prevention and scientific research for the future should be provided. There is a great opportunity to save large sums of money for the health system if age-related diseases could be prevented by appropriate health motivations. In particular, older people could profit from prevention, since age-related diseases are increasing tremendously, leading to considerable problems for welfare systems in Europe and the US. If forced, lifestyle counseling could be realized worldwide, the compression of morbidity and enhancement of life quality could be achieved.

REFERENCES

1. Küpper C. Ernährung im Alter. *Med Welt* 2000; **51**: 393–9.
2. Marz RB. *Medical Nutrition.* (Omni Press: Portland, 1999.)
3. Werbach MR. *Nutritional Influences on Illness*, 2nd edn. (Third Line Press: Tarzana, USA, 1996.)
4. Steinmetz KA, Potter JD. Vegetables, fruit and cancer prevention: a review. *J Am Diet Ass* 1996; **96**: 1027–39.
5. Olgun A, Akman S, Serdar MA, Kuluay T. Oxidative phosphorylation enzyme complexes in caloric restriction. *Exp Gerontol* 2002; **37**: 639–45.
6. Lee C-K, Klopp RG, Weindruch R, Prolla TA. Gene expression profile of aging and its retardation by caloric restriction. *Science* 1999; **285**: 1390–3.
7. Weindruch R. How does dietary restriction retard diseases and aging? *Prog Clin Biol Res* 1989; **287**: 97–103.
8. Blüher M, Kahn BB, Kahn CR. Extended longevity in mice lacking the insulin receptor in adipose tissue. *Science* 2003; **299**: 572–3.
9. Walford RL, Mock D, Verdery R, MacCallum T. Calorie restriction in Biosphere 2: alterations in physiologic, hematologic, hormonal, and biochemical parameters in humans restricted for a 2-year period. *J Gerontol* 2002; **57A**: B211–B224.
10a. Drinkwater BL. Osteoporosis and exercise. In: (Rippe JM, ed) *Lifestyle Medicine.* (Blackwell Science: London, 1999) 237–41.
10b. Matulonis UA. Breast cancer: modifiable lifestyle risk factors. In: (Rippe JM, ed) *Lifestyle Medicine.* (Blackwell Science: London, 1999) 322–31.

11a. Holmes MD, Hunter DJ, Colditz GA et al. Association of dietary intake of fat and fatty acids with risk of breast cancer. *JAMA* 1999; **281:** 914–20.

11b. Leaf A. Dietary prevention of coronary heart disease. The Lyon Heart Study. *Circulation* 1999; **99:** 733–5.

12. Willett WC. Diet and cancer: one view at the start of the millennium. *Cancer Epidemiol, Biomarkers Prev* 2001; **10:** 3–9.

13. Howe GR, Hirohata T, Hislop TG et al. Dietary factors and risk of breast cancer: combined analysis of 12 case-control studies. *J Natl Cancer Inst* 1990; **82:** 561–9.

14. Hunter DJ, Spiegelman D, Adami HO et al. Cohort studies of fat intake and the risk of breast cancer: a pooled analysis. *N Engl J Med* 1996; **334:** 356–61.

15. Kaaks R. Nutrition, hormones and breast cancer: is insulin the missing link? *Cancer Causes Control* 1996; **7:** 605–25.

16. Giovannucci E, Willett WC. Dietary factors and risk of colon cancer. *Ann Med* 1994; **26:** 443–52.

17. Giovannucci E, Rimm EB, Stampfer MJ et al. Intake of fat, meat, and fiber in relation to risk of colon cancer in men. *Cancer Res* 1994; **54:** 2390–7.

18. Hu FB, Stampfer PJ, Manson JE et al. Dietary fat intake and the risk of coronary heart disease in women. *N Engl J Med* 1997; **337:** 1491–9.

19. Gaard M, Tretli S, Loken EB. Dietary factors and risk of colon cancer: a prospective study of 50,535 young Norwegian men and women. *Eur J Cancer Prev* 1996; **5:** 445–54.

20. Rippe JM, O'Brien D, Taylor K. Lifestyle strategies for risk factor reduction and treatment of coronary artery disease: an overview. In: (Rippe JM, ed) *Lifestyle Medicine.* (Blackwell Science: London, 1999) 54–66.

21. Salmeron J, Manson JE, Stampfer MJ et al. Dietary fiber, glycemic load and risk of non-insulin-dependent diabetes mellitus in women. *JAMA* 1997; **277:** 472–7.

22. World Cancer Research Fund, and American Institute for Cancer Research. *Food, Nutrition and the Prevention of Cancer: A Global Perspective.* (American Institute of Cancer Research: Washington DC, 1997.)

23. Michels KB, Giovannucci E, Johipura KJ et al. Fruit and vegetable consumption and colon cancer risk in men and women. *J Natl Cancer Inst* 2000; **92:** 1740–52.

24. Wolfram G. Stoffwechsel und Ernährung. In: (Platt D, ed) *Altersmedizin.* (Schattauer-Verlag: Stuttgart, 1997) 2–12.

25. Harman D. Aging: a theory based on free radical and radiation chemistry. *J Gerontol* 1956; **11:** 298–300.

26. Iha P, Flather M, Lonn E et al. The antioxidant vitamins and cardiovascular disease: a critical review of epidemiologic and clinical data. *Ann Int Med* 1995; **123:** 860–72.

27. Lonn EM, Yusuf S. Is there a role for antioxidant vitamins in the prevention of cardiovascular disease: an update on epidemiological and clinical trials data. *Can J Cardiol* 1997; **13:** 957–65.

28. GISSI–Prevenzione Investigators. Dietary supplementation with n-3 polyunsaturated fatty acids and vitamin E after myocardial infarction: results of the GISSI-Prevenzione trial. *Lancet* 1999; **354:** 447–55.

29. Heart Protection Collaborative Group. MRC/BHF heart protection study of antioxidant vitamin supplementation in 20 536 high-risk individuals: a randomised placebo-controlled trial. *Lancet* 2002; **360:** 23–33.

30. Stephens NG, Parsons A, Schofield PM et al. Randomised controlled trial of vitamin E in patients with coronary disease: Cambridge Heart Antioxidant Study (CHAOS). *Lancet* 1996; **347:** 781–6.

31. Yusuf S, Dagenais G, Pogue J et al. Vitamin E supplementation and cardiovascular events in high-risk patients. The Heart Outcomes Prevention Evaluation study investigators. *N Engl J Med* 2000; **342:** 154–60.

32. Loria CM, Klag MJ, Caulfield LE, Whelton PK. Vitamin C status and mortality in US adults. *Am J Clin Nutr* 2000; **72:** 139–45.

33. Enstrom JE. Counterpoint-vitamin C and mortality. *Nutr Today* 1993; **28:** 28–32.

34. Adlercreutz H, Mazur LO. Phyto-estrogens and western diseases. *Ann Med* 1997, **29:** 95–120.

35. Smith-Warner SA, Spiegelman D, Yaun S-S et al. Alcohol and breast cancer in women. A pooled analysis of cohort studies. *JAMA* 1998; **279:** 535–40.

36. Ingram D, Sanders K, Kolybaba M. Case control study of phytoestrogens and breast cancer. *Lancet* 1997; **350:** 990–4.

37. Wu AH, Ziegler RG, Horn-Ross P et al. Tofu and risk of breast cancer in Asian-Americans. *Cancer Epidemiol* 1996; **5:** 901–6.

38. Horn-Ross PL, John EM, Lee M et al. Phytoestrogen consumption and breast cancer risk in a multiethnic population. The Bay area breast cancer study. *Am J Epidemiol* 2001; **154:** 434–41.

39. Pate R, Pratt M, Blair S. Physical activity and public health: a recommendation from the Centers for Disease Control and Prevention and the American College of Sports Medicine. *JAMA* 1995; **273:** 402–7.

40. British Medical Journal (BMJ). *Clinical evidence.* (BMJ Publishing Group, London, 2002.)

41. Leon AS, Connett J, Jacobs DR. Leisure-time physical activity levels and risk of coronary heart disease and death: the Multiple Risk Factor Intervention Trial. *N Engl J Med* 1987; **258:** 2388–95.

42. Paffenbarger RS, Hyde RT, Wing AL. Physical activity, all-cause mortality and longevity of college alumni. *N Engl J Med* 1986; **314:** 605–13.

43. Cook TC, Laporte RE, Washburn RA. Chronic low level physical activity as a determinant of high density lipoprotein cholesterol and subfractions. *Med Sci Sports Exerc* 1986; **18:** 653–7.

44. Albanes D, Blair AA, Taylor PR. Physical activity and the risk of cancer in the NHANES I population. *Am J Public Health* 1989; **79:** 744–50.

45. Bernstein L, Henderson BE, Hanisch R. Physical exercise and reduced risk of breast cancer in young women. *J Natl Cancer Inst* 1994; **86:** 1403–8.

46. D'Avanzo B, Nanni O, La Vecchia C. Physical activity and breast cancer risk. *Cancer Epidemiol Biomarkers Prev* 1996; **5:** 155–60.

47. Gammon MD, John EM, Britton JA. Recreational and occupational physical activities and risk of breast cancer. *J Natl Cancer Inst* 1998; **90:** 100–17.

48. Thune I, Brenn T, Lund E, Gaard M. Physical activity and the risk of breast cancer. *N Engl J Med* 1997; **336:** 1269–76.

49. De Lorgeril M, Salen P, Martin J-L et al. Mediterranean diet traditional risk factors, and the rate of cardiovascular complications after myocardial infarction. Final report of the Lyon Diet Heart Study. *Circulation* 1999; **99:** 779–85.

50. Kohrt WM, Snead DB, Slatopolsky E, Birge Jr SJ. Additive effects of weight-bearing exercise and estrogen on bone mineral density in older women. *J Bone Miner Res* 1995; **10:** 1303–11.

51. Corrao G, Rubbiati L, Bagnardi V et al. Alcohol and coronary heart disease: a meta-analysis. *Addiction* 2000; **95:** 1505–23.

52. White IR. The level of alcohol consumption at which all-cause mortality is least. *J Clin Epidemiol* 1999; **52:** 967–75.

53. Flesch M, Schwarz A, Böhm M. Effects of red and white wine on endothelium-dependent vasorelaxation of rat aorta and human coronary arteries. *Am J Physiol* 1998; **275:** 1183–90.

54. Groenbaek M, Deis A, Sorensen TI et al. Mortality associated with moderate intake of wine, beer or spirits. *BMJ* 1995; **310:** 1165–9.

55. Glanz K, Brekke M, Harper D. Evaluation of implementation of a cholesterol management program in physicians' offices. *Health Educ Res* 1992; **7:** 151–63.

56. Emmons KM, Maggi S. Behavioral approaches to enhancing smoking cessation. In: (Rippe JM, ed) *Lifestyle Medicine.* (Blackwell Science: London, 1999) 520–30.

57. Collaborative Group of the Primary Prevention Project (PPP). Low-dose aspirin and vitamin E in people at cardiovascular risk: a randomised trial in general practice. *Lancet* 2001; **357:** 89–95.

58. Packer L, Witt EH, Tritschler HJ. Alpha-lipoic acid as a biological antioxidant. *Free Radic Biol Med* 1995; **19:** 227–50.

59. Platz EA, Willett WC, Colditz GA et al. Proportion of colon cancer risk that might be preventable in a cohort of middle-aged US men. *Cancer Causes Control* 2000; **11:** 579–88.

60. Wolk A, Manson JE, Stampfer MJ et al. Long-term intake of dietary fiber and decreased risk of coronary heart disease among women. *JAMA* 1999; **281:** 1998–2004.

24

Phytoestrogens

H Adlercreutz

Introduction • Phytoestrogens • Isoflavones and coumestrol • Isoflavones and breast cancer
• Negative effects of phytoestrogens on the breast • Conclusions • References

INTRODUCTION

The menopause in women is associated with a number of symptoms like hot flushes and vaginal dryness, but also with diseases not immediately recognized by the woman like osteoporosis and coronary heart disease. There are numerous drugs used for the prevention of these diseases caused by decreased hormonal levels and for the alleviation of menopausal symptoms. Of these, hormone replacement therapy (HRT) with the combination of an estrogen and a progestin or only estrogen replacement therapy (ERT) with natural synthetic estrogens have been the most effective. The use of HRT (this abbreviation will be used for both HRT and ERT in the following text) varies very much from one country to another and even within the same country, depending on socioeconomic status, information, the medical system and also the patient's physician. However, there seem to be other factors involved because the incidence of menopausal hot flushes, the most annoying menopausal symptom, varies enormously between countries being lowest in Singapore (14%) and other Asian countries, and highest in North America (85%). It was suggested that one factor potentially responsible for these differences could be soy intake, because soy contains phytoestrogens (isoflavonoids) that have estrogenic activity.[1]

However, the majority of postmenopausal women in the Western hemisphere do not want to use estrogens even if they are offered the possibility, one reason being the slightly increased risk of breast cancer. Recently it was also found that HRT has a surprisingly small, if any, effect on risk factors of cardiovascular disease, particularly in healthy women at low risk. Because of the breast cancer risk many women want to try more natural ways of treating their symptoms and soy products and/or isoflavone concentrates in dietary supplements are now more popular in the US than HRT. But is this an option and is it effective, and are there special indications to treat postmenopausal women with soy or isoflavone supplements? In this chapter I try to provide answers to these questions.

PHYTOESTROGENS

The compounds included in the original group of phytoestrogens have changed over time because of the detection of new compounds with weak estrogenic activity in addition to the isoflavones and coumestanes. Such compounds are the mammalian lignans and some flavonoids. The plant lignans have not been shown to have any estrogenic activity but are converted to weakly estrogenic mammalian lignans in the proximal part of the colon. However, because of their low estrogenic activity they have no effect on the most common postmenopausal symptoms but may be of interest in breast cancer prevention.[2]

The main isoflavones are genistein, daidzein and glycitein, which are found in high concentrations in soybeans and soy flour as glycosidic conjugates, and in fermented soy products mainly in the free form. Numerous supplements with high isoflavone concentrations have been produced using extracts of soybeans or clover leaves. The latter contains mainly biochanin A and formononetin with low estrogenic activity, but are converted in the gut to the more estrogenic genistein and daidzein, respectively, and the latter further to equol, which is more estrogenic than daidzein. Smaller amounts have been found in other beans and in some vegetables and fruits.[3–5] The most estrogenic of these compounds are coumestrol, genistein and equol, the latter is produced in larger amounts only by a limited number of people (about 30%) both in Western countries and in Asia. However, all subjects produce a little equol if measured by sensitive methods. Coumestrol, mainly found in alfalfa sprouts and some beans, is not used for the treatment of menopausal symptoms. Equol is produced from daidzein in the gut, the production being higher in subjects on a carbohydrate-rich diet and has been suggested to be asociated with lower breast cancer risk.[6,7] Up to micromolar concentrations of genistein and daidzein have been observed in the plasma of Japanese subjects.[8,9]

Several reviews have discussed the problem of whether soy or isoflavones have any effect on menopausal symptoms and diseases, and whether this is due to the isoflavones, the soy without isoflavones or a combination of the two.[10–13]

ISOFLAVONES AND COUMESTROL

Effect on menopausal symptoms

In 1991, Lock[14] reported that Japanese women have far fewer menopausal symptoms than Western women. In 1992, the present author's group published a paper of results of phytoestrogen determinations in the urine of Japanese, Finnish and American women, which showed that the excretion was 10–100 times higher in Japanese women compared to Western women.[1] We suggested that the lower incidence of menopausal symptoms could be due to intake of soy products with high isoflavone contents. This resulted in many studies on the possible effect of soy product intake or administration of supplements containing isoflavones in menopausal women. The results have been very variable. In one of the first published controlled studies, soy food plus linseed (containing lignans) showed statistically significant effects on hot flushes and vaginal dryness; however, the reduction of total menopausal scores, being greater in the phytoestrogen group, did not reach statistical significance.[15] Because about one-third of the women were spontaneously relieved of their symptoms, the importance of controlling the studies is obvious.

Some of the studies published are presented in Table 24.1. Some studies have revealed only slight or no influence of phytoestrogens on menopausal symptoms.[12,16–19] In other studies effects have been observed, particularly in those with shorter durations or in the first part of the study.[15,20–25] The effects on hot flushes and night sweats may be dramatic at the beginning of soy or isoflavone therapy, but it is possible that some women's tolerance levels are reset over time, resulting in negative results after longer periods of treatment. It is always possible to increase the estrogen dose in HRT, but to increase soy food intake is not possible due to abdominal symptoms. The controversial observations and negative findings have raised the question of whether isoflavone therapy is any better than placebo.[26] However, it is too soon to draw any definite conclusions.[27]

Table 24.1   Studies on the treatment of menopausal symptoms with soy or isoflavones

Author (ref)	Design of study – phytoestrogen or soy product	No.*	Vaginal cytology, endometrium effects	Hot flushes Plasma FSH	Remarks
Wilcox et al[97]	Six weeks treatment in three subsequent 14 day period with either soy flour (45 g/day), red clover sprouts (10 g dry seed daily), or linseed (25 g/day). Latin square design	23	Maturation value increased with soy and linseed	Not studied FSH decreased cumulatively	No washout periods between treatments. No assays
Murkies et al[30]	A 12-week randomized double-blind study in which 45 g soy or unbleached wheat flour was consumed	23+24	No effect on vaginal maturation index	Hot flushes reduced by 40% in soy and 25% in the wheat group FSH, no effect	No difference between the dietary groups†
Baird et al[98]	Soy food comprising one-third of the caloric intake; controls consumed their normal diet, nature of food not known; 4 weeks duration	66+25	Slight nonsignificant effect on maturation index ($P = 0.06$)	Not studied FSH unchanged	Only semiquantitative assay of phytoestrogens in urine
Brzezinski et al[15]	80 g tofu, two glasses of soy drink, 5 g miso and 10 g flaxseed were consumed daily for 12 weeks	78+36	Vaginal dryness score reduction significant	Hot flush score reduction significant	Six phytoestrogens were assayed in plasma, about 100-fold increase
Albertazzi et al[21]	Double-blind randomized study using 60 g/day of soy protein (76 mg isoflavone aglycones) or 60 g of casein for 12 weeks	40+39	Not studied	45% reduction with soy and 30% reduction with placebo	
Dalais et al[16]	A 12-week double-blind, randomized, crossover study with soy, linseed or a wheat diet	44	Soy increased maturation index (103%)	Linseed (41%) and wheat (51%) reduced hot flushes, but not soy	Four phytoestrogens to creatinine ratios were measured‡ Bone mineral content increased (5.2 %) by soy

Table 24.1 continued

Author (ref)	Design of study – phytoestrogen or soy product	No.*	Vaginal cytology, endometrium effects	Hot flushes Plasma FSH	Remarks
Washburn et al[20]	Double-blind study in which women were randomized to three different diets during 6-week periods. Control diet, 20 g complex carbohydrates: diet 2, 20 g soy protein supplement containing 34 mg of isoflavones once per day; diet 3, the same as diet 2 but divided into two equal portions	42	Not studied	Significant reduction of hot flush severity with diet 3. No effect on number	No assays in plasma or urine
Baber et al[24]	A randomized, placebo-controlled crossover study using one tablet per day of Promensil and red clover supplement containing 40 mg of isoflavones	43+44	No effect	At 4 and 12 weeks a a substantial, but nonsignificant reduction of hot flushes, but no difference at 12 weeks. No effect on Greene scores at any time	HPLC assay of phytoestrogens in urine§
Upmalls et al[23]	Soy isoflavone extract (50 mg isoflavone glycosides per day = about 30 mg aglycones/day) Randomized, double-blind study over 12 weeks	89+86	No effect on vaginal maturation index No stimulation of endometrium	Significant effect after 6 weeks ($P = 0.03$), after 12 weeks almost ($P = 0.08$) significant FSH, no change	No assays in plasma or urine
Scambia et al[22]	Soy extract (50 mg of isoflavones per day) in a double-blind randomized study during 6 weeks	20+19	No effect on vagina or endometrium	Significant reduction after 6 weeks ($P < 0.01$)	Plasma levels of genistein and daidzein measured
Quella et al[17]	Double-blind crossover study using 50 mg soy isoflavone tablets given three times per day to breast cancer survivors (4 weeks)	149	Not studied	No effect	Most subjects were treated with Tamoxifen. No assays

Study	Intervention	Number of subjects			
Somekawa et al[18]	Dietary records and calculation of isoflavones in diet; mean intake 54.3 mg/day‡	478	Not investigated	High isoflavone intake associated with less palpitation and back No difference with regard to hot flushes	Assays of urinary phytoestrogens in the first 51 women
St Germain et al[19]	Double-blind 24-week study. Soy protein isolate with (80.4 mg aglycones/day) and without isoflavones (4.4 mg/day aglycones) and a whey protein control	24+24+21	Not investigated	Decreased in all groups in the same way. No difference between groups	Urine phytoestrogens measured
Van Patten et al[28]	Randomized, placebo-controlled, soy beverage containing 90 mg of isoflavones (12 weeks) All subjects had breast cancer	59+64	Not investigated	Decreased significantly in both groups. No difference between groups	Mean serum genistein in soy group 610 nmol/l, in placebo group 430 nmol/l[||] No difference for daidzein
Han et al[25]	Randomized, double-blind, placebo-controlled trial with 100 mg isoflavones (tablets)/day over 4 months	40+40	Not investigated, transvaginal sonographic results unchanged	All symptoms included in the Kupperman index significantly reduced	Estradiol increased and FSH decreased significantly

* Number of subjects completing study if known; second number = controls.

† Urinary excretion of daidzein was relatively high in both groups at baseline (soy group 2.13 µmol/day and wheat group 1.71 µmol/day) and equol excretion was also relatively high in the wheat group (0.58 µmol/day). After treatment at 12 weeks the urinary daidzein was very high in the soy group (44.9 µmol/day) but had also almost doubled in the wheat group (3.02 µmol/day). This latter level is higher than the mean level we observed in Japanese women (2.6 µmol/day[1,58]). This could explain why no difference was observed between the groups.

‡ The diet compositions were based on experience obtained in the above study in which the wheat diet caused a high excretion of daidzein in urine and also equol values increased (not measured in this study). Because spot urines were used and the phytoestrogen/creatinine ratios were presented in a figure (scale erroneous and assays not carried out at 8 and 12 weeks of wheat treatment?), it is not possible to get an exact view of the phytoestrogen concentrations, but the daidzein values also seem high in this study, which could explain the peculiar result that the wheat diet significantly reduces hot flushes. The authors suggest that larger studies should be carried out.

§ In accordance with the other studies with subjects living in Australia it is reported that many of the control subjects showed high isoflavone excretion at the end of the time points. It is obvious that it is difficult to keep an isoflavone-free diet in Australia. The most interesting observation was that when the controls and treated subjects were analyzed together the sum of the measured isoflavones in urine (genistein, daidzein, formononetin and biochanin A) correlated negatively with the percentage change in hot flushes. This was particularly true for daidzein excretion.

|| The values in the control group are very high, higher than mean values in Japanese women, which could explain the negative result.

FSH, Follicle-stimulating hormone, HPLC, high-performance liquid chromatography.

There is some evidence that daidzein may be the most effective isoflavone,[24] but it also seems that it may be better to consume a whole product also containing soy protein than to take pills containing isoflavones alone. In a review, Eden[10] concludes that about two-thirds of menopausal women may benefit from phytoestrogenic products, but that the effect on vaginal dryness is uncertain. In other studies with positive results the placebo effect has been great (about 25–30%) and only about 15% of the women, in addition to those who would have improved without therapy anyway, felt a positive effect of the soy or isoflavones.

How can these controversial results be interpreted? It seems that the effect may depend on the endogenous estrogen production and level of sex hormone-binding globulin (SHBG), as well as on the isoflavone plasma levels in the controls, which may be relatively high.[24,28] Women with high estrogen levels may not see any improvement but women with low estrogen production due to low peripheral conversion of androgens to estrogens probably benefit more. Moderately obese and obese women produce more estrogens than slim women and may not recognize any positive effects of weak estrogens. However, nobody has made any evaluation or discussed the effects of isoflavones or soy in relation to the endogenous hormone levels. In a recent study the controls had high isoflavone plasma levels[28] and no effect of a soy beverage on postmenopausal symptoms was observed (Table 24.1). However, the plasma levels of isoflavones in the controls were higher than in Japanese women.[29] This could explain the negative results. In another study there was high urinary excretion of isoflavonoids at baseline,[30] which could have caused the negative results. It is also possible that women producing equol from daidzein benefit more due to the conversion of daidzein to equol. Evidence from rat studies indicate that equol is concentrated in certain areas of the brain (frontal lobe and cerebellum) – and has anxiolytic effects in rats.[31–33] Supplements contain very variable amounts of isoflavones and their composition also varies considerably.[34,35] The results of therapy with tablets containing clover extracts is influenced by the effectiveness of the metabolism of biochanin A and formononetin to more estrogenic isoflavonoids (genistein, daidzein, equol), but biochanin A may have some effects on itself. Some supplements contain little genistein and more daidzein and glycitein, and these may have different effects compared to soy food or tablets prepared from whole soy with the same distribution of isoflavones as in the soybean. However, soy protein with isoflavones may be more efficient than only isoflavones. It has also been shown that women have different thresholds for the effect of estrogens on menopausal symptoms and this may change with therapy. Women with a high threshold will probably not benefit from intake of the relatively weak plant estrogens.

It is important to measure both estrone and estradiol levels in plasma with a good chromatographic method before treatment, and to relate the values to the effect of the isoflavones or soy. The determination of equol in plasma during therapy would also give important information, but other phytoestrogens should also be assayed both in the controls and the treated subjects before and during treatment. A recent study found that Japanese women with the highest soy or isoflavone intake had 53 and 58%, respectively, reduced risk of hot flushes compared to the group with lowest intake,[36] which supports the original hypothesis.[1] However, this does not show that the effect was due to the isoflavones. Japanese women are seldom obese compared to Western women and because of that the effect of soy may be better in the former population. These results also suggest that rather moderate intake of isoflavones may have an effect in slim women, because in the cited study in Japanese women the mean intake of genistein was 30 mg/day and that of daidzein 16 mg/day.[29] In one study with no effect on menopausal symptoms,[17] most of the breast cancer patients were also treated with Tamoxifen, which may have caused the negative result. Thus, it can be concluded that numerous factors may have influenced the results obtained and more thorough studies are required taking into account the above considerations. A rather good approach was shown by the van de Weijer group in a poster presented at the North American Menopause Society's 12th Annual Meeting in New Orleans, October 4–6, 2001. In that study 30 women received first a single-blind placebo for 4 weeks and were subsequently randomized, double-blind to placebo or 80 mg isoflavones from clover. During the single-blind run-in month the frequency of hot flushes decreased by 14% but during the subsequent double-blind phase a further 44% decrease was observed in the isoflavone group but no additional effect in the placebo group. In this way the placebo effect was eliminated before the real study began. This approach seems quite good and should be repeated.

Effects on the brain

The possible effects of isoflavones on brain function is interesting. Studies in rats by Lephart et al[33] show that in particular equol is concentrated in the brain in the frontal cortex and cerebellum, where other scientists have found an abundance of estrogen receptor-beta (ERβ). Soy treatment seemed to have various effects on the rats, the most interesting in this regard being the anxiolytic effect.[33] Eating soy seems to improve human memory and mental flexibility, and perhaps reduces tension.[37] Positive effects on the brain may, therefore, explain why soy and isoflavone supplements have such wide usage among postmenopausal women.

Effects on bone

The most estrogenic soy phytoestrogens are genistein and the daidzein metabolite equol, but their estrogenic activity is still low compared to estradiol. Coumestrol, a coumestan, has higher estrogenic activity but occurs in very low amounts in the human diet. The isoflavones bind weakly to ERα and somewhat better to ERβ, and are about 500–1000 times less estrogenic than estradiol.[38–40] Because of their estrogenicity one could, in an environment of low estrogen concentration, expect a positive effect on bone metabolism. In fact, in numerous animal studies carrying out experiments in ovariectomized animals soy phytoestrogens have been shown to conserve bone, i.e. both decreasing bone loss and increasing bone mass. However, in postmenopausal women only a few studies have been done and so far only moderate beneficial effects of soy isoflavones have been observed and really only with regard to the lumbar spine (see review by Anderson and Garner[41]). In later studies effects have been observed,[42,43] also using isoflavonoids from red clover leaves,[44] in agreement with the conclusions made by Anderson and Garner.[41] In tissue cultures daidzein has anabolic effects[45] on cortical bone and in rats daidzein is more effective than genistein in preventing ovariectomy-induced bone loss.[46] A synthetic isoflavone called ipriflavone is metabolized to daidzein and has significant treatment effects on osteoporosis,[47] but the doses are high and these results have not been confirmed in a recent human study.[48] The authors conclude that 'ipriflavone does not prevent bone loss or affect biochemical markers of bone metabolism'. Additionally, ipriflavone induces lymphocytopenia in a significant number of women.

In a study in The Netherlands it was found that a high rate of bone loss is associated with high enterolactone excretion,[49] but in Korean postmenopausal women with osteoporosis urinary enterolactone was lower than in the controls.[50] In the Korean women, bone mineral density (BMD) of L2–L4 and of the femoral neck and Ward's triangle correlated positively with urinary enterolactone. Vegetarians with a high fiber diet resulting in high enterolactone excretion[51,52] tend to have more osteoporosis than omnivoros women, which would fit with the results in The Netherlands. Korean women consume soy products but no relation was found to the isoflavones in urine. However, the very different diets in the two countries may affect the results. In one study with moderate effect of treatment of menopausal symptoms, a combination of soy and linseed was administered.[15] It is, therefore, not impossible that a high level of both enterolactone and isoflavones is more effective than isoflavones alone.

Effects on the cardiovascular system and lipids

Soy intake modulates favorable plasma lipids,[53] but there is controversy with regard to which component – the protein or the isoflavonoids or both – is responsible for the effect. Recently, in premenopausal normocholesterolemic women a favorable dose-dependent effect on plasma cholesterol and the lipid profile of the isoflavones has been observed.[54] In these experiments the amount of protein was kept constant. However, in other studies in monkeys, isoflavones combined with casein-lactalbumin seemed not to have any effect but intact soy protein with isoflavones had significant favorable lipid effects.[55] Furthermore, isoflavones from red clover extracts seemed not to have any effect on plasma lipids in postmenopausal women.[56,57] However, approximative calculations of total isoflavonoid excretion from Table 24.1 in the first-mentioned study reveals that the isoflavonoid excretion (total > 9 μmol per day) before treatment in these subjects was similar to that observed in Japanese men and women,[58] so an additional effect could, in the present author's opinion, not be expected. However, other studies in male or ovariectomized monkeys reveal that it is mainly the isoflavones which have the antiarteriosclerotic effects, but soy protein also seems to contribute.[59,60] The relation of isoflavones to cardiovascular disease has recently been excellently reviewed by Clarkson.[61] He concludes that there is no definite experimental evidence to establish that the cardiovascular benefits of soy protein are accounted for by its isoflavones.

The possible protective effect on arteriosclerosis may have other mechanisms because we and others have observed that soy phytoestrogens increases the resistance of low-density liproprotein (LDL) against oxidation or reduces oxidized LDL.[62–64] Furthermore, isoflavone phytoestrogens consumed in soy decrease F2-isoprostane concentrations in plasma.[65] An interesting new line of research is studies on the role of phytoestrogen fatty acid esters as possible inhibitors of LDL oxidation.[66] Negative results with regard to protection of LDL against oxidation have, however, also been obtained.[67,68]

It has also been shown in experimental studies that isoflavones may have favorable effects on endothelial function,[69] but recently no effects on lipoprotein levels or endothelial function could be found in healthy postmenopausal women with evidence of endothelial dysfunction.[70] Soy isoflavone improves flow-mediated arterial dilation[61] of postmenopausal women. Thus, the field is exciting but quite controversial, like that with regard to the protection of coronary vascular disease using ERT,[71] and further studies are definitely needed. The cardiovascular and lipid effects have recently been discussed in several reviews[13,61,63,72–74] where additional information may be found.

ISOFLAVONES AND BREAST CANCER

Isoflavonoids occur particularly in soybean products that are regularly consumed in Asian countries such as Japan, China, Korea and Indonesia. These countries had, until recently, very low incidences of the most common cancers in the Western world, like breast, prostate and colon cancer, and the incidence of coronary heart disease was also low.[75] However, the incidence is steadily increasing due to changes in dietary habits and lifestyle. Many other types of beans, including peanuts, contain isoflavonoids, and in countries with high legume consumption the incidence of Western diseases is lower than in, for example, some north European countries with low intake of beans. However, it must be kept in mind that many studies indicated that soybean products may prevent cancer long before it was suggested that this could be due to their content of phytoestrogens. In these studies it was proposed that protease inhibitors, phytic acid or β-sitosterol could be the active component(s).[76,77] It is therefore very likely that many different compounds participate in disease prevention.

The role of phytoestrogens in breast cancer has recently been reviewed.[2] Publications dealing with the possible association between isoflavonoids or isoflavonoid-rich or lignan-containing diets and breast cancer risk in women are shown in a table published on the website (http://oncology.thelancet.com).[2] There is some evidence, although relatively modest, for a protective effect of a diet containing soybean products, but low consumption of lignan-rich food and fiber (which contains lignans) seems more consistently related to higher risk, even though controversial results exist.[78] In this regard, lignans and breast cancer risk will not be further discussed. In some studied populations soy consumption was very low and may not give an accurate picture of the situation. A large prospective study in Japan did not find any effect of soy consumption on breast cancer risk in Japanese women.[79] The reason for the many negative results with regard to soy consumption may be that dietary intake was studied in adult women, but the effect of a soy diet may be most significant prepubertally or during adolescence.[80,81]

Studying Asian immigrants in California and Hawaii it was found that when immigration occurred later in life, rates for breast cancer were substantially lower than when migration occurred earlier.[82] This and other studies[83,84] confirmed earlier observations on increased disease risks after immigration from Asia to the United States. Our observation that the urinary excretion of phytoestrogens of recent Oriental immigrants to Hawaii is very low within 6 months after immigration from Asia to Hawaii, similar to the levels found in American and Finnish omnivores, supports the view that phytoestrogens may be involved. These immigrants still consumed a very low-fat diet. The amounts of isoflavonoids excreted by the immigrants is roughly one-tenth of the amounts found in urine of Japanese women.[75] Many other studies in various populations and in vegetarians show that high excretion of phytoestrogens is associated with low breast cancer risk.[75] Chimpanzees in captivity are very resistant to breast cancer and excrete enormous amounts of isoflavonoids (but also lignans) in urine and the relative amounts of equol are very high.[85,86]

NEGATIVE EFFECTS OF PHYTOESTROGENS ON THE BREAST

There is evidence that high endogenous estrogen levels prenatally may increase breast cancer

risk in women,[87] and there is some experimental support in rats for the view that phytoestrogens may negatively affect breast cells during pregnancy.[88] However, in this study, parenteral administration of genistein was employed, which has a much stronger effect than after oral dosage because some phytoestrogens will circulate in the unconjugated form. Furthermore, equol is the main isoflavone metabolite in the rat and is much more estrogenic than daidzein from which it is derived. Both in newborn Japanese children and in their mothers at birth high levels of phytoestrogen are found,[89] implying that Asian women should have a higher breast cancer incidence, but it is, in fact, the opposite. The problem is controversial and complicated and has recently been well reviewed.[90] Very few human studies are available.

Isoflavone-rich soy protein isolate consumed by adult surgically postmenopausal macaques did not have any stimulatory effect on the mammary gland.[91] Chimpanzees in captivity are very resistant to experimental breast cancer and excrete enormous amounts of equol (and enterolactone) in their urine.[86] Recently, an approximately 14-day course of 60 g of soy protein containing about 45 mg of isoflavones per day was given to premenopausal patients with various breast diseases including cancer.[92] No differences in the thymidine labeling index, Ki67 labeling index, estrogen and progesterone receptor labeling indices, apoptotic and mitotic indices, and Bcl-2 mean optical density, but higher pS2 levels – an indication of an estrogenic effect – were found in the soy-treated subjects compared to controls when the menstrual cycle and age was controlled for. This does not exclude long-term effects. Long-term treatments will, however, also affect the endogenous estrogen[93] and SHBG levels,[94] thus reducing biological activity of the endogenous estrogens.

CONCLUSIONS

Treatment of menopausal symptoms, and prevention or treatment of osteoporosis and cardiovascular disease, with soy isoflavones or isoflavone supplements is less effective than ordinary HRT. It is unlikely that such therapy with normal dosage can cause breast cancer, but negative effects on the breast cannot yet be completely excluded, although they are most likely less than with ordinary HRT. There is no convincing evidence to indicate that soy intake or administration of isoflavones during adult life would protect a woman living in the Western hemisphere against breast cancer. However, there is evidence suggesting that life-time soy intake could be protective. To conclude, from the literature available, that these compounds have no better effect than placebo and may involve dangers seems to be an exaggeration.[26,95] Many results are controversial but some of the negative results seem to be due to poor experimental conditions and some may probably be explained when even more careful studies are carried out. Keeping the isoflavone dose between 20 and 100 mg/day in postmenopausal women is, according to present views, safe. Soy or isoflavones have beneficial effects on bone preservation, at least in the lumbar spine, in postmenopausal women, but compared to present commercially available drugs for prevention of osteoporosis they are less effective. The improvement of vascular compliance seems to be one beneficial effect of isoflavones in women, as well as the antioxidant activity and reduction of oxidated fatty acids. Favorable effects on cognitive function and memory have also been observed. There is, however, no doubt that more studies are needed taking into consideration the discussion above. Among other data, more information about the differences between endogenous estrogens and isoflavonoids with regard to their genomic effects is needed, because of their different binding to ERα and ERβ;[96] in addition, careful clinical studies with known possible interfering variables are also required. Because there will always be women who want to avoid synthetic estrogens it would be good to identify among these women those which may particularly benefit from phytoestrogens. Such groups may be those who are slim and/or on a low-fat diet, or with low estrogen levels or high equol. We should also consider a combination of low-dose synthetic estrogens with isoflavones.

REFERENCES

1. Adlercreutz H, Hämäläinen E, Gorbach S, Goldin B. Dietary phyto-oestrogens and the menopause in Japan. *Lancet* 1992; **339:** 1233.
2. Adlercreutz H. Phyto-oestrogens and cancer. *Lancet Oncol* 2002; **3:** 32–41.
3. Mazur W. Phytoestrogen content in foods. In (Adlercreutz H, ed) *Phytoestrogens.* (Baillière Tindall: London, 1998) 729–42.
4. Liggins J, Bluck LJC, Runswick S et al. Daidzein and genistein content of fruits and nuts. *J Nutr Biochem* 2000; **11:** 326–31.
5. Liggins J, Bluck LJC, Runswick S et al. Daidzein and genistein contents of vegetables. *Br J Nutr* 2000; **84:** 717–25.
6. Martini MC, Dancisak BB, Haggans CJ et al. Effects of soy intake on sex hormone metabolism in premenopausal women. *Nutr Cancer* 1999; **34:** 133–9.
7. Duncan AM, Merz-Demlow BE, Xu X et al. Premenopausal equol excretors show plasma hormone profiles associated with lowered risk of breast cancer. *Cancer Epidemiol Biomark Prev* 2000; **9:** 581–6.
8. Adlercreutz H, Markkanen H, Watanabe S. Plasma concentrations of phyto-oestrogens in Japanese men. *Lancet* 1993; **342:** 1209–10.
9. Morton M, Arisaka O, Miyake A, Evans B. Analysis of phyto-oestrogens by gas chromatography–mass spectrometry. *Environ Toxicol Pharmacol* 1999; **7:** 221–5.
10. Eden J. Phytoestrogens and the menopause. In: (Adlercreutz H, ed) *Phytoestrogens.* (Baillière Tindall: London, 1998) 581–7.
11. Messina M. Soy, soy phytoestrogens (isoflavones), and breast cancer. *Am J Clin Nutr* 1999; **70:** 574–5.
12. Vincent A, Fitzpatrick LA. Soy isoflavones: are they useful in menopause? *Mayo Clin Proc* 2000; **75:** 1174–84.
13. Glazier MG, Bowman MA, A review of the evidence for the use of phytoestrogens as a replacement for traditional estrogen replacement therapy. *Arch Intern Med* 2001; **161:** 1161–72.
14. Lock M. Contested meanings of the menopause. *Lancet* 1991; **337:** 1270–2.
15. Brzezinski A, Adlercreutz H, Shaoul R et al. Short-term effects of phytoestrogen-rich diet on post-menopausal women. *Menopause* 1997; **4:** 89–94.
16. Dalais FS, Rice GE, Wahlqvist ML et al. Effects of dietary phytoestrogens in postmenopausal women. *Climacteric* 1998; **1:** 124–9.
17. Quella SK, Loprinzi CL, Barton DL et al. Evaluation of soy phytoestrogens for the treat-

ment of hot flashes in breast cancer survivors: a North Central Cancer Treatment Group trial. *J Clin Oncol* 2000; **18**: 1068–74.

18. Somekawa Y, Chiguchi M, Ishibashi T, Aso T. Soy intake related to menopausal symptoms, serum lipids, and bone mineral density in post-menopausal Japanese women. *Obstet Gynecol* 2001; **97**: 109–15.

19. St Germain A, Peterson CT, Robinson JG, Alekel DL. Isoflavone-rich or isoflavone-poor soy protein does not reduce menopausal symptoms during 24 weeks of treatment. *Menopause* 2001; **8**: 17–26.

20. Washburn S, Burke GL, Morgan T, Anthony M. Effect of soy protein supplementation on serum lipoproteins, blood pressure, and menopausal symptoms in perimenopausal women. *Menopause* 1999; **6**: 7–13.

21. Albertazzi P, Pansini F, Bonaccorsi G et al. The effect of dietary soy supplementation on hot flushes. *Obstet Gynecol* 1998; **91**: 6–11.

22. Scambia G, Mango D, Signorile PG et al. Clinical effects of a standardized soy extract in post-menopausal women: a pilot study. *Menopause* 2000; **7**: 105–11.

23. Upmalis DH, Lobo R, Bradley L et al. Vasomotor symptom relief by soy isoflavone extract tablets in postmenopausal women: a multicenter, double-blind, randomized, placebo-controlled study. *Menopause* 2000; **7**: 236–42.

24. Baber RJ, Templeman C, Morton T et al. Randomized placebo-controlled trial of an isoflavone supplement and menopausal symptoms in women. *Climacteric* 1999; **2**: 85–92.

25. Han KK, Soares JM, Haidar MA et al. Benefits of soy isoflavone therapeutic regimen on meno-pausal symptoms. *Obstet Gynecol* 2002; **99**: 389–94.

26. Davis SR. Phytoestrogen therapy for menopausal symptoms? There's no good evidence that it's any better than placebo. *BMJ* 2001; **323**: 354–5.

27. Husband AJ. Phytoestrogens and menopause – published evidence supports a role for phyto-estrogens in menopause. *BMJ* 2002; **324**: 52.

28. Van Patten CL, Olivotto IA, Chambers GK et al. Effect of soy phytoestrogens on hot flushes in postmenopausal women with breast cancer: a randomized, controlled clinical trial. *J Clin Oncol* 2002; **20**: 1449–55.

29. Arai Y, Uehara M, Sato Y et al. Comparison of isoflavones among dietary intake, plasma con-centration and urinary excretion for accurate estimation of phytoestrogen intake. *J Epidemiol* 2000; **10**: 127–35.

30. Murkies AL, Lombard C, Strauss BJG et al.

31. Dietary flour supplementation decreases post-menopausal hot flushes: effect of soy and wheat. *Maturitas* 1995; **21**: 189–95.

31. Lephart ED, Adlercreutz H, Lund TD. Dietary soy phytoestrogen effects on brain structure and aromatase in Long-Evans rats. *Neuroreport* 2001; **12**: 3451–5.

32. Lund TD, West TW, Tian LY et al. Visual spatial memory is enhanced in female rats (but inhib-ited in males) by dietary soy phytoestrogens. *BMC Neurosci* 2001; **2**: 20.

33. Lephart ED, West TW, Weber KS et al. Neurobehavioral effects of dietary soy phyto-estrogens. *Neurotoxicol Teratol* 2002; **24**: 5–16.

34. Setchell KDR, Brown NM, Desai P et al. Bioavailability of pure isoflavones in healthy humans and analysis of commercial soy isoflavone supplements. *J Nutr* 2001; **131**: 1362S–1375S.

35. Nurmi T, Mazur W, Heinonen S et al. Isoflavone content of the soy based supplements. *J Pharmac Biomed Anal* 2002; **28**: 1–11.

36. Nagata C, Takatsuka N, Kawakami N, Shimizu H. Soy product intake and hot flashes in Japanese women: results from a community-based prospec-tive study. *Am J Epidemiol* 2001; **153**: 790–3.

37. File SE, Jarrett N, Fluck E et al. Eating soya improves human memory. *Psychopharmacology* 2001; **157**: 430–6.

38. Mayr U, Butsch A, Schneider S. Validation of two in vitro test systems for estrogenic activities with zearalenone, phytoestrogens and cereal extracts. *Toxicology* 1992; **74**: 135–49.

39. Markiewicz L, Garey J, Adlercreutz H, Gurpide E. In vitro bioassays of non-steroidal phytoestro-gens. *J Steroid Biochem Molec Biol* 1993; **45**: 399–405.

40. Kuiper GGJM, Lemmen JG, Carlsson B et al. Interaction of estrogenic chemicals and phyto-estrogens with estrogen receptor beta. *Endocrinology* 1998; **139**: 4252–63.

41. Anderson JJB, Garner SC. Phytoestrogens and bone, In: (Adlercreutz H, ed) *Phytoestrogens* (Baillière Tindall: London, 1998) 543–57.

42. Alekel DL, StGermain A, Pererson CT et al. Isoflavone-rich soy protein isolate attenuates bone loss in the lumbar spine of perimenopausal women. *Am J Clin Nutr* 2000; **72**: 844–52.

43. Horiuchi T, Onouchi T, Takahashi M et al. Effect of soy protein on bone metabolism in post-menopausal Japanese women. *Osteoporos Int* 2000; **11**: 721–4.

44. Atkinson C, Compston JE, Robins SP, Bingham SA. The effect of isoflavone phytoestrogens on bone: preliminary results from a large

randomised controlled trial. *Endocr Soc Ann Meet Program Abstr* 2000; **82:** 43.

45. Gao YH, Yamaguchi M. Anabolic effect of daidzein on cortical bone in tissue culture: comparison with genistein effect. *Molec Cell Biochem* 1999; **194:** 93–7.

46. Picherit C, Coxam V, Bennetau-Pelissero C et al. Daidzein is more efficient than genistein in preventing ovariectomy-induced bone loss in rats. *J Nutr* 2000; **130:** 1675–81.

47. Agnusdei D, Bufalino L. Efficacy of ipriflavone in established osteoporosis and long-term safety. *Calcif Tissue Int* 1997; **61:** S23–S27.

48. Alexandersen P, Toussaint A, Christiansen C et al. Ipriflavone in the treatment of postmenopausal osteoporosis – a randomized controlled trial. *JAMA* 2001; **285:** 1482–88.

49. Kardinaal AF, Morton MS, Bruggemann-Rotgans IE, van Beresteijn EC. Phyto-oestrogen excretion and rate of bone loss in postmenopausal women. *Eur J Clin Nutr* 1998; **52:** 850–5.

50. Kim MK, Chung BC, Yu VY et al. Relationships of urinary phyto-oestrogen excretion to BMD in postmenopausal women. *Clin Endocr* 2002; **56:** 321–8.

51. Adlercreutz H, Fotsis T, Heikkinen R et al. Excretion of the lignans enterolactone and enterodiol and of equol in omnivorous and vegetarian women and in women with breast cancer. *Lancet* 1982; **2:** 1295–9.

52. Adlercreutz H, Fotsis T, Bannwart C et al. Determination of urinary lignans and phytoestrogen metabolites, potential antiestrogens and anticarcinogens, in urine of women on various habitual diets. *J Steroid Biochem* 1986; **25:** 791–7.

53. Anderson JW, Johnstone BM, Cooknewell ME. Meta-analysis of the effects of soy protein intake on serum lipids. *N Engl J Med* 1995; **333:** 276–82.

54. Merz-Demlow BE, Duncan AM, Wangen KE et al. Soy isoflavones improve plasma lipids in normocholesterolemic, premenopausal women. *Am J Clin Nutr* 2000; **71:** 1462–9.

55. Greaves KA, Wilson MD, Rudel LL et al. Consumption of soy protein reduces cholesterol absorption compared to casein protein alone or supplemented with an isoflavone extract or conjugated equine estrogen in ovariectomized cynomolgus monkeys. *J Nutr* 2000; **130:** 820–6.

56. Howes JB, Sullivan D, Lai N et al. The effects of dietary supplementation with isoflavones from red clover on the lipoprotein profiles of post menopausal women with mild to moderate hypercholesterolaemia. *Atherosclerosis* 2000; **152:** 143–7.

57. Dewell A, Hollenbeck CB, Bruce B. The effects of

soy-derived phytoestrogens on serum lipids and lipoproteins in moderately hypercholesterolemic postmenopausal women. *J Clin Endocr Metab* 2002; **87:** 118–21.

58. Adlercreutz H, Honjo H, Higashi A et al. Urinary excretion of lignans and isoflavonoid phytoestrogens in Japanese men and women consuming traditional Japanese diet. *Am J Clin Nutr* 1991; **54:** 1093–100.

59. Anthony MS, Clarkson TB, Bullock BC, Wagner JD. Soy protein versus soy phytoestrogens in the prevention of diet-induced coronary artery atherosclerosis of male cynomolgus monkeys. *Arterioscler Thromb Vasc Biol* 1997; **17:** 2524–31.

60. Anthony MS, Clarkson TB, Williams JK. Effects of soy isoflavones on atherosclerosis: potential mechanisms. *Am J Clin Nutr* 1998; **68:** 1390S–1393S.

61. Clarkson TB. Soy, soy phytoestrogens and cardiovascular disease. *J Nutr* 2002; **132:** 566S–569S.

62. Tikkanen MJ, Wahala K, Ojala S et al. Effect of soybean phytoestrogen intake on low density lipoprotein oxidation resistance. *Proc Natl Acad Sci USA* 1998; **95:** 3106–10.

63. Tikkanen MJ, Adlercreutz H. Dietary soy-derived isoflavone phytoestrogens could they have a role in coronary heart disease prevention? *Biochem Pharmacol* 2000; **60:** 1–5.

64. Jenkins DJA, Kendall CWC, Vidgen E et al. Effect of soy-based breakfast cereal on blood lipids and oxidized low-density lipoprotein. *Metabolism* 2000; **49:** 1496–500.

65. Wiseman H, O'Reilly JD, Adlercreutz H et al. Isoflavone phytoestrogens consumed in soy decrease F-2-isoprostane concentrations and increase resistance of low-density lipoprotein to oxidation in humans. *Am J Clin Nutr* 2000; **72:** 395–400.

66. Helisten H, Hockerstedt A, Wahala K et al. Accumulation of high-density lipoprotein-derived estradiol-17 beta fatty acid esters in low-density lipoprotein particles. *J Clin Endocr Metab* 2001; **86:** 1294–300.

67. Hodgson JM, Puddey IB, Croft KD et al. Isoflavonoids do not inhibit in vivo lipid peroxidation in subjects with high-normal blood pressure. *Atherosclerosis* 1999; **145:** 167–72.

68. Samman S, Wall PML, Chan GSM et al. The effect of supplementation with isoflavones on plasma lipids and oxidisability of low density lipoprotein in premenopausal women. *Atherosclerosis* 1999; **147:** 277–83.

69. Squadrito F, Altavilla D, Squadrito G et al.

Genistein supplementation and estrogen replacement therapy improve endothelial dysfunction induced by ovariectomy in rats. *Cardiovasc Res* 2000; **45**: 454–62.

70. Simons LA, von Königsmark M, Simons J, Celermajer DS. Phytoestrogens do not influence lipoprotein levels or endothelial function in healthy postmenopausal women. *Am J Cardiol* 2000; **85**: 1297–301.

71. Manson JE, Martin KA. Clinical practice. Postmenopausal hormone-replacement therapy. *N Engl J Med* 2001; **345**: 34–40.

72. Humfrey CD. Phytoestrogens and human health effects: weighing up the current evidence. *Nat Toxins* 1998; **6**: 51–9.

73. Lissin LW, Cooke JP. Phytoestrogens and cardiovascular health. *J Am Coll Cardiol* 2000; **35**: 1403–10.

74. Setchell KDR, Soy isoflavones – benefits and risks from nature's selective estrogen receptor modulators (SERMs). *J Am Coll Nutr* 2001; **20**: 354S–362S.

75. Adlercreutz H. Epidemiology of phytoestrogens, In: (Adlercreutz H, ed) *Phytoestrogens*. (Baillière Tindall: London, 1998) 605–24.

76. Kennedy AR. The evidence for soybean products as cancer preventive agents. *J Nutr* 1995; **125**: S733–S743.

77. Messina MJ, Persky V, Setchell KDR, Barnes S. Soy intake and cancer risk – a review of the in vitro and in vivo data. *Nutr Cancer* 1994; **21**: 113–31.

78. den Tonkelaar I, Keinan-Boker L, Van't Veer P et al. Urinary phyto-oestrogens and breast cancer risk in a Western population. *Cancer Epidem Biomarker Prev* 2001; **10**: 223–8.

79. Key TJ, Sharp GB, Appleby PN et al. Soya foods and breast cancer risk: a prospective study in Hiroshima and Nagasaki, Japan. *Br J Cancer* 1999; **81**: 1248–56.

80. Lamartiniere CA. Protection against breast cancer with genistein: a component of soy. *Am J Clin Nutr* 2000; **71**: 1705S–1707S.

81. Shu XO, Jin F, Dai Q et al. Soyfood intake during adolescence and subsequent risk of breast cancer among Chinese women. *Cancer Epidem Biomarker Prev* 2001; **10**: 483–8.

82. Ziegler RG, Hoover RN, Pike MC et al. Migration patterns and breast cancer risk in Asian-American women. *J Nat Cancer Inst* 1993; **85**: 1819–27.

83. Stanford JL, Herrinton LJ, Schwartz SM, Weiss NS. Breast cancer incidence in Asian migrants to the United States and their descendants. *Epidemiology* 1995; **6**: 181–3.

84. Tominaga S, Kuroishi T. Epidemiology of breast cancer in Japan. *Cancer Lett* 1995; **90**: 75–9.

85. Adlercreutz H, Musey PI, Fotsis T et al. Identification of lignans and phytoestrogens in urine of chimpanzes. *Clin Chim Acta* 1986; **158**: 147–54.

86. Musey PI, Adlercreutz H, Gould KG et al. Effect of diet on lignans and isoflavonoid phytoestrogens in chimpanzees. *Life Sci* 1995; **57**: 655–64.

87. Ekbom A, Trichopoulos D, Adami HO et al. Evidence of prenatal influences on breast cancer risk. *Lancet* 1992; **340**: 1015–18.

88. Hilakivi-Clarke L, Cho E, Onojafe I et al. Maternal exposure to genistein during pregnancy increases carcinogen-induced mammary tumorigenesis in female rat offspring. *Oncol Rep* 1999; **6**: 1089–95.

89. Adlercreutz H, Yamada T, Wahala K, Watanabe S. Maternal and neonatal phytoestrogens in Japanese women during birth. *Am J Obstet Gynecol* 1999; **180**: 737–43.

90. Bouker KB, Hilakivi-Clarke L. Genistein: does it prevent or promote breast cancer? *Environ Health Perspect* 2000; **108**: 701–8.

91. Foth D, Cline JM. Effects of mammalian and plant estrogens on mammary glands and uteri of macaques. *Am J Clin Nutr* 1998; **68**: 1413S–1417S.

92. Hargreaves DF, Potten CS, Harding C et al. Two-week dietary soy supplementation has an estrogenic effect on normal premenopausal breast. *J Clin Endocr Metab* 1999; **84**: 4017–24.

93. Nagata C, Kabuto M, Kurisu Y, Shimizu H. Decreased serum estradiol concentration associated with high dietary intake of soy products in premenopausal Japanese women. *Nutr Cancer* 1997; **29**: 228–33.

94. Adlercreutz H. Human health and phytoestrogens. In: (Korach KS, ed) *Reproductive and Developmental Toxicology*. (Marcel Dekker, Inc: New York, (1998) 299–371.

95. Sirtori CR. Dubious benefits and potential risk of soy phyto-oestrogens. *Lancet* 2000; **355**: 849.

96. Pettersson K, Gustafsson JA. Role of estrogen receptor beta in estrogen action. *Ann Rev Physiol* 2001; **63**: 165–92.

97. Wilcox G, Wahlqvist ML, Burtger HG, Medley G. Oestrogenic effects of plant foods in postmenopausal women. *BMJ* 1990; **301**: 905–6.

98. Baird DD, Umbach DM, Lansdell CL et al. Dietary intervention study to assess estrogenicity of dietary soy among postmenopausal women. *J Clin Endocr Metab* 1995; **80**: 1685–90.

25

Possible risks of hormone replacement therapy (HRT): venous thromboembolism (VTE)

I Greer

What is the risk of VTE with HRT? • **How does HRT increase the risk of VTE?** • **How do we manage the risk of VTE with HRT?** • **References**

WHAT IS THE RISK OF VTE WITH HRT?

Estrogen-containing oral contraceptive pills have long been recognized to carry an excess risk of VTE.[1,2] HRT, however, was not,[3–6] until recently, considered to be a risk factor for VTE. However, many of the initial studies assessing the risk had limited statistical power or methodological limitations. Recently, a series of case control studies have shown a modest increase in the relative risk of VTE in women using estrogen-containing HRT (Table 25.1). A North American population-based nested case control study reported that women with idiopathic VTE had a relative risk of 3.6 [95% confidence interval (CI) 1.6–7.8] for VTE with current use of estrogen compared to non-users.[7] The absolute risk was estimated at 9 per 100,000 women per year in non-users compared to 32 per 100,000 women per year in users. A UK hospital-based case control study[8] assessed 45–64 year old women with idiopathic VTE. This study found an odds ratio for current HRT use, compared to non-users, of 3.5 (95% CI

1.8–7.0). Furthermore, the risk appeared to be highest among short-term current users. The estimate of absolute risk was 11 per 100,000 women per year for non-users and 27 per 100,000 women per year for current users. The Nurses Health Cohort study estimated the adjusted relative risk of primary pulmonary embolism to be 2.1 (95% CI 1.2–3.8) for current HRT users.[9] The General Practice Research Database in the UK was used to conduct a population-based case control study and found an adjusted odds ratio of VTE for current users of 2.1 (95% CI 1.4–3.2) relative to non-users.[10] In this study, the increase in risk was restricted to the first year of use with an odds ratio of 4.6 (2.5–8.4) during the first 6 months. An Italian case control study reported that there was a 2.3 times (95% CI 1.0–5.3) increase in risk with the effect restricted to the first year of use.[11] The Heart and Estrogen/progestin Replacement Study (HERS), a large randomized controlled trial on the secondary prevention of coronary artery disease using HRT (containing equine

Table 25.1 Epidemiologic studies showing the risk of VTE with HRT		
Authors (ref)	**Study design**	**Relative risk**
Jick et al[7]	Population-based nested case control study in USA	2.1–6.9 dependant on estrogen dose for current users for idiopathic VTE
Daly et al[8]	Hospital-based case control study	3.5 (95% CI 1.8–7.0) for idiopathic VTE in current HRT users
Grodstein et al[9]	Questionnaire study on Nurses Health Cohort in USA	2.1 (95% CI 1.2–3.8) for idiopathic primary PTE in current HRT users
Gutthann et al[10]	Population-based nested case control in (UK GP research Database)	2.1 (95% CI 1.4–3.2) for current HRT users for idiopathic VTE
Varas-Lorenzo et al[11]	Italian case control study	2.3 (95% CI) for current HRT users for idiopathic VTE
Grady et al (HERS)[12]	Randomized, double-blind, placebo-controlled trial of HRT for secondary prevention of coronary heart disease	VTE: 2.7 (95% CI 1.4–5.0) DVT: 2.8 (95% CI 1.3–6.0) PTE: 2.8 (95% CI 0.9–8.7) for current HRT users for VTE
Hoibraaten et al[13]	Population-based case control study	3.54 (95% CI 1.54–8.2) in first 12 months of HRT use but 1.22 (95% CI 0.76–1.94) overall

CI, Confidence interval: DVT, deep vein thrombosis; HRT, hormone replacement therapy; PTE, pulmonary thromboembolism; VTE, venous thromboembolism.

conjugated estrogens and medroxyprogesterone acetate), reported an increase in risk of coronary events in women in the first 4 months of use followed by a reduction in risk over the last 2 years of this trial, which was conducted over 4.1 years. An increase in relative risk of VTE of 2.7 (95% CI 1.4–5.5.1) was also reported.[12] A Scandinavian population-based case control study reported that HRT preparations containing only estradiol had no overall association with VTE with an adjusted odds ratio of 1.22 (95% CI 0.76–1.94).[13] However, stratification by duration of exposure found that there was a significantly increased risk in the first year (odds ratio 3.54; 95% CI 1.54–8.2) reducing after the first year of use (odds ratio 0.66; 95% CI 0.39–1.10). This study differed from the others in several respects. It studied only estradiol-containing HRT and, in contrast with other studies that had excluded cases with presumed risk factors such as surgery, previous VTE and bed rest. It did not select the women except for excluding cancer-related VTE. While this study differed from the others with regard to the overall risk of VTE, it was consistent with regard to an excess risk occurring in the first year of use (Table 25.2).

Thus, the evidence consistently shows an

Table 25.2   VTE with duration of use of HRT over 1 year

Authors (ref)	Duration of use (months)	Relative risk	95% Confidence interval
Jick et al[7]	<12	6.7	1.5–30.8
	12–60	2.8	0.6–11.7
Daly et al[8]	<12	6.7	2.1–21.3
	13–24	4.4	1.6–11.9
	25–60	1.9	0.5–7.8
	>60	2.1	0.8–6.1
Gutthann et al[10]	<6	4.6	2.5–8.4
	7–12	3.0	1.4–6.5
	>12	1.1	0.6–2.1
Hoibraaten et al[13]	<12	3.5	1.5–8.2
	>12	0.7	0.4–1.1

increased relative risk of VTE, although the absolute risk, particularly in the absence of other risk factors, is low. For example, in the study Jick et al,[7] the absolute risk was estimated at 9 per 100,000 women per year in non-users, compared to 32 per 100,000 women per year in users. The absolute risk was much higher in the HERS study (current users 6.2 versus non-users 2.3 per 1000 women-years), but the population was at much greater risk of VTE. The dose of estrogen may also be a factor, as Grodstein et al[9] reported that the relative risk of VTE increased from 3.3 (95% CI 1.4–7.8) with 0.625 mg 2 estrogen to 6.9 (95% CI 1.5–33.0) with 1.25 mg estrogen. Similar data were reported by Daly et al.[8] Furthermore, transdermal therapy may carry a lower risk, although data are very limited. For example, Daly et al[8] reported a relative risk of 4.6 (95% CI 2.1–10.1) with oral therapy compared to 2.0 (95% CI 0.5–7.6) for transdermal. Epidemiologic studies do have limitations such as diagnostic suspicion bias or patient selection bias, possibly due to the established association between the Pill and VTE, restricting prescription of HRT in women with thrombotic risk fac-tors. However, the consistency of the data appear to indicate that this is a real increase in risk.

HOW DOES HRT INCREASE THE RISK OF VTE?

The menopause provokes several changes in hemostasis such as increased Factor VII, Factor VIII and fibrinogen, factors that are established risk factors for vascular disease, and an increase in antithrombin and protein C.[14,15] Oral HRT is associated with reduced plasma levels of fibrinogen, Factor VII and von Willebrand's Factor antithrombin, but fibrinolysis is enhanced.[16–21] Interestingly, there is an established association between resistance to activated protein C (APC) and venous thrombosis, and HRT is known to provoke an increase in resistance to activated protein C.[20,21] These effects are associated with increased thrombin generation.[21] Some of these hemostatic effects appear beneficial while others appear detrimental in terms of VTE risk. Inflammation is also a recognized vascular risk factor and plasma C-reactive protein (CRP) levels (an inflammatory marker produced by the liver) are increased with estrogen-containing HRT.[22,23] Thus, resistance to activated protein C and increased inflammation may be potential mechanisms underlying the association between HRT and VTE.

Oral preparations undergo first-pass hepatic metabolism and, therefore, have a greater effect on coagulation factors produced by the liver than do transdermal preparations, which avoid the first-pass effect. A large cross-sectional study in women aged 40–59 years found that oral HRT, but not transdermal, was associated with increased plasma levels of Factor IX, APC resistance and CRP, and with reduced levels of tissue plasminogen activator and plasminogen activator inhibitor.[23]

The risk of VTE increases with age.[7,8,24,25] The incidence of VTE in postmenopausal women is around double that of premenopausal women, but the risk of VTE is higher in the first year of HRT exposure. Thus, the interaction of age and HRT cannot be responsible for the increased risk of VTE, but it does raise the possibility of HRT unmasking heritable or acquired thrombophilias. Heritable thrombophilias, when considered together, have an underlying prevalence of between 15 and 20% in Western European populations (Table 25.3), and additional risk factors are usually required for a clinical event to occur. Antithrombin, protein-C

and protein-S deficiencies, Factor V Leiden and prothrombin 20210A are known to cause particular problems in pregnancy,[26,27] where physiologic hyperestrogenism occurs along with procoagulant alterations in hemostatic and fibrinolytic systems. Hyperhomocysteinemia is a risk factor for venous and arterial thrombosis. It is frequently the result of a combination of genotype [homozygotes for the so-called thermolabile (C677T) variant of methylene tetrohydrofolate reductase, which is present in over 10% of European populations who are thus at risk] and acquired factors, namely, dietary deficiency in B vitamins. As estrogen-containing HRT reduces serum homocysteine, this is unlikely to explain the excess risk of VTE on HRT.[28]

Lowe et al,[30] in a case control study using women from the study by Daly et al,[8] determined whether a thrombophilic phenotype was associated with the risk of clinical VTE when combined with HRT. VTE was significantly associated with HRT use, APC resistance, low antithrombin and high Factor IX. Overall, this study found that regardless of the underlying prothrombotic tendency, HRT resulted in around a threefold increase in risk. When multiple risk factors are present, such as HRT and one or more prothrombotic states, there is substantial increase in risk with an estimated odds

Table 25.3   **Prevalences of heritable thrombophilia in Western European populations**

Heritable thrombophilia	Underlying prevalence in the general population (%)	Unselected consecutive patients with first VTE exhibiting the thrombophilia (%)
Antithrombin deficiency	0.02	1
Protein-C deficiency	0.3	3
Protein-S deficiency	Unknown	1
Factor V Leiden	3–15	20
Factor II 20210A	2–3	6

ratio of 153 (95% CI 23.5–1001) for a woman on HRT with increased Factor IX, APC resistance and low antithrombin.[30] Thus, multiple acquired and/or inherited risk factors, including use of HRT, are necessary for a clinical VTE to occur, and a combination of a genetic susceptibility and physiologic, pathologic or pharmacologic factors such as pregnancy, surgery and the Pill or HRT is likely to be important in the clinical expression of thrombophilias.[31] Risk factors, other than thrombophilia – such as age, obesity, varicose veins, previous VTE, deep venous insufficiency, immobility, trauma or surgery, malignancy, cardiac failure, paralysis of lower limbs, infection, inflammatory bowel disease and nephrotic syndrome – must also be considered.[32] HRT should now be added to the list of established risk factors for VTE. Varas-Lorenzo et al[11] looked at the relative risk of various risk factors for VTE and found that obesity and varicose veins carried a greater risk than HRT (Table 25.4), so putting the relative risk in context. Nonetheless, potentially large interactions between risk factors can occur. A randomized double-blind placebo-controlled trial of HRT (2 mg estradiol plus 1 mg norethisterone) in 140 women with a previous confirmed VTE found that the incidence of VTE was 10.7% in the HRT group and 2.3% in the placebo group within 262 days of starting therapy.[33] The groups were balanced for additional risk factors including underlying thrombophilia.[33]

HOW DO WE MANAGE THE RISK OF VTE WITH HRT?

There is insufficient evidence to support universal screening for thrombophilia prior to starting or continuing HRT in the woman with no personal history of VTE and no family history of thrombophilia. We have limited information on the natural history of thrombophilia in asymptomatic kindred and the absolute risk of VTE with HRT is usually low. In general terms, it may be prudent to discuss the small risk of VTE with the woman, but it should be set in the context of her particular case.

It is important to assess for the presence of other risk factors for venous thrombosis,[32–34] specifically a personal history of VTE or a history of VTE in a first- or second-degree relative. Screening for thrombophilia should be offered if a woman has such a personal or family history of VTE, and in women over 50 years of age with a recent VTE, consideration should be given to the possibility of underlying malignancy or connective tissue disease. In the presence of multiple risk factors for VTE, HRT, which is an additional risk factor, should probably be avoided, but the woman's overall situation should be taken into account.[35] In particular, where the woman has had a previous VTE, regardless of whether she has a known thrombophilia, oral HRT should usually be avoided because of the relatively high risk of recurrence. If HRT is considered necessary for such a patient, transdermal therapy may be best as it has less effect on the hemostatic system than oral HRT. She should be made aware of the risk of recurrent VTE. Strategies such as anticoagulant 'cover' can be considered while HRT is required, but the risk of hemorrhage associated with anticoagulant therapy must be taken into account. Women on long-term anticoagulation because of a thrombotic problem need not avoid HRT and, again, transdermal

Table 25.4 Examples of odds ratios for VTE with various risk factors (from Varas-Lorenzo et al[11])

Risk factor	Adjusted odds ratio
Varicose veins	6.9
Obesity	4.6
Osteoarthritis	2.4
Age (65–80 versus 45–64 years)	2.3
HRT (current use)	2.3
Diabetes	1.9

HRT, Hormone replacement therapy.

therapy may be best. These situations merit specialist advice from clinicians with expertise in the management of thrombophilia.

Women with a thrombophilia picked up through screening because of a family history of VTE require individual assessment. HRT should be avoided in high-risk situations such as antithrombin deficiency and with combinations of heritable or acquired thrombophilic defects, e.g. Factor V Leiden homozygotes or women with Factor V Leiden combined with prothrombin 20210A or protein-C deficiency. For asymptomatic carriers of thrombophilia, such as Factor V Leiden heterozygotes or prothrombin 20210A heterozygotes with no other risk factors for VTE, HRT could be considered, but it is important to recognize that these women will have a several-fold increase in relative risk of VTE. These women can present difficult management problems and should, therefore, be referred to a clinician with special expertise in thrombophilia.

Some clinicians have considered HRT a risk factor for postoperative VTE, although there are no data to support this. Nonetheless, in view of the data linking VTE and HRT, it seems reasonable to consider HRT a risk factor for postoperative VTE, just as we do with established risk factors such as obesity, varicose veins and immobility when assessing patients preoperatively. This risk from HRT alone is likely to be small and virtually all women on HRT will meet the criteria for perioperative thromboprophylaxis as set out in guideline documents.[32,34] The practice of routinely stopping HRT prior to surgery is not evidence based and provided appropriate thromboprophylaxis, such as low-dose or low-molecular-weight heparin with or without thromboembolic deterrent stockings are used,[32,34] HRT may be continued.

REFERENCES

1. Carter C. The pill and thrombosis: epidemiological considerations. In: (Greer IA, ed.) *Thromboembolic Disease in Obstetrics and Gynaecology. Baillière's Clin Obstet Gynaecol* 1997; **11:** 565–86.

2. Spitzer WO, Lewis MA, Heinemann LAJ et al. Third generation oral contraceptives and risk of venous thromboembolic disorder: an international case control study. *BMJ* 1996; **312:** 83–8.

3. Carter C. Pathogenesis of thrombosis. In: (Greer IA, Turpie AGG, Forbes CD, (eds.) *Haemostasis and Thrombosis in Obstetrics and Gynaecology.* (Chapman & Hall: London, 1992) 229–56.

4. Devor M, Barrett-Connor E, Renvall M et al. Estrogen replacement therapy and the risk of venous thrombosis. *Am J Med* 1992; **92:** 275–84.

5. Pettiti DB, Wingerd J, Pellegrin F, Ramcharan S. Risk of vascular disease in women. *JAMA* 1979; **242:** 1150–4.

6. Nachtigall LE, Nachtigall RH, Nachtigall RD, Beckman EM. Estrogen replacement therapy II A prospective study in the relationship to carcinoma and cardiovascular and metabolic problems. *Obstet Gynecol* 1979; **54:** 74–79.

7. Jick H, Derby LE, Myers, MW et al. Risk of hospital admission for idiopathic venous thromboembolism among users of postmenopausal oestrogens. *Lancet* 1996; **348:** 981–93.

8. Daly E, Vessey MP, Hawkins MM et al. Case control study of venous thromboembolism risk in users of hormone replacement therapy. *Lancet* 1996; **348:** 977–80.

9. Grodstein F, Stampfer MJ, Goldhaber SZ et al. Prospective study of exogenous hormones and risk of pulmonary embolism in women. *Lancet* 1996; **348:** 983–7.

10. Gutthann SP, Garcia Rodrigues LA, Castallsague J, Oliart AD. Hormone replacement therapy and risk of venous thromboembolism: population based case control study. *BMJ* 1997; **314:** 796–800.

11. Varas-Lorenzo C, Garcia-Rodriguez LA, Cattaruzzi C et al. Hormone replacement therapy and the risk of hospitalization for venous thromboembolism: a population based study. *Am J Epidemiol* 1998; **147:** 387–90.

12. Grady D, Wenger NK, Herrington D et al. Postmenopausal hormone therapy increases risk for venous thromboembolic disease. The heart and estrogen/progestin replacement study. *Ann Intern Med* 2000; **132:** 689–96.

13. Hoibraaten E, Abdelnoor M, Sandset PM. Hormone replacement therapy with estradiol and risk of venous thromboembolism. *Thromb Haemostas* 1999; **82:** 1218–21.

14. Meade TW, Dyer S, Howarth DJ et al. Antithrombin III and procoagulant activity: sex differences and effects of the menopause. *Br J Haematol* 1994; **74:** 77–81.

15. Lowe GDO, Rumley A, Woodward M et al. Epidemiology of coagulation factors, inhibitors

and activation markers: the third Glasgow MONICA Survey 1 illustrative reference ranges by age, sex and hormone use. *Br J Haematol* 1997; **97:** 775–784.

16. Lindoff C, Peterson F, Lecander I et al. Transdermal oestrogen replacement therapy: beneficial effects on haemostatic risk factors for cardiovascular disease. *Maturitas* 1996; **24:** 43–50.

17. The Writing Group for the Oestradiol Clotting Study. Effects on haemostasis of hormone replacement therapy with transdermal oestradiol and oral sequential medroxyprogesterone acetate: a one-year double-blind placebo-controlled study. *Thromb Haemostas* 1996; **75:** 476–80.

18. Lip GYH, Blann AD, Jones AE, Beevers DG. Effects of hormone replacement therapy on hemostatic factors, lipid factors and endothelial function in women undergoing surgical menopause: implications for prevention of atherosclerosis. *Am Heart J* 1997; **134:** 764–71.

19. Koh KK, Mincemoyer R, Bui MN et al. Effects of hormone-replacement therapy on fibrinolysis in postmenopausal women. *N Engl J Med* 1997; **336:** 683–90.

20. Lowe GDO, Rumley A, Woodward M et al. Activated protein C resistance and the FV:R506Q mutation in a random population sample associations with cardiovascular risk factors and coagulation variables. *Thromb Haemostas* 1999; **81:** 918–24.

21. Douketis JD, Gordon M, Johnston M et al. The effects of hormone replacement therapy on thrombin generation, fibrinolysis inhibition, and resistance to activated protein C: prospective cohort and review of the literature. *Thromb Res* 2000; **99:** 25–34.

22. Ridker P, Hennekens C, Rifai N et al. Hormone replacement therapy and increased plasma concentration of C-reactive protein. *Circulation* 1999; **100:** 713–16.

23. Lowe GDO, Upton MN, Rumley A et al. Different effects of oral and transdermal hormone replacement therapies on factor IX, APC resistance, t-PA, PAI and C-reactive protein. A cross-sectional population survey. *Thromb Haemostas* 2001; **86:** 550–6.

24. Jick H, Jick SS, Gurewich V et al. Risk of idio-pathic cardiovascular death and nonfatal venous thromboembolism in women using oral contraceptives with differing prostagen components. *Lancet* 1995; **346:** 1589–93.

25. PEPI (The Postmenopausal Estrogen/Progestin Interventions Trial) Writing Group. Effects of estrogen/progestin regimens on heart disease risk factors in postmenopausal women. *JAMA* 1995; **273:** 199–208.

26. Walker ID. Congenital thrombophilia. In: (Greer IA, ed) *Thromboembolic Disease in Obstetrics and Gynaecology. Ballière's Clin Obstet Gynaecol* 1997; **11:** 431–45.

27. Greer IA. Thrombosis in pregnancy: maternal and fetal issues. *Lancet* 1999; **353:** 1258–65.

28. Van der Mooren MJ, Vouters GAJ, Blom JH et al. Hormone replacement therapy may reduce high serum homocysteine in postmenopausal women. *Eur J Clin Invest* 1994; **24:** 733–6.

29. Hellgren M, Svensson PJ, Dahlback B. Resistance to activated protein C as a basis for venous thromboembolism associated with pregnancy and oral contraception. *Am J Obstet Gynecol* 1995; **173:** 210–13.

30. Lowe GDO, Woodward M, Vessey M et al. Thrombotic variables and risk of idiopathic venous thromboembolism in women aged 45–64 years. *Thromb Haemostas* 2000; **83:** 530–5.

31. Rosendaal F. Venous thrombosis: a multicausal disease. *Lancet* 1999; **353:** 1167–73.

32. Lowe GDO, Greer IA, Cooke TG et al. Thromboembolic Risk Factors (THRIFT) Consensus Group. Risk of and prophylaxis for venous thromboembolism in hospital patients. *BMJ* 1992; **305:** 567–74.

33. Hoibraaten E, Qvigstad E, Arnesen H et al. Increased risk of recurrent venous thromboembolism during hormone replacement therapy. *Thromb Haemostas* 2000; **84:** 961–967.

34. Greer IA, Walker ID. Hormone replacement therapy and venous thromboembolism. *Climacteric* 1999; **2:** 1–8.

35. Whitehead M, Godfree V. Venous thromboembolism and hormone replacement therapy. In: (Greer IA, ed) *Thromboembolic Disease in Obstetrics and Gynaecology. Ballière's Clin Obst Gynaecol* 1997; **11:** 587–99.

26

Gallbladder, liver, pancreas

H Kuhl

Hepatic metabolism   •   Pancreas   •   References

HEPATIC METABOLISM

Like many steroids, natural estrogens are metabolized by hepatic cytochrome P-450-dependent enzymes which are responsible for hydroxylation, oxidation and reduction processes. As this enzyme family is also involved in the metabolism of many endogenous and exogenous compounds, the clearance of estrogens can be influenced by medications and many xenobiotics ingested advertently and inadvertently by diet, smoking, alcohol, etc. Estrogen metabolism can be stimulated by smoking, and increased or inhibited by many drugs. Conversely, estrogens can also modify metabolism, clearance and serum levels of various medications and other xenobiotics. The chronic enhancement of estrogen inactivation by, for example, smoking, may have consequences for lipid and bone metabolism and endometrial proliferation.

There a numerous isoenzymes of the cytochrome P-450 enzyme family which are localized in close proximity on microsomal membranes. Hepatic cytochrome P-450 enzymes undergo a rapid turnover with half-lives between 12 and 24 hours. They consist of two components, apoprotein and haem, which are regulated separately by induction and feedback mechanisms. The apoprotein couples with one haem molecule which is freely available (the so-called haem pool) within the hepatocytes, becoming an active cytochrome P-450 enzyme. A decrease in free haem causes a rise in the δ-aminolevulin acid synthesis and the resulting protoporphyrin is transferred to haem after uptake of an iron atom. Many drugs including natural and synthetic sex steroids can act as enzyme inducers. The rate-limiting step in the haem synthesis is the δ-aminolevulinic acid synthetase, and among the potent inducers of cytochrome P-450 mono-oxygenase are barbiturates, carbamazepin, diazepam and rifampicin, but also some synthetic progestogens like norethisterone and medroxyprogesterone acetate, but not chlormadinone acetate.

There are many natural and synthetic compounds which can inhibit cytochrome P-450 irreversibly. Mono-oxygenases can oxidatively activate the ethinyl group into a very reactive intermediate which immediately reacts with a nitrogen atom of haem. This causes release of the iron and an irreversible inactivation of the haem to an alkylated porphyrin. As in this way the enzyme contributes to its own destruction, the process is called suicide-inhibition or mechanism-based inactivation of the enzyme. These mechanisms may explain the higher impact on the liver of steroids containing an ethinyl group as compared to natural steroid hormones.

After oral administration, the absorbed estrogen and its metabolites and conjugates are transferred to the liver via the portal vein. During this first liver passage, the estrogens and estrogen metabolites may reach high concentrations in the portal circulation which are four- to five-fold higher than the peripheral serum levels. Consequently, oral treatment with estrogens is associated with a pronounced influence on hepatic metabolism, which includes not only lipid and lipoprotein synthesis, uptake, degradation and excretion in the bile, but also carbohydrate metabolism and various enzymes and other proteins including hemostasis factors. These metabolic changes can both be regarded as adverse and beneficial. As compared to parenteral administration, estrogens taken orally cause more pronounced changes in many hepatic serum parameters which are dependent on the type and dose of the estrogen (Table 26.1). The most potent estrogen is ethinylestradiol which is degraded at a much lower rate than estradiol. The weaker effectiveness of estriol is due to the lower binding affinity to the estrogen receptor, while estrone sulfate becomes active after conversion to estradiol via estrone. The higher hepatic effect of conjugated estrogens is partly due to the effect of equilin which is converted to the active estrogen 17β-dihydroequilin.

The serum levels of various proteins synthesized in the liver, e.g. sex hormone-binding globulin (SHBG), corticosteroid-binding globulin (CBG), thyroxine-binding globulin (TBG), and angiotensinogen, increase during oral treatment with estrogens. Progestogens with androgenic properties may counteract the estrogenic effect, e.g. on SHBG but not on CBG. The liver is also the key organ of lipid metabolism and plays an important regulatory role in hemostasis. Cholesterol is synthesized in hepatocytes and the rate-limiting enzyme is the 3-hydroxy-3-methylglutaryl coenzyme A (HMG-CoA) reductase. Cholesterol is packaged in the very-low-density lipoprotein (VLDL) particles, which also consists of triglycerides, phospholipids and apolipoproteins produced in the liver. Estrogens stimulate the production of apolipoproteins, triglycerides and VLDL, while progestogens have the opposite effect. Inhibition of HMG-CoA reductase by statins reduces cholesterol synthesis and, hence, increases receptor-mediated uptake of low-density lipoprotein (LDL) from the circulation. Estrogens may also increase the receptor-mediated uptake of remnants and LDL. The degradation of triglycerides and phospholipids in the liver is catalyzed by the hepatic triglyceride hydrolase, the activity of which is reduced by estrogens and stimulated by progestogens.

The synthesis of many hemostasis factors can

Table 26.1 Relative potency of various orally administered estrogens with respect to some clinical and metabolic parameters

Estrogen	HF	FSH	HDL-CH	SHBG	CBG	ANG
Estradiol	100	100	100	100	100	100
Estriol	30	30	20			
Estrone sulfate		90	50	90	70	150
Conjugated estrogens	120	110	150	300	150	500
Equilin sulfate			600	750	600	750
Ethinylestradiol	12,000	12,000	40,000	50,000	60,000	35,000

HF, Hot flushes; FSH, follicle-stimulating hormone; HDL-CH, high-density lipoprotein-cholesterol; SHBG, sex hormone-binding globulin; CBG, corticosteroid-binding globulin; ANG, angiotensinogen.

be increased by potent estrogens, e.g. ethinyl-estradiol, while estradiol barely influences co-agulation and fibrinolysis factors. Progestogens with androgenic properties may slightly modulate the estrogen-induced changes. Certain progestogens with glucocorticoid activities, e.g. medroxyprogesterone acetate, may upregulate the synthesis of the thrombin receptor and tissue factor in the vessel wall.

The differences between the hormonal potency of various estrogens are only partly dependent on the binding affinity to the estrogen receptor. More important is the bioavailability and a delayed enzymatic inactivation which can be brought about by substituents in the steroid skeleton.

After oral administration, estradiol is extensively metabolized in the intestinal mucosa and during the first liver passage, resulting in a poor bioavailability. A large proportion of the dose is converted to estrone, estrone sulfate and estrone glucuronide, which are circulating in high concentrations and serve as a hormonally inert reservoir, as they can be reconverted to estradiol (Fig. 26.1). After daily ingestion of 2 mg estradiol valerate a steady state is reached with 0.3 nmol/l estradiol, 1.5 nmol/l estrone and 55 nmol/l estrone sulfate, while the concentration of estradiol sulfate is 1 nmol/l and of estrone glucuronide 15 nmol/l.[1] The reversible interconversion between estradiol, estrone,

estrone sulfate and estradiol sulfate prevents the rapid decline in estradiol levels after reaching the serum maximum as observed with estriol, ethinylestradiol or progestogens, and maintains a relatively constant estradiol level for many hours. After intake of conjugated estrogens, a small part is directly absorbed in the gut, while the major proportion of the dose is hydrolyzed and, after absorption, rapidly resulfated. The circulating estrogen sulfates are cleared at a much slower rate than the unconjugated estrogens. Estrogens and estrogen metabolites are excreted mainly in form of glucuronides, in the urine and bile, but can also be reabsorbed after hydrolysis of estrogen conjugates in the colon by bacterial enzymes. This enterohepatic circulation contributes considerably to the serum levels and the efficacy of estrogens. Therefore, a meal may increase estrogen levels, while antibiotics may decrease serum estrogens.

Besides this reversible metabolism, estrogens are irreversibly inactivated by hydroxylation at C16alpha resulting in the formation of estriol or at C2 and C4 yielding the so-called catecholestrogens which can further be methylated.

Liver function

It has been demonstrated that the human liver contains estrogen receptors, but the liver differs from other target organs in so far as it responds to natural estrogens with activation of nuclear estrogen receptors only at high local concentrations.

Long-term estrogen deficiency may be associated with elevated serum liver enzymes. Women with Turner's syndrome are at increased risk of developing chronic liver disease such as liver cirrhosis. Many patients with Turner's syndrome have elevated alkaline phosphatase, ASAT, and γ-glutamyl transferase, while bilirubin and albumin levels are generally normal. In most patients, normalization of elevated liver enzymes can be observed after 3 months of treatment with oral or transdermal estradiol and additional progestogen. In these patients, conjugated estrogens or ethinylestradiol should be avoided as there are reports on deterioration of the liver function.

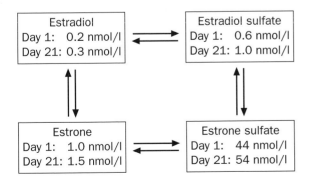

Figure 26.1 Mutual interconversion and serum concentrations of 17β-estradiol, estrone, estrone sulfate and estradiol sulfate in postmenopausal women on day 1 and day 21 of oral treatment with 2 mg estradiol valerate (after Aedo et al[1]).

In postmenopausal women, the activity of serum alkaline phosphatase increases due to an increased bone resorption and can be normalized by HRT. In general, estrogen deficiency is associated with a reduction in γ-glutamyl transpeptidase and lactate dehydrogenase, while ASAT and ALAT are not altered. The available data show that in healthy postmenopausal women, hormone replacement therapy (HRT) does not deteriorate liver function tests like ASAT (serum glutamic–oxaloacetic transaminase: SGOT), ALAT (serum glutamic–pyruvic transaminase: SGPT), 5-nucleotidase and total bilirubin.[2] Oral estrogens may increase hepatic production of C-reactive protein by 100%, but reduce serum levels of other inflammation markers. The serum levels of urea, bilirubin and creatinine are influenced neither by estrogen deficiency nor by HRT.

Liver disease

The liver plays a central role in the metabolism of estrogens and other sex steroids, particularly of synthetic compounds. After oral administration, there is a marked metabolism already in the intestinal mucosa, but after absorption, the serum concentration of estrogens during the first liver passage is four to five times higher than in peripheral serum. Moreover, much higher levels of estrone and estrogen conjugates, as well as other metabolites, are circulating through the liver. Therefore, the hormonal and pharmacologic impacts on the metabolic capacity of the liver are high, particularly after oral intake of estrogens of non-human origin or synthetic estrogens like ethinylestradiol, the degradation of which is slowed down.

In women with acute severe liver disease, prescription of HRT should be postponed until the acute phase has improved and liver function normalized. In women with chronic liver disease with a strong indication for HRT, caution is recommended and an excessive burden of the liver's metabolic capacity must be avoided. Therefore, transdermal treatment with estradiol should be preferred. Concerning the various progestogens which are indicated for endometrial protection, there are no long-term

safety studies. It can, however, be assumed that vaginal progesterone has the least impact on a lesioned liver. In patients with severe liver disease, liver function tests should be carried out before and after 3 months of treatment.

Cholestasis

The pathogenesis of intrahepatic cholestasis is not clarified. It has been suggested that an increased sensitivity of the hepatic excretory system to estrogens is the underlying defect, while progestogens appear to be inconspicuous. Estrogens appear to reduce the excretory capacity for bilirubin, bile salts, steroids, porphyrins and bromsulfophthalein. The change in the composition of bile leads to an elevated concentration of cholesterol, which impairs permeability and function of canalicular membranes and causes a reduced bile flow due to a loss of membrane fluidity. In the majority of women, these effects are without clinical relevance, but may cause pruritus and jaundice in predisposed women who already have a reduced excretory capacity.

The occurrence of idiopathic recurrent jaundice of pregnancy not associated with hepatitis or primary biliary tract disease indicates an excretory dysfunction of the liver which is accompanied by elevated levels of serum conjugated bilirubin and nonspecific alkaline phosphatase. As it becomes manifest during the third trimester, when serum estradiol reaches a level up to 20 ng/ml, a causal relationship cannot be excluded. The symptoms of intrahepatic cholestasis, which is characterized by centrilobular bile staining of hepatocytes and canalicular bile plugs but without portal inflammation or parenchymal injury, disappear after delivery but tend to recur in subsequent pregnancies. About 50% of women with jaundice occurring during treatment with oral contraceptives have a history of cholestasis during pregnancy. In patients who suffered from pruritus or jaundice during pregnancy, treatment with high doses of ethinylestradiol may cause recurrence of the symptoms, while 20 mg/day medroxyprogesterone acetate does not.

Treatment of postmenopausal women with

high doses of estradiol and estriol reduced hepatic excretion of bromsulfophthalein and caused a significant rise in serum transaminase. As the liver has a large reserve capacity for excretion of bilirubin, jaundice does not usually appear before the excretory capacity is 10% below the normal range. In cases of cholestasis induced by exogenous estrogens, jaundice mostly appears within the first 6 months of treatment and is accompanied by pruritus, pale stools and dark urine. Bilirubin is elevated but mostly not above 5 mg/dl, serum alkaline phosphatase and aminotransferase are normal or slightly elevated.[3] After discontinuation of treatment, complete recovery can be expected within 2 months. A genetic predisposition has been suggested and women with a history or family history of cholestasis during pregnancy or oral contraception may be at increased risk. Therefore, these patients must be closely monitored during HRT.

Porphyria

Hepatic porphyrias are caused by defective haem synthesis leading to an overproduction of porphyrins. Acute intermittent porphyria is caused by defective uroporphyrinogen I synthetase (porphobilinogen deaminase), which is associated with a secondary overproduction and urinary excretion of δ-aminolevulinic acid and porphobilinogen. Acute attacks can be precipitated by cyclical endogenous hormone changes or by exogenous steroids or alcohol. Sex steroids may induce cytochrome P-450 and consequently an increased haem consumption. This may lead to a haem deficiency and an excessive rise in porphyrinogens. In predisposed women, attacks may be triggered during the luteal phase by progesterone. The formation of porphyrinogens can be increased by fasting and decreased by treatment with carbohydrates.

Most of the patients who develop subclinical or clinical chronic porphyria cutanea tarda show a hereditary defect of uroporphyrinogen decarboxylase. The manifestation can be triggered by a further reduction in the activity of this liver enzyme by estrogens or alcohol. There is no increase in 5-amino levulinic acid or porphyrinogens, but the accumulation of porphyrins in the skin leads to characteristic skin symptoms. In postmenopausal women with phlebotomy-induced remission of porphyria cutanea tarda, no relapse or other adverse effects occurred during transdermal replacement therapy with 50 µg estradiol.[4]

Cholelithiasis

Estrogens are suggested to be a promoting factor in the pathophysiology of gallstones. The prevalence of gallstones in women is two to three times higher than in men, and the relative risk increases during oral contraception and HRT. As compared with controls, the relative risk of surgically confirmed gallbladder disease is 2.5 in postmenopausal women treated with estrogens, i.e. 13 additional cases per 10,000 women-years.[5] On the other hand, the prevalence of gallstones increases in women not on HRT by 20% between the ages of 40 and 74, and about 20% of postmenopausal women have microscopic cholesterol crystals in their bile.[6]

The pathophysiology of cholelithiasis is not totally clarified, but includes a higher cholesterol saturation index of bile in older women. Gallstones consist of 60–90% cholesterol and are the result of enhanced saturation of bile with cholesterol, rapid nucleation of solid cholesterol crystals in bile which then grow. Moreover, mucous glycoprotein in bile may have a triggering function on nucleation. In general, the solubility of cholesterol in bile is maintained by bile acids and phospholipids. Moreover, disorders of postprandial gallbladder contraction and reduced bile flow appears to be involved in the development of gallstones. The sensitivity of the gallbladder to cholecystokinin decreases with age.

While estrogens did not influence the contractility of the gallbladder, it was reduced by progestogens, and both during the luteal phase and pregnancy, gallbladder emptying is delayed.[7] Estrogens are thought to promote the formation of gallstones by increasing cholesterol saturation of the bile as a consequence of an alteration of the composition of bile acids, and by reducing bile flow.

The alterations of various serum parameters during oral HRT reflect a pronounced impact on hepatic metabolism due to high local estrogen concentrations during the first liver passage. Therefore, it was believed that oral HRT increases the risk of cholelithiasis more than transdermal HRT. It could, however, be demonstrated that treatment of postmenopausal women with either 100 µg estradiol transdermally or 1.25 mg conjugated estrogens orally increased biliary cholesterol saturation and decreased the time required to form cholesterol crystals in bile to the same degree, even though oral HRT had a much higher impact on lipids and SHBG.[8]

The estrogen-induced enhancement of LDL receptor- and remnant receptor-mediated uptake of LDL and VLDL remnants increases the cholesterol content of hepatocytes, and consequently the excretion of cholesterol in bile. The results suggest that the risk of gallstone formation during transdermal HRT is not lower than during oral HRT. In women with a history of gallstones, treatment with estrogens may cause cholelithiasis irrespective of the route of administration.

Venous thrombosis in the liver

It is now established that HRT increases the relative risk of venous thromboembolic diseases and, therefore, may also concern the risk of hepatic vein and portal vein thrombosis. This may be related to the procoagulatory effect of estrogens, particularly in women with thrombophilia, but may also be influenced by certain progestogens which may upregulate the thrombin receptor due to their glucocorticoid activity.[9]

Liver tumors and hepatic vascular changes

HRT does not increase the incidence of hepatocellular carcinoma but rather may decrease it.[10,11] The relative risk of hepatocellular adenoma, which is a very rare disease, is increased by oral contraceptives but there are no data on the effect of HRT. The benign tumors are usually asymptomatic, but may rupture and cause intraperitoneal hemorrhage. In most, but not all, cases they regress after discontinuation of treatment.[3] Ethinylestradiol has been implicated as the major cause of development of benign tumors and vascular changes in the liver which may lead to spontaneous hepatic rupture, while in predisposed patients natural estrogens may at most be active in high doses. In postmenopausal women with a history of hepatocellular adenoma, parenteral HRT may be taken into consideration, e.g. transdermal estradiol and vaginal progesterone. As the incidence of focal nodular hyperplasia is not increased during treatment with oral contraceptives, it is in all probability also not influenced by HRT. In some cases of pre-existing focal nodular hyperplasic lesions, intake of ovulation inhibitors may cause an increase in size.

It cannot be excluded that pre-existing liver hemangioma enlarge during HRT. There are two case reports on the development of hepatic hematoma and hepatic peliosis which ruptured during treatment with 1.25 or 2.5 mg conjugated estrogens.[12]

Acute and chronic liver disease

In many women with chronic liver disease, successful pregnancies have been reported with no deleterious effects on liver function. Therefore, in women with chronic liver disease HRT is not absolutely contraindicated, but transdermal HRT should be preferred.

Cirrhosis
In women with primary biliary cirrhosis the risk of bone fractures is high because of a pronounced loss of bone mass and density. This is probably due to a premature estrogen deficiency caused by disturbance of the hypothalamo–pituitary–ovarian function as a consequence of hepatic dysfunction or certain medications. Treatment with cyclosporine A decreased significantly the serum levels of estradiol in postmenopausal women with primary biliary cirrhosis, but did not influence those of other hormonal parameters. In women with nonalcoholic cirrhosis the serum levels of SHBG are elevated.[13,14]

Estrogens can inhibit the deleterious effects of glucocorticoids and cyclosporine on bone. Treatment of these patients with 50 µg estradiol transdermally and 5 mg medroxyprogesterone acetate orally (10 days) increased bone mineral density without a deterioration of hepatic function tests.[15] The prevalence of gallstones in patients with liver cirrhosis is elevated but it is not clarified whether it is influenced by treatment with estrogens. In women with alcohol-induced liver cirrhosis, the serum levels of estradiol and estrone are elevated, while those of testosterone, leuteinizing hormone (LH), follicle-stimulating hormone (FSH) and estrone sulfate are significantly lower.[16]

Hepatitis

There is no reason for stopping use of HRT during acute viral hepatitis. Patients with chronic active hepatitis require treatment with glucocorticoids and have, therefore, a high risk of osteoporosis. In cases of menopausal symptoms, treatment with transdermal estradiol 50 µg and norethisterone 1 mg may improve both climacteric symptoms and bone mineral density.[17]

Autoimmune hepatitis is believed to be a disease of young women, but can also occur in older women. The patients often present with acute icteric hepatitis and partly with definite or incomplete cirrhosis. Complete remission was achieved with glucocorticoid therapy. As the presentation and course of the disease does not differ between younger and older age, HRT might be an option in selected cases.

Sarcoidosis

In a postmenopausal woman with hepatic sarcoidosis, HRT improved her liver function, which possibly reflects a prevention of progression of the disease. Although long-term studies are required, it appears that in carefully selected patients with sarcoidosis, HRT may possibly be suitable for the prevention of corticosteroid-induced osteoporosis.

Liver transplantation

Cholestatic reactions appear to occur not more frequently in a transplanted liver. Therefore, there is no contraindication for HRT, except for patients transplanted for the Budd–Chiari syndrome that is associated with thrombophilia.

Due to immobility and immunosuppressant medications, e.g. glucocorticoids or cyclosporine A, patients with liver transplantation are at increased risk for development of osteoporosis due to estrogen deficiency. Within 1 year after liver transplantation there is a high incidence of vertrebral fractures.

As estrogens may prevent bone loss without adverse effects on liver function, transdermal HRT may be possible after liver transplantation. In this population, however, no data from controlled studies are available.

PANCREAS

Pancreatic growth is regulated by gastrointestinal hormones, e.g. cholecystokinin and secretin, while somatostatin inhibits growth of normal and malignant pancreatic cells. With respect to pancreatic function, there is probably a common regulatory mechanism for estrogens and somatostatin, which inhibits exocrine secretion in the pancreas.

In the luteal phase the serum concentrations of somatostatin and motilin are significantly elevated and correlate with serum progesterone. In contrast, the levels of secretin and vasoactive intestinal peptide (VIP) correlate with that of estradiol. No association to sex steroid levels was found regarding pancreatic polypeptide concentration.

Although the pancreatic gland is not a typical estrogen target organ, the presence of estrogens appear to play an essential role in the synthesis and secretion of pancreatic digestive enzymes. Treatment with estrogens increases the activity of amylase and lipase in pancreatic juice as well as the concentration of triglycerides and total lipids in pancreatic tissue. Estrogens are taken up and retained in the pancreas due to binding to a specific estrogen binding protein. Estradiol accumulates in the pancreas much more than in the other nonreproductive organs. In contrast to estrogen receptors, which are present at low concentrations, the pancreas-specific estrogen-binding protein occurs in high concentrations, in the pancreatic tissue, particularly in the islets of Langerhans. Treatment of women with estrogens increases glucose-induced insulin secretion, and progesterone was also observed to enhance insulin secretion in response to a glucose load.

Pancreatitis

Oral treatment with estrogens is known to increase triglyceride serum levels by stimulating VLDL production, while progestogens may increase hepatic lipoprotein lipase activity. Therefore, an estrogen-induced increase in triglyceride serum levels is counteracted by progestogen, particularly those with androgenic properties. Patients with primary familial hypertriglyceridemia (> 750 mg/dl) or hyperchylomicronemia are at high risk for estrogen-induced pancreatitis. In patients with type IV or V hypertriglyceridemia, treatment with conjugated estrogens resulted in an excessive elevation of serum triglycerides and caused severe acute pancreatitis.[18] A similar response was also observed during treatment with tamoxifen. Discontinuation of estrogens, diet and treatment with gemfibrozil and omega-3 fatty acids may normalize triglyceride levels. In patients with serum triglycerides > 300 mg/dl oral estrogens should not be prescribed, with levels > 750 mg/dl oral estrogens are contraindicated. In these cases, transdermal estradiol might be considered as a suitable alternative as it does not increase triglyceride levels. Patients with high triglyceride levels who begin HRT should be followed-up 2 weeks after starting treatment.

The additional administration of progestogens with pronounced androgenic properties (e.g. norethisterone or levonorgestrel) may attenuate or prevent the estrogen-induced hypertriglyceridemia and pancreatitis in patients with type IV or V hyperlipoproteinemia, but not with hyperchylomicronemia. This appears to be associated with a reduction in triglyceride synthesis and an increase in the activity of hepatic lipoprotein lipase.

In contrast, oral treatment with estrogens of women with type III hyperlipoproteinemia may normalize the high serum levels of cholesterol and trigycerides. This disturbance of lipid metabolism is caused by an impaired receptor-mediated hepatic uptake of VLDL and chylomicron remnants, which will be improved by oral estrogens.[19]

Pancreatic cancer

Although estrogen, progesterone and androgen receptors were found in tissue of pancreatic cancers, neither menopause nor HRT has any influence on the incidence of pancreatic cancer.[11,20] It has been suggested that in pancreatic cancers containing estrogen receptors, growth may be inhibited by tamoxifen, but this could not be confirmed in a randomized study.

REFERENCES

1. Aedo AR, Landgren BM, Diczfalusy E. Pharmacokinetics and biotransformation of orally administered oestrone sulphate and oestradiol valerate in postmenopausal women. *Maturitas* 1990; **12:** 333–43.
2. Moore B, Paterson M, Sturdee D. Effect of oral hormone replacement therapy on liver function tests. *Maturitas* 1987; **9:** 7–15.
3. Dourakis SP, Tolis G. Sex hormonal preparations and the liver. *Eur J Contracept Reprod Health Care* 1998; **3:** 7–16.
4. Bulaj ZJ, Franklin MR, Phillips JD et al. Transdermal estrogen replacement therapy in postmenopausal women previously treated for porphyria cutanea tarda. *J Lab Clin Med* 2000; **136:** 482–8.
5. Boston Collaborative Drug Surveillance Program. Surgically confirmed gallbladder disease, venous thromboembolism, and breast tumors in relation to postmenopausal estrogen therapy. *N Engl J Med* 1974; **290:** 15–19.
6. Marks JW, Uhler ML, Bonorris GG et al. Nucleation of biliary cholesterol, arachidonate, prostaglandin E2, and glycoproteins in postmenopausal women. *Gastroenterology* 1997; **112:** 1271–6.
7. Wedmann B, Schmidt G, Wegener M et al. Effects of age and gender on fat-induced gallbladder contraction and gastric emptying of a caloric liquid meal: a sonographic study. *Am J Gastroenterol* 1991; **86:** 1765–70.
8. Uhler ML, Marks JW, Voigt BJ et al. Comparison of the impact of transdermal versus oral estrogens on biliary markers of gallstone formation in

postmenopausal women. *J Clin Endocr Metab* 1998; **83:** 410–14.

9. Herkert O, Kuhl H, Sandow J et al. Sex steroids used in hormonal treatment increase vascular procoagulant activity by inducing thrombin receptor (PAR-1) expression – role of the glucocorticoid receptor. *Circulation* 2001; **104:** 2826–31.

10. LaVecchia C. HRT and the risk of neoplasma other than in the breast. *Eur Menopause J* 1996; **2:** 232–6.

11. Persson I, Yuen J, Bergkvist L et al. Cancer incidence and mortality in women receiving estrogen and estrogen–progestin replacement therapy – long-term follow-up of a Swedish cohort. *Int J Cancer* 1996; **67:** 327–32.

12. Lundell CJ. Spontaneous hepatic rupture in postmenopausal women receiving oral estrogen replacement. *J Vasc Intervent Radiol* 1993; **4:** 245–9.

13. Becker U, Gluud C, Farholt S et al. Menopausal age and sex hormones in postmenopausal women with alcoholic and non-alcoholic liver disease. *J Hepatol* 1991; **13:** 25–32.

14. Pearce S, Bassendine M, Dowsett M. Sex hormone binding globulin and non-protein-bound oestradiol in postmenopausal patients with primary biliary cirrhosis and normal controls. *J Steroid Biochem Molec Biol* 1993; **44:** 273–6.

15. Olsson R, Mattsson LA, Obrant K et al. Estrogen–progestogen therapy for low bone mineral density in primary biliary cirrhosis. *Liver* 1999; **19:** 188–92.

16. Gavaler JS, van Thiel DH. Hormonal status of postmenopausal women with alcohol-induced cirrhosis: further findings and a review of the literature. *Hepatology* 1992; **16:** 312–19.

17. Clements D, Rhodes J. Hormone replacement therapy in chronic active hepatitis; a case report. *Gut.* 1993; **34:** 1639–40.

18. Glueck CJ, Lang J, Hamer T et al. Severe hypertriglyceridemia and pancreatitis when estrogen replacement therapy is given to hypertriglyceridemic women. *J Lab Clin Med* 1994; **123:** 59–64.

19. Kushwaha RS, Hazzard WR, Gagne C et al. Type III hyperlipoproteinemia: paradoxical hypolipidemic response to estrogen. *Ann Intern Med* 1977; **87:** 517–25.

20. Kreiger N, Lacroix J, Sloan M. Hormonal factors and pancreatic cancer in women. *Ann Epidemiol* 2001; **11:** 563–7.

27

Carcinogenesis and the role of hormones: promotion and prevention

HPG Schneider

Introduction • Hormones and the developmental process of cancer • Estrogens and cancer
• Glandular breast and hormone-dependent cancer • Adjuvant endocrine impact on tumor development
• Conclusions • References

INTRODUCTION

Apparently, more than 40% of all newly diagnosed female cancers are hormone dependent. In addition to endometrial cancer, these mainly are breast and ovarian cancer. What is our current view on the way hormones influence the oncogenetic cascade? This cascade of carcinogenesis is related to an accumulation of intracellular genetic mutations as well as epigenetic abnormalities in controlled gene expression. Hormones can indeed influence the development of various cancers, as demonstrated by clinical experiments and epidemiology. Hypotheses have been formulated to show a relation of specific female reproductive tumors to hormonal signaling; the same holds true for the prostate gland of men. Parturition has been shown to be related to the morphogenesis of ovarian cancer. Breast cancer, with its incremental incidence, is epidemiologically associated with family history as well as reproductive and environmental factors. Early menarche, late menopause and nulliparity have been defined as risk factors; loss of ovarian function at younger age appears to be protective as does the first full-term pregnancy at a younger age. Primiparity beyond 35 years of age certainly increases breast cancer risk. Such epidemiologic information, very often of borderline significance, requires intensified research in order to provide a basis for biological plausibility of the importance of any of those inferred epidemiological impacts.

HORMONES AND THE DEVELOPMENTAL PROCESS OF CANCER

In 1947, Gusberg[1] defined adenomatous hyperplasia as a morphologic precursor lesion of endometrial cancer. In a prospective follow-up investigation, Gusberg and Kaplan[2] described 191 patients with adenomatous hyperplasia, of whom 90 were immediately hysterectomized. In these surgical specimens, 20% of the cases had co-existent cancer, in 30% borderline lesions were detected. Among the remainder of 101 women, eight (11.8%) developed endometrial cancer within an average follow-up of 5.3 years. In the control group of 202 women with postmenopausal bleeding, when without any sign of hyperplasia or cancer in the primary breast cancer specimen, only one woman experienced endometrial cancer within the same time period. Gusberg and Kaplan[2] calculated a cumulative risk of a transition of adenomatous hyperplasia to develop into endometrial cancer to be one-third within 9–10 years, a concept that was contradicted by others. Fearon and Vogelstein[3] demonstrated convincingly that carcinogenesis can be considered a developmental process of hyperplasia to adenomatosis to in situ cancer to infiltrating cancer depending on specific and multiple genomic defects, as demonstrated with colon cancer. Kurman et al[4] looked at 'untreated' hyperplasia of endometrial cancer in 170 women and demonstrated hyperplasia and neoplasia to represent two separate and biologically different phenomena; the morphologic discriminant is cellular atypia.

Cellular proliferation, apoptosis and angiogenesis are interdependent determinants of tumor growth. Experimental experience with control and quantitation of apoptosis has provided a growing insight into the development of hormone-dependent tumors.[5] Apoptosis is the genetically programmed process of active cellular self-destruction, clearly distinguishable from necrosis. Apoptosis is under the control of intrinsic and extrinsic factors (hormones, growth factors); it can be activated in tissues, during embryonic development or in association with normal cyclicity of endocrine-related organs. Loss of apoptotic mechanisms can foster tumor development.[6] Key experiments in order to gain some insight into the dependence of programmed cell death from estrogenic stimuli have been done in hamsters with kidney tumor transplants. When diethylstilbestrol (DES)-pretreated hamsters are inoculated with cellular suspensions of estrogen-induced kidney tumors, within 2–3 weeks these hamsters develop solid tumors. If DES is withdrawn, the tumor in the recipient animal will regress within a few days by 80–90% of its mass. Following this estrogen withdrawal, tumor regression occurs within 4 days. The key morphologic event was demonstrated to be apoptosis. Within a period of 24 hours, the mitotic activity of these tumors, returned to the level of what it was before DES withdrawal. The extent of areas of necrosis remained unchanged during the experiment. The inoculated tumor regained its original volume within 2 days after reuptake of DES treatment. Indeed, there is a clear dependence of apoptosis in kidney tumors from the estrogen signal in an inhibitory and,

following its discontinuation, supportive manner. Functional and morphologic variation characterizes the typical demise of tumor cells as apoptosis. These observations can also be interpreted as indicating an important mechanism in which, independent of its mitogenic capacities, estrogenic hormones can alter tumor growth.

ESTROGENS AND CANCER

It was in the early 1940s that rodent experiments with estradiol and progesterone demonstrated a promoting impact on experimental breast tumor development. Since that time, the debate on whether or not sex steroids may be involved in breast cancer has never been silenced.

The role of catechol estradiol metabolites in the process of experimental carcinogenesis

Estradiol administration to rodents by oral or subcutaneous routes may increase the incidence of mammary, pituitary, uterine, cervical, vaginal, testicular, lymphoid, and bone tumors (mice). Estradiol also induced tumors when administered orally in the drinking water or in rodent chow. The various animal tumor models have been developed using pharmacologic doses of estradiol with the aim of examining the tumor-promoting activity of this hormone in a relatively short period of time.[7] Such biological studies in animals identify estradiol as a carcinogen. In humans, long-term exposure to elevated endogenous or therapeutic estrogens appears to cause increased breast or uterine cancer risk.[8] Combined estrogen and progestin, in the randomized controlled trial of the Women's Health Initiative,[9] accounted for a 26% increase in the diagnosis of breast cancer after 5.2 years of follow-up. The estrogen-alone arm of this investigation, however, did not produce this effect. This is in line with most of the observational data, showing increased risk of breast cancer with estrogen–progestogen combination therapy (mostly medroxyprogesterone acetate (MPA)) for more than 5–10 years. The absolute risk, however, is small with about one additional breast cancer case per 100 women of 60 years of age who have taken estrogen for at least 10 years.

The biological investigation in animals and epidemiologic studies in humans appear to identify estradiol as a potential carcinogen or co-carcinogen in rodents. Tumors can be induced in small groups of animals with pharmacologic doses of estradiol in a short period of time. On the other hand, in humans we do find a dependence of breast and endometrial cancer incidence on estrogens and progestogens.[10] However, potential carcinogenic or co-carcinogenic activity can, if correct, only be very weak, because estrone and estradiol and other steroidal estrogens are physiologic endogenous hormones at low picomolar levels and stronger carcinogenicity would have provided severe evolutionary disadvantages to humans and other species. Experimental and clinical experience suggest that the in vivo co-carcinogenic activity of estradiol catechol metabolites is facultative, as it will only affect a small proportion of cancer-prone individuals, who are characterized by special, already existing, genetic or metabolic and reproductive conditions as a prerequisite.

Contributions of estradiol to the course of breast cancer

What then are the discernible contributions of estradiol to carcinogenesis? Ever since Beatson,[11] a Scottish surgeon, reported in 1896 about his experience of a remission of breast cancer following bilateral oophorectomy in premenopausal women, the possible relationship of ovarian function and mammary tumor development never escaped our clinical conscience. From a recent critical review of the results of population-based case control studies in the US and Europe, as well as prospective cohort studies or nationwide American breast cancer screening programs,[12] it was quite apparent that estrogen-alone regimens of hormone therapy in postmenopausal women did not result in a significantly increased risk of breast cancer, even with increasing duration of use up to more than 15 years [odds ratio = 1.06;

confidence interval (CI) 0.97–1.15]. Studies that detect an increased risk of breast cancer in hormone users nevertheless indicate a paradoxical better outcome. It is established that screening facilitates the early detection of breast cancer which might otherwise remain clinically silent for many years. Mammography, our most effective screening tool, advances the time of diagnosis such that in women exposed to estrogens and progestins, screening would likely have resulted in the selective identification of an excess of cases that might otherwise not have been diagnosed, or only after the studies were completed. However, lower grade tumors are present even when there is no difference in the prevalence of mammography when hormone users and non-users are compared or when the data are adjusted for the method of detection.[13–15] The American breast cancer detection project reported an association of hormone use with a 40–60% reduction in breast cancer mortality of 12 years after diagnosis.[13] This effect persisted even after correction for cases detected at screening intervals and when in situ tumors were excluded, indicating the exclusion of detection or surveillance bias. This project also presented data on protection against breast cancer mortality associated with hormone use that could not be attributed to tumor size, age at diagnosis, body mass index (BMI), tumor histology or node status. What may be affected is grade of disease, tumor differentiation and aneuploidy. An excess of grade I tumors has been seen both in users of estrogen alone and of combined estrogen and progestin.[16]

GLANDULAR BREAST AND HORMONE-DEPENDENT CANCER

The breast is the only immature primate organ at birth. Its further growth and development is related to sexual maturation. The glandular breast may therefore serve as the most intricate model organ of hormone dependence.

Estrogen and carcinogenesis of glandular tissue of the breast

Estrogens exert their physiologic effects on reproductive and nonreproductive organs by binding to their specific receptors, estrogen receptors (ER) alpha or beta.[17] While there is no doubt that receptor-mediated processes play an important role in the development and growth of cancer, accumulating evidence suggests that specific oxidative metabolites of estrogens, by reacting with DNA, can act as endogenous carcinogens by causing mutations leading to cancer.[18–20]

The most intensely investigated reproductive organ as related to potential hormone-dependent carcinogenesis is the glandular breast. That is why the focus should be on the discussion of our experience with 'cancerization' of the breast.

In general, the risk of breast cancer could be determined by the cumulative exposure of breast tissue to estrogen.[21] The biological consequences of terminal pregnancy for cellular differentiation of breast tissue, in addition the preventive character of lactation with its promotion to type IV lobules that will regress at a later phase,[22,23] give rise to a plausible experimental model of breast carcinogenesis. The further differentiated the glandular breast will be, the less prone it is to experimental cancerization[10] Contributing factors to individual variation in exposure to estrogens are obesity in postmenopausal women, and differences in exercise and dietary intake of certain nutrients. Among the latter, studies of intakes of alcohol, fat, antioxidant vitamins and fiber have produced conflicting results. Phytoestrogens, with their structural similarity to physiologic estrogens when ingested, have both estrogen-agonist and -antagonist effects in humans. Flaxseed, a source of mammalian lignanes and α-linoleic acid, has been shown to exert anti-estrogenic effects by binding to ER and inhibiting the binding of endogenous estrogens. The incidence of breast cancer is lowest in regions where the intake of soy, an abundant source of phytoestrogens, or flaxseed is high; whether or not this inverse relation is direct or only indicative of other influencing factors is a matter of debate.[24]

What is the evidence for individual variation of local tissue estrogen exposure or genetic variation responsible for the production of oxidative metabolites of estradiol which induce mutations?

There is significant information showing that breast cancer tissues contain all the enzymes necessary for the formation of estradiol from circulating precursors, including aromatase, sulfatase and 17β-hydroxysteroid dehydrogenase (17β-HSD). Two main pathways are implicated in estradiol formation in normal breast and breast cancer tissues. The 'aromatase pathway' that transforms androgens into estrogens, and the 'sulfatase pathway' that converts estrone sulfate into estrone, which is then transformed into estradiol by the reductive 17β-HSD activity.

The fact that estradiol levels in breast tumors of postmenopausal women remain as high as in the premenopasue, while plasma levels decrease, clearly points to the discrepancy between these two components. It would implicate the necessity of mechanisms that require local factors. In addition, the hypothesis has been confirmed that local production of estradiol within the breast is the main source of estrogen at breast tissue level.[25] By the same token, the androstenedione was found at lower concentrations in the tumor as compared to fatty tissues of all quadrants, whereas testosterone did not show this difference. Finally, estrone sulfate is highly concentrated in the tumor.

The precise mechanism controling estrogen production in postmenopausal women as is not yet fully understood. Both cytochrome CYP-17 (encoding P-450 17α-hydroxylase) and cytochrome CYP-19 (encoding P-450 aromatase) are involved in estrogen biosynthesis; polymorphisms of both genes have been identified in the general population.[26,27] Women who are heterozygous or homozygous for cytochrome CYP-17 polymorphism have been shown to produce high serum estradiol concentrations; however, this polymorphism is not unequivocally associated with increased risk of breast cancer.[24] There are, however, ongoing studies demonstrating a link between polymorphisms of the P-450 aromatase gene with increased risk of breast cancer.[26] The aromatase gene may act as one of the many oncogenic, mutagenic factors and radicals which stimulate tumor formation and promotion in cancer-receptive breast tissue. Estrogen production may also be influenced by variation in tissue-specific promoters of aromatase gene expression.[28] A change of promoter I.4 in normal breast tissue to promoter P-II and P-I.3 in breast cancer has been demonstrated in a detailed investigation of the expression of aromatase in human breast tumors,[29] these promoter changes may result in increased synthesis of aromatase mRNA. Such promoter functional studies are essential for a clear understanding of the control of aromatase expression in breast tumors and its role in cancer development, and may involve transcription factors specific to breast cancer cells. In fact, the aromatase gene may act as an oncogene that initiates tumor formation in breast tissue.[24]

Breast tissue sensitivity to estrogen

Estrogen may diffuse passively through cellular and nuclear membranes. On the other hand, specific cells and tissues express ER to which estrogen would bind and form a ligand–receptor complex in order to activate specific sequences in the regulatory region of genes responsive to estrogen, known as estrogen-response elements. These genes, in turn, regulate cell growth and differentiation.

Estrogens behave differently from tissue to tissue and from cell to cell, but there are also variations among individual women. Physiologically active doses in one individual may produce less of an effect in another. ER levels are low in normal breast tissue and high levels have been directly correlated with an increased risk of breast cancer.[29] Receptor levels increase with age in some ethnic groups and apparently are higher in white women as compared to Black or Japanese women. This phenomenon may be related to the function of a tumor-suppressor gene, the loss of which may

result in failure to downregulate ER with resultant defects of the cell cycle, finally promoting breast carcinoma development.[30]

The human ER belongs to the nuclear receptor superfamily of ligand-inducible transcription factors. The recent identification of ERβ has indicated that the cellular responses to ER ligands are far more complex. ERα and ERβ interact with the same DNA response elements and exhibit similar, but not identical, ligand-binding characteristics. ERβ binds estrogens with a similar affinity to ERα and activates the expression of reporter genes containing estrogen-response elements in an estrogen-dependent manner. In vitro, ERα and ERβ form heterodimers with each other, and ERβ decreases the sensitivity of estrogen, thereby acting as a physiologic regulator of the proliferative effects of ERα.[31]

In order to evaluate the role of differentiated ER in breast cancer, the expression of both ER isoforms in normal and malignant breast tissue has been investigated.[32] In normal breast tissue, expression of ERβ predominated, with 22% of samples exclusively expressing ERβ; this was not observed in any of the breast tumor cells. Most tumors expressed ERα, either alone or in combination with ERβ.

Metabolism of estrogens and genotoxicity

Estrogens are catabolized predominantly by hydroxylation with a resultant formation of 2-hydroxyestrone, 2-hydroxyestradiol, 4-hydroxyestrone and 4-hydroxyestradiol, 16α-hydroxyestrone and 16α-hydroxyestradiol (Fig. 27.1).[33] The 2-hydroxy and 4-hydroxy metabolites are converted to anticarcinogenic methoxylated metabolites (2-methoxyestrone and 2-methoxyestradiol, 2-hydroxyestrone and 2-hydroxyestradiol-3-methylether, 4-methoxyestrone and 4-methoxyestradiol, 4-hydroxyestrone and 4-hydroxyestradiol-3-methylether) by catechol-O-methyltransferase (COMT). The catechol metabolites of estrogens are implicated in the carcinogenic and cytotoxic effects of these compounds (Fig. 27.2).[33] They can be further metabolized to electrophilic quinoids, such as o-quinones, which can isomerize to their tautomeric p-quinone metides; the roles of these

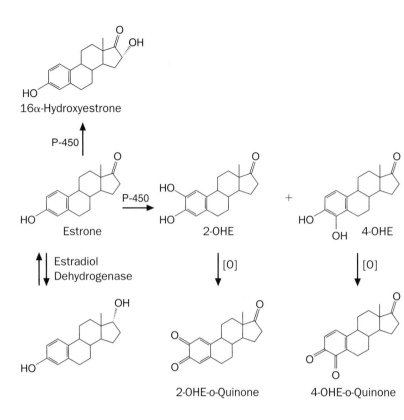

Figure 27.1 Major metabolites of estrone and 17β-estradiol.[33]

quinoids in mediating the adverse effects of estrogens have not been investigated in detail. It is possible for these electrophilic and redox active quinoids to cause damage within cells by a variety of pathways. Catechol estrogen-mediated redox cycling can cause lipid peroxidation, consumption of reducing equivalents, oxidation of DNA and DNA single-strand breaks.[33]

Postmenopausal women with a variant allele that codes for COMT with low activity have a higher risk of breast cancer than women with a wild-type allele.[34] On the other hand, 17β-HSD activity is higher in breast tumors than in normal breast tissue.[25] Taking these tissue-specific variations of estrogen production and catabolism into consideration, there is reason to believe that cumulative exposure to estrogen and its metabolites may vary distinctly within individual women. Polymorphisms of cytochrome CYP-17, CYP-1A1 and COMT are found to be associated with increased risk of breast cancer (Table 27.1).[27] To identify high-risk genotypes in women may delineate the individual at increased risk of breast cancer. Russo et al[35] have demonstrated the preponderance of the 2- and 4-OH-catechol estrogens in human breast cancer tissue.

Biological demonstration of estrogenic carcinogenicity in the human breast

Having given supporting arguments for the experimental and biological potential of estradiol as a weak genotoxic and mutagenic agent[7] what is the biological proof in humans? If estrogen is carcinogenic in the human breast through the above-mentioned pathways, it would induce transformation phenotypes indicative of neoplasia in human breast epithelial cells (HBEC) in vitro and also induce genomic alterations similar to those observed in spontaneous malignancies, such as DNA amplification and loss of genetic material that may represent tumor-suppressor genes. To test this hypothesis, Russo et al[35] evaluated the transforming potential of estradiol on the

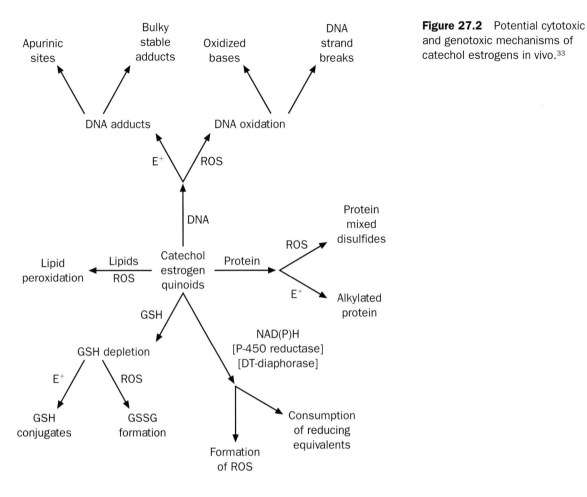

Figure 27.2 Potential cytotoxic and genotoxic mechanisms of catechol estrogens in vivo.[33]

Table 27.1 Genotype polymorphisms of estrogen-metabolizing genes and risk of breast cancer[27]*		
Risk factor	**Odds ratio**	**95% CI**
CYP-17	1.23	0.67–2.28
Encoding P-450 17α-hydroxylase		
CYP-1A1	1.79	0.86–3.78
Encoding cytochrome P-450 1AI		
COMT	4.02	1.12–19.08
Two putative high-risk genotypes	3.52	1.06–12.4

* Association higher with prolonged estrogen exposure years.
CI, Confidence internal; COMT, catechol-O-methyltransferase.

spontaneously immortalized HBEC MCF-10F in vitro.[36,37] This cell line lacks both ERα and ERβ. The same phenotype and characteristics by these MCF-10F cells transformed by the chemical carcinogen benzo(a)pyrene and oncogenes were expressed in estradiol-treated cells. Estradiol-transformed cells exhibited loss of heterozygocity in loci of chromosome 11, known to be affected in spontaneously occurring breast lesions, such as ductal hyperplasia, carcinoma in situ and invasive carcinoma. This MCF-10F cell line thereby provides an excellent model to study estradiol-induced transformation and mutation.

To mimic the intermittent exposure of HBEC to endogenous estrogens, MCF-10F cells were exposed to various doses of estradiol at different time intervals. The ductulogenesis, the number of ductules per 10,000 cells plated, decreased with increasing estradiol doses. Also, solid masses were formed in a dose-dependent manner (Fig. 27.3).[35] The ductulogenic capacity of these cell cultures was also significantly decreased by other compounds such as diethylstilbestrol (DES), 4-OH-estradiol or 16α-estradiol, but 4-OH-estradiol was the most efficient in inducing the transformation phenotypes. By the some token, it could be demonstrated that estradiol, DES and the catechol estrogens would induce phenotypes of cell transformation in ER-negative HBEC. While 4-OH-estradiol was shown to be the most efficient inductor of transformation phenotypes, these data demonstrate transforming properties of these hormones in human breast epithelial cells

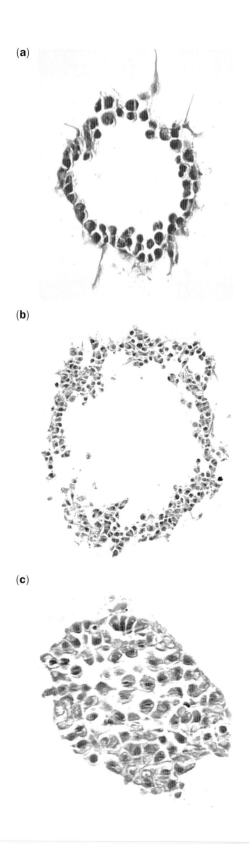

Figure 27.3 Histologic section of cell growing in collagen gel. The cells have been fixed in buffered formalin, embedded in paraffin and the sections stained with hematoxylin and eosin. (**a**) MCF-10F cells treated with solvent (dimethyl sulfoxide) forming well-defined ductular structures lined by a single cuboidal layer of cells; (**b**) MCF-10F cells treated with 0.007 nmol/l of 17β-estradiol forming ductular structures lined by multiple layers of cells; (**c**) 70 nmol/l of 17β-estradiol induces the formation of spherical masses formed by large cuboidal cells. Bright field × 10.[35]

by a mechanism which is ER independent but related to genomic changes with resultant metabolic variation.

ADJUVANT ENDOCRINE IMPACT ON TUMOR DEVELOPMENT

Almost 40 years ago, the first clinical selective ER modulator (SERM), tamoxifen, came into use. It was approved by the Food and Drug Administration (FDA) in 1978 for secondary prevention of breast cancer. Tamoxifen now is the most widely prescribed antineoplastic drug worldwide, having more than 10 million women-years of use. The Early Breast Cancer Trialists' Collaborative Group presented an overview of randomized trials of tamoxifen for early breast cancer.[38] A total of 37,000 women from 55 randomized trials had 5 years of therapy with a median follow-up of 10 years. As compared to placebo, tamoxifen reduced tumor recurrence by 47% and mortality by 26%.

Because of this clinical experience, in 1992 a total of 13,388 women, considered to be at increased risk for the development of breast cancer, were randomized to receive either tamoxifen 20 mg/day or placebo. The plan of this Breast Cancer Prevention Trial (BCPT) was to follow these women for 5 years. However, the study was stopped early because it demonstrated a great decrease in the incidence of both noninvasive and invasive breast cancer. Tamoxifen reduced the incidence of invasive breast cancer by 49% ($P < 0.00001$) and noninvasive breast cancer by 50% ($P = 0.002$).[39]

While this BCPT was progressing, unusual ultrasonic appearances of the uterus were noted in patients on tamoxifen. These were the first hints as to an increased risk of endometrial cancer depending on the cumulative dose of tamoxifen. In 1998, Schwartz et al[40] described asymptomatic postmenopausal women on tamoxifen presenting 27% polyp formation, and 4% endometrial carcinoma. These lesions were different from estrogen-induced endometrial carcinoma. One possible alternate etiology was thought to be the tamoxifen-related induction of the angiogenic peptide adrenomedullin. Adrenomedullin increases angiogenesis and

stimulates direct carcinoma cell growth. These actions may work in concert to cause endometrial cancer.

In the MORE Trial,[41] a study on prevention of bone loss, it was noted that after 48 months there was a marked decrease in breast cancer incidence in the raloxifene-treated group compared to placebo; the relative risk was calculated to be 0.38 (95% CI 0.24–0.58). The same investigation, using both transvaginal sonography and saline infusion sonohysterography, did not find any evidence of endometrial proliferation. Conservative biopsy showed atrophic endometrium in all 43 patients who had already presented endometrial atrophy at the beginning of the study. It appears that although raloxifene has favorable tamoxifen-like effects on breast, bone and lipids, it has none of tamoxifen's stimulatory effects on the endometrium.

These effects of tamoxifen as a preventive agent clearly demonstrate yet again the hormone dependence of reproductive cancer. Women under 50 years of age who have had lobular or ductal carcinoma in situ and atypical hyperplasia on breast biopsies probably also fit the preventive criteria of tamoxifen.

In terms of new cancers, 5 years of adjuvant tamoxifen decrease the incidence of contralateral breast cancer by a factor of approximately 2 (26 per 1000 versus 47 per 1000) and increase the incidence of endometrial cancer by a factor of approximately 4 (11 per 1000 versus 3 per 1000). In terms of cause-specific deaths, for every 1000 patients treated for 5 years with raloxifene, 80 deaths from breast cancer are prevented at the price of two excess deaths from endometrial cancer and one excess death from thromboembolic disease.[38]

Hormonal therapy has also advanced to the initial therapy of choice for women with ER-positive metastatic breast cancer. The new generation of aromatase inhibitors have been demonstrated to be superior to megestrol acetate, aminoglutethimide and tamoxifen. Letrozole was initially compared with both megestrol acetate and aminoglutethimide following tamoxifen failure. In a double-blind randomized trial, 363 patients received either megestrol acetate or letrozole at a daily dose of either 0.5 or 2.5 mg. Letrozole 2.5 mg was superior to megestrol acetate with respect to response rate (24 versus 16%; $P = 0.04$), response duration ($P = 0.01$), time to treatment failure (5.1 versus 3.9 months; $P = 0.04$), quality of life and deterioration in performance status, as well as drug-related serious adverse events ($P < 0.05$). Overall survival also favored letrozole.[42]

Letrozole was later compared with tamoxifen in a randomized, double-blind, crossover phase III study of 907 patients of whom 65% had ER-positive disease (the remainder had unknown ER status and no prior hormonal therapy for metastatic disease). Letrozole was shown to be superior to tamoxifen in terms of response rate (30 versus 20%; $P < 0.001$), clinical benefit (49 versus 38%; $P < 0.001$), time to progression (41 versus 26 weeks; $P < 0.0001$) and time to treatment failure (40 versus 25 weeks; $P < 0.0001$).[43] Anastrozole, when compared with tamoxifen in two double-blind, placebo-controlled studies, while not showing any statistically significant difference in the overall population of 1021 patients, the subgroup of patients with ER- or progestogen-receptor (PR)-positive tumors had a longer time to progression (10.7 versus 6.4 months; $P = 0.022$).[44,45]

Exemestane has also been compared with tamoxifen in a randomized phase II study. In an interim report of the first 63 patients, the response rate (42 versus 16%), complete response rate (10 versus 3%), clinical benefit (58 versus 31%) and time to progression (8.9 versus 5.2 months) all favored exemestane.[46]

All of the aromatase inhibitors resulted in significantly less weight gain than megestrol acetate. The most detailed study of toxicity found more headaches, hair loss, insomnia, nausea and diarrhea for letrozole, but less increase in appetite, vaginal bleeding and dyspnea than megestrol acetate.[47] No other significant differences in toxicities have been noted and there is no clear difference in toxicity profile between the different aromatase inhibitors. Progestins such as megestrol acetate and medroxyprogesterone are now reserved for use as third-line hormonal therapy following failure of tamoxifen and aromatase inhibitors.

The aromatase inhibitors letrozole, anastrozole and exemestane continue to be studied in clinical trials in the adjuvant setting but no data are yet available. As aromatase is the enzyme that converts testosterone to estrogen, and with mounting evidence that aromatase exists in high concentrations in the cytosole of hormonally responsive breast cancer, intratumoral aromatase levels are therefore a potential predictive factor for aromatase inhibitors. Again, this type of hormonal intervention proves effective in interfering with reproductive tumors.

CONCLUSIONS

There are many ways to demonstrate hormone dependence of tumors in human reproductive organs. Proven clinical experience derives from hormone therapy in cancer patients (Table 27.2). The question as to whether estrogen is associated with tumor development or with its initiation has been exemplified along the lines of current clinical research.

The multiple forms of DNA damage induced by catechol estrogen metabolites after metabolic activation to quinone-reactive intermediates support the conclusion that such metabolites of natural estradiol may, under certain conditions, act genotoxically via metabolic conversion to catechol estrogens and formation of quinones. Initial experimental evidence exists as to the transforming property of estrogen metabolites in human breast epithelial cells independent of ER signalling.

Human data are in line with animal carcinogenicity and cell-culture data. They are also in agreement with the more moderate levels of DNA modification by estrogen compared with the substantial genotoxicity of potent carcinogens such as benzopyrene or dimethylbenzanthrazene. As yet, it has to be demonstrated that the possible weak mutagenic activity of some estradiol metabolites is of clinical relevance in humans, in addition to the many other exogenous and endogenous mutagens and carcinogens taking part in the process of carcinogenesis and the preconditions for them to be active. The human species would not have

Table 27.2 Hormone therapy in postmenopausal women with estrogen receptor-positive breast cancer	
Adjuvant	Steroidal anti-estrogen
	Tamoxifen
First-line metastatic	Nonsteroidal aromatase inhibitors
	Anastrozole, letrozole
Second-line metastatic	Steroidal aromatase inhibitors
	Exemestane
Other	Steroidal anti-estrogens
	Faslodex
	Progestins
	Megestrol acetate, Medroxyprogesterone acetate

survived 2 million years, had there been a high mutagenic and carcinogenic activity of estradiol. It appears that genetic polymorphism paves the way to individual susceptibility to such hormone-dependent carcinogenicity. The absolute cancer risks that women have to face from estradiol and its metabolites are, however, rather limited.

REFERENCES

1. Gusberg SB. Precursors of corpus carcinoma, estrogens, and adenomatous hyperplasia. *Am J Obstet Gynecol* 1947; **54**: 905.
2. Gusberg SB, Kaplan AL. Precursors of corpus cancer. *Am J Obstet Gynecol* 1963; **87**: 662.
3. Fearon ER, Vogelstein B. A genetic model for colorectal tumorigenesis. *Cell* 1990; **61**: 759–67.
4. Kurman RJ, Kaminski PF, Norris HJ. The behavior of endometrial hyperplasia. A long-term study of 'untreated' hyperplasia in 170 patients. *Cancer* 1985; **56**: 403–12.
5. Bursch W, Liehr JG, Sirbasku DA et al. Control of cell death (apoptosis) by diethylstilbestrol in an estrogen-dependent kidney tumor. *Carcinogenesis* 1991; **12**: 855–60.
6. McCloskey, DE, Armstrong DK, Jackisch C, Davidson NE. Programmed cell death in human breast cancer cells. *Rec Prog Horm Res* 1996; **51**: 493–508.
7. Liehr JG. Is estradiol a genotoxic mutagenic carcinogen? *Endocr Rev* 2000; **21**: 40–54.
8. Schneider HPG, Jackisch C. Reproductive cancer and hormone replacement. In: (Fischl FH, Huber JC, eds) *Menopause–Andropause.* (Krause & Pachernegg GmbH: Gablitz, 2001) 173–203.
9. Writing Group for the Women's Health Initiative. Risks and benefits of estrogen plus progestin in healthy postmenopausal women. *JAMA* 2002; **288**: 321–33.
10. Jackisch C, Schneider HPG. Biological effects of estrogens and progestogen on human breast cancer carcinogenesis. *Menopause Rev* 1997; **2**: 26–34.
11. Beatson GT. On the treatment of inoperable cases of carcinoma of the mamma: suggestions for a new method of treatment, with illustrative cases. *Lancet* 1896; **2**: 104–7.
12. Speroff L. Postmenopausal estrogen–progestin therapy and breast cancer: a clinical response to epidemiological reports. *Climacteric* 2000; **3**: 3–12.
13. Schairer C, Gail M, Byrne C et al. Estrogen replacement therapy and breast cancer survival in a large screening study. *J Natl Cancer Inst* 1999; **91**: 264–70.
14. Jernström H, Frenander J, Fernö M, Olsson H. Hormone replacement therapy before breast cancer diagnosis significantly reduces the overall death rate compared with never-use among 984 breast cancer patients. *Br J Cancer* 1999; **80**: 1453–8.
15. Bilimoria MM, Winchester DJ, Sener SF et al. Estrogen replacement therapy and breast cancer: analysis of age of onset and tumor characteristics. *Ann Surg Oncol* 1999; **6**: 200–7.
16. Harding C, Knox WF, Faragher EB et al. Hormone replacement therapy and tumor grade

in breast cancer: prospective study in screening unit. *BMJ* 1996; **312**: 1646–7.

17. Paech K, Webb P, Kuiper GG et al. Differential ligand activation of estrogen receptors ERalpha and ERbeta at AP1 sites. *Science* 1997; **277**: 1508–10.

18. Cavalieri E, Frenkel K, Liehr JG et al. Estrogens as endogenous genotoxic agents: DNA adducts and mutations. In: (Cavalieri E, Rogan E, eds) *JNCI Monograph 27: Estrogens as Endogenous Carcinogens in the Breast and the Prostate.* (Oxford Press: Oxford, 2000) 75–93.

19. Yan Z-J, Roy D. Mutations in DNA polymerase P mRNA of stilbene estrogen-induced kidney tumors in Syrian hamster. *Biochem Molec Biol Int* 1997; **37**: 175–83.

20. Zhu BT, Bui QD, Weisz J. Conversion of estrone to 2- and 4-hydroxyestrone by hamster kidney and liver microsomes: implications for the mechanism of estrogen-induced carcinogenesis. *Endocrinology* 1994; **135**: 1772–9.

21. Pike MC, Spicer DV, Dahmoush L, Press MF. Estrogens, progestogens, normal breast cell proliferation, and breast cancer risk. *Epidemiol Rev* 1993; **15**: 17–35.

22. Russo J, Russo IH. Biological and molecular bases of mammary carcinogenesis. *Lab Invest* 1987; **57**: 112–37.

23. Russo J, Gusterson BA, Rogers AE. Comparative study of human and rat mammary tumorigenesis. *Lab Invest* 1990; **62**: 244–78.

24. Clemons M, Goss P. Estrogen and the risk of breast cancer. *N Engl J Med* 2001; **344**: 276–85.

25. Blankenstein MA, Maitimu-Smeele I, Donker GH et al. On the significance of in situ production of estrogens in human breast cancer tissue. *J Steroid Biochem Molec Biol* 1994; **41**: 891–6.

26. Sigelmann-Danieli N, Buetow KH. Constitutional genetic variation at the human aromatase gene (Cyp19) and breast cancer risk. *Br J Cancer* 1999; **79**: 456–63.

27. Huang CS, Chern HD, Chang KJ et al. Breast cancer risk associated with genotype polymorphism of the estrogen-metabolizing genes CYP17, CYP1A1, and COMT: a multigenic study on cancer susceptibility. *Cancer Res* 1999; **59**: 4870–85.

28. Harada N, Utsumi T, Takagi Y. Tissue-specific expression of the human aromatase cytochrome P-450 gene by alternative use of multiple exons I and promoters, and switching of tissue-specific exons I in carcinogenesis. *Proc Natl Acad Sci USA* 1993; **90**: 11,312–16.

29. Khan SA, Rogers MA, Obando JA, Tamsen A. Estrogen receptor expression of benign breast epithelium and its association with breast cancer. *Cancer Res* 1994; **54**: 993–7.

30. Shoker BS, Jarvis C, Clarke RB et al. Estrogen receptor-positive proliferating cells in the normal and precancerous breast. *Am J Pathol* 1999; **155**: 1811–15.

31. Hall JM, McDonnell DP. The estrogen receptor beta-isoform (ERbeta) of the human estrogen receptor modulates ERalpha transcriptional activity and is a key regulator of the cellular response to estrogens and anti-estrogens. *Endocrinology* 1999; **140**: 5566–78.

32. Speirs V, Parkes AT, Kerin MJ et al. Coexpression of estrogen receptor α and β: poor prognostic factors in human breast cancer? *Cancer Res* 1999; **59**: 525–8.

33. Bolton JL, Pisha E, Zhang F, Qiu S. Role of quinoids in estrogen carcinogenesis. *Chem Res Toxicol* 1998; **11**: 1113–27.

34. Lavigne JA, Helzlsouer KJ, Huang HY et al. An association between the allele coding for a low activity variant of catechol-O-methyltransferase and the risk for breast cancer. *Cancer Res* 1997; **57**: 5493–7.

35. Russo J, Lareef HM, Russo IH. The pathway by which estrogens induce breast cancer. In: (Schneider HPG, ed) *Menopause: The State of the Art – In Research and Management.* (Parthenon: London, 2002) 58–64.

36. Soule HD, Maloney TM, Wolman SR et al. Isolation and characterization of spontaneously immortalized human breast epithelial cell line, MCF-10. *Cancer Res* 1990; **50**: 6075–86.

37. Tait L, Soule H, Russo J. Ultrastructural and immunocytochemical characterizations of an immortalized human breast epithelial cell line MCF-10. *Cancer Res* 1990; **50**: 6087–99.

38. Early Breast Cancer Trialists' Collaborative Group. Tamoxifen for early breast cancer: an overview of the randomised trials. *Lancet* 1998; **351**: 1451–67.

39. Fisher B, Costantino JP, Wickerham DL et al. Tamoxifen for prevention of breast cancer: report of the National Surgical Adjuvant Breast and Bowel Project P-1 Study. *J Natl Cancer Inst* 1998; **90**: 1371–88.

40. Schwartz LB, Snyder J, Horan C et al. The use of transvaginal ultrasound and saline infusion sonohysterography for the evaluation of asymptomatic postmenopausal breast cancer patients on tamoxifen. *Ultrasound Obstet Gynecol* 1998; **11**: 48–53.

41. Cummings SR, Eckert S, Kruger KA et al. The effect of raloxifene on risk of breast cancer in postmenopausal women: results from the MORE randomized trial. *JAMA* 1999; **281**: 2189–97.

42. Dombernowsky P, Smith I, Falkson G et al. Letrozole, a new oral aromatase inhibitor for advanced breast cancer: double-blind randomized trial showing a dose effect and improved efficacy and tolerability compared with megestrol acetate. *J Clin Oncol* 1998; **16**: 453–61.

43. Mouridsen H, Gershanovich M, Sun Y et al. Superior efficacy of letrozole versus tamoxifen as first-line therapy for postmenopausal women with advanced breast cancer: results of a phase III study of the International Letrozole Breast Cancer Group. *J Clin Oncol* 2001; **19**: 2596–606.

44. Buzdar A, Nabholtz JM, Robertson JF et al. Anastrozole (Arimidex) versus tamoxifen as first-line therapy for advanced breast cancer in postmenopausal women – combined analysis from two identically designed multicenter trials.

Proc Am Soc Clin Oncol 2000; **19**: 154a (abstract 609D).

45. Nabholtz JM, Buzdar A, Pollak M et al. Anastrozole is superior to tamoxifen as first-line therapy for advanced breast cancer in postmenopausal women: results of a North American multicenter randomized trial. Arimidex Study Group. *J Clin Oncol* 2000; **18**: 3758–67.

46. Paridaens R, Dirix LY, Beex L et al. Exemestane is active and well tolerated as first-line hormonal therapy of metastatic breast cancer patients: results of a randomized phase II trial. Proceedings of the American Society of Clinical Oncology. *J Clin Oncol* 2000; **19**: 83a (abstract 316).

47. Buzdar A, Douma J, Davidson N et al. Phase III, multicenter, double-blind, randomized study of letrozole, an aromatase inhibitor, for advanced breast cancer versus megestrol acetate. *J Clin Oncol* 2001; **19**: 3357–66.

28

Strategies for the prevention of breast and gynecologic cancer

C Lauritzen

Introduction • Incidences and mortality rates • Basis of prevention • Mammary cancer • Endometrial cancer • Ovarian cancer • Colon cancer • References

'An ounce of prevention is better than a pound of treatment'

INTRODUCTION

The prevention of gynecologic cancers is possible.[1–10,28,45,54,59,63,64,91,93,115] Regrettably, this fact is too little known to lay people and even to the medical profession, and the possibilities of prevention are hardly profitably used in practice. The future will however, without doubt, be dominated by prevention and less by reparative medicine, which is currently in use. The potential of prevention for economical saving is considerable but presently completely unused.

Authoritative cancer researchers[2] claim that up to 70% of all cancerous diseases could be prevented by prophylactic measures and a quarter of expenses of the health service might be saved by prevention, which itself must not be expensive. Much human suffering could also be avoided.

The number of worldwide studies concerning cancer prevention is so considerable that complete comprehension is nearly impossible. A careful selected critical overview of the present knowledge is therefore strongly indicated. Medicine can no longer afford to neglect this important issue.

Ideally, every medical practice should in the future become a center of prevention. This chapter will, corresponding to the scope of this book, deal only with cancers that are dependent on estrogen promotion and respond to hormonal or lifestyle changes, i.e. mammary, ovarian, endometrial and colon cancer. The data given in this chapter are intended to give the therapeut a basis for counseling his/her patients in practice.

INCIDENCES AND MORTALITY RATES

About 10% of all women in Western countries will develop mammary cancer – (20–400 per 100,000, dependent on age and country. The mean incidence for Germany is 126 per 100,000), 6.6% will develop ovarian cancer (2–50, mean of 10 per 100,000); 2.6% will develop endometrial cancer (2–80, mean of 20 per 100,000), 8.5% will develop colon cancer (about 15 per 100,000).[11] The mortality of mammary cancer is about 40 per 100,000, ovarian cancer 8 per 100,000, endometrial cancer about 3 per 100,000 and colon cancer 11 per 100,000).[11]

It is one of the most important tasks of science to characterize beforehand that group of the female population, about 3–10% for each of these cancers, who will be attacked by these cancerous diseases during their lifetime. This knowledge would help us to get a handle on prevention, early diagnosis and early treatment for the benefit of our patients.

BASIS OF PREVENTION

The main risks for mammary, genital and colon cancer are: female sex, familial genetic disposition and increasing age. Carcinogenesis begins with a genetic change within the cell, caused mostly by exogenous harmful carcinogenic substances or by exogenous substances that are metabolized to carcinogens in the organism. This occurs if the multistage guardian system of proto-oncogenes and tumor repressors, DNA repair and the immunologic system are defective.[13,16] Cancer will become manifest when about five or six genetic defects of basic growth regulation have developed.[2,3,13,16,168] Known inborn mutations such as BRCa 1 and 2 account for only 5% of all breast and genital cancer cases.[15]

Certainly, there are more still unknown genetic defects which are causal for carcinogenesis. The carcinogenic process can be promoted by exogenous harmful substances, by lifestyle factors[89,90] and by factors of reproduction. It must also be stressed that cancer appears to be the price to be paid for a modern lifestyle.[14,18,21]

The most important promoting factors for cancerogenesis of breast and genital cancers are being overweight, faulty nutrition,[14,18,21] metabolic syndrome, hormones and other substances that stimulate proliferation and growth, such as insulin-like growth factor (IGF) and epidermal growth factor (EGF).[16,33,70] Moreover ionizing radiation,[17,18,39,68,101] sterility or late first pregnancy,[19,20,32,84] and a refrain from postpartal breast feeding also promote cancer. Prevention must accordingly try to eliminate these promoting factors.

MAMMARY CANCER

The prevention of mammary cancer should eliminate those established risk factors which cause or stimulate the initiation and manifesta-

tion (promotion, progression) of breast cancer (Table 28.1).

Risk profile

It would be ideal if we were able to identify women most at risk for mammary cancer as early as possible, to establish for each person an individual risk profile and to develop, on this basis, an individual program of prevention. This has been attempted (Table 28.2) but not all of the data required are available. The necessary practical experience concerning the real preventive effectivity of the risk concept is still lacking. It should be an aim to solve this problem by research over the coming decades. The following summary will to give the basis of a determination of risk as a model.

Genetic defects

The most important factor for mammary cancer risk is a family history of accumulation of breast, genital and colon cancer. Therefore, the taking of a family history is of utmost importance; a history of cancer in the family is always a relative contraindication for hormone replacement therapy (HRT). Besides the known genetic defects, there are presumably other still unknown genetic anomalies and polymorphisms that are causes of cancerogenesis.[15,27,158] It is to be hoped that markers of such genetic defects can be developed for future practice.

Having a mother with breast cancer raises the relative lifetime risk for this disease 1.4-fold if the disease in the mother or her sister occurred after age 60. If the disease manifested at an earlier age, the relative risk (RR) may increase 9.0-fold. Multiple cases of breast cancer in the family signify a still higher risk.[11] The RR from a multiple familial cancer load is up to 6.8 (Gail model, Table 28.3) and is still higher in combination with other risk factors like late first pregnancy or the number of diagnostic biopsies from the breast.[24] Thus, the age at first delivery becomes relevant only in combination with the number of first-degree relatives with a history of mammary cancer. The risk increases still further if mammary cancer occurred at an early

Table 28.1 Factors which increase the risk of diagnosis of mammary cancer (data from the world literature)	
Risk factor	**Relative risk (RR)**
Family history of cancer (breast, endometrium, ovary, colon)	3.0–4.0
BRCa 1 and 2	8.0
Mammary cancer in first-degree relatives (mother, sister, aunt)	9.0
Mother having breast cancer before the age of 40	3.0
Mother having breast cancer after the age of 60	1.4
Breast cancer in two first-degree relatives	4.0–6.0
Previous breast, endometrial, ovarian or colon cancer	6.0–8.0
Benign proliferative mastopathia	1.6
Atypical proliferative mastopathia	3.0–8.0
Early menarche, late menopause	0.8–1.3
Long-term anovulatory cycles	3.8–5.4
Luteal insufficiency, polycystic ovary syndrome	2.0
Sterility, no completed pregnancy	1.9–4.0
Late first pregnancy (25 years or older)	1.3–3.0
High-calorie diet, overweight	2.0–4.0
Tallness, large breasts	1.4
Diabetes, metabolic syndrome	2.0–4.0
Alcohol, dependent on dose and duration of abuse	1.4–4.4
Nicotine > 10 cigarettes/day, dependent on age and duration of misuse	1.3–1.8
Ionizing radiation (repeated X-ray thorax)	1.5–2.0
Exposure to atomic bomb radiation	3.0
Estrogens > 5 years	0.6–1.0
> 5 years, depending on age and duration	0.8–1.5
Estrogen–progestogen	0.4–2.1

age and was bilateral. If alcohol abuse is added, the risk for an occurrence of mammary cancer is very high.[25–29] These patients should be included in an individual counseling and prevention program. For such patients routine estrogen substitution is relatively contraindicated.

The inherited defect of the genes BRCa 1 and 2 concerns about 5% of the population with breast cancer, led to an 80% probability of manifestation of the disease.[15] At present, in Germany and other European countries, these cases are counseled by an association between gynecologic university hospitals and special consultations.

The carrying out of a preventive mastectomy in such cases is controversial[30] and, in my opinion, not recommended because the result is not absolutely safe and the operation is unnecessary given the good chance of a cure under careful control and early diagnosis. It is an interesting fact that the usual risk factors for breast cancer become less apparent and important under estrogen replacement therapy.[23,31]

Table 28.2   Profile of risk in the form of a breast cancer (BC) score*

Risk	Risk factors	Consequences
Low risk (about 85% of the population)	Healthy, normal weight women without risk factors for BC without conspicuous local findings and with normal mammographies	Estrogen–progestogen substitution, probably without risk, also in long-term medication
Increased risk (about 10% of population)	Family history for BC, genital and colorectal cancer Overweight of abdominal type High calories and fat consumption Underweight (estrogen takers) Metabolic syndrome, diabetes mellitus High alcohol consumption and smoking No deliveries. Late first pregnancy (> 30 years of age) No or too short breastfeeding Reduced physical activity Questionable suspect mammography Tallness Voluminous breasts Early menarche and late menopause	Estrogens–progestogens for treatment of climacteris complaints for 3–5 years If necessary further treatment with phytoestrogens or SERM
High risk (about 2% of population)	Histologically verified proliferative mastopathia Questionable or suspect mammography BC history in family Multiple risk factors Breast biopsies Breast cancer T1–2 N0 M0, no relapse for 5 years Endometrial, ovarian and/or colorectal cancer	If substitution, SERM or phytoestrogens If heavy complaints: estrogens possible, when estrogen-receptor negative
Very high risk (about 3% of population)	Mother and sister BC, especially before 40th year of life and on both sides BRCa-Gen Status after mammary cancer T2 N1 M0 or higher Multiple grave risk factors	SERM or phytoestrogens

* As a basis for assessment of indication and contraindications for a substitution with estrogens–progestogens in the peri–postmenopause (after Scheele et al[85])
In all cases, advise lifestyle counseling, refrain from alcohol and smoking, recommend a healthy diet, including radical scavengers, regular check-ups and mammographies, and observe risk markers.

Table 28.3   Calculation of the relative risk (RR) for breast cancer according to the Gail model[24]

Risk factor		RR
Age at menarche	> 14 years	1.00
	12–13	1–10
	< 12	1.21
	Number of biopsies	
Age < 50 years	no	1.00
	1	1.70
	>2	2.88
Age > 50 years	no	1.00
	1	1.27
	> 2	1.62
Age at first delivery	No. of first-degree relatives with mammary cancer	
Age < 20 years	no	1.0
	1	2.61
	> 2	6.80
Age 20–24 years	no	1.24
	1	2.68
	> 2	5.78
Age 20–29 years	no	1.66
	1	2.76
	> 2	4.91
> 30 years	no	1.93
	1	2.83
	> 2	4.17

The basis of possible preventive measures

Early menarche

The significance of early menarche (RR 0.8–1.3) as a risk factor must be seen in connenction with the period of time from menarche up to the first completed pregnancy. Each year of prolongation of the interval between menarche and first completed pregnancy increases the risk of breast cancer by 4%.[19] A delay of menarche seems theoretically possible, for example, by intensive sports during premenarche in cases of established familial risk. Such a post-poning of menarche is, however, not practically feasible and the risk is relatively small.

Significance of the first full-term pregnancy and sterility

A completed pregnancy before the 25th year of life ensures relative protection against mammary cancer of about 70%.[11,19,22,32,101] Childlessness increases the risk for breast, endometrial and ovarian cancer with a RR of about 2 (1.9–4.0). This RR increases in combination with other risk factors.

In pre- and postmenopausal women who are nulliparous, lobular mammary structures prevail, which are regressive and prone to malignant degeneration (lobular type 1 and 2 of the terminal ductal unit after Russo). These exhibit a higher proliferative activity than the stages lobular type 3 and 4 of parous women. Lobular type 1 has the highest percentage of estrogen receptors and is the site of origin of breast cancer.[22,35]

The increase of risk following treatment for sterility is probably linked to childlessness or late first completed pregnancy. Between the ages of 30 and 40, genetic defects or premalignant stages may already be present. The probability of faulty copies of genes increases with age.

It is apparent that the sociological facts of long education, professional career and late marriage as a cause of late pregnancy can scarcely be influenced. The knowledge of these facts is however very limited in the women concerned. Perhaps awareness of these facts would influence, in a few cases, the decision to accept an early otherwise unwanted pregnancy in cases of a high familial risk for breast cancer, much more so as an induced abortion possibly may increase cancer risk. This last point is however controversial.

Breast feeding and mammary cancer

The American Cancer Society stated, in 1989, that refraining from breastfeeding or breastfeeding for less than 6 months will increase the risk for breast cancer significantly (RR 1.4–2.0). Less importantly, feeding with only one breast will increase the risk of breast cancer.[2,3,19]

If women who feed for less than 3 months would feed for more than 12 months, then their breast cancer risk would decrease by 11%, breastfeeding for 24 months would result in a 25% decrease. The mechanism of this preventive effect of breastfeeding is not completely known. A possibility is full ripening of the epithelium of the breast or a decrease of estrogen receptors in the breast during pregnancy, an influence of placental (hCG, hPrl), inhibin or pituitary hormones (prolactin?)[22,35] and, lastly,

the resting of ovarian ovulatory function during pregnancy and breastfeeding. Transmission of a virus by breastfeeding, like in animal experiments (Bittner's factor), has not been shown for humans.

Therefore, long-term breastfeeding should emphatically be recommended to all women, not only for the health of the child but also because of its preventive effect against breast cancer.

Benign changes in the breast

Less than 10% of women who have benign changes of the breast will develop a mammary cancer in later years (RR 1.6–1.8). Less than 20% of women having breast cancer show a history of a breast biopsy. In cases of mild epithelial hyperplasia, the RR of breast cancer is 2.3–3.6 [confidence interval (CI) 2.0–6.4] and increases to 3.0–8.0 in marked hyperplasia.[11,36,37] HRT does not further increase the risk of mammary cancer in cases of benign changes of the breast.[36,37]

When an atypia has been proven, the surgical extirpation is mandatory. The presence of a familial history of breast, endometrium, ovary or colon cancer, a late first pregnancy or childlessness will increase the risk to RR 11.0. Also, carcinomata in situ are to be extirpated.

Size of the breast

The greater the size of the breast, the greater the risk of mammary cancer.[8,40] The RR in the literature is about 1.2–3.7. For such women the prevention by nutrition and lifestyle, as well as check-ups at regular intervals, is especially important. As mammary cancer occurs in 60% of cases in the upper outer quadrant of the breast, a reduction operation should preferably reduce this quadrant. Tallness of a woman is also a risk factor for mammary cancer, which, of course, cannot be influenced.[43]

Mammographic density

Of 19 studies dealing with this question, 14 came to the conclusion that there is a connection between mammograhic density and breast cancer risk. The RR is estimated to be 2.0.[6,34,216,217] Mammographic density is especially intensive in cases of estrogens plus medroxy-progesterone acetate (MPA) when given combined and continously without interruption. In cases of increased mammographic density, I recommend a lower dose of estrogen and a change of progestogen, preferably to progesterone or the diuretic progestogen drospirenon or to tibolone. A short withdrawal of HRT of about 1–2 weeks before a mammography could, in certain cases, give an improvement in mammographic diagnostics.

Hormones

Oral hormonal contraception

The intake of the contraceptive pill (i.e. the Pill) does not apparently influence breast cancer rates significantly. The RR is estimated to be 1.24 and, therefore, well within bias range. It has been suspected that intake of the Pill in young girls before the first full-term pregnancy could increase the risk for breast cancer after an interval of 25–35 years (RR 1.72). After withdrawal of the Pill the risk will decrease within 5–10 years to a RR of 1.07.[47]

Breast tumors occurring under oral hormonal contraception are usually more localized, do not metastasize and show a better prognosis than control cases.

Young girls, before having been pregnant, should therefore probably use other nonhormonal methods of contraception or should take the Pill only under good indication and not for a long period of time. Probably, however, each method that prolongs the time between menarche and the first full-term pregnancy slightly increases the breast cancer risk. However, as stated above, the prognosis of breast cancer following the intake of oral hormonal contraceptives is relatively favorable. In addition, it should be taken into consideration that the long-term intake of oral hormonal contraceptives decreases the risk of benign breast changes and of endometrium and ovarian cancer, and also for many years after withdrawal of hormones. This is an important fact

to consider when making an overall evaluation. There exists no epidemiologic experience with an aimed prevention of ovarian, endometrial and colorectal cancer by prescribing the Pill in cases at risk for these cancers.

Selective estrogen receptor modulators (SERM)

Estrogen and progesterone receptors are the only known members of the family of steroid receptors that have multiple subtypes. The estrogen receptor (ER) is thought to have protein–protein interactions with the DNA-bound AP-1 complex without having direct contact with DNA itself. This diversity of ER offers unique possibilities for the modulation of estrogen-responsive genes.

While estradiol stimulates alpha and beta ER, most SERM stimulate preponderately ERβ, which prevail in heart and bone and inhibit ERα.

SERM inhibit the stimulatory effects of estradiol at its target organs. Tamoxifen exerts a estrogen-antagonistic effect upon the breast, while it exerts estrogen-agonistic effects upon the endometrium, such that the risk of endometrial cancer increases by its intake. The second-generation SERM, raloxifene and toremifene, are estrogen antagonistic with regard to the breast and endometrium. These second-generation SERM do not stimulate the breast or the endometrium and do not, therefore, provoke uterine bleeding, and will not increase the risk of endometrial and breast cancer. However, they do increase climacteric complaints. Both SERM have estrogen-agonistic effects on lipids and bone metabolism. However, they also slightly increase the risk of phlebothrombosis (3.1%).

Studies have shown that SERM exert a preventive effect upon the incidence of mammary cancer in cases at risk.[1,48,49] The reduction of risk has been shown to be about 65% with 60 and 120 mg raloxifene.[49] In high-risk cases for mammary cancer, preventive treatment with SERM at early postmenopause may thus be indicated. Primary prevention of a breast cancer of the contralateral breast following mammary cancer treatment is also possible. The reduction of risk may amount to –58% by tamoxifen. Similar or even better results can be achieved by aromatase inhibitors (ATAC study).

Apparently, SERM have a similar effect to estrogens on wellbeing. Osteoporosis seems to be prevented by SERM after 1–2 years' use.[49] The effect on lipids, however, seems to be less beneficial than with natural estrogens. Controlled studies concerning the prevention of atherosclerosis and myocardial infarction are still lacking. In animal experiments in cynomolgous monkeys, a preventive action of SERM on atherosclerosis was shown.[50] Whether the designer hormone tibolone may exert an inhibiting effect upon the promotion of breast cancer has to be further investigated. (See The One Million Women Study.)

Phytoestrogens

Phytoestrogens stimulate preponderately ERß. Mammary cancer shows a lower incidence in countries where the consumption of soya containing phytoestrogens, is high.[50–52] The blood levels of phytoestrogens (genistein, daidzein) are low in women with mammary cancer.[51,52] Migration of Japanese women to Hawaii, experiencing a change of environment and an influence of Western nutrition, increased the risk for breast cancer, especially for the second generation immigrants (Table 28.4). This underlines

the importance of environment and lifestyle on cancer risk.

It has been claimed that a high consumption of phytoestrogens may decrease the risk for breast cancer.[51,52] However, so far there is only meager circumstantial epidemiologic evidence for this assumption from observational studies (see Chapter 24).

Oophorectomy

The presence of the ovaries is without doubt partly responsible for the level of incidence of breast cancer by promoting growth of existing cancer cell clones. Premature oophorectomy, performed before the age of 40, is said to afford a 50% reduced risk as compared to normal menopause.[53,83] On the other hand, castration will promote precocious osteoporosis and atherosclerosis. Preventive measures against these diseases, other than estrogen–progestogen, should be considered.

In selected cases of high breast cancer risk, an oophorectomy before occurrence of the natural menopause could be considered, e.g. in cases of premenopausal big and multiple ovarian cysts or cases of ovarian endometriosis. The extent of accessible prevention by early oophorectomy is show in Table 28.5.

The indication for a post-oophorectomy

Table 28.4 Increase of breast, endometrial, ovarial and colorectal cancer		
Localization of cancer	**Incidence per 100,000 women**	
	Japan	**Hawaii**
Esophagus	4.1	0.3
Stomach	40.1	21.8
Colorectal	5.4	18.8
Lung	7.0	7.7
Breast	13.0	44.2
Cervix	13.8	7.6
Endometrium	1.3	15.6
Ovary	2.8	6.9

Decrease of esophagus, cervical cancer and cancer of the stomach in the following generation as consequence of emigration from Japan to Hawaii. These changes in cancer incidences demonstrate the importance of lifestyle, nutrition and environment for carcinogenesis. Incidence standardized for age per 100,000 Japanese and Hawaiian women. (See also Ziegler et al[97]).

Table 28.5 Lifetime breast cancer risk in hysterectomized, oophorectomized women who received a short-term HRT compared to women who received a lifelong HRT[83]

Age at hysterectomy/ oophorectomy (years)	Increase of the lifetime risk for breast cancer (%)	
	Estrogens to the age of 50	Estrogens lifelong
30	0.5	1.2
35	0.7	1.7
40	0.9	2.3
45	1.1	2.7

estrogen substitution would be critical in breast cancer risk cases. Probably, one would not choose mammotropic estrogens like conjugated estrogens and estradiol. An indicated substitution could be tried with SERM or phytoestrogens, and for osteoporosis with calcium, vitamin D and bisphosphonates. However, SERM will not abolish typical climacteric complaints but may instead strengthen them. Therefore, these compounds are best indicated postmenopause or in patients without climacteric complaints. Phytoestrogens are not sufficiently effective against more severe climacteric symptoms but may, as far as is known, be given without disadvantages. Accumulation of further experience is necessary: there is no experience concerning a combination of small doses of estrogens with SERM or phytoestrogens.

Age at menopause

Every year increment in the age of menopause is said to bring an approximately 3% increased risk of mammary cancer.[54,56] This fact could be of importance for an extended indication for oophorectomy in women at risk of mammary cancer.[53] Gonadotropin-releasing hormone (GnRH) medications could, in theory, be given to anticipate the menopause, but would be very expensive.

Exogenous estrogens

Some studies indicate a 1.2–1.4-fold increase in the RR of breast cancer in patients under long-term postmenopausal HRT, and even slightly higher in older women. There was no increase within 5 years of intake.[55–58] Five meta-analyses showed no significant increase in risk, except in a few cases of long-term ERT or HRT. Diagnostic bias of cases and additional alcohol consumption may have exaggerated the risk. Other studies did not find an increase when contraindications and risks were adequately considered and competent individual management and supervision was given.[19,55,59–66]

Lando et al[65] found, in a national representative cohort study of 5761 postmenopausal women (73,253 person-years), 219 mammary cancers. The RR of mammary cancer was 0.8 with no increase in RR over more than 10 years.

Bush,[66] in a meta-analysis of 45 studies of long-term estrogen intake, (all peer-reviewed papers), showed a decreased RR of less than 0.9 in 20% of the studies, no increased risk with a RR between 0.9–1.1 in 47% of the studies and a slight increase with a RR greater than 1.1 in 30% of the studies, all well below a RR of 2.0. In the 20 studies of long-term combined estrogen–progestogen intake (mostly a small number of cases), two studies showed a significant increased risk and three a significant decreased risk. Thus, an estrogen–progestogen substitution (HRT) did not apparently increase breast cancer risk. In all five studies, also dealing with mortality, the death rate was decreased significantly in four cases. All six studies showed a prolonged survival rate and life expectancy, five of them significantly.

Speroff[67] came to the conclusion that an increased breast and ovarian cancer risk had still not conclusively been shown and that a RR in all studies was well within the range of bias.

In this group's study from 1968 to 1992, only 5–15% of the women with mammary cancer took estrogens,[55,64] which means that in about 90% of cases an exogenous medication of estrogens played no role in the promotion of mammary carcinogenesis. Contraindications for ERT are regrettably not always fully investigated and respected, especially concerning a family history of cancer. The strict observation of the contraindication 'history of cancer in the family' is claimed to reduce breast cancer risk by about 5%, and in some cases will postpone the risk to a higher age with the effect that it may not even become clinically manifest.[55,59–64] Autopsy findings in women who died from other causes show that in about 2% of cases an undiagnosed mammary cancer will be found.[68] In another investigation of 90 women who had died from other causes, carcinomata in situ were found in 14% of cases and invasive mammary cancers in 5% of cases.[12] Promotional factors, like an estrogen medication, may stimulate these cancers to clinical appearance.

The possible slight increase in risk of mammary cancer by ERT in some subgroups is offset by the decrease in osteoporotic fractures and the reduced risk for colorectal cancer, and the increased cure rate and decreased mortality in all mammary and genital cancer cases in estrogen-treated women. In the Nurses Health Study, the mortality of mammary cancers was 0.71 (0.56–1.02).

The all-cancer mortality RR was 0.71 (0.62–0.81). Whether the dose of exogenous estrogens plays a role for the promotion of early cancer clones is controversial. In any case, I would recommend prescription of the lowest effective estrogen dose. The duration of estrogen medication, i.e. the total sum of ERT received, is probably of greater importance. Therefore, the decision of whether ERT or HRT is to be continued should be discussed at each check-up, and especially after 5 years of ERT or HRT. Further treatment after about 5 years, when the climacteric symptoms have disappeared, using SERM or phytoestrogens should be considered in high-risk cases.

Selection of the progestogen

Progestins stimulate the cyclin D1 mRNA-expression and lead the mitotic cycle into the S phase.[70,71,72,94] This effect is transient and further application of most progestins will suppress the cyclins, arresting the breast cell division in the G0 or the early G1 phase. Selection of the optimal progestogen is a question of utmost importance if a uterus is present. Ideally, a progestogen should: not increase the cell proliferation of the breast epithelium; not additionally stimulate the promotional effect of estrogens on breast cancer clones; not increase sulfatase activity within the breast (stimulate the production of estrone/estradiol from estrone sulfate); and, of course, not weaken the positive effect of estrogens on lipids and the nitric oxid (NO)-mediated organ perfusion. Progesterone comes nearest to these demands. Some progestogens exert in vitro unwanted mitogenic effects upon the breast epithelium, bind to corticosteroid receptors (such as MPA), show disadvantageous effects upon glucose/insulin metabolism, antagonize the positive effect of estrogens on lipids and organ perfusion, and exert prothrombotic effects. Some progestogens can be metabolically converted to estrogens (e.g. nortestosterones).

In my opinion, only such progestogens should be used in long-term substitution, which will not increase breast cancer risk and will not antagonize the positive effects of estrogens on lipids and organ perfusion. Ideally they should inhibit the interconversion of estrone to estradiol, inhibit the enzymes aromatase and sulfatase in the body, especially within the breast, and should not stimulate the production of the proto-oncogenes c-myc and c-fos, cathepsin D and the relevant growth factors. In this respect there is much basic research to do.

The pharmacogic research will, without doubt, develop products which would selectively modulate the progesterone receptors in order to remove unwanted effects. In some clinical studies (e.g. Magnusson et al,[72] Schairer et al[23]) it was shown that women who received a long-term substitution with estrogens and artificial progestogens postmenopause developed a higher breast cancer incidence than women who received estrogens alone or estrogens and natural progesterone, or closely related compounds. Although these results are not well secured, I recommend, on the basis of these findings and on the grounds of fundamental considerations, the use of natural progesterone, preferably applied near the target organ in vaginal or rectal application, to avoid rapid inactivation during the first liver passage. Such preparations are on the market. The research teams of large pharmaceutic companies have been requested to create a progesterone derivative, that is resorbed from the intestine by the intestinal lymph vessels and is therefore not submitted to the first liver passage, as is the case with the testosterone undecanoate, which circumvents the primary liver passage by lymphatic transport.

Interesting possibilities of local application of progestogens are the intrauterine device, which secretes small amounts of levonorgestrel directly onto the endometrium, leading to atrophy, and local transdermal application of prog-esterone gel over the breasts, causing significant inhibition of mitosis of the breast epithelium.

Prevention of breast cancer by diet

The selection of daily food can apparently exert an inhibiting or a promoting effect on causation and development of cancer.[3,8,9,42,51,52,73–86,88,91–93]

According to Doll and Peto,[2] 35% of cancer mortality may be caused by a poor diet; while Wynder and Gori[89a] estimated mortality of about 40%. Breast cancer would probably be less frequent if all women consumed sufficient amounts of fruit and vegetables, at least five portions per day.[90] Numerous studies in vitro, animal experiments and epidemiologic research recommend a health-promoting diet – low in calories, high in fruit and vegetables, and rich in fibers[5,7–9,73,79,,86–89,91,92] and substances that act as radical scavengers (Table 28.6). In the Western world, currently about 11 g of fibers per day is consumed: according to the guidelines of the US National Cancer Institute intake

---

Table 28.6 Judgment of the Research Group Food, Nutrition and the Prevention of Cancer. World Cancer Research Fund and American Institute of Cancer Research 1997 – the possibilities of prevention of breast cancer, evaluation of the world literature

Evidence	Decreased risk	No influence	Increased risk
Convincing		Coffee	Rapid growth during youth, large adults.
Probable	Fruit, vegetables, fiber substances, carotenoids	Cholesterin in plasma	High BMI, weight increase, alcohol
Probable effect	Physical activity	Monounsaturated fat, polyunsaturated fatty acids, retinol, vitamin E, poultry, black tea	Total fat consumption, saturated animal fats, red meat, caloric hyperalimentation
Insufficient evidence	Vitamin C, isoflavones, lignans, fish	Animal proteins, DDT residues	

should be 30 g per day. The diet should contain ample secondary plant substances and should cover the individual needs of vitamins, minerals and trace elements.[84] Such a diet would have the advantage not only of being preventative toward breast and other cancers, but also offer protection from cardiovascular dieases.

Consumption of fruit and vegetables
Their protective effect for breast cancer has a RR of 0.7–1.0, which is not very impressive.[7,8,73,74,86–89,91,92]

Consumption of fat
The main point of dietary recommendations is the restriction of animal fat and the preference of intake of omega-3 fatty acids, e.g. in fish oil.[76] The ratio of multiple unsaturated fatty acids to saturated fatty acids is 0.20 in the Western world. However, it should be 0.6–1.0. Consumption of fish twice a week is to be recommended. Fat supplies the highest amount of calories per gram of nutrient – 38.9 KJ (9.3 kcal) per gram. In postmenopausal women, fat consumption should not amount to more than 60 g per day, comprising not more than 30% of the total calories.[7,73,76,77,80,81,88–89,91,92]

A high amount of animal fat is thought to play a causal role in the genesis and promotion of breast, endometrial and colon cancer. Animal fat should be substituted by plant fats and oils, as well as by fish oils with a high content of omega-3 fatty acids.[5,8,52,76,80,83,88]

Currently, it is suspected that a high total amount of calories and the preferred intake of hardened fats, including a reduced intake of omega-3 fatty acids, fruit, vegetables and fiber, will result in a moderate increase of the breast cancer risk (RR 1.2–1.8). The increased risk in the higher social classes is apparently dependent on their higher intake of calories and animal fats. The amount of fat intake may also influence the recurrence of cancers and their outcome.[92]

The World Cancer Research Fund[92] came, after evaluation of all the available evidence, to the conclusion that 'a diet rich in total fat will increase the breast cancer risk. A diet rich in multiple unsaturated and plant fats shows in contrast no secure preventive effect on the incidence of breast cancer.' Interventions using adjuvant dietary fat intake reduction have been tried in the management of breast cancer patients;[76] however, success is difficult to prove.

In summary: a high consumption of olive oil (single unsaturated fatty acids) shows a clear preventive effect. A diet rich in fruit, vegetables and fiber decreases the risk of breast cancer. A high-protein diet probably increases the risk, although the preferential consumption of fish probably decreases the risk of breast cancer. Diet counseling is therefore an important part of cancer prevention.

Some studies did not find an association of fat consumption and breast cancer risk. However, they only accounted for the fat intake in old age, not in childhood, adolescence and maturity.

In which stage of carcinogenesis will the prevention of breast cancer by diet be effective?

Initiation
Most hints concerning connections between nutrition and cancer point to the phase of initiation of cancer on the basis of a primary influence of cancer-generating substances (carcinogens). The most susceptible phase for pre-neoplastic and neoplastic processes is still the undifferentiated lobulus I stage of the terminal ducts of the breast epithelium during adolescence and early maturity.[22,35,46,93] Normally, tumor-suppressor genes (p 21, p 53, BRCa, FRB, MTS), proto-oncogenes and the sentinel substances in the cell cycle will signal genetically defective cells, and induce DNA repair and apoptosis. Thus, normally tumor-suppressor genes, signal transmitters and the immune system exert a controling influence upon the further development of precancerous cells and the first cancer clones, and will mostly induce their destruction, at least if the harmful substances and the radical influence is not too massive. A disordered proliferation is only possible if genetic mutations have taken place in this multiple system of protection.[11,13,15] Radical scavengers in the diet prevent the occurrence of

oxidative cell damage. How this damage becomes manifest will depend on the specific function of the tissue concerned. If all guardian and regulating factors fail, the process will move into the second phase.

Promotion

In this second phase of cancer development, increased mitotic activity of the cancer clones begins, including the passing on of faulty information. Their growth will be stimulated by hormones like insulin, IGF, estrogens and some artificial progestogens. Also during this phase of carcinogenesis the organism still has the possibility to inhibit further development of cancer, when the influence of promotors is blocked by tumor suppressors and immunologic mechanisms.

Progression

In this phase the initiated and promoted cancer cells will be stimulated, largely uncontrollably, promoting factors to accelerate their cell doubling rate and growth. This stage can no longer be controlled by the body's other defense mechanisms such as diet or bioactive inhibitors. Only selective receptor modulators or receptor blockers can exert a partial effective inhibiting and dilatory influence upon further development of the established cancer.

Alcohol

Abuse of alcohol apparently plays a causal role for the genesis of breast, endometrium and colon cancer.[25–29,41,95,96,99,214,221] According to a meta-analysis of 50 epidemiologic studies, alcohol intake is a dose-dependent causal factor for the risk of developing breast cancer.[25,41,95,98] Alcohol is a strong generator of radicals, a cell poison and a metabolic carcinogen (Table 28.7). According to Colditz et al,[58] only women under ERT who consume alcohol show an increased risk for breast cancer (RR 2.5): the relative risk for ERT alone was 1.3–1.7. That is, after those women who consume alcohol were removed from consideration, Colditz et al[58] concluded that ERT did not increase the risk of breast cancer (RR 0.99).

Zumoff[99] also suggested that an increased risk of breast cancer is only seen among HRT users who drink alcohol. Women who postmenopausally take estrogens also appear to consume more alcohol.[100,100a]

The breast cancer risk caused by alcohol is especially high in young girls and young women (RR 2.6), and decreases after the age of 35 to a RR of 1.8.[41,95,96] This fact underlines the importance of prevention in early life. To reduce the risk of breast cancer significantly, alcohol abuse should therefore be suspended at young ages.[41,95,96] The literature contains six apparently reliable prospective studies concerning alcohol and breast cancer showing clear connections. A meta-analysis of 30 epidemiologic studies yielded the result that even one drink per day will increase the risk for breast cancer. The increase is linear, dependent on the increase of the dose of alcohol consumed.[96]

Alcohol intervenes with the metabolism of estrogens, increasing the blood level of estradiol by up to 300%,[26] but not in all individuals. Genetic factors such as polymorphism of the cytochrome P-450c-17-alpha gen (CYP 17) may therefore play a role.

Misuse of alcohol is defined as a regular consumption of more than 5 g/day. This dose is the starting point for the increase of breast cancer risk in most studies.[41,95,96] Women who take estrogens consume more alcohol per day than comparable controls: this as shown by Colditz et al.[58] Gapstur et al[25] and the IOWA Women's Health Study[29,53] have repeatedly drawn attention to the importance of alcohol consumption for the causation of mammary cancer. Their RR for breast cancer was 1.88 (CI 1.30–2.72) in consumers of alcohol. Studies on estrogens and breast cancer risk which do not record alcohol consumption, and thus do not extract or separate these patients from the RR data of other patients, will probably calculate overall risks that are too high.

Of most interest is the finding that the substitution of sufficient doses of folic acid reduces the risk for breast cancer caused by alcohol.[98] If this is confirmed, it may allow insight into the mechanism of carcinogenesis caused by alcohol.

Table 28.7   Cohort studies concerning the influence of alcohol consumption upon the relative risk (RR) of breast cancer [RR (95% CI) in relation to the daily alcohol consumption]

Studies	Nondrinking women	5–< 15 g $n = 727$	15–< 30 g $n = 360$	30–60 g $n = 194$	> 60 g $n = 30$	P trend
Canadian	1.0	0.94	1.39	1.89	0.96	0.23
National Breast Screening Study		(0.64–1.37)	(0.90–2.13)	(1.02–3.49)	(0.37–2.50)	
IOWA Women's Health Study		0.97 (0.73–1.29)	1.37 (0.94–1.98)	1.74 (1.12–2.70)	1.74 (0.49–6.15)	0.007
The Netherlands Cohort Study		1.28 (0.90–1.83)	1.20 (0.76–1.91)	1.79 (0.93–3.45)	0.89 (0.11–8.83)	0.27
New York State Cohort		0.93 (0.63–1.38)	0.69 (0.39–1.21)	1.28 (0.63–1.76)	4.16 (0.71–24.39)	0.53
Nurses' Health Study 1988		1.12 (0.93–1.35)	1.34 (1.07–1.68)	1.29 (0.95–1.76)	0.94 (0.44–2.01)	0.02
Nurses' Health Study 1995		1.01 (0.81–1.25)	0.95 (0.75–1.26)	1.20 (0.85–1.70)	1.64 (0.76–3.43)	0.23
Sweden Mammography Cohort		1.13	1.03	Not investigated	0.23	
TOTAL		1.06 (0.96–1.17)	1.16 (0.98–1.38)	1.41 (1.18–1.69)	1.31 (0.85–1.98)	< 0.001

Multivariate RR: adjusted for age at menarche, age at first delivery, menopause, oral hormonal contraceptives, estrogen substitution, benign breast diseases, family history, breast cancer, smoking, education, BMI, consumption of fiber, intake of calories. See refs 25,95,96,214,221.

Smoking

In the past, a decrease of breast cancer risk by heavy smoking was suspected. This finding was attributed to a decrease in estrogen levels caused by smoking via induction of estrogen-metabolizing enzymes in the liver. Later, the generation of noxious radicals and the direct carcinogenic effect of smoking was demonstrated. Palmer et al,[44] in a meta-analysis of all then available studies, concluded that smoking more than 10 cigarettes per day will increase the risk of breast cancer (RR 1.3). Alcohol combined with smoking increases the risk further.[41,103] The carcinogenic effect is especially high during postpuberty, ado-lescence and early sexual maturity, i.e. in phases of high rates of mitosis of the epithelium of the breast and before the first pregnancy. Young women who smoke more than 25 cigarettes per day before the age of 16 have an increased breast cancer risk of RR 2.8.[41,44]

Xenoestrogens

These are artificial substances that bind to ER and exert strong proliferative effects (xenopro-liferines). They mostly exert direct mutagenic and carcinogenic effects. They cause, for instance, mutation of the p53 gene, and damage to tumor repressors, cyclins and sentinel proteins. They have a clear influence upon the causation and development of breast and other cancers. Their avoidance is difficult because they are found in food (e.g. mykestrogens) and drinking water. Their reduction would be possible only by general hygienic and environmental measures, enforced by a general and firm political intent.

Residues of DDT, DDE and their metabolites in food most likely increase the risk for cancer, including breast cancer. They have been found in increased concentrations in the breast tissue of women with mammary cancer (Table 28.8).

The concentration of these harmful substances in food and the environment is fortunately decreasing. These substances are however stored in the breast and some glandular tissues. Their avoidance seems possible by a preference of indigenous, home-made bioproducts.

Ionizing radiation and electromagnetic fields

Surviving persons from the atomic bomb radiation in Hiroshima showed an increased risk of mammary cancer when at the time of radiation exposure they were between the ages of 4 and 40. Radiation doses higher than 0.5 Gray will increase the breast cancer risk.[20,39,68] The age at the time of radiation exposure is significant. At 10–14 years of age the breast cancer risk in the doses stated amounted to a RR of 4.46, between the ages 15 and 24 the RR is 1.77, in women older than 35 years of age it is 1.1 and no longer to be discriminated from the risk of controls without radiation. The breast cancer will become manifest 25–34 years after the radiation load. In girls suffering from morbus Hodgkin or tuberculosis, which included radiation in the breast area, the RR was 4.1.[68] Doses used in radiodiagnostics and radiotherapy today will be associated with little, if any, increased risk, except perhaps in young girls.

Whether exposure to electromagnetic fields will increase the risk for breast cancer is controversial. Loomis[106] found an increase of 1.4–2.2. Further results must be awaited.

Weight, weight increase and decrease

A high body weight during youth, maturity and in the pre- and postmenopause, e.g. a high Quetelet's Index or a Body Mass Index (BMI) of

Table 28.8 Level of carcinogenic organic polychlorides in normal breast tissue, in cancerous breast tissue, in surrounding tissue and in fat tissue of the breast (ng/g tissue)[235,236]

	Carcinogens in tissue from cancerous breasts		
	Cancer tissue	Surrounding tissue	Fat tissue
pp DDT	4.39	1.42	0.75
	CI 1.3–6.4	CI 0.3–2.8	CI 0.1–1.4
Total PCB	9.1	2.7	0.9
	CI (4.3–14.2)	CI 1.3–4.2	CI 0.2–1.4

	Carcinogens in fat tissue from cancerous and normal breasts		
	Cancer tissue		Controls
	ER positive	ER negative	(normal breast tissue)
DDE	2132±2,050	609±339	765±527
Total PCB	405±131	332±75	397±162

more than 28, brings an increased risk for benign breast changes[42,43] and breast cancer.[3,8,9,85] The risk is even higher in women who were slim earlier and adipous at the time of diagnosis of the breast cancer. Prevention of adiposis during adolescence will reduce mammary cancer incidence during postmenopause.[23] Especially risky is the fat distribution of the androgenic type (abdomino-visceral fat). The prognosis of mammay cancer worsens with increasing body weight, and therefore can be improved by weight reduction.[7,28]

However, if women receive ERT, being underweight seems to increase the breast cancer risk.[22] With respect to the small body volume of such women, the usual estrogen doses probably mean an overdosage. The estrogen metabolism of slim women moreover deviates from that of women of normal weight.

Prevention by physical activity: sport

A decrease in the risk for breast and genital cancer in female athletes in comparision to controls was shown by Frisch et al.[107] Physical activity, apparently by reduction of weight and by positive influences on the levels of glucose/insulin and on energy metabolism, decreases the risk for breast cancer by up to 80%.[7,107–109] Also, the prevention of internal and orthopedic postmenopausal diseases by physical activity is considerable.

Prevention by vitamins

Constant protection against free radicals is necessary, since the organism is continuously exposed to their detrimental effect, which may induce cell changes, aging and cancer. Scavengers of radicals are among other substances in food, some vitamins, mainly ascorbic acid (vitamin C) and vitamin E. Obviously, an unhealthy lifestyle, including an insufficient amount of radical scavengers, is corrected by an intelligent selection of food and positive lifestyle changes rather than by an intake of medicaments or vitamin preparations.[75,77,79,92]

The separate discussion of singular vitamins is essentially artificial, as vitamins act best in combination and within their natural environment, together with the other secondary substances in natural food.

However, it is a fact that the vitamin supply of many older people is deficient. On the other hand, the amounts of vitamins which must be taken for certain suggested pharmacologic effects are not accessible by food selection only.

Vitamin A
The supply of vitamin A (200–1200 IE/day) seems to exert a certain protection against breast cancer. In any case, the Nurses' Health Study showed a moderate protective effect (RR 0.8). A similar protective effect resulted from a cohort study from New York and from Canada (RR 0.8). β-Carotene (provitamin A) seems to exert similar beneficial effects on breast and colon cancer. Retinoids (vitamin A analogs) exhibit a clear chemopreventive effect against mammary cancer.[8]

Folic acid
The supply of folic acid in a daily amount of 0.4 mg/day seems (as stated in the Alcohol section above) to inhibit the carcinogenic effect of alcohol.[98] Women in Europe consume, on average, only 0.2 mg/day of folic acid. In addition to the above, folic acid also exhibits a beneficial effect in the prevention and treatment of cervical dysplasia.

Vitamin C
Ascorbic acid is a strong scavenger of free radicals, especially together with vitamin E. The preventive effect of ascorbic acid is categorized as 'possible' by the World Cancer Research Fund[8,79,92] when 1000 mg/day of ascorbic acid is taken. The breast cancer risk between the highest and lowest quintiles of ascorbic acid levels in plasma is 0.69. An intake of ascorbic acid-rich fruit and vegetables to an amount equivalent to 380 mg/day was calculated to result in a risk reduction of 16% for mammary cancers.[92]

Vitamin D
A deficiency of vitamin D is a risk factor for the development of mammary cancer in rodents. Vitamin D inhibits the growth of breast cancer

cells in vitro. In clinical studies, however, a preventive effect of vitamin D could not be shown up to doses of 0.01 mg/day. However, vitamin D receptor-positive breast cancer patient show a longer disease-free interval. The presence of vitamin D receptors is therefore a positive prognostic factor for breast cancer. Palliative effects using very high doses of vitamin D in advanced breast cancer cases have been described.[21,79]

Vitamin E

Vitamin E is a strong antioxidant. The results of preventive studies using 800–1200 IE/day are controversial. Some show a protective effect, others not. In the Nurses' Health Study the protective effect of vitamin E disappeared if a correction for vitamin A levels was performed.[75,92]

Recommendations for the primary prevention of breast cancer

If the risk factors listed cause or promote mammary carcinogenesis, then the avoidance of these factors should prevent the genesis of breast cancer. Modification of lifestyle may be the most important point for prevention. Prevention apparently is most effective in phases of high proliferative activity of the breast epithelium, as in puberty and adolescence.[62,110] Therefore, young girls should refrain from alcohol and smoking. Normal body weight should be maintained and weight increase avoided. A diet rich in fruit, legumes and vitamins should be recommended, eventually with an addition of a vitamin/mineral/trace element preparation.

Physical activity should be regularly maintained. Ionizing radiation should be kept to a minimum, especially in breast and abdominal areas. The importance of early pregnancy and of having more children should be made known to every young woman, although it seems questionable whether a change of reproductive behavior can, or should, be achieved. The use of HRT should be carefully indicated. Low doses of estrogens and a suitable progestogen, not stimulating breast epithelium growth, should be selected.

Of all the contraindications for HRT, a family history of cancer and the presence of cancer risk factors should be respected and regarded as relative or absolute contraindications according to a competent treatment.

After 5 years' perimenopausal HRT and after disappearance of climacteric complaints, the use of SERM, phytoestrogens or designer hormones, not stimulating the endometrium and breasts, should be considered, if indicated. Clinical research should collect experiences concerning the combination of small doses of natural estrogens with SERM, phytoestrogens or designer hormones. In late postmenopausal women, if an indication for treatment is given, an organ-near and organ-specific application of hormones should be preferentially used, e.g. progesterone gel applied to the breast or vagina or progestogen directly to the endometrium.

ENDOMETRIAL CANCER

Basic facts

Endometrial cancer is the second most common gynecologic cancer. In Western countries, the cumulative incidence rates range from 1 to 2% (10.9 per 100,000) up to 75 years of age. The standard mortality rate is declining in most countries down to 3.0 per 100,000. Endometrial cancer has a favorable clinical outcome, the 5-year survival rate being 76%. The cure rate is even higher in women who develop endometrial cancer during estrogen intake (95%).[11,111,112]

Estrogens stimulate the proliferation and angiogenesis of the endometrium. This effect is mediated by production of ER and by growth factors and cytokines, which can act in a juxtacrine, paracrine and autocrine fashion, from and upon epithelial cells and the extracellular matrix.[13,70]

Risk factors

The principal risk factors for endometrial cancer relate to reproductive function and reproductive history. Observations on familial aggregation of genital and mammary cancer show that the disease has an important genetic component. The risk profile is almost identical to that of mammary cancer.[11]

The incidence of endometrial cancer begins to increase at about 40 years of age, rising to a maximum at about 65–70 years of age.[113–116]

Estrogens

Endometriotropic estrogens, by their effect on endometrial growth factors,[117] can promote endometrial cancer by enhanced proliferative stimulation of the endometrial cells. Such a one-sided effect will, after some months, result in hyperplasia and, in some cases, neoplasia if the counteraction by progesterone is missing after repeatedly prolonged (more than 14 days) stimulation for many months or years.

Estrogen monotherapy has not been used in Europe as frequently as in the US. In Europe, early in the introduction of estrogen substitution, progestogen is also added.

Endogenous or exogenous estrogens are partly causal for the so-called type I estrogen-related endometrial carcinoma.[113] Some endometrial cancers can however arise from an atrophic endometrium (type II).[114]

Endogenous estrogens

The endometrium is controlled by ovarian estrogens and progesterone. Anomalies of the normal biphasic ovarian regulation, as during the perimenopause, will show up in histopathology of this target organ and in uterine bleeding anomalies. In addition, the endometrium is an endocrine gland with its own prodution and metabolism of active substances. Postmenopause, residual endogenous estrogen production, mostly derived from aromatization of androgens, influences endometrial histology and endometrial thickness. Low estrogen levels will leave the endometrium atrophic. Endogenous estrogen production leading to significant estradiol levels will, in due course, cause endometrial hyperplasia and, in some especially predisposed cases, cause endometrial cancer.

The polycystic ovary syndrome is characterized in most cases by a protracted production of

significant amounts of estrogens, a loss of ovulation and of progesterone production, and an increase of ovarian androgens. Newer investigations have shown that the metabolic syndrome hyperinsulinemia and a decrease in insulin sensivity plays a central role in the genesis of this disease. Estrogen-producing ovarian tumors (estroblastomata, granulosa cell tumors) are associated with an increased risk for endometrial cancer.[118,119]

Exogenous hormones

Contraceptive pill

The use of the contraceptive estrogen–progestogen combined contraceptive pill has been shown to reduce endometrial cancer risk by about 40–50%. This risk reduction persists for years or even decades after discontinuation of the Pill. The addition of an effective progestogen, causing endometrial secretion and stopping proliferation during the 3 or 4 weeks of estrogen medication, is probably responsible for the preventive effect. Sequential treatment, using a weak progestogen for 7 days, weakly increased the incidence of endometrial cancer.[46,47,123,124] Therefore, medication of a potent progestogen for at least 12 days per month is necessary.

HRT

A duration-dependent increase of the incidence of hyperplasia and endometrial cancer is documented for women taking estrogens only (unopposed estrogens). The RR increased up to eightfold in Europe when high doses and a long-term substitution was given. Predominantly early, well-differentiated tumors, most of them noninvasive, resulted.[113,115,116,120–145]

The histologic differentiation between endometrial cancer and the pre-stages may be difficult in some cases. Experts do not always agree on the diagnosis of malignancy.[146,147] Unopposed estrogen medication played no role in Europe (as in the US) since mostly a sequential estrogen–progestogen medication for more than 10 days was given. The addition of a potent progestogen for more than 10 days, optimal 14 days or more, will reduce the risk to null, and possibly to even lower RR, depending on the strength of the progestogen and the duration of medication.[132,135,140,143–145,148,148a,149] In some studies,[138,140,142] the RR went down to 0.2–0.4, especially with a continuous low-dose combined HRT.[148–150]

Thus, an appropriate progestin, used for most days of a cycle, may exert nearly complete protection against endometrial cancer. The cure rate of and survival from endometrial cancer is improved in patients under ERT or HRT.[126,127,132,134–143,145,148,151–153]

In some cases of reduced tolerance to progestogens, a progestogen medication for 12–14 days every 3 months,[154–157] or according to ultrasonic measurement of the endometrial thickness (> 8 mm) was tried. This procedure may be an alternative for a short time. However, the question of effective prevention of endometrial cancer when using an additional progestogens medication every 3 months only is controversial.[155–157]

Tamoxifen has been classified as an endometrial carcinogen, as it increases the incidence of endometrial cancer. It apparently exerts a selective estrogen-antagonistic effect on the breast and an agonistic estrogenic effect on the endometrium.[158–160] This endometrial effect seems to be missing with raloxifen[160] and with some designer estrogens, perhaps including tibolone and 17α-estradiol.

Parity
There is an inverse relationship between parity and endometrial cancer risk. Sterility and nulliparity will cause an increased risk, especially when caused by long-standing anovulatory sterility, i.e. by long-term loss of the progestative phases.[11,113–115]

Age at menopause
An early menarche and a late menopause are markers for a premenopausal prolonged period of exposure to estrogens unopposed by progesterone. Such a one-sided estrogen effect will result in endometrial overstimulation. The influence of early menarche is controversial and must be viewed in connection with age at first pregnancy. However, females who experience menopause after the age of 50 have about a 2.5 times higher risk for endometrial cancer than females whose menopause occurs before the age of 50.[11,113]

Overweight
Adult obesity is a consistently reported risk factor, especially the androgenic type of obesity. Extreme obesity may increase the risk of endometrial cancer up to 10-fold. [11,114,115,161,162,222] It has been hypothesized that the factor behind this increased risk is the aromatization of androgens to estrogens in the peripheral fat tissue. However, much more important is an apparently disturbed insulin/glucose metabolism (metabolic syndrome).[11]

Diabetes
Noninsulin-dependent diabetes mellitus (Type 2) has been shown to be an independent risk factor for endometrial cancer. This relationship is independent of the BMI insulin, glucose and IGF-1 are basic for the proliferation of the breast epithelium and for many growth and proliferative actions (IGF binds to insulin receptors). In addition, in such cases, often elevated androgens and lowered sex hormone-binding globulin (SHBG) levels are found.[11,113–115,132]

Hypertension
Hypertension is not an independent risk factor. Data from recent studies indicate that hypertension is caused by a metabolic syndrome, which is associated with an increased endometrial cancer risk.[11,132]

Alcohol
As in mammary cancer, alcohol consumption (> 5 g/day) increases the risk for the occurrence of endometrial cancer to a RR of about 1.5.[163]

Smoking
Some studies seem to show that cigarette smoking may reduce the risk of endometrial cancer by upregulating the estrogen-metabolizing liver enzymes, resulting in reduced estrogen levels and an early menopause. Of course, smoking cannot be recommended as a measure to prevent endometrial cancer in the small group of

women at risk because of its many carcinogenic and disadvantageous cardiovascular effects.[11]

Recommendations for the primary prevention of endometrial cancer

Treatment of cycle disturbances caused by anovulation should be carefully performed by medication of progesterone in the second 14 days of a cycle. The risk of nulliparity and late first pregnancy should be brought to the attention of the female population, especially women most at risk.

Early treatment of sterility, avoiding obesity, and early treatment of metabolic syndrome and diabetes are all advisable. Restriction of calories, preference of fruit and legumes, a diet rich in vitamins, trace elements and minerals, physical activity and maintainance of normal body weight is to be recommended. An important benefit of oral hormonal contraceptives is the long-lasting reduced risk for endometrial, ovarian and colorectal cancer. In selected cases, long-term estrogen–progestogen combined oral contraception should be discussed in terms of reducing endometrial cancer risk for many years. The optimal progestogen to be added to the estrogen for the optimal time in post-menopausal women reducing endometrial cancer without exerting unfavorable metabolic effects, must still be exactly ascertained. Tubal ligation, which has been shown to reduce endometrial cancer risk, and hysterectomy are to be considered in high-risk cases when an additional indication is given. A SERM like raloxifen, phytoestrogens and (partly) tibolone will not stimulate endometrial growth.

OVARIAN CANCER

Ovarian cancer is the fifth most common cancer (6.6%) and one of the most frequent genital cancers in women. In Western societies 1.0–1.4% of women will develop this disease. The incidence rates are highest in affluent Western societies and lowest (but fastest growing) in Asian countries. The age-standardized mortality rate is 7.0–15.3 per 100,000. Death from ovarian cancer is the most common fatal cancer in the Western world[195] and the fourth leading cause of death in Germany.[11,164] Most cases are still diagnosed too late at an advanced stage.

The ER and progesterone receptors, which are found in 30–70% of ovarian cancers, are probably inactive. Therefore, ovarian cancer is not really an estrogen-dependent or even a hormone-dependent tumor.[165] Accordingly, clinical course, prognosis, rate of remission and occurrence of relapse are not influenced by receptor status, and the outcome is not significantly influenced by an endocrine treatment with estrogens, progestogens, anti-estrogens, androgens and luteinizing hormone releasing hormone (LHRH) analogs.[164] Also, luteinizing hormone (LH), hCG and androgen receptors have been found, and are apparently without clinical importance in the therapy of the disease. Treatment with high doses of progestogens results in a remission rate of 7%; for tamoxifen it is 11%. Androgens are ineffective. GnRH analogs cause a remission rate of between 0 and 10% (German Cancer Society: Frauenarzt 41,2000,999).

Etiologic hypotheses

The strongest correlated factor is genetically determined risk.[11,165] Regarding the mechanism of ovarian carcinogenesis, there are three hypotheses under discussion.

1. *Incessant ovulation*: it is suggested that each ovulation traumatizes the ovarian epithelium and that the healing process entails increased mitotic activity and an increased likelihood for entrapment of epithelial cells in the ovarian stroma, which is rich in growth factors.[11] It has been shown that a high number of ovulations may be associated with increased amounts of of proliferation of ovarian epithelium, associated DNA damage and an increased overexpression of p53.[166]

2. The high postmenopausal gonadotropin levels could increase ovarian cancer risk by stimulating the mitotic activity of the ovarian epithelium,[1,164,167] thus increasing the statistical risk of mutations by exogenous

harmful substances or of faulty gene copies promoted by increasing age.

3. Newer hypotheses suggest that retrograde menstruations may carry carcinogens or endometrial growth factors to the ovaries,[168] that estrogens may exert direct stimulatory effects upon the ovarian epithelium and that, on the other hand, progesterone may clear away premalignant cells, induce apoptosis and reduce ER and epithelial proliferation.[11,169] Furthermore, influences of sexual hormones on growth factors like IGF and EGF in the ovarian epithelium must be considered.[164]

Risk factors

Genetic factors

Familial and genetic factors play a prominent role concerning the incidence of ovarian cancer.[166] Patients showing a familial history of mammary, genital and/or colorectal cancer exhibit an increased risk for ovarian cancer.[11,164,165,168]

Reproduction

Some studies found a small increase in risk of ovarian cancer with early menarche, others did not.[171] A role of androgens and of missing progesterone was discussed.[167] An increase in cases of late menopause was suspected in retrospective studies, but this was not confirmed in cohort studies.[11,169,171]

A popular hypothesis, although of weak evidence, is that the number of ovulations during a lifetime is related to ovarian cancer risk. Married women, whose number of ovulations may be reduced by pregnancies and lactation, exhibit a lower risk for this disease.[11]

Parity and lactation

This would fit the supposition of the significance of parity, age at first pregnancy and lactation, as all lead to a reduction of risk for ovarian cancer. The preventive effect of a full-term pregnancy is well documented. Parous women have a 30–70% lower risk of developing ovarian cancer than nulliparous women.[164,172,174,178a]

Lactation, especially of long duration, may bring an additional protective effect. The hypothesis also fits well with the protective effect of the inhibition of ovulation by oral hormonal contraception.[11,172]

Tubal ligation and hysterectomy

These operative procedures may partly protect against ovarian cancer. It has been suggested that ovarian perfusion and hormone production may be compromised by these operations, or that the number of ovulations is reduced.[11]

Exogenous hormones

Combined oral contraceptives

These effect a substantial and long-lasting reduction of ovarian cancer incidence. Protection is registered after only a few years of intake, regardless of age at diagnosis. Prevention has not clearly been shown for special types of tumors, such as borderline and mucinous ovarian tumors. A meta-analysis of available studies has revealed that a 5-year intake of the combined pill will be associated with a 50% reduced risk of ovarian cancer, persisting for at least 10–15 years after withdrawal of the hormones.[11,175] The mechanism of reduction of ovarian cancers by estrogen–progestogen substitution is thought to be suppression of ovulation, reduction of gonadotropin levels and the induction of apoptosis by progestogens.

Estrogen replacement

As concerns studies on the influence of hormone substitution upon the incidence of ovarian hormones, unopposed estrogen (ERT) and estrogen–progestogen substitution (HRT) must be considered separately.

Rodriguez et al,[176] in a prospective cohort study using questionnaires, found a basal incidence of 26.4 ovarian cancer cases per 100,000 women and of 36.4 for earlier estrogen takers. The incidence of actual ERT users was 64.4 per 100,000 women. The RR for mortality during ERT was 1.51 (1.16–1.96), increasing to 2.2 (1.53–3.17) after more than 10 years' medication.

However Coughlin[177] in a meta-analysis of 15

case control studies of ERT detected no increase in RR. Carg,[171] in a survey of the literature from 1966 to 1977, found a slight, but not significant, increase following ERT after more than 10 years [RR 1.27 (1.0–1.61)].

As concerns estrogen–progestogen substitution (HRT), Persson et al,[169] in a Swedish study of 22,597 participants, could not find any correlation to HRT [RR 0.9 (0.8–1.1)]. Also, Purdie et al,[178] in a case control study with 793 cases of epithelial ovarian cancer and 855 controls, came to the conclusion that there was no association between HRT and ovarian cancer. However, they found a slightly increased risk of endometrioid and clear-cell cancer of the ovaries in unopposed ERT.

Thus, most studies show no significant influence of HRT on ovarian cancer incidence under ERT and HRT.[170–172,174,178–180,195a] In a recent meta-analysis, nine epidemiologic studies were analyzed.[190] Two showed an increased risk of about 70% after more than 10 years' estrogen medication, while the remaining seven showed a non-significant reduction or no change of risk. Thus, it is uncertain whether a risk or a preventative effect of estrogen medication exists concerning postmenopausal ERT and HRT. Sequential and especially combined estrogen–progestogen medication, given over a long period of the postmenopause, may reduce the risk of ovarian cancer.[60] ERT and HRT after treated ovarian cancer seems not to increase the risk of a relapse.[181]

Treatment of sterility

Studies conducted in the US suggest an increase in ovarian cancer in women exposed to ovulation-inducing drugs. This is particularly the case when no subsequent pregancy and birth results. Three investigations of younger women who received in vitro fertilizations with the usual stimulation protocol found no effect on ovarian cancer risk.[167,176,178,182,183] Probably, the increased risk found in some studies is a consequence of childlessness or of a late first pregnancy. In any case, infertile patients having received fertility drugs show a similar risk for ovarian cancer as do untreated infertile women.

Dietary factors

Three of four studies reviewed by Block et al [184] demonstrated a preventive effect of the consumption of fruit and vegables and a 1.8-fold increased risk associated with a low dietary intake of fruit and vegetables.

Adipositas

Overweight during youth and postmenopause is a risk factor for ovarian cancer.[170]

Alcohol

Consumption of high amounts of alcohol (> 15g/day) may slightly increase the risk of ovarian cancer.[177]

Recommendations for primary prevention of ovarian cancer

Patients with a family history of genital, breast and/or colon cancer are also at higher risk of ovarian cancer development. Thus, in such cases special considerations for prevention and early diagnosis are necessary.

The most important preventive factor is pregnancy, especially a young age at first pregnancy. The use of oral hormonal contraceptives is clearly preventive for epithelian ovarian cancer. Both factors should be considered in counseling patients at risk. Recent research suggests that the type and the estrogen–progestogen content of HRT plays a role in ovarian cancer risk. An early beginning and a protracted use of an estrogen with a potent progestogen in sequential, or better in combined, form may reduce postmenopausal risk of ovarian cancer.[59,60] The optimal combination, probably with a strong inhibiting effect on gonadotropins and stimulation of apoptosis, has still to be found. A high consumption of fruit and vegetables, as well as physical activity, may lead to a decreased risk. Alcohol consumption should be dissuaded. The early diagnosis of ovarian cancer is an important unsolved problem. Its determination by ultrasonography and tumor markers must be further improved.[185]

COLON CANCER

Worldwide, this is the second most frequent cancer in women: the cumulative incidence rate varies between 3.1 and 6.7%, or 27.9 per 100,000 for females in Germany (19,000 cases per year). In the last decades an increased incidence has been observed. The mortality has, however, been decreasing – 15.3 per 100,000.[11,186–188]

Risk factors

An adenomatous polyposis predisposes for colon cancer. Such multiple intestinal polyps progress in 60–70% of cases to cancer. Familial inherited mutations in the DNA repair and the APC genes account for 1–5% of all colon cancers. A familial adenomatous polyposis accounts for 60–70% of all colorectal tumors. Five to six genetic mutations must happen before colon cancer becomes manifest.[11,188,189]

Sex

The incidence of colon cancer is equal in men and women up to the age of 50. At higher ages women show a lower incidence of the disease compared to men.[11]

Nulliparity

Some studies have shown an increased risk of colon cancer in nuns. Effects of parity could however not be shown in subsequent studies.[189–192]

Physical activity

Several studies have demonstrated an increased risk of colon cancer in sedentary occupations. High levels of physical activity have been shown to reduce the risk of adenomatous polyps and colon cancer by 50%. This fact suggests an effect of physical activity in the early stages of carcinogenesis.[193–195]

The preventative effects of physical activity are: a shortening of the gastrointestinal transit time, a reduction of insulin levels and a normalization of glucose metabolism, inducing a favorable influence on the metabolic syndrome. Finally, there is a positive influence on prostaglandin metabolism.[11,189]

Obesity

Obesity is associated with an increased risk of colon polyps and colon cancer. Possible mechanisms are hyperinsulinemia, insulin resistance, the metabolic syndrome and the effect of elevated growth factors associated with obesity.[11,196]

Diet

Preference for fruits and vegetables,[184,197–199] high-fiber foods[215] and the use of multivitamin drugs[197] seems to reduce the risk of colon cancer by up to 50%. In 27 previous epidemiologic studies reviewed by Block et al,[184] 20 of these studies showed a protective effect, while three did not, but did not suggest any increased risk. Suggested mechasnisms are reduction of proliferative stimuli, antioxidation, induction of enzymes inactivating carcinogens, an increase in stool bulk and a shortening of the intestinal transition time.

A high-fat diet is considered to be a risk factor. Willett et al[200] found an association with total fat consumption, but closer scrutiny singled out animal fat consumption as the most important factor. On the other hand, high intake of red meat increases the risk of colon cancer. Red meats (beef, pork and veal) seem to be associated with the greatest risk while white meats (poultry and fish) seem to be associated with lowest or no risk. This is posibly due to the presence of carcinogens in roasted or very strongly heated, salted and grilled meats[201–203] due to the presence of heterocyclic amines or the presence of high concentrations of divalent iron, generating free radicals. Willett et al investigated the role of dietary fiber and was unable to demonstrate an effect on the incidence of colon cancer. Today it is believed that the positive effect of fiber in colon cancer incidence, which has been recognized in many studies, is due not only to the effect of fiber on intestinal functions but also to the presence of vitamins, minerals and other secondary substances in fiber-rich foods.[197,203]

Antioxidant vitamins

Provitamin A, folic acid, and vitamins C and E may neutralize radicals. The antioxidants alone will probably not reduce the risk of colorectal cancer, however, together with the intake of fruit and vegetables and their additional effective substances, antioxidants may help to reduce risk.[194]

Alcohol and tobacco misuse

There is an association between the amount of alcohol intake and an increased risk of colon cancer. In some studies a dose–response curve was shown. Francheschi et al,[193] in a survey study of 15 cohort and 19 case control studies found a RR of < 2. Long-term cigarette smoking may increase the risk of both polyposis and colon cancer, especially in combination with alcohol.[193]

Use of hormones

Hormonal contraception
Oral hormonal contraception reduces the risk of colon cancer by about 20–50%.[194] The reduction increases with the duration of hormone intake and the effect lasts for many years after withdrawal of the hormones.

ERT and HRT
Replacement of estrogens and estrogens–progestogens may be beneficial against colon cancer. The reduction of risk amounts to 50%. A meta-analysis of the studies made showed a reduction of risk of 20% for women who had ever taken estrogens. The protective effect was greatest with actual or recent intake, and exhibited a further preventive effect for some years after withdrawal of hormones. An increase of the preventive effect with the duration of hormone intake was suggested.[189–192,195–199] In addition, the cure rate and the mortality rate of colon cancer is improved in estrogen users.[189]

The hypotheses of the preventive mechanisms consider an alteration of the bile acid production and metabolism on DNA methylation and a beneficial influence on hyperinsulinism, and a decrease of growth factors like IGF–1 by oral estrogens.

Nonsteroidal antirheumatics

It has been shown that the use of aspirin and other antirheumatics decreases the risk of ovarian and colon cancer.[200,201] This fact may give an insight on the genesis of these cancers.

Recommendations for the prevention of colon cancer

Effective measures for the prevention of colon cancer include: physical activity, increased consumption of fruit, vegetables and fibers, intake of multivitamins, a decreased intake of calories, a reduction of body weight, refraining from red, salted and grilled meats, and refraining from alcohol and smoking.

HRT and hormonal contraception may also be protective against polyposis and colon cancer. Fecal blood detection and regular 2-year colposcopies in high-risk cases may secure early detection, treatment and cure.

It is well established that a change of lifestyle and population-based colon cancer screening would result in a substantial reduction of colon cancer incidence.

REFERENCES

1. Beckmann MW, Untch M, Rabe T et al. (Chemo)Prävention des Mammakarzinoms. *Der Gynäkologe* 1999; **32:** 150–7.
2. Doll R, Peto R. The causes of cancer: quantitative estimates of avoidable risks of cancer in the United States today. *Natl Cancer Inst* 1981; **66:** 1196–305.
3. Harvard Report on Cancer Prevention. *Volume I: Causes of Human Cancer.* Cancer Causes Control (Suppl 1) 55–8.
4. Henderson BED, Ross RK, Pike MC. Hormonal prevention of breast cancer in women. *Science* 1993; **259:** 633–8.
5. Newell GR, Vogel VG. Personal risk factors – what do they mean? *Cancer* 1988; **62:** 1695–701.
6. Persson I, Thurfjell E, Holmberg L. Effects of estrogen and estrogen–progestin replacement regimens on mammographic breast parechchymal density. *J Clin Oncol* 1997; **125:** 3201–7.
7. Stoll B. Diet and exercise regimens to improve breast carcinoma prognosis. *Cancer* 1996; **78:** 2465–70.

8. Pence BC, Dunn DM. *Nutrition and Women's Cancer.* New York: CRC Press, 1998.

9. Vorherr H. *The Breast.* (Academic Press: New York, 1974.)

10. Wolf AS. Phytoestrogene. Stellenwert und Sinnhaftigkeit in der Menopause. In: (Fischl FH, Huber JC, eds) *Menopause–Andropause.* (Krause a. Pachernegg: Gablitz, 2000) 51–60.

11. Becker N, Wahrendorf J. *Krebsatlas der Bundesrepublik Deutschland. 3. Aufl.* (Springer; Heidelberg, 1998.)

12. Murphy GK. Undetected cancer. *JAMA* 1977; **237:** 786–8.

13. Beckmann MW, Hanstein B, Niederacher R et al. Wirkungsmechanismus ovarieller Steroidhormone und Antiestrogene in der Karzinogenese der Mamma und des Endometriums. *Geburtsh Frauenheilk* 2000; **60:** 712–6.

14. LaVecchia C. Nutritional factors and cancer of the breast, endometrium and ovary. *Eur J Cancer Clin Oncol* 1989; **25:** 1945–51.

15. Chang Claude J, Eby N, Becher H. Die Bedeutung genetischer Faktoren für die Entstehung von Brustkrebs. *Zbl Gynaek* 1994; **116:** 660–9.

16. Dickson RB, Lippman ME. Growth factors in breast cancer. *Endocr Rev* 1995; **16:** 559–89.

17. Lower EE, Blau R, Gazder P, Stahl DL. The effect of estrogen usage on the subsequent hormone receptor status of primary breast cancer. *Breast Cancer Res Treat* 1999; **58:** 205–11.

18. Miller AB, Berrino F, Piteionen P et al. Diet in the etiology of cancer. A review. *Eur J Cancer* 1994; **30:** 207–20.

19. Ewertz M, Duffy SW, Adami HO et al. Age at first birth, parity and risk of breast cancer: Meta-analysis of 8 studies from Nordic countries. *Int J Cancer* 1990; **46:** 597–603.

20. Mabuchi K, Soda M, Ron E et al. Cancer incidence in atomic bomb survivers. Part I: Use of the Tumor Registries in Hiroshima and Nagasaki for Incidence Studies. *Radiat Res* 1994; **137:** 1–16.

21. Negri E, La Vecchia C, Franchesci E et al. Intake of selected micronutritients and the risk of breast cancer. *Int J Cancer* 1996; **45:** 140–6.

22. Russo J, Russo IH. Role of hormones in human breast development; the menopausal breast. In: (Wren B, Ed) *Progress in the Management of the Menopause.* (Parthenon: New York, 1997) 184–93.

23. Schairer C, Lubin J, Troisi R et al. Menopausal estrogen and estrogen–progestin replacement therapy and breast cancer risk. *JAMA* 2000; **283:** 485–91.

24. Gail MH, Brinton LA, Bayar DP et al. Projecting individual probability in developing breast cancer for white females, who are being examined annually. *J Natl Cancer Inst* 1999; **82:** 1879–86.

25. Gapstur SM, Potter JD, Sellers TA, Folsom AR. Increased risk of breast cancer with alcohol consumption in postmenopausal women. *Am J Epidemiol* 1992; **136:** 1221–31.

26. Ginsburg EL, Mello NK, Mendelson JH et al. Effects of alcohol ingestion on estrogens in postmenopausal women. *JAMA* 1996; **276:** 1747–51.

27. Lichtenstein P, Holm NV, Pia K et al. Environmental and heritable factors in the causation of cancer – analysis of cohorts of twins from Sweden, Denmark and Finland. *N Engl J Med* 2000; **343:** 78–85.

28. Stoll BA, Love S. *Reducing Breast Cancer Risk in Women.* (Kluwer Acacemic: Dordrecht, 1995.)

29. Willett WC. Diet, nutrition and avoidable cancer. *Environ Health Perspec* 1995; **103** (Suppl 8)**:** 165–70.

30. Eldar S, Meguid MM, Beatty JD. Cancer of the breast after prophylactic subcutaneous mastectomy. *Am J Surg* 1984; **148:** 691–3.

31. World Cancer Research Fund and American Institute of Cancer Research. *Food, Nutrition and the Prevention of Cancer.* (Washington, 1997).

32. Kalache AY, Maguire A, Tompson SG. Age at first full term pregnancy and risk of breast cancer. *Lancet* 1994; **341:** 33–6.

33. Musgrove LA, Sutherland LA. Steroidal control of cell proliferation in the breast and breast cancer. In: (Wren B, ed) *Progress in the Management of the Menopause.* (Parthenon: New York, 1977) 194–202.

34. Rosenberg RD, Hunt WC, Williamson MR et al. Effects of age, breast density, ethnicity and estrogen replacement therapy on screening mammographic sensivity and cancer stage at diagnosis. Review of 183 134 screening mammograms in Albuquerque, New Mexico. *Radiology* 1998; **209:** 511–18.

35. Russo J, Russo IH. Biological und molecular basis of mammary carcinogenesis. *Lab Invest* 1987; **57:** 112–37.

36. Dupont WD, Parl FF, Hartmann WH et al. Breast cancer risk associated with proliferative breast disease and atypical hyperplasia. *Cancer* 1993; **71:** 1258–65.

37. Dupont WD, Page DL, Parlö FF et al. Estrogen replacement therapy in women with a history of proliferative breast disease. *Cancer* 1999; **85:** 1277–83.

38. Persson I, Yuen J, Bergkvist L, Schairer C. Cancer incidence and mortality of women receiving estrogen-progestin replacement therapy: long-term follow-up of a Swedish cohort. *Int J Cancer* 1996; **67:** 327–32.

39. Tokunaga M, Norman JE, Agano M. Malignant breast tumors among atomic bomb survivors in Hiroshima and Nagasaki. 1959–1974. *J Natl Cancer Inst* 1979; **62:** 1347–52.

40. Vogel VG, Yeomans A, Higginbotham E. Clinical management of women at increased risk for breast cancer. *Breast Cancer Res Treat* 1993; **28:** 195–200.

41. Adami HO, Lund E, Bergström R, Meirik O. Cigarette smoking, alcohol consumption and risk of breast cancer. *Br J Cancer* 1988; **58:** 832–7.

42. Baghurst PA, Rohan TE. Dietary fiber and risk of benign proliferative epithelial disorders of the breast. *Int J Cancer* 1995; **63:** 481–5.

43. Cold S, Hansen S, Overrad K, Rose C. A woman's build and the risk of breast cancer. *Eur J Cancer* 1998; **34:** 1166–74.

44. Palmer JR, Rosenberg L, Clarke EA et al. Breast cancer and cigarette smoking. A hypothesis. *Am J Epidemiol* 1991; **134:** 1–13.

45. Pike MC, Spica DV. The chemoprevention of breast cancer by reduction of sex steroids. Experimental perspectives for epidemiology. *J Cell Biochem* 1993; **17:** 26–36.

46. Schindler AE. Menopauseforum Tuohilampi. *Frauenarzt* 1999; **38:** 1–3.

47. Collaborative Group on Hormonal Factors. Breast cancer and oral contraceptives. *Lancet* 1996; **347:** 1713–27.

48. Cunnings SX R, Norton L, Eckert SX et al. Raloxifen reduces risk of breast cancer and may decrease the risk of endometrial cancer in postmenopausal women. *Proceedings of the 34th American Association of Clinical Oncology Proc* Abstract 3.

49. Early Breast Cancer Trialists Collaborative Group: Tamoxifen for early breast cancer: an overview of the randomized trials. *Lancet* 1998; **351:** 1451–6.

50. Adams MR, Scott A, Washburn JA et al. Estrogen deficiency and effects of hormone replacement. In: (Lobo R, ed). *Treatment of the Postmenopausal Woman. Basic and clinical aspects.* (Raven Press: New York, 1994): 243–50.

51. Adlercreutz H, Hämalainen E, Gorbach S, Goldin B. Dietary phytoestrogens and cancer: in vitro and in vivo studies. *J Steroid Biochem Molec Biol* 1992; **41:** 331–7.

52. Wirtensohn G, Petri, Kaffenberger E, Altwein JE. Diät und Mammakarzinom. *Frauenarzt* 1998; **39:** 1558–68.

53. Mayer ME. Hormone replacement and breast cancer. Implications of the Iowa Women's Health Study. *Cleve Clin J Med* 1999; **66:** 613–17.

54. Kuschel B, Aba F, Lux M et al. Mammakarzinom. Ermittlung des individuellen Erkrankungsrisikos und Möglichkeiten der Prävention. *Z: aerztl. Fortb Qual sich* 2000; **94:** 231–7.

55. Lauritzen C. Östrogen-Gestagensubstitution und Risiko für Endometrium- und Mammakarzinom. In: (Lauritzen C, ed) *Menopause. Hormonsubstitution heute,* edition. informed. (München, 1991) 26–31.

56. Beral V, Reeves G, Bull D et al. Breast cancer and hormone replacement therapy: putting the risk into context. In: (Birkhäuser M, Rozenbaum H, eds) *IV European Congress on Menopause.* (Eska: Paris, 1998) 267–7.

57. Burger CW, Koonen J, Peters NAJB et al. Postmenopausal replacement therapy and cancer of the female genital tract and breast. *Eur Menopause J* 1997; **4:** 33–6.

58. Colditz GA, Stanpfer GJ, Willet C et al. Prospective study of estrogen replacement therapy and risk of breast cancer in postmenopausal women. *JAMA* 1990; **264:** 264–8.

59. Fentiman IS. Future prospects for the prevention and cure of breast cancer *Eur J Cancer* 2000; **36:** 1085–8.

60. Lauritzen C. Östrogensubstitution vor und nach behandeltem Genital- und Mammakarzinom. In: (Lauritzen C, ed) *Menopause. Hormonsubstitution heute,* Aesopus, Basel, 1993) 76–88.

61. Lauritzen C. Einige Gedanken zum Problem Estrogene und Mammakarzinom. *Menopause-Praxis* 2001; **6:** 2–35.

62. Lauritzen C. Die präventive Estrogen-Gestagen Langzeitsubstitution. *Frauenarzt* 2001; **42:** 1230–67.

63. Lauritzen C. Prävention mit Phytoestrogenen. *Zbl Gynaekol* 2002; **124:** 262.

64. Lauritzen C. Möglichkeiten der Praevention des Mammakarzinoms. *Zbl Gynaekol* 2002; **124:** 269–79.

65. Lando JF, Heck KE, Brett KM. Hormone

replacement therapy and breast cancer risk in a national representative cohort. *Am J Prev Med* 1999; **17**: 176–80.

66. Bush T, Whitman M, Flaws JA. Hormone replacement therapy and breast cancer: a qualitative review. *Obstet Gynecol* 2001; **98**: 498–507.

67. Speroff L. Ovarian cancer and estrogens. *Obstet Gynecol Clin Alert* 2001; **18**: 1–8.

68. Miller AB, Home GR, Sherman GR et al. Mortality from breast cancer after irradiation during fluoroscopic examinations in patients being treated for tuberculosis. *N Engl J Med* 1989; **321**: 1285–9.

69. Nanda K, Bastian LA, Schulz K. Hormone replacement therapy and risk of death from breast cancer: a systematic review. *Am J Obstet Gynecol* 2002; **186**: 325–34.

70. Knabbe C. In: (Braendle W, Schulz KD, eds) *Hormone und Mammakarzinom. Steroide und Wachstumsfaktoren in der Proliferationskontrolle von Mammakarzinomen.* (Zuckschwerdt: München, 1999) 6–14.

71. Kutenn F, Malet C, Leygue E et al. Antiestrogen action of progestogens on human breast cells. In: (Berg G, Hammar M; eds) *The Modern Management of the Menopause.* (Parthenon: New York, 1994) 419–33.

72. Magnusson C, Holmberg L, Norde T et al. Prognostic characteristics in breast cancers after hormone replacement therapy. *Breast Cancer Res Treat* 1996; **38**: 325–34.

73. Armstrong BK, Doll R. Environmental factors, cancer incidence and mortality in different countries with special reference to dietetical practices. *Int J Cancer* 1975; **15**: 617–31.

74. Block G, Patterson B, Subar AS. Fruit, vegetables and cancer prevention a review of the epidemiologic evidence. *Nutr Cancer* 1992; **18**: 1–29.

75. Blot WJ, Li JY, Taylor PR, Guo W. Nutrition intervention trials in Linxian, China, with specific vitamin/mineral combinations, cancer incidence and disease-specific mortality in the general population. *J Natl Cancer Inst* 1993; **85**: 1483–92.

76. Cargill CPJ, Charlett A, Hill MJ. Fat, fish, fish oil and cancer *Br J Cancer* 1996; **74**: 159–64.

77. Chlebowski RT, Rose D, Buzzard IM et al for the Woman's Intervention Nutrition Study (WINS). Adjuvant dietary fat intake reduction in postmenopausal breast cancer patient management. *Breast Cancer Res Treat* 1991; **20**: 73–84.

78. Gerber M. Fiber and breast cancer: another piece of the puzzle. But still an incomplete picture. *J Natl Cancer Inst* 1996; **86**: 857–8.

79. Hunter DJ, Manson JE, Colditz GA et al. A prospective study of consumption of vitamin CEA and breast cancer. *N Engl J Med* 1993; **329**: 234–40.

80. Hunter DJ, Spiegeman D, Adami H-O et al. Cohort studies of fat intake and the risk of breast cancer. *N Engl J Med* 1996; **334**: 356–61.

81. Ingram D, Sanders K, Kolyhaba M, Lopez D. Case-control study in fat intake and the risk of breast cancer. *Lancet* 1997; **350**: 99–104.

82. Lauritzen C, Meier F. Risk of endometrial and mammary cancer morbidity and mortality in long-term estrogen treatment. In: (Herendaal et al, eds) *The Climacteric. An Update.* (MTP Press: Lancaster, 1984) 207–16.

83. Meier WT, van Lindert ACM. Prophylactic oophorectomy. *Eur J Obstet Gynecol Reprod Biol* 1992; **47**: 59–65.

84. Negri E, La Vecchia C, Franchesci E et al. Age at first and second birth and breast cancer risk in biparous women. *Int J Cancer* 1990; **45**: 428–35.

85. Scheele F, Burger CW, Kenemans P. Postmenopausal hormone replacement in the woman with reproductive risk factors for breast cancer. *Maturitas* 1999; **33**: 291–6.

86. Steinmetz KAS, Potter JD. Vegetables, fruits and cancer. *Cancer Causes Control* 1991; **2**: 325–57.

87. Willis DB, Calle EE, Miracle-McHill HL et al. Estrogen replacement therapy and risk of fatal breast cancer in a prospective cohort of postmenopausal women in the United States. *Cancer Causes Control* 1996; **7**: 449–57.

88. Wirtensohn G, Griffiths K, Altwein JE. Beeinflusst die Ernährungsweise die Entstehung des Mamma- und Prostatakarzinoms? *Onkologe* 1996; **23**: 401–8.

89. Wynder EL, Gory GB. Contribution of the environment to cancer incidence: an epidemiological exercise. *J Natl Cancer Inst* 1977; **58**: 825–32.

90. German Institute of Nutrition. Gerber B. Persönlicher Lebensstil und Brustkrebsrisiko. *J F Menop* 2003; **10**: 7–14.

91. Kleine Gunke B. Brustkrebs-Prophylaxe. Welche Rolle spielt die Ernährung? *Gynäkol Nachr* 1999; **11**: 11–14.

92. World Cancer Research Fund and American Institute of Cancer Research (WCRF/AICR).

'Food, nutrition and the prevention of cancer. A global perspective. (WCRF/AICR; Washington 1997).

93. Schindler AE. Prävention und Lebensführung in der Gynäkologie und Geburtshilfe: ein Überblick. *Zbl Gynäkol* 2002; **124:** 258–61.

94. Clarke CL, Sutherland RL. Progestin regulation of cellular proliferation. *Endocr Rev* 1990; **11:** 266–73.

95. Bowling SJ, Leske C, Varma A et al. Breast cancer risk and alcohol consumption: results from a large case-control study. *Int J Epidemiol* 1997; **236:** 915–23.

96. Smith-Wartner SA, Spiegelman D, Yaun SS et al. Alcohol and breast cancer in women. A pooled analysis of cohort studies. *JAMA* 1998; **279:** 535–40.

97. Ziegler RG, Hoover RN, Pike MC et al. Migration pattern and cancer risk in Asian-American women. *J Natl Cancer Inst* 1993; **85:** 1819–27.

98. Zhang S, Hunter DJ, Hankinson SE. A prospective study of folate intake and the risk of breast cancer. *JAMA* 1999; **281:** 1632–7.

99. Zumoff B. The critical role of alcohol consumption in determining the risk of breast cancer with postmenopausal estrogen administration *J Clin Endocr Metab* 1992; **82:** 1656–8.

100. Matthews KA, Wing RR, Kuller LH et al. Influence of natural menopause on psychological characteristic and symptoms of middle ages women. *J Cons Clin Psychol* 1880; **58:** 345–51.

100a. Darby DN, Glaser S, Wilkson DTL. Characteristics of people adopting particular styles of health care. In: (Darby DN, ed). *Health Care and Lifestyle.* (University Press: NWS, 1991).

101. MacMahon B, Cole P, Lin T et al. Age at first pregnancy and breast cancer risk. *Bull WHO* 1970; **43:** 209–20.

102. Zhang S, Folsom AR, Saellers TA et al. Better breast cancer survival for postmenopausal women who are less overweight and eat less fat. *Cancer* 1995; **76:** 275–83.

103. Ortmann O, Schulz KD, Diedrich K. Hormonelle Substitutionstherapie und Mammakarzinomrisiko. *Gynäkologe* 1996; **31:** 885–90.

104. Thune I, Brenn T, Lund E, Gaard M. Physical activity and the risk of breast cancer. *N Engl J Med* 1997; **336:** 1269–75.

105. Armstrong K, Erisen A, Weber B. Assessing the risk of breast cancer. *N Engl J Med* 2000; **342:** 564–71.

106. Loomis DP, Savitz DA, Amanth CV. Breast cancer mortality among female electrical workers in the United States. *J Natl Cancer Inst* 1994; **86:** 921–5.

107. Frisch RE, Wyashak G, Albright TE et al. Lower prevalence of breast cancer and cancers of the reproductive system among former college athletes compared to non-athletes. *Br J Cancer* 1985; **52:** 108–13.

108. Bernstein L, Henderson BE, Hanisch R et al. Physical exercise and reduced risk of breast cancer *J Natl Cancer Inst* 1994; **86:** 1403–8.

109. Friedenreich CM, Thune I, Brinton LA, Albames D. Epidemiologic issues related to the association between physical activity and breast cancer. *Breast Cancer* 1998; **83:** 600–120.

110. Pickard J. Endometrial risks for hormone replacement therapy. In: (Studd J, ed). *The Management of the Menopause. Annual Review.* (Parthenon: London, 1998): 111–20.

111. Chu J, Schweid AL, Weis NS. Survival among women with endometrial cancer. *Am J Obstet Gynecol* 1982; **143:** 569–73.

112. Collins J, Donner A, Allen LH, Adams O. Oestrogen use and survival in endometrial cancer. *Lancet* 1980; **8201:** 961–4.

113. Gambrell Jr RD. Pathophysiology and epidemiology of endometrial cancer. In: (Lobo RA, ed) *Treatment of the Postmenopausal Woman.* (Raven Press: New York, 1994) 355–61.

114. Grady D, Ernster V. Endometrial cancer. In: Schottenfield D, Fraumeni JF (eds) *Cancer Epidemiology and Prevention*, 2nd edn. (Oxford University Press: New York 1997) 1058–89.

115. Kelsey JL, Whittemore AS. Epidemiology and primary prevention of cancers of the breast, endometrium and ovary. *Ann Epidemiol* 1994; **4:** 89–95.

116. MacDonald TW, Anbnegers JF, O'Fallon WM et al. Exogenous estrogens and endometrial carcinoma: case-control and incidence study. *Am J Obstet Gynecol* 1977; **127:** 572–9.

117. Gurpide E, Murphy LJ. Effects of hormones and growth factors on human endometrial cell proliferation. In: (Lobo RA, ed) *Treatment of the Postmenopausal Woman.* (Raven Press: New York, 1994) 363–7.

118. Björkholm E, Petterson F. Granulosa-cell and theca-cell tumors. The clinical picture and long-term outcome for the Radiumhemmet series. *Acta Obstet Gynaecol Scand* 1980; **59:** 3651–5.

119. Weiss NS, Bersford SA, Voigt LF et al. Unresolved issues in endometrial cancer and

postmenopausal hormone therapy. In: (Wren B, ed) *Progress in the Management of the Menopause.* (Parthenon: New York, 1997) 236–40.

120. Antunes CM, Strolley PD, Rosenheim NB et al. Endometrial cancer and estrogen use. Report of a large case-control study. *N Engl J Med* 1979; **300:** 9–13.

121. Hammond CB, Jelovsek FR, Lee K et al. Effects of long-term estrogen replacement therapy. II Neoplasia. *Am J Obstet Gynecol* 1979; **1233:** 537–47.

122. Horwitz RI, Feinstein AR. Estrogens and endometrial cancer. Responses to arguments and current status of an epidemiologic controversy. *Am J Med* 1989; **81:** 503–10.

123. Jick S, Walker A, Jick H. Estrogens, progestogens and endometrial cancer. *Epidemiology* 1993; **4:** 20–4.

124. Beresford SA, Weiss NS, Voigt LF, McNight B. Risk of endometrial cancer in relation to use of oestrogen combined with cyclic progestogen therapy in postmenopausal women. *Lancet* 1997; **349:** 458–61.

125. Brinton L, Hoover R. Estrogen replacement and endometrial cancer risk. *Obstet Gynecol* 1993; **81:** 265–71.

126. Gelfand MM, Ferenczy A. A prospective 1-year study of estrogen and progestin in postmenopausal women: effects on the endometrium. *Am J Obstet Gynecol* 1989; **74:** 398–402.

127. Gambrell RD, Massey FM, Castenada TA et al. Reduced incidence of endometrial cancer among postmenopausal women treated with progestogens. *J Am Geriatr Soc* 1979; **27:** 389–94.

128. Grady D, Gebretsadik T, Kerlikowske K et al. Hormone replacement therapy and endometrial cancer risk: a meta-analysis. *Obstet Gynecol* 1995; **85:** 304–13.

129. Grady D, Rubin SMN, Petitti DB et al. Hormone therapy to prevent disease and prolong life in postmenopausal women. *Ann Intern Med* 1992; **117:** 1016–37.

130. Gray LS, Christophersen WM, Hoover RN. Estrogens and endometrial carcinoma. *Obstet Gynecol* 1977; **49:** 385–9.

131. Jelovsek FR, Hammond CB, Woodward BH et al. Risk of exogenous estrogen therapy and endometrial cancer. *Am J Obstet Gynecol.* 1980; **137:** 85–91.

132. Lauritzen C. Hormonsubstitution und Endometriumkarzinom. In: (Römer T, Straube W, eds) *Klimakterium und Hormonsubstitution.* (Pia Verlag: Nürnberg, 1996) 56–62.

133. Lauritzen C. Critical comment on the paper of Beresford et al. *Lancet* 1997; **349:** 458–61 and *Maturitas* 1998; **30:** 90–2.

134. Lauritzen C, Meier F. Risk of endometrial and mammary cancer morbidity in long term oestrogen treatment. In: (Herendael et al, eds) *The Climacteric, An Update.* (MTP Press: Lancaster, 1984) 207–16.

135. Lauritzen C, Wolf AS, Strabl A. A retrospective study concerning postmenopausal estrogen therapy and endometrial cancer. In: (Brush, King, Taylor, eds) *Endometrial Cancer.* (Baillière Tindall: London, 1977) 39–44.

136. Lauritzen C. Östrogensubstitution in der Postmenopause vor und nach behandeltem Genital- und Mammakarzinom. In: (Lauritzen C; ed) *Menopause. Hormonsubstitution heute. Bd. 6.* (Aesopus: Basel, 1993) 76–88.

137. Lauritzen C. Oestrogen-Gestagensubstitution und Risiko für Endometrium-und Mammakarzinom. In: (Lauritzen C, ed) *Menopause. Hormonsubstitution heute.* (München, 1991) 26–31.

138. Lauritzen C, Meier F. Risk of endometrial cancer morbidity and mortality in long term oestrogen treatment. In: (van Herendaal FE, Riphagen HB, eds) *The Climacteric. An Update.* (MTP Press: Lancaster, 1984) 207–16.

139. Mack TM, Pike MC, Henderson BE et al. Estrogen and endometrial cancer in a retirement community. *N Engl J Med* 1976; **294:** 12,621–7.

140. Nachtigall LE, Nachtigall RH, Nachtigall RD, Beckman EM. Estrogen replacement therapy II: a prospective study in the relationship to carcinoma and cardiovascular and metabolic problems. *Obstet Gynecol* 1979; **32:** 74–9.

141. Paganini-Hill A, Ross R, Henderson B. Endometrial cancer and patterns of use of oestrogen replacement therapy in a cohort study. *Br J Cancer* 1989; **59:** 445–7.

142. Persson IR, Adami HO, Bergkvist L et al. Risk of endometrial cancer after treatment with estrogens alone or in conjunction with progestogens: results of a prospective study. *BMJ* 1989; **298:** 147–51.

143. Voelker W. Oestrogentherapie und Endometriums-Carzinom. *Geburtsh u Frauenheilk* 1978; **38:** 735–9.

144. Voigt LF, Weiss NS, Chu J et al. Progestogen supplementation of exogenous oestrogens and risk of endometrial cancer. *Lancet* 1991; **3:** 274–7.

145. Weiderpass E, Adami H-O, Baron JA et al. Risk of endometrial cancer following estrogen replacement with and without progestins. *J Natl Cancer Inst* 1999; **91:** 1131–7.
146. Lignieres de B, Moyer DL. Influence of sex hormones on hyperplasia/carcinoma risks. In: (Lobo RA, ed) *Treatment of the Postmenopausal Woman* (Raven Press: New York, 1994) 375–9.
147. Whitehead MI, Pickar JH. Variations among pathologists in the reportings of endometrial histology with combination oestrogen/progestogen therapies. *Proceedings of the British Medical Society* Exeter UK, July 1996.
148. Comerci Jr JT, Fields AR, Runowicz CD, Goldberg GL. Continuous low-dose combined hormone replacement therapy and the risk of endometrial cancer. *Gynecol Oncol* 1997; **64:** 4235–340.
148a. Pike MC, Peters RK, Cozen W et al. Estrogen–progestin replacement therapy and endometrial cancer. *J Natl Cancer Inst* 1997; **89:** 1110–16.
149. Grady D, Gebretsadik T, Kerlikowski K et al. Hormone replacement therapy and endometrial cancer: a meta-analysis. *Obstet Gynecol* 1995; **85:** 304–13.
150. MacLennon AH, MacLennon A, Wenzel S et al. Continuous low-dose oestrogen and progestogen in postmenopausal hormone replacement therapy. *Med J Aust* 1993; **159:** 102–6.
151. Petitti DB, Pearlman JA, Sidney S. Noncontraceptive estrogens and mortality: long-term follow-up of women in the Walnut Creek Study. *Obstet Gynecol* 1987; **70:** 2389–93.
152. Rabe Th, Vladescu E, Heinemann L, von Holst Th. Endometriumkarzinom. OC (orale hormonale Kontrazeptiva), HRT (Oestrogen. Gestagen-Therapie) und Tamoxifen. *Onkologe* 1999; **5:** 432–43.
153. Rose DP, Boyar AP, Wynder EL. International comparisons in mortality rate for cancer of the breast, ovary, prostate and colon, and per capita food consumption. *Cancer* 1986; **58:** 2363–71.
154. Boerogter PJ, Van der Weijer PHM, Baak JPA. Endometrial response in a replacement therapy, quarterly combined with a progestogen. *Maturitas* 1996; **124:** 63–71.
155. Williams DB, Voigt BJ, Yao FU et al. Assessment of less than monthly progestin therapy in postmenopausal women given estrogen replacement. *Obstet Gynecol* 1994; **81:** 787–93.
156. Heikkinen J, Kyllonen E, Kurttila Matero E et al. Comparision of bleeding patterns and endometrial histology between a three monthly and monthly cycle HRT. *Acta Obstet Gynecol Scand* 1997; **76:** P76.33.
157. Hirvonen E, Salmi T, Puolakka J et al. Can progestin be limited to every third month only in postmenopausal women taking estrogen? *Maturitas* 1995; **21:** 39–44.
158. Andersson M, Storm HH, Mouridsen HT. Incidence of new primary cancers after adjuvant tamoxifen therapy. *J Natl Cancer Inst* 1991; **83:** 1013–17.
159. Breckwoldt M, Karck U. Tamoxifen for breast cancer prevention. *Exp Clin Endocr Diabetes* 2000; **108:** 243–6.
160. Boss SM, Huster WJ, Neild JA et al. Effects of raloxifen hydrochloride on the endometrium of postmenopausal women. *Am J Obstet Gynecol* 1997; **177:** 1458–64.
161. Levi F, La Vecchia CL, Parazzini Francheschi S. Body mass at different ages and subsequent endometrial cancer risk. *Int J Cancer* 1992; **50:** 567–71.
162. Sherman, ME, Sturgeon S, Brinton LA et al. Risk factors and hormonal levels in patients with serious and endometrioid uterine carcinomas. *Med Pathol* 1997; **10:** 963–8.
163. Newcomb PA, Trentham-Dietz A, Storer BE. Alcohol consumption in relation to endometrial cancer risk. *Cancer Epidemiol Biomark Prev* 1997; **6:** 775–8.
164. Emons G, Kavanagh JJ. Hormonal interactions in ovarian cancer. *Hematol Oncol Clin North* 1999; **13:** 145–61.
165. Booth M, Beral V, Smith P. Risk factors for ovarian cancer: a case control study. *Br J Cancer* 1989; **60:** 592–8.
166. Beller FK. Verursacht die postmenopausale Östrogentherapie Ovarialkarzinome? *Frauenarzt* 2000; **42:** 8.
167. Jacobs IJ, Skates SJ, MacDonald N et al. Screening of ovarian cancer: a pilot randomized controlled study. *Lancet* 1999; **353:** 1207–10.
168. Claus EB, Schildkraut JM, Thompson WD, Risch NJ. The genetic attributable risk of breast and ovarian cancer. *Cancer* 1996; **77:** 2318–24.
169. Persson IR. Cancer diseases in the menopause. Causes and prevention. In: (Aso T, Yanaihara T, eds) *The Menopause at the Millennium.* Parthenon New York, 1999) 54–64.
170. Rossmanith, WG: Substitutionstherapie und Ovarialkarzinom. *Frauenarzt* 1997; **38:** 1108–9
171. Garg PP, Kerlikowski K, Subak L, Grady D.

Hormone replacement therapy and the risk of epithelian ovarian cancer. *Obstet Gynecol* 1998; **32:** 472–9.

172. Adami HO, Hsieh CC, Lambe M et al. Parity, age at first birth and risk of ovarian cancer. *Lancet* 1994; **344:** 250–4.

173. Garg PP, Kerlikowski K, Subak L, Grady D. Hormone replacement therapy and the risk of epithelial ovarian carcinoma: a meta-analysis. *Obstet Gynecol* 1998; **92:** 472–9.

174. Risch HA. Estrogen replacement therapy and risk of ovarian cancer. *Gynecol Oncol* 1996; **63:** 354–7.

175. Cramer DW, Xu H. Epidemiological evidence of uterine growth factors in the pathogenesis of ovarian cancer. *Ann Epidemiol* 1995; **5:** 310–14.

176. Rodriguez C, Calle EE, Coates RJ et al. Estrogen replacement therapy and fatal ovarian cancer. *Am J Epidemiol* 1995; **141:** 828–35.

177. Coughlin SS, Giustozzi A, Smith SJ, Lee NC. A meta-analysis of estrogen replacement therapy and risk of epithelial ovarian cancer. *J Clin Epidemiol* 2000; **53:** 367–85.

178. Lacey JV, Mink P. Menopausal hormone replacement therapy and risk of ovarian cancer. *JAMA* 2002; **17:** 3288–334.

178a. Purdie D. Reproductive and other factors and risk of epithelial ovarian cancer: an Australian case-control study. *Int J Cancer* 1995; **62:** 678–84.

179. Mosgaard BJ, Lidegaard O, Kjaer SK et al. Infertility, fertility drugs, and invasive ovarian cancer: a case control study. *Fertil Steril* 1997; **67:** 1005–12.

180. Risch HA. Hormonal etiology of ovarian cancer, with a hypothesis concerning the role of androgens and progesterone. *J Natl Cancer Inst* 1998; **90:** 1774–86.

181. Eales E. Estrogen-progestogen replacement after ovarian cancer. *Brit Med J* 1881; **309:** 259–62.

181a. Whittemore AS, Harris R, Intire J. The Collaborative Ovarian Cancer Group. Characteristics relating to ovarian cancer risks. Collaborative analysis of 12 US case-control studies. II. Invasive epithelial ovarian cancer in white women. *Am J Epidemiol* 1992; **136:** 1184–1203.

182. Hankinson SE, Colditz GA, Hunter DJ et al. A prospective study of reproductive factors and risk of epithelial ovarian cancer. *Cancer* 1995; **76:** 284–90.

183. Riman T, Persson I, Nilsson S. Hormonal aspects of epithelial ovarian cancer: review of epidemiological evidence. *Clin Endocr* 1998; **69:** 695–707.

184. Rossouw JE, Anderson GL, Prentice RL et al. Risks and benefits of estrogen plus progestin in healthy postmenopausal women: Principal results From the Women's Health Initiative randomized controlled trial. *JAMA* 2002; **288**(3): 321–33.

185. Gwinn ML, Webster LA, Layde PM, Rubin GL and the Cancer and Steroid Hormone Group. Original contributions: alcohol consumption and ovarian cancer risk. *Am J Epidemiol* 1986; **123:** 759–66.

186. Longnecker MP, Gerhardson de Verdier M, Frumkin H, Carpenter C. A case-control study of physical activity in relation to risk of cancer of the right colon and rectum. *J Epidemiol* 1995; **24:** 42–50.

187. Steinmertz KA, Potter JD. Vegetables, fruits and cancer. II. Mechanisms. *Cancer Causes Control* 1991; **2:** 427–42.

188. Whittemore ASD, Wu-Williams AH, Lee M et al. Diet, physical activity and colorectal cancer among Chinese in North America and China. *J Natl Cancer Inst* 1990; **82:** 915–26.

189. Gerhardson de Verdier M, Steineck G, Hagman, U et al. Physical activity and colon cancer. A case referent study in Stockholm. *Int J Cancer* 1990; **46:** 985–9.

190. Fernandez E, La Veccchia C, D'Avanzo, B et al. Oral contraceptives, hormone replacement therapy and the risk of colorectal cancer. *Cancer Epidemoiol Biomark Prev* 1998; **7:** 329–33.

191. Gerhardson de VM, London S. Reproductive factors, exogenous female hormones, and colorectal cancer by subsite. *Cancer Causes Control* 1992; **3:** 355–60.

192. Lauritzen C. Reduziert die langzeitige Öestrogensubstitution das Risiko für die Entstehung des Kolonkarzinoms? In: (Lauritzen C, ed) *Menopause. Hormonsubstitution heute. Bd.5.* (PMS Cedip: München, 1994) 89–92.

193. Francheschi S, La Vecchia C. Alcohol and the risk of cancers of the stomach and colon-rectum. *Dig Dis* 1994; **12:** 276–89.

194. Greenberg ER, Baron JA, Tosteson TD et al. A clinical trial of antioxidant vitamins to prevent colorectal adenoma. *N Engl J Med* 1994; **331:** 141–7.

194a. Willett WC, Stampfer MJ, Colditz GA et al. Relation of meat, fat and fiber intake to the risk of colon cancer in a prospective study among women *N Engl J Med* 1990; **323:** 1664–72.

195. Rose DP, Boyar AP, Wynder EL. International comparisons of mortality rates for cancer of the breast, ovary, prostate, and colon, and per capita food consumption. *Cancer* 1986; **58:** 2363–72.

195a. Whittemore AS, Harris R, Intyre J. Characteristics relating to ovarian cancer risk: collaborative analysis of 12 US case-control studies. IV. The pathogenesis of epithelial ovarian cancer. Collaborative Ovarian Cancer Group. *Am J Epidemiol* 1992; **136:** 1212–20.

196. Block G, Patterson B, Subar A. Fruit, vegetables, and cancer prevention. A review of epidemiological evidence. *Nutr Cancer* 1992; **18:** 1–29.

196a. Grodstein F, Newcomb PA, Stampfer MJ. Postmenopausal hormone therapy and the risk of colorectal cancer: a review and meta-analysis. *Am J Med* 1999; **106:** 574–82.

197. Gann PH, Manson JE, Glynn, RJ et al. Low dose aspirin and incidence of colorectal tumors in a randomized trial. *J Natl Cancer Inst* 1993; **85:** 1220–4.

197a. Gerhardsson de Verdier M, Hagman U, Peters RK et al. Meat, cooking methods and colorectal cancer. A case referent study in Stockholm. *Int J Cancer* 1991; **49:** 520–5.

198. Hebert-Croteau N. A meta-analysis of hormone replacement therapy and colon cancer in women. *Cancer Epidemiol Biomark Prev* 1995; **7:** 653–59.

198a. Newcomb PA, Storer BE. Postmenopausal hormone use and risk of large bowel cancer. *J Natl Cancer Inst* 1995; **87:** 1067–71.

199. Potter JD. Hormones and colon cancer. *J Natl Cancer Inst* 1995; **87:** 1039–40.

199a. Steinmetz KA, Potter JD. Vegetables fruits and cancer. I. Epidemiology. *Cancer Causes Control* 1991; **2:** 325–7.

200. Calle EE, Hiracle-McMahill HL, Thun MJ, Heath CW. Estrogen replacement therapy and risk of colon cancer in a prospective cohort of postmenopausal women. *J Natl Cancer Inst* 1995; **87:** 517–23.

201. Marchand L, Wilkens LR. MI.MP: Obesity in youth and middle age and risk of colorectal cancer in men. *Cancer Causes Control* 1992; **3:** 349–54.

201a. Venn A, Watson L, Lumley J et al. Breast and ovarian cancer incidence after infertility and in vitro fertilization. *Lancet* 1995; **346:** 995–1000.

202. Franceschi S, La Vecchia C. Colorectal cancer and hormone replacement therapy: an unexpected finding. *Eur J Cancer Prev* 1998; **7:** 427–38.

203. Smalley W, Ray WA, Daugherty J, Griffin MR.

204. Potter J, McMichael AJM. Large bowel cancer in women in relationship to reproductive and hormonal factors. *J Nat Cancer Inst* 1983; **71:** 703–9.

205. Benson K, Hartz AJ. A comparison of observational studies and randomized clinical trials *N Engl J Med* 2000; **342:** 1878–80.

206. Bondy ML, Vogel VG, Halaby S et al. Identification of an increased risk for breast cancer in a population based screening program. *Cancer Epidemiol Biomark Prevent* 1992; **1:** 143–7.

207. Byrne C, Conolly JL, Colditz GA, Schnitt SJ. Biopsy confirmed benign breast disease, postmenopausal use of exogenous female hormones and breast cancer risk. *Cancer* 2000; **89:** 2046–52.

208. Collins J, Donner A, Allen LH, Adams O. Oestrogen use and survival in endometrial cancer. *Lancet* 1980; **961:** 4.

209. Dorgan JF. Physical activity and breast cancer. *J Natl Cancer Inst* 1998; **90:** 1116–19.

210. Hall K, Isola J, Cuzik J. Low biological aggressiveness in breast cancer in women using hormone replacement therapy. *J Clin Oncol* 1998; **16:** 3115–20.

211. Houlihan MJ, Goldwyn RM. Mastectomy for cancer prevention. In: (Stoll BA, Love SM, eds) *Reducing Breast Cancer Risk in Women.* (Kluwer Academic Publishers: Dordrecht, 1995) 69–80.

212. Hulka BS, Brinton LA. Hormones and breast and endometrial cancers. Preventive strategies and further research. *Environ Health Perspe.* 1995; **103** (Suppl 8): 185–9.

213. Jernstrom H, Frenander J, Ferno M, Olsson H. Hormone replacement therapy before breast cancer diagnosis significantly reduces the overall death rate compared with never use among 984 breast cancer patients. *Br J Cancer* 1999; **80:** 1453–8.

214. Longnecker MP, Berloin JA, Orza MJ, Chalmers TC. A meta-analysis of alcohol consumption in relation to the risk of breast cancer. *JAMA* 1988; **260:** 652–6.

215. Nixon D. Anti-Krebs-Diät. Düsseldorf: *Econ* 1996.

216. Schoultz von B. Postmenopausale Hormonbehandlung und mammographische Dichte. *Gyne* 2001; **22:** 237–8.

217. Schoultz von B, Soederquist G, Cline M et al.

Use of nonsteroidal antiinflammatory drugs and incidence of colorectal cancer: a population based study. *Arch Int Med* 1999; **159:** 161–6.

Estrogen–progestogen effects on the breast. In: (Roemer Th, Straube W, eds) *Klimakterium und Hormonsubstitution*. (Pia Verlag: Nürnberg, 1996) 63–5.

218. Stellungnahme der Kommission Steroid-toxikologie zum Thema Antiöstrogene und SERMs. *Endokrinologie Inf* 2000; **24:** 168.

219. Stellungnahme der Kommission Steroid-toxikologie zur Thema. Karzinogene Eigenschaften von 17β-Estradiol. *Endokrinologie Inf* 2000; **24:** 181–6.

220. Swanson CA, Coates RJ, Malone KE et al. Alcohol consumption and breast cancer risk among women under age 45 years. *Epidemiology* 1997; **8:** 231–7.

221. Willett WC, Stampfer MJ, Colditz GA et al. Moderate alcohol consumption and the risk of breast cancer. *N Engl J Med* 1987; **316:** 1174–80.

222. Goodman RT, Weilkens LR, Hankin JH et al. Association of soy and fiber consumption with the risk of endometrial cancer. *Am J Epidemiol* 1997; **146:** 294–306.

223. IARC. Hormonal contraception and post-menopausal hormone therapy. *IARC Monographs on the Evaluation of Carcinogenic Risk to Humans*. (IARC: Lyon, 1999) Volume 72.

224. Leathahy A, Farquhar C, Sartkis A et al. Hormone replacement therapy in post-menopausal women. Endometrial hyperplasia and irregular bleeding (Cochrane Review). In: *The Cochrane Library 2000, issue 2.* (Oxford update software: www.update-software com/abstracts/ab 000402.htm.)

225. Luciano AA, De Souzam MJ, Roy MP et al. Evaluation of low-dose estrogen and progestin therapy in postmenopausal women. *Eur J Clin Invest* 1991; **21:** 601–7.

226. The Writing Group for PEPI-Trial. Effects of hormone replacement on endometrial histology in postmenopausal women. The Postmenopausal Estrogen/ Progestin Intervention (PEPI) Trial. *JAMA* 1996; **275:** 370–5.

227. Weiderpass E, Adami H, Baron J et al. Use of oral contraceptives and endometrial cancer risk. *Cancer Causes Control* 1999; **10:** 277–84.

228. Wenderlein JM. HRT – eine preiswerte Präventivmedizin. *Frauenarzt* 1999; **40:** 1130–2.

229. Hankinson SE, Colditz GA, Hunter DJ. A quantitative assessment of oral contraceptive use and risk of ovarian cancer. *Obstet Gynecol* 1992; **80:** 708–14.

230. Rossing MA, Daling JR, Weiss NS, Moore DE. Ovarian tumors in a cohort of infertile women. *N Engl J Med* 1994; **331:** 771–6.

231. Augustsson K, Skog K, Jagerstad M et al. Dietary heterocyclic amines and cancer of the colon, rectum, bladder and kidney. *Lancet* 1999; **353:** 703–7.

232. Writing Group for the Women's Health Initiative Investigators. Risks and Benefits of Estrogen Plus Progestin in Healthy Postmenopausal Women. *JAMA* 2002; **288:** 321–33.

233. Yu H, Harris RE, Gao YT et al. Comparative epidemiology of cancers of the colon, rectum, prostate and breast in Shanghai, China versus United States. *Int J Epidemiol* 1991; **20:** 76–81.

234. Zylka-Menhorn V. Verbundprojekt, Familiärer Darmkrebs. *Dtsch Ärzteblatt* 2000; **97:** C182.

235. Falck F, jr, Ricci A, jr, Wolff MS et al. Pesticides and polychlorinated biphenyl residues in human breast lipids and their relation to breast cancer. *Arch Environm Health* 1995; **143:** 143–7.

236. Wolff ME, Toniolo PG, Lee EW et al. Blood levels of organichlorine residues and risk of breast cancer. *J Natl Cancer Inst* 1993; **85:** 648–52.

29

Benefits, risks and costs of estrogen and hormone replacement therapies

C Lauritzen

Established principles of estrogen (ERT) and hormone (HRT) replacement therapies • Problems of long-term treatment • Impacts of ERT and HRT: lifetime risks, morbidity and mortality • Consequences of longevity • Basic considerations concerning benefit–risk determinations and costs • WHI study results • Objection of healthy user bias • Benefits and risks in the opinion of patients • Objective ultimate measures of effectivity and limitations • Estimations of benefit–risk and cost-effectiveness • Benefits of ERT • Risk, benefits and costs of estrogen–progestogen sequential treatment (HRT) • Costs • Prevention of osteoporosis and fractures • Hypertension • Coronary heart diseases • Prevention of stroke • Prevention of dementia • Prevention of colon cancer • Prevention of urogenital atrophy • Prevention of other diseases • Socioeconomic effects • Quality of life • Hospital admissions • Decrease of mortality (life expectancy) • Cost savings • New preparations • Possible risks: the Minimax concept • Endometrial cancer • Ovarian cancer • Breast cancer • Gallbladder diseases • Deep vein thrombosis and thromboembolism • Postmenopausal bleeding, curettage, hysterectomy • General impact of estrogen–progestogen on health life years • Total impact of costs • Screening costs • General remarks • Summary of the results of the benefit–risk assessment • References

In every treatment the benefits of a recommended medication must clearly surpass the possible side effects and risks. The costs of a regimen must be in reasonable relation to the benefits which can be expected. This principle is even more important if a preventive long-term treatment is given to healthy women who may, however, be at risk for certain diseases which could possibly be avoided by interventional medicopharmacologic measures. Innumerable variables influence the conditions of a disease, its prevention and treatment, and these will, in addition, vary individually and by country and region. This is why an answer to any question concerning risks and benefits is so difficult. Many attempts have been made to critically address the problem to an exact as possible analysis using mathematical tools,

with the aim of making physicians' recommendations more scientific, which so far have mainly been subjective and empirical. After all, the very nature of medical activity comprises the evaluation of the risk and benefits of a treatment where the physican acts as an arbitrator for his/her patient.

A positive benefit:risk ratio justifies a well-founded medical recommendation to the client. The recommendation includes advice on which form of treatment would be the most advantageous for the individual needs of the patient in question, having the least side effects in her special situation. The answer will promote the decision of whether the regimen justifies the expenditure.

Moreover, analysis of the benefit:risk ratio may give the basis for professional guidelines, disease management programs and for the decision to prioritize allocation of financial resources. To obtain the preventive long-term benefits of hormone replacement therapy (HRT), women must maintain long-term compliance. Honest counseling concerning benefits and risks of HRT based on well-founded facts will promote adherence of the client to therapy. The cost factor must regrettably be a point for recommendation or dissuasion, although ideally should not be decisive. However, it has become clearer that there is a limit to the amount of money available for health care, which concerns large numbers of the population; therefore, priorities have to be established. Evaluation of the efficiency of available health care resources and therapies is therefore of increasing interest for the decision-makers in health services. Fortunately, estrogen–progestogen medication is not expensive, but may become so when extended to greater parts of the population, who will possible not absolutely need substitution.

A science of health economics has been established. Well-conducted trials using the methods of evidence-based medicine can contribute to clarification of an increase or reduction in risk by a regimen and to the elimination of ineffective or even dangerous regimens.

ESTABLISHED PRINCIPLES OF ESTROGEN (ERT) AND HORMONE (HRT) REPLACEMENT THERAPIES

Medical intervention with hormones during the perimenopausal years has the following major goals: (1) to treat or to prevent unwanted and severe, quite unnecessary, climacteric complaints; thereby (2) prolonging the period of maximal physical energy and of optimal mental and social activity with a good quality of life; (3) to detect early major chronic diseases such as osteoporosis, cardiovascular diseases, hypertension, metabolic syndrome, diabetes mellitus, and gynecologic and colorectal cancer. Also, impairments of vision and hearing should be detected early and treated, thus securing successful aging. The general aim is to help a perimenopausal women to traverse the climacteric

and late postmenopausal period of life as smoothly as possible without unnecessary and pointless complaints, and probably fatal diseases, to achieve a compression of morbidity.

Some peri- and post-menopausal women do not experience climacteric complaints and it is not recommended that such patients receive HRT.

According to current medical consensus, severe perimenopausal cycle disturbances and climacteric complaints, which restrict the quality of life, are treated for as long as they last, mostly for 3–5 years, by estrogen + sequential progestogen substitution. This is the usual time of duration of climacteric complaints and therefore the regimen for the majority of all postmenopausal women with an indication for treatment. This treatment is extremely successful and will generally not include any adverse side effects or risks. The small possible risk for thromboembolism (3/10,000) found in recent studies can be virtually excluded by taking the family history of thromboembolic events, by exploring the relevant individual history and by counseling the patient with the aim of avoiding events which could trigger thrombosis. Low-dose treatment with ERT or HRT, and possibly parenteral application as well as a co-treatment of existing varicosis and of being overweight, may add to the safety of ERT and HRT in this respect.

In older women with atrophic urogenital changes a local estrogen application is mostly sufficient to abolish all complaints. Transdermal low-dose substitution as opposed to oral treatment is generally to be preferred in older women.

PROBLEMS OF LONG-TERM TREATMENT

Long-term ERT or HRT is defined as a treatment maintained for more than 5 years. After the phase of symptomatic treatment of the climacteric syndrome, the practical problem of the therapeut is who should he/she select for long-term substitution.

Of course, the wishes of the patient and her experiences with hormones so far are the most important factors against or for a decision in favor of long-term substitution. The problem is how do we identify women at increased risk for complications or even of dying from hormone-promoted breast cancer rather than benefiting from the antiosteoporotic and cardioprotective effect of HRT? Risk factors are regrettably not always reliable or helpful for prediction of future real risk.

HRT can be maintained for additional years if the climacteric complaints persist, if atrophic genital changes and corresponding symptoms still occur, and if the patient will probably benefit from the antiosteoporotic and antiatherosclerotic effects of estrogens. The supposition of a prospective benefit may be made by personal or family history, and pertinent medical, physical and laboratory findings. This could be familial or personal risk factors for osteoporosis or low bone density, constitutional characteristics (such as being under- or overweight), laboratory findings like high low-density lipoprotein (LDL) and liproprotein (a) [Lp(a)] increased levels of homocysteine, and of C-reactive protein for the cardiovascular risk.

The necessary prerequisite for a long-term substitution is that the patient has no problems with subjective side effects or the possible treatment risks of HRT.

To be effective, long-term treatment must not start later than at the time of menopause and should use well-proven estrogen and progestogen preparations in low doses and an optimal mode of application for the individual patient. For instance, a continuous combined estrogen–progestogen therapy with medroxyprogesterone acetate (MPA) is apparently not suited for primary cardiovascular prevention (e.g. HERS, ERA and WHI studies) and is disputed concerning an increased risk of breast cancer.

The effects of long-term estrogen substitution therapy thus includes the elimination of troublesome climacteric complaints, of atrophic urogenital changes and the overall improvement of cognitive functions and of quality of life, which secure the social competence and the dignity of an aged woman.

Favorable preventive influences of estrogens on atherosclerosis, coronary infarction and, in some studies, stroke have been amply demonstrated for long-term estrogen substitution by experimental, clinical and epidemiologic studies. This controversial topic is, however, still under discussion, as the success of prevention is dependent on a strict indication, careful consideration of contraindications and existing risk factors, on a competent individual treatment and careful regular supervision. Moreover, as stated before, a prerequisite of success is beginning the prevention before atherosclerotic changes have had chance to become established. Competent treatment again means selection of the best-suited estrogen, the optimal dose and, in particular, selection of the best-suited progestogen. Finally, the optimal application technique of the hormone must be found, appropriate to the individual needs and wishes of the patient.

Problems of studies

Study results concerning the problems of prevention by estrogen treatment have sometimes been misleading, as they did not always investigate the relevant age groups at recruitment (50–55 years of age, peri–postmenopausal healthy women) and because they used inadequate diagnostic tools, hormone application and progestogens, and inappropriate groups for comparison and inappropriate endpoints of success. Some of them were because of their design far from practical relevance.

Undisputed effects of HRT

Undisputed is the preventive and therapeutic effect of estrogens on climacteric complaints, urogenital disorders, osteoporosis and bone fractures in all parts of the body, and their preventive effect on colon cancer.

Possible risks

The possible risks comprise a slight promotion of mammary, ovarian(?) and endometrial cancer (when estrogen is given unopposed by a progestogen), the slightly increased incidence of thromboembolism (mostly in the first year of treatment) and of cholecystitis/cholelithiasis.

These risks are nearly all preventable, especially by observing the contraindications, like mammary, endometrial and colon cancer in the family, the family and patient history of myocardial infarction, stroke, thromboembolism, severe liver or gallbladder diseases, and by giving preventive lifestyle counseling or an additional preventive treatment directed to the specific individual risk of the patient.

The group that will experience manifestation of one or the other of these risks is relatively small and it makes the art of treatment to anticipate and to prevent these risks as outlined above by a strict observation of indications, contraindications, as well as a prudent choice of hormones, doses and modes of application. If meaningful, appropriate additional medical measures can be performed, this will add to the safety of substitution.

IMPACTS OF ERT AND HRT: LIFETIME RISKS, MORBIDITY AND MORTALITY

To weigh the impact of risks of ERT and HRT, it is first necessary to consider the postmenopausal real lifetime risks for morbidity and, as the endpoint of judgment, that of mortality of the expected postmenopausal diseases.

Ten per cent of all women of a high age may develop breast cancer, 50% osteoporosis and about 35% cardiovascular diseases. The risk of a 50-year-old woman to die from a hip fracture is about 2.8%, that of mortality from coronary disease is as high as 31%. The risk of dying from breast cancer is, in contrast, relatively low at 2.5%, and the risk of dying from endometrial cancer amounts to 0.7%.[1] These data must be kept in mind when considering the evaluation of the risk:benefit ratio and of cost-effectiveness for prevention.

CONSEQUENCES OF LONGEVITY

The prolongation of life expectancy poses severe problems to society. In this regard, ERT and HRT are not a major problem as they will only slightly prolong life expectancy. The problem is a general one of population development, caused by better life conditions and progress in medicine. Who will pay the very high costs for the care of the steadily increasing number of elderly people and who will care for them in the nursing homes? If we prevent diseases, we will spare money for some time; but if we prolong life, we will postpone the costs to a later time and will, on the whole, prolong and increase the expense. As nearly everybody wishes to live longer in good quality, and indeed has a longer life expectancy, government policies must find ways to solve the monetary and human problems.

BASIC CONSIDERATIONS CONCERNING BENEFIT–RISK DETERMINATIONS AND COSTS

Methods of analysis include *risk:benefit ratios*, *cost–benefit analyses* and pure *cost calculations*. Estrogen and estrogen–progestogen sequential substitution must each be dealt with separately, as many investigations concern unopposed estrogen therapy. Moreover, the main positive actions of hormone substitution on lipids, organ perfusion and bone metabolism are to be attributed to estrogen effects and certain progestogens may attenuate some of the many wanted beneficial effects of estrogens. Some progestogens may increase breast cancer risk.

Unopposed estrogen therapy was not used in Europe, except in hysterectomized women. Therefore, the errors and confusions concerning unopposed ERT in the US in the 1970s, causing harm to the idea of hormone treatment, were not applicable to Europe. Only some 25% of the patients in the US studies under unopposed estrogens were also hysterectomized and therefore not at risk for uterine cancer.

The consideration of risk of mammary cancer under ERT must discriminate between less than 5 years use of unopposed estrogens [e.g. relative risk (RR) 0.99] and more than 5 years of use (e.g. RR 1.34). The risks for breast cancer and cardiovascular diseases seem slightly higher when a progestogen like MPA or nortestosterone is added (RR of 1.53 for breast cancer).[125,137]

It is not well documented as to how far conjugated estrogens are principally similar in action, side effects and risks to micronized estradiol or to estradiol valerate, estrogen preparations that were preferentially used in Europe.

All the benefit–risk considerations so far concern oral medication. However, oral medication may not be the optimal method of treatment with estrogens when liver/gallbladder load, primary liver passage with early inactivation and unwelcome metabolism of estrogens, effects on hepatic coagulation factors and unphysiologically high levels of estrone in plasma and breast are considered. On the other hand, do the accentuated positive effects of estrogen on lipids go together with oral medication of estrogen?

Prerequisite and necessary requirement of an optimal HRT is, I repeat, the use of a well-suited progestogen. At present too many different progestogens are used and some of them may be disadvantageous for the beneficial actions of estrogens.

Regrettably, very little data are available on the combination of estradiol with natural progesterone, which is, in my opinion, the optimal combination and would probably improve risk:benefit ratios, especially when progesterone is given rectally or vaginally, which is, as concerns metabolism, nearer to physiologic ovarian secretion.

WHI STUDY RESULTS

Concerning the WHI study,[2] is to be stressed again, that the start of ERT or HRT with the aim of prevention of osteoporosis and cardiovascular diseases should begin as early as possible, i.e. at latest at the perimenopause or menopause, and possibly in overall healthy women. In the WHI study most probands were too old for primary prevention, many of them were not healthy, presented contraindications, had been taking estrogens for some years and in addition to estrogens had received other medicaments. It can be learned from the WHI study that a late start of prevention or treatment of patients older than 60 years may give poor results. It is apparently too late for primary prevention with estrogens, particularly in

women who already have organic atherosclerotic lesions in their vessels.[3,4]

Indications, contraindications, risk factors and conditions of practice should be observed in strictly controlled trials, which was not the case in the WHI study. The results of the WHI study show that a combined continuous oral treatment with conjugated estrogens 0.625 mg and progestogen MPA 2.5 mg is apparently not well suited for primary prevention of cardiovascular diseases, as the daily addition of this progestogen attenuates the beneficial effects of estrogens. This has been shown in many investigations. However, sequential addition of MPA in the second half of the cycle seems not to have significant disadvantageous effects. While in the sequential regimen estrogens act unopposed in the first phase of the cycle and a monthly dose of only 25 mg MPA is given during the second half of the cycle, in the combined continuous regimen 75 mg MPA per cycle is given, which certainly represents considerable permanent antiestrogenic and corticoid-like activity.

In summary, it is clear that the description given in this chapter of earlier benefit–risk studies with oral ERT and HRT may reflect treatment in the past up to recent times but not current actual treatment and definitely not that of the future. The following elaboration must therefore be seen under *time-conditioned restrictions*. Regrettably, only scanty data are available for transdermal and other parenteral treatments, as well as for estrogen–androgen preparations, designer hormones and selective estrogen receptor modulators (SERM).

OBJECTION OF HEALTHY USER BIAS

It has been argued that the beneficial effects of estrogens might be caused by a 'healthy user bias'. This means that patients receiving or demanding estrogens may be healthier and more health conscious than controls who do not receive estrogens. Therefore, the better long-term results of patients receiving ERT or HRT were suspected to be possibly spurious and only seemingly beneficial. There are however some studies where this possibility has been excluded by a very homogenous population, by matched pairs, special calculations or by randomization. A comparison of more than 150 uncontrolled observational studies with a similar number of controlled randomized studies showed that the results were identical in both groups.[5]

The Centers for Disease Control, after analysis of the problem, came to the conclusion that there are no substantial differences between HRT users and nonusers as concerns health before treatment and risky lifestyle. Healthy user bias therefore seems not to play a role in the causation of long-term benefits of estrogens.

BENEFITS AND RISKS IN THE OPINION OF PATIENTS

Perimenopausal patients have their own fears and reservations concerning ERT/HRT. These are mostly caused by diagreeable articles in the media. The expected or experienced benefit is the improvement of climacteric complaints,

mainly flushes, depressive mood and sleep disturbances, urogenital complaints and the improvement of overall quality of life. The most prominent fear is due to recent discussions of mammary cancer. Endometrial and colon cancer play a minor role, as do cardiovascular diseases, because they are discussed less (Table 29.1).

Patients in nursing homes see the greatest benefits in the prevention of osteoporosis, coronary disease and cognitive function. Drawbacks of HRT are considered to be withdrawal bleedings, increased risk of breast and endometrial cancers, and thrombosis.

Guenther,[6] reported, after questioning 100 patients, that 92% felt that HRT was beneficial for them, i.e. Only 8% saw more drawbacks than benefits. The author found that women wanted as low a dosage of estrogen as possible. Benefits of HRT were the relief of climacteric complaints (49%), general wellbeing, improvement in the quality of life (31%), prevention of osteoporosis (14%), fever wrinkles (3%), greater

Table 29.1 Benefits and drawbacks of HRT in the opinion of late postmenopausal patients in a nursing home[10]

	Greatest					Least
	1	2	3	4	5	6
Benefits						
Prevention of osteoporosis	79	10	7	0	4	0
Improvement of memory loss	3	35	21	14	14	0
Prevention of urinary infection	0	3	29	25	32	4
Decrease of coronary artery disease	17	41	18	14	14	0
Prevention of depression	0	7	21	39	21	7
Decrease of wrinkling	0	0	0	0	7	82
Drawbacks						
Withdrawal bleeding	22	19	15	11	11	19
Increase in breast cancer	37	22	22	0	19	0
Increase in endometrial cancer	11	33	22	7	4	19
Mood swings	11	0	11	22	27	30
Increase in blood pressure	4	4	11	33	26	19
Increase of thrombosis	15	19	15	22	15	11

tolerance (70%) and no uterine bleedings (2%). These effects were important for compliance.

In the opinion of the probands, drawbacks of HRT were weight increase (20%), breast complaints (22%), cancer risk (21%), aversion to medicaments (13%), thrombosis and varicosis (6%) and uterine bleedings (2%). Patients demanded from the treatment good tolerability (79%), reliable effectivity (30%), no weight increase (15%), individualization (6%) and simplicity in application (4%). The opinions of what the patients thought to be important for treatment were quite different to those of gynecologists.[7]

OBJECTIVE ULTIMATE MEASURES OF EFFECTIVITY AND LIMITATIONS

Some important criteria of effectivity of ERT/HRT are subjective and are expressed by the patient or her doctor only on questioning. A personal inquiry is, however important, far from objective.

An ideal objective measure of the effectivity of a treatment or prevention needs to be *outcome orientated* over many years. Useful parameters would be: (1) *the length of life* (years of life gained); (2) frequency and duration of *hospitalization*; (3) *mortality* (4) the *quality of life*: (1)–(3) are easily and exactly determined, but (4), although for most women highly important, is difficult to assess and is mostly subjective. Quantitative measurement tools of quality of life have been elaborated and evaluated [e.g. menopause rating scale (MRS) I and II]. Another factor that needs to be incorporated into the analysis is the *balance between present and future health benefits*, the latter of which is, of course, difficult to anticipate.

In preventive medicine the costs are immediate, some of the benefits may be actual but others will (or will not) materialize only in the future. Not every benefit–risk analysis can, in spite of using mathematical tools, be exact, and only approximations can be made. The components of the equations used to have to be individualized and updated continuously with advancing knowledge.

ESTIMATIONS OF BENEFIT–RISK AND COST-EFFECTIVENESS

So far, scientific data dealing with the benefit–risk of ERT/HRT are based on data of retrospective and a few longitudinal epidemiologic studies and on subjective experiences with routine HRT. Benefit–risk determinations can be found readily in the literature.[8–27]

The opinion of the patient is, of course, and should remain, the most important criterion of benefits and success. The benefit of a prevention or treatment in older publications were measured, as outlined above, by well-controled data, as the influence of ERT/HRT on morbidity, mortality, frequency of hospitalization, quality of life and years of life gained.

The mostly frequently used weighting schemes or health status indices (Lambda S = disability weight) are those of Bush et al[28] and Weinstein and Stason,[29] assigning a numerical weight between 0 and 1 to differentiate full health (0) from varying degrees of disability or discomfort (maximum = 1). The greater the number, the greater the disability: 0 would accordingly indicate perfect health and 1.0 would imply a patient's worst condition with death imminent. Thus, the health status is calculated as $1 - P$.

BENEFITS OF ERT

The benefits of ERT and HRT are summarized in Box 29.1. In the following studies only unopposed ERT was considered, although in a few sequential addition of a progestogen (based on a small number of cases) was also mentioned. Since 1980 there have been at least a dozen published reports that have estimated the impact of ERT on overall health, as measured by changes of 'disease event rates' and changes in overall 'life expectancy.'

Weinstein[30] first considered the impact of unopposed estrogen substitution in 50 to 55-year-old women, followed up for 10–15 years. He included effects on climacteric symptoms, heart diseases, risks of endometrial hyperplasia and cancer, hip and wrist fractures, and gallbladder disease. Mammary cancer risk was not

---

Box 29.1 BENEFITS AND RISKS OF ERT AND HRT

Benefits

Improvement or elimination of climacteric complaints, hot flushes, sweating, palpitations, depressive mood, sleep disturbances

Improvement of vigilance and cognitive functions, of psychic stability, fatigue, anxiety, nervousness, irritability

General improvement of organ perfusion, including coronaries and brain

Improvement or maintenance of quality of life

Regulation of premenopausal menstrual cycle disturbances (estrogen + progestogen)

Improvement of skin, hair, teeth, mucous membranes and conjunctivae, their structure and function (esthetic medicine)

Prevention or improvement of atrophic urogenital complaints.

   Dry vagina (lubrication), atrophic vulvitis, colpitis, cohabitation problems, pollakisuria strangury, nocturia, urinary incontinence, urogenital infections

Improvement of muscles and joints (osteoarthritis)

Prevention of osteoporosis, spine (back pain), wrist and hip fractures

Prevention of disability and nursing home care

Primary prevention of atherosclerotic changes and of some of its sequelae, such as angina pectoris, coronary infarction and stroke(?)

Reduction of hospitalization rate

Reduction of the capability to work

Partial prevention of colorectal cancer

Prevention of or postponing Alzheimer's disease (still questionable)

Improvement of cancer cure and survival rates

Decrease of cancer and cardiovascular mortality

Small increase in life expectancy

The benefits of estrogens can be optimally secured by strict observance of indication, early beginning of preventive medication and by individualization of treatment

Risks

Small increase of breast cancer diagnoses(?)

Small increase of deep phlebothrombosis

Small increase of cholecystitis/cholelithiasis

The possible risks are mostly preventable by strict observance of indication and by prudent counseling

considered, as at that time an increased risk had not been clearly shown. Life expectancy, quality of life and costs were considered. Effects on climacteric symptoms and quality of life were found to be decisive for the judgment of benefit. When measured in terms of quality of years of life (QALY), Weinstein came to a positive benefit:risk ratio for ERT; the costs were estimated to be comparatively minor. A small net prolongation of life expectancy was reported for women over 50 years of age, amounting to 0.04 years after 10 years of treatment and 0.06 years after 15 years of treatment.

This work was later extended and updated to assess treatment with estrogen and estrogen + sequential progestogen in 50-year-old women, followed up for 5–15 years.[31] Again, a positive risk:benefit ratio was found, positively influenced also by the reduction of fractures and endometrial cancer risk by addition of a progestogen. The beneficial influence of estrogen on heart disease was not substantially reduced by sequential addition of a progestogen in low doses. A small increase in life expectancy for women receiving long-term estrogen substitution was also found. The costs of estrogen–progestogen therapy were estimated to be low in comparison to the treatment of preventable diseases.

The formula of health costs of Weinstein and Stason[29] was the following:

$$\text{Delta C} = \text{Delta RX} + \text{Delta SE} - \\ \text{Delta C Benef} + \text{Delta RX} + \text{Delta LE}$$

where Delta C is the net health care costs, Delta RX is all direct costs (drugs, physicians, etc.), Delta SE is all health costs due to side effects of treatment, Delta C Benef is the benefits and savings in health care costs due to prevention of diseases, and Delta LE is the change in life expectancy.

Henderson et al[32] considered 10 years unopposed ERT and estrogen–progestogen replacement therapy (HRT) in relatively old women (65–74 years of age). They estimated as the endpoint the reduction of mortality per 100,000 late postmenopausal women compared with women of the same age group without intervention, including the impact of ERT and HRT

on fractures, ischemic heart disease, and breast and endometrial cancer mortality. A reduction of mortality of 230 lives saved per 100,000 women/year was estimated for women with a uterus receiving ERT. For hysterectomized women an even higher reduction of mortality of 256 lives saved per 100,000 women/year was estimated: for estrogen + progestin medication a reduction of only 163 lives saved per 100,000 women/year was calculated. Thus, the difference in mortality was due to the better effect of estrogens only, while the addition of a progestin (MPA) reduced the beneficial effect of estrogens on mortality from 48 to 31%, apparently caused by the antiestrogenic effect of the progestogen, affecting preponderantly cardiovascular diseases.

RISK, BENEFITS AND COSTS OF ESTROGEN–PROGESTOGEN SEQUENTIAL TREATMENT (HRT)

In the studies discussed below unopposed ERT was not considered. Tosteson et al[33] included in their risk–benefit estimate fractures, heart diseases, and breast and endometrial cancer in 50-year-old women treated and followed up for 5–15 years. Life expectancy, quality of life and costs were calculated. The findings were similar to their former investigations and thus thought positive.

Tosteson et al[34] (from the Weinstein group) investigated the use of estrogen–progestogen sequential replacement in 50-year-old women with an intact uterus. The HRT group and the controls were followed for 5 years to life-long. Analysis included hip fractures, and mortality from ischemic heart diseases and from breast cancer, and estimated a net increase in life expectancy, which ranged from 0.14 to 0.24 years for 10–15 years of HRT. Quality of life was greatly improved and therefore the cost was low compared to treatment costs of the diseases prevented. The balance was therefore positive overall.

The following risk–benefit analyses are near to actual conditions. Daly et al[35] considered treatment of hysterectomized women with ERT and of women with a uterus under sequential

HRT. The start age was 50, and treatment and follow-up lasted for 10 years. Included in this paper were fractures, ischemic heart diseases (50% reduction after 10 years HRT), cerebrovascular diseases (25% reduction with ERT and 12.5% reduction with HRT) and breast cancer (0% increased risk at 5 years, 30% at 10 years, 50% at 15 years of treatment). The authors assumed a 25% probability of curettage and hysterectomy. They found a reduced death rate of 6% and a reduced hospital admission rate of 1% (evidencing reduction of morbidity) in estrogen-substituted women in 5-year age bands. A less favorable (3%) reduction of death rate resulted (compared to British mortality rates) when estrogens were combined with a progestogen (MPA), and, in addition, an elevated hospital admission rate of 1% was found with addition of a progestogen. The quality of life was substantially improved by both ERT and HRT. The health care cost included lifetime costs of therapy and monitoring, expected costs of treating side effects, expected saving of costs from reduced morbidity and expected costs of treating patients during an increased life expectancy. Details of all assumptions must be read in the original paper (Table 29.2).

Cheung and Wren[36] combined Australian data with data from the epidemiologic literature. They evaluated both unopposed and opposed replacement in symptomatic and asymptomatic women. Their benefit–risk analysis included hip and wrist fractures, and endometrial and breast cancers. The benefits prevailed significantly when mortality, and life quality and expectancy were considered. They estimated 377 cases of additional mammary cancers in the estrogen–progestogen-treated group for Australia per year in a total of 1577 breast cancer cases – an additional 33%. No increase of endometrial cancer but minus 1583 cases of myocardial infarction and minus 558 cases of stroke were calculated. Thus, 1764 precocious deaths per year in their population were assumed to be prevented by ERT.

Grady et al,[37] in a most comprehensive study, estimated the impact of long-term ERT and HRT on asymptomatic postmenopausal women 50 years of age. Improvement of climac-

Table 29.2   Range of health service costs (1992/93) in pounds sterling per hospital admission or per case (for fractures)[35]

Disease	Costs* (£ sterling)
Breast cancer	1950–6910
Ischemic heart disease	1540–4750
Cerebrovascular disease	4000–12,010
Hysterectomy	1610–3810
Dilatation and curettage	350–1300
Hip fracture	2230–6210
Vertebral fracture	170–420
Wrist fracture	170

* Includes inpatient costs, outpatient costs, radiotherapy, physiotherapy, general practitioner consultations and drugs costs.

teric complaints and quality of life was accordingly not considered. It was the aim of the authors to quantify risk and benefits of long-term ERT and HRT for prevention of diseases such as osteoporosis and coronary heart diseases which are influenced by estrogens. Endometrial and breast cancer risks were included. The second endpoint was the possibility of prolonging life. Meta-analysis was used to estimate the RR and benefits of HRT, and for their calculation all relevant literature from 1979 to 1992 was taken into account (the source of these data must be checked in the original paper).

The reduction of coronary diseases, stroke, femoral cervical fracture, and the influence of ERT and HRT on endometrial and mammary cancer with the reduction of total RR (including that for hysterectomized women) can be seen in Tables 29.3 and 29.4. Also, the probabilities of occurrence of postmenopausal diseases in women who are at risk was calculated. Again, a prolongation of life expectancy of 0.9 years was estimated for women receiving ERT and 1.0 year for HRT. HRT (addition of a progestogen) was assumed to reduce coronary heart disease

Table 29.3   Probability for the occurrence of postmenopausal diseases during lifetime in 50-year-old women under long-term ERT/HRT[37]

Disease	No treatment	Estrogens	Estrogen + progestogen*	Estrogen + Progestogen†
Coronary heart disease (%)	46.1	34.2	34.4	30.0
Stroke (%)	19.8	20.2	20.3	129.3
Femoral cervical fracture (%)	15.3	12.7	12.8	12.0
Breast cancer (%)	10.2	13.0	13.0	19.7
Endometrial cancer (%)	2.6	19.7	2.6	2.6
Life expectancy (years)	82.8	83.7	83.6	82.9

* Under the assumption that the addition of a progestogen will not influence the relative risk (RR) of ERT, except for reduction of endometrial cancer risk (RR of 1.0).
† Under the assumption that addition of a progestogen reduces the benefits of ERT concerning coronary heart diseases by one-third. The RR for coronary heart diseases is taken as 0.8 and for breast cancer as 2.0.

Table 29.4   Relative risk (RR) for all clinical subtypes of stroke under long-term substitution with estrogens and estrogen + sequential progestogen in the postmenopause and senium[165]*

Hormones	All strokes	Acute stroke	Subarachnoidal bleeding	Intracerebral bleeding	Thromboembolic stroke
Estrogens only†	0.79	0.72	1.24	0.57	0.78
Estradiol valerate + levonorgestrel	0.61	0.56	0.83	0.20	0.57

* Number of women, 23,088; number of cases of cerebrovascular diseases, 361; follow-up, 5.8 years.
† Conjugated estrogens and estradiol valerate.
Significance of the positive estrogen effect only apparent at 60 years of age or older, increasing with age and duration of ERT/HRT. Estriol was not effective.

by 66% and to increase the risk of breast cancer twofold (RR 2.0), the overall life expectancy, compared to no intervention, was still prolonged but reduced to 0.1 years.

In women at risk for cardiovascular diseases, life expectancy under ERT was increased for 2.1 years and prolonged even in patients with mammary cancer. However, addition of a progestogen reduced the life expectancy to 0.6 years. Also, in cases with risk for osteoporosis and coronary infarction, assuming an increase in mammary cancer, the benefits of risk reduction and prolongation of life prevailed. Even in patients with increased risk for endometrial and mammary cancers the life expectancy was shown to be increased by 0.7 years if these diseases occur. The benefit of HRT will only vanish if a progestogen preparation is added continuously, which counteracts the positive effects of the estrogens.

In their latest study, Tosteson et al[33] analyzed two groups of patients who were 50 years of age postmenopausal. For hysterectomized women they evaluated 10 and 15 years of ERT with 0.625 mg conjugated estrogens daily. Women with a uterus received 0.625 mg conjugated estrogens + 5–10 mg of MPA sequentially for 13 days/month. Net effectiveness was measured as Delta LE or as quality-adjusted life expectancy (Delta QALE) for patients treated by HRT, which were then compared with untreated controls.

The components of Delta LE were correlated with breast cancer, coronary heart disease and osteoporotic fractures of the hip, denoted as + Delta LE BRCA, + Delta LE CHD and + Delta LE HIP.

For the quality of life expectancy components of quality of life were considered that were associated with morbidity due to hip fracture, symptom relief and side effects associated with treatment. These were denoted as + Delta Q HIP, + Delta Q Sympt and + Delta Q Side. Quality of life was generally improved by ERT or HRT.

Costs associated with HRT, long-term nursing home care, breast cancer, hip fracture and coronary heart disease treatment were denoted as + Delta C HRT, + Delta C NH, + Delta C BRCA, + Delta C HIP and + Delta C CHD. (The quality of life adjustments are shown later in this chapter.)

The ratio of additional cost (AC) to additional health benefits, when HRT is compared with no intervention, is expressed by the following equation:

Delta AC/Delta LE = (+ Delta C HRT + Delta C NH + Delta BRCA + Delta C CHD)/ (+Delta LE HIP + Delta E BRCA + Delta E CHD)

Symptom relief was found to be nearly complete. Life expectancy of good quality was slightly increased, morbidity of hip fractures was decreased by about 50%. Nursing home admission was totally prevented by HRT. The costs associated with intervention were about 40% of the cost when no intervention was made. The overall benefits were significant.

Notelovitz,[21] considering urogenital atrophy, reduction of fractures, cardiovascular diseases and colon cancer, and improvement of cognitive functions against breast and endometrial cancer risks, concluded from his assessment of benefits and risks that the benefits greatly outweigh the possible side effects. This holds true for both morbidity and mortality related conditions that can have a negative impact on postmenopausal life.

COSTS

Costs have been considered in some of the previously cited papers (see above). Twenty per cent of the expense for total medical care of women is spent in the postmenopause in those who suffer from a disease that is in some way linked to estrogen deficiency.[38] By a preventive long-term substitution with estrogen–progestogen 40% of these expenses could be saved.[7]

The cost-effectiveness, including the quality of life considerations, is expressed in the following equation:[33]

Delta C/Delta QALY = (+ Delta C HRT + Delta HIP + Delta NH + Delta BRCA + Delta C CHD)/(+ Delta LE HIP + Delta LE BRCA + Delta LE CHD + Delta Q Hip+ Delta Q Sympt + Delta Q SIDE)

The analysis of costs of Wren[39] resulted in a clear prevailing of benefits and a reduction of costs by estrogen–progestogen prevention.

In Germany, 37% of women take estrogens for 2–5 years, 15% more than 5 years and 8% more than 8 years.[40,41] Wenderlein[27,42] calculated the costs in Germany for HRT per person and per year to be 113 DM. The total costs of use of sexual hormones came to 250 million DM for women between the ages 60 and 69, to 530 million DM for those between the ages of 50 and 59, alternative treatments were much more expensive. The cost of statins, cardiovascular medicaments and antidementia came to 735 million DM between the ages of 50 and 59 and 1434 million DM between the ages of 60 and 69 (data from the Scientific Institute of the German Health Insurance 1996).

PREVENTION OF OSTEOPOROSIS AND FRACTURES

The lifetime risk for hip fractures is 3% in women who have a lifespan of 75 years and 11% for those with a lifespan of 85 years. In Germany 3.17 million women per year suffer hip fractures. The mean hospital stay of these patients is 34.2 days and the necessary rehabilitation is expensive. Nearly all elderly women are thereafter invalids. Post-fracture mortality is as high as 22%.

The incidence of osteoporosis increases in later decades. Osteoporosis in its beginning is slowed or stopped in women receiving ERT and HRT. Estrogen therapy should begin at early menopause and continue for at least 10–15 years for a significant decrease in hip fractures. Fractures are prevented in 50–60% of cases in 54% for femoral (see Michaelsson et al[43] and WHI study) and 50–90% for spinal fractures. One-hundred-and-three hip, wrist and vertebral fractures/1000 women are preventable. Nortestosterone–progestogens act synergistically to estrogens against osteoporosis in prevention and treatment. After withdrawal of HRT, decreases in bone density will continue.

The potential benefit of prevention of osteoporosis can be calculated as shown in Table 29.5. The costs for the acute care of a patient

with a hip fracture was calculated in the US to be US$17,440–20,590 year.[29] Alternatives like bisphosphonates are more expensive as compared to estrogen; calcium, vitamin D and physical activity are, although basic for prevention and treatment, not alone sufficient.

The probability of death from hip fractures was estimated to be 0.06 for women aged 50–59, 0.03 for women aged 60–69, 0.06 for women aged 70–79 and 0.11 for women aged 80 and over. Persons who survive a hip fracture usually require long-term placement in a nursing home. The probability of remaining in a nursing home at 1 year following hip fracture ranges from 0 for women aged 50–59 to 0.30 in women aged 85 and over. Quality of life is diminished accordingly. The quality weights reflect acute and chronic morbidity following a fracture. The estimate for uncomplicated fractures is 0.95, for a disabling hip fracture 0.76 and for long-term nursing home placement 0.36. The lower the number, the higher the loss of quality of life.

In other calculations 0 was defined as death and 1.0 as perfect health, which seems more logical. The risk–benefit of long-term ERT and HRT for hip fractures in cases at risk for coronary heart diseases, from the calculation of Grady et al,[37] can be seen in Table 29.5.

In Germany, Ringe and Steinhagen-Thiessen[44] have calculated that the costs for prevention of osteoporosis by HRT were 384,850 DM/year, while the treatment of osteoporosis

---

Table 29.5   Potential benefit of prevention of osteoporosis[37]

Condition	P
Radiologic osteoporosis, no disability	0.1
Occasional discomfort on exertion	0.35
Fractured wrist	0.55
Femoral neck or vertebral compression fracture	0.85
Totally bedridden, disabled, intractable pain	1.0

P, Probability of death; 1 – P, disability weight; Lambda y_{osteo} in quality of years of life.

amounted to 4.5 million DM/year. Thus, by prevention with estrogens most of these expenses could be saved. Invalidity will cost about 300 million DM/year.

HYPERTENSION

There is anxiety about the use of hormones and the possible development of hypertension. When blood pressure increases during HRT, most therapeuts will withdraw estrogens. Many papers have shown that estrogens do not increase normal blood pressure and that a slightly increased blood pressure may even be decreased by estrogens. In a few cases with a disturbance or renin–angiotensin–aldosterone metabolism, oral conjugated estrogens may increase blood pressure.

Accordingly, HRT is safe in hypertensive women who should not therefore be denied ERT/HRT if they complain of menopausal symptoms.[45] In questionable cases, transdermal estradiol and vaginal progesterone, avoiding the first liver passage, may be preferred.

CORONARY HEART DISEASES

Epidemiologic studies have consistently found that women receiving ERT are at lower risk of coronary heart disease.[47–50] Recent meta-analyses have reported a decrease in the RR by estrogens for ischemic heart diseases of 0.50–0.65 [confidence interval (CI) 0.43–0.71].[37,51] The reduction of mortality under ERT has been shown in various studies to have a RR of 0.21–0.81.[14,32,51–58] This fact has to be stressed in counseling patients who are considering HRT.

Prevention must start early, at about 50 years of age, when the atheriosclerotic changes have not yet been irreversibly established. In surgically postmenopausal hominid monkeys, estrogen inhibits the development of atherosclerosis, where the disease is not yet established; however, a preventive effect of estrogen was not observed in monkeys with established atherosclerotic disease.[59]

Innummerable positive effects of estrogens on lipids, cardiac function and blood vessels have been documented experimentally and clinically (so-called surrogate parameters). Sequential addition of a progestogen may attenuate the effect on lipids and on organ perfusion. MPA is apparently not a suitable progestogen when given daily combined with the estrogen continuously without interruption. In such a combination the positive estrogen effect may be completely eliminated. Estrogen + sequential MPA seems not to be disadvantageous, as unopposed estrogen acts sufficiently beneficially during the first half of the cycle.

Selective drug usage, sufficiently high doses of estrogen, sequential addition of genuine progesterone or of a suitable progestogen (e.g. medrogestone) and an individualization of application is therefore of utmost importance for a positive benefit:risk ratio.

The most comprehensive benefit–risk calculation, including the effect of ERT and HRT on coronary heart disease, is that of Grady et al.[37] The substantial reduction of the probability of occurrence of postmenopausal diseases, such as coronary heart disease and stroke, is shown in Table 29.3. A possible reduction of the beneficial estrogen effects on cardiovascular diseases by some progestogens is also taken into account in Grady et al.[37]

Primary and secondary prevention of cardiovascular diseases as the only indication for estrogens

An indication of ERT/HRT for primary or secondary prevention of cardiovascular diseases alone was never practiced in Europe by gynecologists or internists. Climacteric complaints in the present author's experience are in about 80% of women. Prevention of osteoporosis is an additional reason to treat climacteric symptons in 59% of cases; the remainder are mostly indicated by treatment of urogenital complaints.

Therefore, the ongoing discussion on the topic of primary or secondary prevention of cardiovascular diseases as a primary indication is far removed from practice. The cardiovascular benefit found mostly in American epidemiologic studies was welcome information for European gynecologists as an additional factor in a symptomatic estrogen therapy and in counseling of patients concerning risks–benefits, and as an additional argument for a long-term treatment.

Costs of coronary disease claim 1.3% of all expenses for diseases, some of which could possibly be prevented by estrogens.[60] Secondary prevention with estrogens in older patients is not indicated, as atherosclerotic changes are mostly already present and because cardiovasular events have occurred before (HERS and ERA studies). In such cases statins seem to be indicated.

PREVENTION OF STROKE

Stroke is the third leading killer after heart diseases and cancer of women in developed countries. It leaves many survivors mentally and physically impaired. Stroke is therefore an important aim of primary prevention. Several studies suggested that ERT might reduce the risk of stroke (see Table 29.4). About 30 studies have produced controversial results. The Nurses' Health Study found a decrease of stroke incidence of RR 0.68 (0.39–1.16).[46,51] The majority of results suggest that long-term ERT does not increase the risk of stroke and results in a moderately reduced risk of fatal stroke (RR 0.15–0.68),[47,48,50,55,56,58] and that estrogens may improve survival (meta-analysis of 51, 52, 54). Because of the uncertainties in the summary of studies with different results, stroke is not included in the risk–benefit considerations. The costs of stroke claim 7.1% of all costs, some of which may be prevented by estrogen therapy for postmenopausal women.[60] A secondary prevention of stroke by estrogens is not indicated.

PREVENTION OF DEMENTIA

Ten per cent of women older than 65 years of age and nearly half of those over the age of 85 have Alzheimer's disease. A person with Alzheimer-type dementia will live on average for about 20 years from the onset of symptoms and for 8 years after its full development. More than 70% of people with Alzheimer's disease live at home, but half of those who are nursing home residents suffer from morbus Alzheimer.[61] The number of people with the disease will steadily increase in the coming decades and will thus become a grave medicosocial problem. An effective means of prevention would therefore be of great importance.

There are some observational studies, small retrospective cohort studies and one prospective study suggesting the possibility of an early primary prevention of atherosclerotic and Alzheimer-type dementia by estrogen substitution. Henderson[62,65] concluded, from 14 epidemiologic studies in a meta-analytic evaluation, a 45% reduction of risk. Estrogens improve cerebral blood flow, induce cellular markers of memory function in neurons critical to memory, and vulnerable to negative effects of aging and Alzheimer disease. They inhibit the production of the β-amyloid which is causal for the disease.[63] In addition, estrogen significantly and potently protects neurons against toxic insults associated with morbus Alzheimer.[64]

The epidemiologic data are however still inadequately secured. Therefore the possible reduction of this disease can at present not be safely included in a risk–benefit equation. The saving of expenses and of human suffering, if the prevention should be effective, would be very high as the costs of caring for dementia are the highest of all diseases which could be prevented by estrogens, e.g. 19.2% of all costs in The Netherlands.[60] A 5-year delay of onset of Alzheimer's disease would generate savings of at least 55 billion Euro/year worldwide. A 1-month delay in nursing home placement would save 1.1 billion Euro/year.[64]

However, some cognitive functions like vigilance, concentration, recall of names and short-term memory can certainly be improved by ERT and HRT, and this effect will improve the patient's quality of life considerably.

PREVENTION OF COLON CANCER

Recent use of HRT is associated with a 33% reduction incidence of colon cancer (RR 0.67; CI, 0.59–0.77[46]). The duration of use was not significantly effective concerning RR. The mortality from colon cancer in estrogen users was reduced by 28% (RR 0.72; 95% CI, 0.64–0.81) in comparision to nonusers[46,161,166] (meta-analysis of Nanda et al[66]; see also WHI study).

PREVENTION OF UROGENITAL ATROPHY

Between 25 and 56% of postmenopausal woman suffer from atrophic and degenerative disorders of the urogenital tract. As the number of old women will increase, the incidence of these problems can be expected to grow in future. Estrogen loss affects the vulva, clitoris, vaginal wall, urethra, bladder, and pelvic floor muscles and ligaments. The most common complaints are itching, dry vagina, problems in intercourse, urgency (20%), pollakiuria/dysuria, strangury (14%), urinary incontinence (16–29%) (frequently during intercourse), urethral prolapse, vaginal prolapse and recurrent urethrocystitis. Abundant estrogen receptors have been found in all the structures of the urogenital tract. Hormone replacement successfully treats or prevents the changes and complaints listed above. ERT and HRT are effective in increasing maximal urethral pressure and transmission of intra-abdominal pressure to the urethra, in decreasing urinary loss, in increasing cystometric capacity, reducing micturition, and improving the bulbocavernosum reflex. About 70% of treated women report general improvement of dysuria and urge incontinence.[67,68] Local treatment using estriol (suppositories or ring) is usually sufficient. In some cases estradiol–testosterone combinations may be optimal to improve the complaints. Many women are treated unsuccessfully for a long time with antibiotics or urinary disinfectants before the basic reason, i.e. atrophy, is recognized and treated successfully by hormone substitution.

PREVENTION OF OTHER DISEASES

The Study of Women's Health Across the Nation in the US showed that pre-, peri- and postmenopausal women more frequently had high blood pressure, diabetes, heart attacks/angina pectoris, arthritis, osteoporosis and cancer than younger women.[69] In contrast, patients receiving postmenopausal HRT had less hypertension, less diabetes, fewer heart attacks/angina pectoris, less arthritis, less osteoporosis, and fewer total cancer diseases and deaths than comparable controls, i.e. there was no healthy user effect!

The frequent increase in weight is not promoted but rather prevented by estrogen use. There is evidence that estrogen prevents skin atrophy and improves hair growth. The depth of wrinkles has been shown in double-blind studies against placeco to be improved by local estrogen application to the face. Hirsutism can be improved by an estrogen–antiandrogen combination. Subcutaneous connective tissue is also strengthened. The effectiveness of these benefits on self-esteem and quality of life has not been investigated, but will probably be high.

SOCIOECONOMIC EFFECTS

In an untreated menopausal women, incapability to perform daily tasks was found in 5% of cases, a reduced working capacity in 20% and a reduction of earning quota in 25%. Under this presupposition, a reduction of income of 4.25 million DM/year was estimated. A corresponding reduction of the gross social product of 4.25 million DM was found.[1]

QUALITY OF LIFE

Many papers have dealt with this subject.[6,9,33,41,70–93] The WHO definition of quality of life is used here, including physical, psychologic, social and environmental factors, and interpersonal relations, which are certainly not all estrogen dependent (Box 29.2).

Nevertheless, the improvement in quality of life is one of the most important effects of long-term estrogen substitution, as most of the criteria of it can only be enjoyed if the mind is well balanced. Quality of life is a subjective parameter and therefore direct questioning of the patient is necessary. There exist standardized questionnaires which try to record all aspects of quality of life. Among the most widely used are

(see Chapter 8)

Box 29.2   Criteria of quality of life according to the World Health Organization (WHO) 1991

Physical domain
   Pain and discomfort
   Energy and fatigue
   Sexual activity, etc.

Psychologic domain
   Work capacity
   Thinking, memory and concentration
   Self-esteem, etc.

Level of independence
   Mobility
   Activities of daily living
   Dependence on medical substances and
   medical aids, etc.

Social relationships
   Personal relationships
   Practical social support
   Activities of provider/supporter

Environment
   Physical safety and security
   Home environment
   Work satisfaction, etc.

Spirituality/religion/personal beliefs

being, the best methods available for determining quality of life (see Chapter 8).

Heavy sweating, cardiac irregularities, sleep disturbances and depressive mood are all important determinants of quality of life in peri- and postmenopausal women, and can all be safely eliminated by estrogen substitution.

A considerable limitation of quality of life and the general feeling of wellbeing, and of several body functions, was shown to accompany sleep disturbances.[84] Estrogen substitution improved quality of life from QOL 57 to 76 and the feeling of wellbeing from 58 to 77. Fears, depression and extraversion were improved as a consequence of the amelioration of sleep quality by estrogens.

Urogenital problems in postmenopausal women also have a major impact on quality of life. Urinary incontinence, together with urging and pollakiuria/strangury are most debilitating for postmenopausal women, as are lower genital tract disorders, inflammations and infections. These increase with age, according to the increasing atrophic changes. Local estrogen therapy is the most widely used and effective measure (e.g. Hudita)[105] against the negative impact of urogenital aging on quality of life.

Minor symptoms like decreased vitality, exhaustion, lack of concentration and general wellbeing will also be improved by estrogens. In the secondary evaluation of the HERS study, wellbeing and improvement of depressive mood under estrogen treatment were determining factors for the quality of life.

Quality of life adjustments

- Climacteric symptoms count: minus 0.01 QALY of symptom suffering (1%); under ERT/HRT the quality adjusted life expectancy (QALE) will increase by 0.01 QALY, equivalent to about 4 days/year.
- Spinal fractures count: minus 0.01 QALY for each year of remaining life expectancy (1%).
- Hip fracture count: minus 0.05 QALY for each year of life expectancy (5%).
- Mammary cancer counts: minus 1 QALY of remaining life expectancy (0.2 year for an average of 5 years).

the Sickness Impact, the Nottingham Health Profile,[94] the Quality of Well Being Scale,[81] the 35 Item Short Form Health Survey (SF 37) and the French Qualifemme. Hunter[95] developed the Women's Health Questionnaire as a menopause-specific instrument, which consists of 37 items making up nine scales. The Clinical Mensi Questionnaire, with a score of between 0 and 38, contains 29 questions.[96] The Utian Quality of Life Index[88,97–100] and the Menopause Rating Scale I and II[41,85,101–104] are, for the time

Wiklund et al[89,90,106] gave an example of the highly significant improvement of quality of life under HRT. It was shown that patients who received HRT had a similar quality of life to normal premenopausal patients without complaints (score of 105). Postmenopausal patients receiving no estrogens showed a score of 87.

Tieffenberg[107] found in his Satisfaction Index a mean of 88 points in women under ERT versus 66 points in nonhormonally treated patients. A worsening of climacteric symptoms of 2.4% was seen in patients under ERT/HRT, but in 44.1% of nonhormonally treated patients. Combination of estrogen with testosterone esters may in special cases additionally improve libido, orgasm, concentration, apathic depression and fatigue, and will thus increase the quality of life considerably.

HOSPITAL ADMISSIONS

Hospital admissions can be used as a measure of morbidity. In the study of Daly et al,[12,35] an overall reduction of hospital admissions was seen under ERT in hysterectomized women to 22/1000, which corresponds to a reduction of 1% against untreated controls. However, under estrogen–progestogen sequential treatment (HRT) the hospital admission rate increased by 1% against controls.

DECREASE OF MORTALITY (LIFE EXPECTANCY)

The mortality from osteoporotic fractures alone is higher than that of endometrial and mammary cancers taken together.[32,56,57] The mortality from cancer and from other diseases decreases under estrogen intake: American cohort studies found a significant decrease in fatal breast cancer deaths (RR 0.53–0.84).[32,56,57,78,109–111] A Swedish randomized study (Jernström et al;[110] see also Sourander et al[58]) showed a longer survival and a mortality reduction of 27% (RR 0.73) in mammary cancer patients under HRT (see Table 29.6). In cases of osteoporosis and cardiovascular events, when occurring under ERT or HRT, a significant reduction of mortality was also seen. The literature shows that

more than 5000 cases of premature unnecessary deaths/100,000 postmenopausal women/year can be prohibited by long-term ERT or HRT.

ERT increases the life expectancy (see above) for 0.2–1.1 years, increasing with the duration of estrogen substitution. Even if the patient develops a breast cancer during ERT or HRT, the use of estrogen is associated with a decrease of mortality of that disease: RR 0.84 (CI 0.75–0.94.)[111] Addition of a progestogen to the estrogen reduces the years of life gained about half.[35]

COST SAVINGS

Many studies on this subject have appeared in the literature.[12,29,76,111–119] Daly et al[35] found costs for ERT of £310/5 years, increasing to £660/20 years ERT. The direct cost for HRT were about 80% higher than for ERT. The cost savings of HRT will accordingly be lower. The range of health service costs for diseases that were not prevented can be seen in Table 29.2.[35] These greatly exceed the costs of ERT.

In Germany, Schneider[26] calculated the cost for the treatment of female osteoporosis as 4 billion DM. The treatment of 2 million postmenopausal women (total of 8 million menopausal women in Germany) receiving estrogen–progestogen substitution cost 100 million DM/year. That would be considerably less than the expenses necessary for the treatment of osteoporosis and fractures alone. The cost–benefit effect, when other savings associated with HRT were included, was calculated to be plus 2.53 billion DM.

NEW PREPARATIONS

For SERM, special application methods of estrogens (e.g. nasal, transdermal), estrogen–androgen combinations, designer hormones and phytoestrogens, few data of risks versus benefits had been available until now. Data for tibolone[120] and raloxifene[121] as compared to HRT have been published. It is probable that the different possibilities of application, as well as SERM and designer hormones, will improve the risk:benefit ratio because they will promote

Table 29.6 Decrease of mortality from breast cancer in postmenopausal women under ERT/or HRT				
Authors (ref)	Design of study	Number of breast cancer patients	Relative (95% CI)	P
Burch et al 1975[166]	Cohort	21	0.67	< 0.01
Bergkvist et al 1989[167]	Cohort	2610	0.68 (0.52–0.87)	< 0.01
Gambrell 1987, 1990[168,169]	Cohort	50	0.53 (0.40–0.76)	< 0.007
Hunt et al 1987[170]	Cohort	50	0.55	< 0.05
Henderson et al 1991[32]	Cohort	148	0.81	< 0.06
Criqui et al 1991[171]	Cohort	42	0.73 (0.44–1.22)	< 0.05
Lauritzen 1994[172]	Case control	63	0.55 (0.39–0.81)	< 0.01
Willis et al 1996[111a]	Prospective cohort	1469	0.84 (0.75–0.94)	0.07
Grodstein et al 1997[51]	Cohort	574	0.76 (0.56–1.02)	< 0.05
Sourander et al 1998[58]	Cohort	–	0.57 (0.27–1.20)	< 0.242
Sellers et al 1999[173]	Cohort	–	0.57 HRT 46/100,000 Control 66/100,000	< 0.242
Jernstrom et al 2001[110] prospective, 9 years' follow-up, 18 years' HRT, 25.9% died. Controls, 46.5% died	Randomized	984	0.73 (0.62–0.87)	0.0005

individualization and well-targeted hormonal treatment.

POSSIBLE RISKS: THE MINIMAX CONCEPT

As regards the possible risks of ERT and HRT, authors like Utian[88,98–100] stress the so-called *Minimax concept*; i.e. the art of replacement must achieve minimizing the risks and maximizing the benefits by risk assessment, selective drug usage and individualization of treatment.

As concerns estrogens and cancer, a scientifically correct judgment of the role of estrogens is not possible so long as the normal incidence of pre-existing occult cancers (breast, endometrium) in the normal female population is not known. It is probable that most cancers which occur under ERT and HRT were already present before HRT began and will only grow faster under the influence of the exogenous hormones (promotion effect).

For prostatic cancer it is known that normal males between the ages of 40 and 50 are host to a latent prostatic cancer in 30% of cases, between 50 and 60 years of age this rises to 40%, between 60 and 70 years of age to 60% and between 70 and 80 years of age to 70%, which may grow due to stimulation by androgens. Parallels to endometrial and breast cancers are apparent.

The endometrial cancer rate in aged females who died from other causes and were autopsied was 0.17%; that of mammary cancer was 0.51%.[122] As this population also contained younger women, it must be suspected that the female cancer rate may be even higher postmenopausally. The detected existing cancer rate at autopsy would correspond to the rate of increase of diagnoses of endometrial and breast cancers during long-term HRT. The detection rate of clinically latent cancers by mammographic screening is 8/1000 cases.

ENDOMETRIAL CANCER

Endometrial cancer is increased in unopposed ERT with a RR of 3.1.[123–125] The disease increases with duration of estrogen intake. It would be appropriate to obtain an endometrial biopsy in women with a uterus who have been on estrogen alone replacement for longer than 2 years. The type of cancer produced under estrogen substitution is usually an early stage, localized, well-differentiated endometrial tumor, and is thus readily amenable to cure (> 90%).[126] Women with endometrial cancer had a three times higher likelihood of having been unopposed estrogen users as compared to controls. This fact should be stressed in counseling patients who are considering HRT. Women who developed endometrial cancer on sequential therapy in general received less than the recommended daily doses of progestogens, had less active progestogens or were noncompliant.[127]

An estrogen monotherapy, as previously often used in the US but not practiced in Europe, should not be pursued in women with an intact uterus. The addition of a potent progestogen for at least 10 days (optimal 14 days) or combined continuously will decrease endometrial cancer risk to, or even below, a RR of 1.0[123–125] Table 29.7 demonstrates the use of the Health Status Index to quantify the situation for a potential risk of uterine cancer.

OVARIAN CANCER

Ovarian cancer is apparently not directly estrogen dependent, as the results of an adjuvant treatment with tamoxifen and progestogens is far less successful than in mammary cancer (12% for tamoxifen).[128]

Ovarian cancer cells show estrogen–progesterone receptors only in 50% of cases. There is no substantial increase in the risk of ovarian cancer in estrogen–progestogen-substituted women, except perhaps in a few controversial, disputed studies, after more than 10 years of substitution. RR is generally within the bounds of systemic or confounding bias.[130] Other studies suggested a protective effect of estrogen–progestogen.[131] Most studies and meta-analyses have not found an increase in ovarian cancer under estrogens.[132] In a Swedish cohort study ovarian cancer risk was not observed and need not be incorporated into the analysis of risk versus benefit.[133,134] A re-analysis of European studies was published by Negri et al.[135]

BREAST CANCER

Many studies and most meta-analyses have shown no significant increase in breast cancer risk by estrogens (Table 29.8). Recent representative prospective trials by Sourander et al[58] and

---

Table 29.7 The Health Status Index to determine the risk of potential uterine cancer[29]

Morbidity	P
Early cancer removed, no disability	0.05
Surgery + radiation, minimal disability	0.15
Vaginal stenosis and pain	0.35
Severe pain and recurrence by advanced secondary disease	0.88

The health status is calculated as as 1 – P; lambda × years = Delta Y, Delta y$_{carcinoma}$ in quality of years of life.

Table 29.8 Meta-analyses concerning long-term ERT/HRT and their influence on the risk of breast cancer

Authors (ref) No. of studies	Relative risk (RR)			Risk groups RR
	Estrogens total	Estrogens higher doses	Estrogens long-term	
Armstrong 1988[174] 23 studies	1.01 (0.95–1.08)	1.043 (0.88–1.24)	No effect	1.25, family history of breast cancer
Dupont and Page 1991[175] 28 studies	1.07 (1.0–1.15)	1.10 (0.95–1.25)	Not investigated	1.6, benign breast diseases
Steinberg et al 1991[176] 16 studies	1.0	Not investigated	1.3 (1.2–1.6)	3.4, family history 1.5, nulliparae 1.7, benign breast changes
Sillero-Arenas et al 1992[177] 23 studies	1.09 (1.0–1.12)	Not investigated	1.23 (1.2–1.6)	0.99 estrogen + progestogen (0.72–1.36) 3 studies
Grady et al 1992[178] 35 studies	1.25	Not investigated	Not investigated	Pooled data
Collaborative Group 1997[138] 51 studies	1.023 Increase of risk per year	–	1.35 > 5 years (1.21–1.49) Estrogens ever/never	Weight Body mass Parity Age at first pregnancy
Bush et al 2001[179] 45 studies estrogens	< 0.9 = 20% of studies 0.9–1.1 = 47% > 1.1 = 30% > 2.0 = 0%			All studies decreased mortality
20 studies estrogen + progestogen	RR significantly increased in 2 studies RR significantly decreased in 3 studies		5 studies: decreased mortality, 4 significant 6 studies life expectancy prolonged, 5 significant	

Lando et al,[136] and other newer studies, found no increase in breast cancer risk under long-term estrogen intake. Our own investigation on 1420 patients and corresponding matched pairs over 25 years found a RR of 0.8.

Nevertheless, the RR of breast cancer is at present mostly estimated to be slightly increased by estrogenic promotion, e.g. RR of 1.25 (CI 1.04–1.51) after more than 5 years substitution.[137,138] The increase in one meta-analysis was 0.2% after more than 5 years (two cases per 1000), 0.5% after 10 years (five cases per 1000) and 1.2% after 15 years (12 cases per 1000).[138] We have adopted these data for a benefit–risk calculation, although this risk is well within the limits of systemic and confounding bias (e.g. alcohol consumption, detection bias). When the data from the Nurses' Health Study were re-evaluated for alcohol consumption, the increased incidence of breast cancer was limited to those estrogen users who consumed substantial amounts of alcohol.[139]

Moreover, it must be considered that the rate of undetected endometrial cancer is 0.17% and of breast cancers 0.51% in autopsies in women who died from other causes,[122] and the rate of breast cancer detections shows a rate of 8/1000 breast cancers in mammographic screening in healthy women between the ages of 50 and 69 years.[140] These are probably the cancers promoted by estrogen use. It must therefore be assumed that most of the cancers diagnosed under ERT/HRT were already preclinically present before the hormone medication was begun and were only induced to faster growth and earlier diagnosis by the hormones. This may result in a spurious cumulative increase. All facts of any weight argue for the assumption that *estrogens are not carcinogenic* but rather facultatively promote mitotic activity only under certain circumstances such as genetic damage, genetic polymorphism, unnatural lifestyle or metabolic anomalies.[141] In addition, the increase in the rate of mitoses may increase the statistical probability of faulty DNA copies.

There are parallels to colon and prostatic cancer, which have a high rate of undetected presence in seemingly healthy persons (65% for 60-year-old males for prostatic cancer). The risk of breast cancer of a woman aged 60 years under continuing ERT may thus, by stimulating pre-existing receptor-positive cancer clones, increase from 1.8 to 3%.

Addition of certain progestogens [medroxyprogesterone acetate (MPA), nortestosterones] may slightly increase the breast cancer risk. Data from France using transdermal estrogen and mostly oral progesterone did not show an increase in breast cancer risk (RR 0.98).[142]

The *actual risk* should be preferred to the RR as it gives the standardized real increase in risk instead of percentages.[143] For breast cancer, if medication starts from age 50, the increase in cancer diagnoses was calculated to be only two more cases per 1000 women per year, three cases after 10 years HRT and 12 (5–20) cases after more than 15 years (if the basic data are correct). All the estrogen takers will have a good prognosis. Patients under estrogen–progestogen will show a 19–41% reduction of death from breast cancer (e.g. Willis et al[111a] and Lauritzen[144]). The reason is that breast cancer under ERT/HRT is characterized by a lower malignancy grade disease, more often localized tumor,[145] and smaller tumor size,[110] lower histologic grading,[145] and therefore a better prognosis, a better survival rate, a reduction of mortality (RR of 0.76),[32,51,56,57,123,146] and a still prolonged life expectancy. The mortality–benefit decreases slightly with the duration of HRT with a RR of 0.56 at less than 5 years to 0.80 after more than 10 years. In addition, the mortality from all cancer diseases is decreased to a RR of 0.71 (0.62–0.81).

Five years after withdrawal of the hormones RR will normalize to 1.0. In cases of long-term substitution and in older women the risk may be slightly higher.[137] Colditz[137] indicated that the positive effects of estrogens on prognosis and mortality may be decreased in older women. The possible increase of mammary cancer, if it occurs, would be computed as minus 1 QALY for the remaining life expectancy with 0.2 year for an average of 5 years.

The risk for mammary cancer can be minimized or even eliminated by respecting contraindications like family history of cancer, child-lessness, underweight, alcohol addiction, diagnostic extirpations of nodules of the breast and suspect or questionable mammographic findings or breast density in mammographies.[144] The costs for non-invasive breast cancer were estimated as US$120,850 per case.[35]

For the benefit:risk ratio it is important to stress that the incidence of total cancers is reduced to 0.71 (0.56–1.02), as stated in the Nurses' Health Study.[137]

GALLBLADDER DISEASES

The risk of gallbladder diseases has been said to be increased 2.5-fold (218/100,000 estrogen users/year versus 87/100,000 year in controls): others did not find such an increase.[123,147,148] The risk is especially increased in overweight patients. The risk can be minimized or even eliminated by respecting contraindications, giving low doses of estrogens, using parenteral medication, reducing weight, eating a fat-reduced diet and by additional treatment for optimizing biliary function. In our study, under these precautions the risk was not significantly elevated.[123]

DEEP VEIN THROMBOSIS AND THROMBOEMBOLISM

Increases in the incidence of thrombosis have been found to amount from 1/10,000/year to 2–3/10,000/year in postmenopausal women.[149] The events occur mostly during the first year of HRT by a demasking of genetic disorders of coagulation. The thrombotic event is estrogen-dose dependent and can apparently be promoted by some progestogens (e.g. MPA). The presence of the Factor V Leiden mutation confers a 50-fold increase in the risk of venous thrombosis, and this mutation exists in 5% of all Caucasian women. The risk can be minimized by a thorough family history of thrombotic events, observing risk factors and contraindications like being overweight, smoking and varicosis, as well as by counseling on how to avoid triggering events for thrombosis and indicating additional treatment of varicosis, e.g. daily gymnastics, local application of heparin–salicylic acid ointment to the calves.

In a clinical randomized prospective study, observing good clinical practice, using 0.625 mg conjugated estrogens and transdermal estradiol (50 µg) + 5 mg sequential medrogeston orally in 42 cases for 3 months no thrombotic complications were seen. The parenteral application of estradiol produced no increase in coagulatory activity. In particular, the acute phase reaction, Factor VII (minus 8.3%), and the fibrinolytical activity (reduction of prothrombin activator inhibitor (PAI) 1) were decreased.[150]

POSTMENOPAUSAL BLEEDING, CURETTAGE, HYSTERECTOMY

The incidence of unscheduled uterine bleedings is increased by a factor of 2.0–3.5 in women under ERT. The incidence of curettage is three-fold and hysterectomies is about three- to ninefold, varying with postmenopausal age categories and decreasing with age.[151] Estrogen–progestogen sequential medication stabilizes the menstrual cycle and reduces unscheduled bleedings. The increase in diagnostic or therapeutic interventions is however a phenomenon which is not necessarily hormone related but is usually associated with intensified regular check-ups by the physicians. The costs of the induced interventions have to be included when calculating the risks and costs of ERT and HRT.[35,93,118] The risks caused by diagnostic interventions and surgery, and the costs, may at present be reduced by ultrasonic measurement of the endometrial thickness, perfusion (color Doppler) and by a therapeutic endometrial ablation. Balanced against the risk/cost factors it must be considered that hysterectomy/oophorectomy may prevent some future uterine and ovarian complications for that particular patient, so that there may later be a benefit in those risks and costs. This argument should, although difficult to quantify exactly, also come into the equation. In general, these are minor and preventable points.

GENERAL IMPACT OF ESTROGEN–PROGESTOGEN ON HEALTH LIFE YEARS

All estrogen–progestogen regimens, when the risk and benefits are considered (Table 29.1), were found to extend life expectancy from 0.06 to 0.24 years.[33,36,37] The best increase in life years was found for women with a uterus who received estrogen–progestogen for 15 years. Estrogen substitution, bringing relief of menopausal symptoms, resulted in a net increase in the quality of life and a gain in life expectancy of 0.11 year.

TOTAL IMPACT OF COSTS

The costs for ERT were US$263/year and for estrogen–progestogen US$340/year in 1994. The largest savings were due to decreased nursing home usage (osteoporotic fractures) and less hospital treatment (coronary heart disease) for persons substituted by estrogens. The costs per year of life saved were about US$15,000–25,000/10 years. The amount of money saved was about threefold higher than the costs of HRT.[35]

Sitruck-Ware and Utian[38] have also dealt with the risks and benefits of HRT. They concluded that if osteoporotic fractures and ischemic heart diseases were each reduced by 50%, as indicated by the pertinent studies, then the reduction in mortality would be almost 41%, although a risk ratio of 2 was considered for endometrial cancer and a RR of 1.1 for mammary cancer. Even if a higher risk of breast cancer of 1.8 was considered, the overall mortality would still be reduced by 31%.

Tieffenberg[107] has analyzed the risk:benefit ratio for Argentinian women in 126 probands in a multicenter prospective study. New patients were randomly assigned to treatment. In 85 cases, the patients took transdermal estradiol and progestin, in 41 cases oral estradiol and sequential progestin, and in 79 cases a nonhormonal symptomatic treatment or no treatment. The number of consulting patients and the necessary treatments were estimated based on the data covering 17,000 women over 50 years of age from the National Home Survey. HRT reduced necessary physican visits by 25% and reduced the number of unnecessary drugs. The Satisfaction Index under HRT was significantly higher than that after symptomatic treatment. Fractures, coronary events and strokes were considered; however, endometrial and mammary cancer were not, as the data at hand at that time showed no increased risk for these cancers. The diseases prevented, the years of life saved and the cost savings per 100,000 patients can be seen in Fig. 29.1.

A very interesting investigation was performed in Sweden. Women in nursing homes show a prevalence of urinary incontinence of nearly 50%.[152] Raven[153] showed that the increased use of treatment with oral estriol from 20 to 100% in a nursing home for old women improved urinary incontinence and urologic infections. Consequently, the costs were reduced for basic care, physican visits, laboratory tests, for treatment with physical measures, medicaments and for use of disposable sanitary material – US$85 million/year could be saved by this preventive estriol medication in Swedish nursing homes for old women.

Wenderlein[27] calculated the costs per day for HRT and came to 113 DM/day for women between the ages of 50 and 54. The costs are slightly increased at 55–59 years of age, as instead of sequential estrogen–progestogen more often a combined continuous substitution or more expensive designer hormones were used (117 DM/day). Thereafter the costs are reduced to 71 DM/day, as mostly local treatment is applied.[154] While the daily costs for HRT amount to 0.80 DM/day, the cost for statins were 2.60 DM/day, for cardiovascular medicaments 1.20 DM/day and for antidementia/antidepressive drugs 2.00 DM/day. Thus, the relation of HRT to the medicaments saved was: 1:3.2:1.5:2.5, respectively.[27]

Recently, Wuttke and Weisspflog[128] have worked out a setting up of the costs of HRT in Germany for the year 1992. Diseases [numbers are those of the International Classification of Diseases (ICD)] were evaluated as follows:

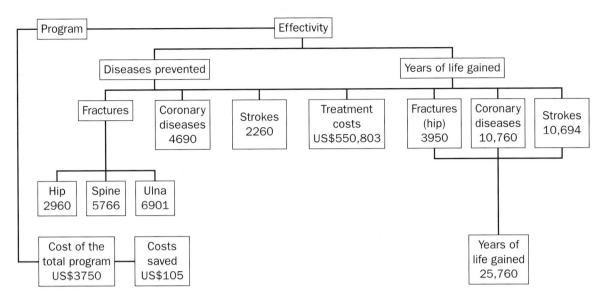

Figure 29.1 Beneficial effects of a long-term substitution with estrogens concerning prevention of diseases, years of life gained and cost savings.[109]

- Climacteric and cerebrovascular complaints
  627 Climacteric and postclimacteric disturbances
- Cardio- and cerebrovascular diseases
  310 Acute myocardial infarction
  412 Postinfarction
  413 Angina pectoris
  414 Forms of ischemic heart diseases
  436 Acute or purely defined cerebral vascular diseases

- Diseases of the urogenital tract
  595 Cystitis
  597 Urethritis, not transmitted by sexual intercourse
  599 Other diseases of the urethra and the urinary tracts
  618 Prolapse of the female inner genitalia
  718 Urologic symptoms

- Diseases of the skeletal system

  733 Affections of bone and cartilage
  805 Fractures of the vertebral spine
  813 Fractures of the radius and ulna
  820 Fractures of the colli femoris

The following factors of costs were considered:

- direct costs: goods and services in the health system that are used for the treatment of diseased persons;
- indirect costs: loss of productivity by incapability to work, early pension and premature death.

The *direct costs* consist of:

- treatment in hospital;[155]
- rehabilitation (calculated from the rehabilitation statistics);
- outpatient treatment with medicaments (calculated from the statistics of the pharmaceutic industry). Note that physicians' services could not be exactly ascertained.

The indirect costs consist of:

- incapability to work;[155]
- early pension (calculated from the pensionists statistics);
- premature death (calculated from the statistics of causes of death).

As most of these diseases are only partly estrogen dependent, a weighting factor was introduced for the calculation of costs of the diseases. For the diseases of the genital tract a factor of 0.2 was adopted (i.e. 20% clearly caused by estrogen deficiency); for cardio- and cerebrovascular diseases a factor of 0.4 was used (i.e. 40% caused by estrogen deficiency); for diseases of the skeleton a factor of 0.5 was taken (i.e. 50% of cases ascribed to estrogen deficiency); for climacteric complaints a factor of 1.0 was used (i.e. 100% estrogen dependent). The costs were then used for calculation of estrogen-dependent costs.

The ascertainment of *direct costs* consists of the following assessment of expenses for the year 1992:

Hospital treatment	376.40 DM/day
Rehabilitation	5674.00 DM/stay
Outpatient treatment, medicaments	40.00 DM/ prescription

The ascertainment of *indirect costs* in working women is based on the following assessment for 1992:

Inability to work	158 DM/day
Early pension	57,800 DM/year
Premature death	57,800 DM/year

The final calculation showed that the direct costs of decreasing estrogen production in post-menopausal women amounted to 3.3 billion DM (unweighted 7 billion DM in the German definition). The main costs were caused by:

Hospital treatment	1.7 billion DM
Outpatient treatment	1.5 billion DM
Cardiovascular diseases	2.2 billions DM
Diseases of the skeleton	1.2 billions DM
Climacteric complaints	0.9 billion DM
Urogenital symptoms	0.3 billion DM

Thus, the total costs of the consequences of postmenopausal estrogen deficiency amounted to 4.5 billion DM/year (10 billion DM unweighted) year. In contrast, treatment with estrogens would cost only 0.67 billion DM/year, i.e. 15% of the calculated total costs and only 15% of the costs for other medicaments.

Wuttke and Weisspflog[128] have not included mammary and endometrial cancer costs, nor the impact of an increased frequency of operations. The inclusion of these items would reduce the advantage in costs by about 1%.

The data for costs per quality adjusted life years gained with ERT in US dollars as compared to no treatment from the data of Weinstein[30] and Weinstein and Stason[29] are given by Zöllner[93] and Zöllner et al.[18] They amount to US$7400 in symptomatic women and US$5500 in women with clinical osteoporosis. Cost per quality of life decreases with duration of treatment and with the positive effects of treatment on the quality of life (the original data must be looked up by the reader in the original papers).

An analysis of the socioeconomics of HRT in Germany by Schmidt-Gollwitzer and Machens[115] determined the annual costs of the postmenopausal women decreased estrogen production to be about US$1400 million in direct costs and US$435 million in indirect costs. A total of US$1050 million is needed for cardio- and cerebrovascular diseases, US$600 for skeletal diseases, US$120 million for urogenital complaints and US$450 million for menopausal and psychovegetative disturbances.

SCREENING COSTS

These have been included as a once-a-year check-up in several studies. They are actually not dependent on ERT/HRT but are generally recommended. The costs of general mammography screening is outside the scope of this chapter.

GENERAL REMARKS

The assessment of the risk:benefit ratio is of utmost importance in judging the suitability of an estrogen–progestogen substitution for the climacteric patient, especially for long-term substitution. An exact determination of the benefits and risks is difficult, as has been shown in this chapter, i.e. only approximations are possible and generalizations are virtually impossible. The judgment of benefits and risks is even difficult and unsafe in well-known individual cases.

Therefore, the severity of the actual complaints and the wishes of the patient following the consultation, which discusses all possible risks and benefits, giving a rough idea as to the expected results, will definitely influence the decision so long as we have no better facts.

SUMMARY OF THE RESULTS OF THE BENEFIT–RISK ASSESSMENT

Well-founded statements can only be made for oral treatment. When general statements have to be given, a differentiation is necessary which discriminates between: (1) an unopposed estrogen monotherapy; (2) an estrogen–progestogen sequential treatment and (3) an estrogen–progestogen combined continuous (uninterrupted) medication. The doses per day of the estrogen and the progestogen component and their mutual relationship may be important for desired beneficial effects and for unwanted side effects. Whether conjugated estrogens exert similar physiopathologic and therapeutic effects and side effects as estradiol or estradiolvalerate is uncertain.

The different progestogens in use exert different effects on target organs and on general metabolism, and cause different side effects and even risks. They may attenuate beneficial effects of estrogens, or influence estrogen metabolism within the breast – an important topic requiring further basic research.

The mode of application of the hormones will influence its metabolism and blood levels. Oral, buccal, nasal, parenteral, rectal, vaginal and transdermal applications are possible. There are, however, no pertinent data on these different modes of application.

Populations in different continents and countries may have different genetic make-ups and may thus react differently to different hormones, doses and application forms. However, the following topics are undisputed.

Short-term treatment of climacteric complaints

Regarding the treatment of climacteric complaints occurring during the 3–5 years after menopause, the benefits of estrogen and estrogen–progestogen therapy are clearly overwhelming, because HRT is successfully able to stabilize the menstrual cycle and eliminate many awkward climacteric symptoms.

In this area the benefit is immediate and very high. This is felt by the patient and has been evidenced by many randomized double-blind studies versus placebo with crossover. Being free from climacteric complaints greatly improves the quality of life, which can be measured by the MRS or the Quality of Life Indices, and is considerable. Most important are the improvement of sleep disturbances and depressive mood. Unwanted side effects are rare and may be caused by too high estrogen doses or by poor compatibility of the progestogen. This can quickly be altered by diminution of doses, change of the progestagen or medication in the evening, so that side effects occur at night. This should occur at latest after 4 weeks of medication.

Thromboembolic or gallbladder diseases usually play no role when the patient's family history and the contraindications are observed, and the treatment is properly and competently performed. Curettage, which may be necessary during perimenopause, are reduced by the cycle-stabilizing effects of sequential estrogen–progestogen medication. Curettage can also be reduced by ultrasonic measurement of endometrial thickness and ascertainment of endometrial shape and a visualization of blood perfusion. Hysterectomies may be reduced by the possibility of endometrial ablation or submucous resection of myomata.

No increase of mammary or genital cancers is to be expected during the 5 years of peri- or postmenopausal treatment (RR of 0.98).[138] However, on the other hand, the highly desired significant preventive effects on osteoporosis, cardiovascular diseases, colon cancer and long-term cerebral functions as well as an impact on mortality, will not occur or cannot be proven during this short-term treatment period.

The costs of ERT/HRT are low compared to other treatment regimens. The best cost–benefit relation is seen in hysterectomized women, where addition of a progestogen is not necessary and uterine bleedings, uterine cancer, curettage or hysterectomy are not problems.

Treatment of atrophic urogenital changes

The very distressing atrophic urogenital changes, which occur in a high percentage of late postmenopausal women, can be safely prevented or abolished by estrogen substitution. In most cases a local treatment with estriol will be sufficient to eliminate these complaints within a short time, a treatment virtually free of side effects and whose costs are low. Both removal of climacteric complaints and of complaints caused by tormenting atrophic urogenital changes will have an important impact on the improvement or the restitution of mental and psychic wellbeing, zest of life and creative abilities, i.e. upon the most important criteria for a good quality of life.

In conclusion, the benefit:risks ratio of the perimenopausal symptomatic treatment of severe climacteric complaints by estrogens and progestogens is highly positive. The costs of ERT/HRT during these few years are relatively low, especially when expenses for alternative treatments such as sedatives, psychotropic medicaments, statins, cardiac glycosides and others are considered. The improvement of quality of life by ERT in the urogenital indication is high and undisputed. There is no increase in cancer incidence within 5 years.

Long-term preventive treatment

Long-term treatment with estrogens–progestogens can be indicated after 5 years of successful ERT/HRT which was well tolerated and free from side effects. Of course, a continuation of treatment must be wanted by the patient. The motivation can be a persistence or recurrence of climacteric complaints or atrophic urogenital changes, or alternatively the aim of prevention of osteoporosis (which needs long-term uninterrupted estrogen medication), cardiovascular diseases or cognitive worsening. Quality of life, esthetic problems of the skin and hair, problems of mucous membranes (e.g. dry eyes) or of

connective tissue may give the motivation for continuation of HRT.

An early loss of ovarian function is, in most cases, a compelling indication for long-term HRT from that time on. Addition of testosterone is then to be discussed because testosterone is greatly reduced following bilateral oophorectomy. The task of the therapeut is to examine the question whether a start or a continuation of the substitution is indicated and can or must even be recommended. Genital and mammographic findings must of course be normal.

Critical remarks concerning the WHI study

The recent randomized controlled trial, the WHI study, which aimed to clarify the impact of long-term ERT/HRT on osteoporotic fractures, cardiovascular diseases and cancer, cannot be taken as a basis for risk–benefit determinations in long-term treatment because this trial is far removed from daily practice. The disadvantageous data were the result of a medication which neglected the general accepted bases of ERT and HRT and of good clinical practice. Most of the probands were too old for primary prevention and the results cannot be transferred to other preparations. This is also the opinion of the WHI authors and of the comments of Fletcher and Colditz.[156] The critical papers about this problem by Beller[3] and Speroff[157] are recommended reading.

What can we learn from this poorly planned, disastrous experiment?

- Estrogens–progestogens must not be given without indication.
- Contraindications and risk factors have to be strictly observed.
- A primary prevention of cardiovascular diseases is only indicated, and possible, when it is begun in high-risk cases during the early menopause (50–56 years of age) before the manifestation of atherosclerosis. Prevention is in most cases no longer effective after the age 60, as at that age active and manifest atherosclerotic changes are mostly already present. Unstable plaques may cause thromboembolic problems. Low transdermal estradiol and a parenteral (vaginal or rectal) progesto-

gen, which is not thrombogenic, should be prescribed with preference in high-risk cases. Probably in such cases a primary treatment with statins would be indicated before estrogens are considered.

- Certain progestogens are not well suited for long-term preventive treatment because of their disadvantageous anti-estrogenic, corticoid, and androgenic activity. This is especially true for the combined continuous long-term HRT (daily estrogen + progestogens), which seems inappropriate for the prevention of cardiovascular diseases and may, in addition, have unwanted effects on the breast.
- Oral medication is not the gold standard for all cases but parenteral medication should preferentially be considered, especially in high-risk cases and older women.
- Older women (more than 65 years of age) should not be treated with the usual normal doses of estrogen and progestogen, lower doses are indicated. Parenteral or local application is to be preferred.
- ERT/HRT must be individualized corresponding to the needs of the patient.
- In addition to therapy, prudent lifestyle counseling together with hormonal substitution is mandatory.
- Randomized controlled studies must be thoroughly assessed. There is a tendency for uncritical reporting of such studies and of accepting their results without checking.[158] Results of papers that are important for patient counseling should not be given prematurely to the public, before experts have had an opportunity for evaluation, analytical comments and well-balanced statements. All papers should state the absolute risk and the number of cases needed to be treated to prove a significant increase of risk or a decrease in the sense of prevention.

Paradigm of good clinical practice

An ideal paradigm of long-term treatment surveillance is the clinical randomized clinical study of Nachtigall et al.[148] Our own report of over 25 years of postmenopausal estrogen–progestogen substitution,[123] the Rancho Bernardo, the Leisure World[22] and the randomized, prospective Walnut Creek long-term study (myocardial infarction RR 0.6, all-case mortality RR 0.8). Optimally, the HRT should follow the stringent scheme of the Minimax Concept, i.e. the achievement of maximal benefit and minimal side effects by prudent indication and care taking.

In our risk–benefit calculations we rely upon the study of Colditz,[137] whose data are generally accepted. This includes a reduction of cardiovascular diseases of about 50% (see also meta-analysis of Grady et al),[37] a reduction of osteoporotic fractures (see also Torgerson et al)[159a] and of colorectal cancer (Lauritzen;[159] see also the prospective study of Calle et al,[160] the meta-analysis of Hebert-Croteau[161] and the WHI study).[158] We take also into account a small increase in mammary cancer which may be partly avoidable by restriction of HRT in high-risk cases.[163] The small increase of thrombosis which has been found can also be avoided by considering contraindications, treating risk factors and avoiding triggering events. In our own investigations we found no significant increase of thromboembolitic cases.[123] Further research should be directed towards characterization of groups at risk and the development of biochemical and genetic risk markers.

No significant influence on endometrial and ovarian cancer is to be expected, but an improvement of cancer cure rate and a reduction of cancer and general mortality has been shown almost unanimously.[137] Finally, a small increase in life expectancy of good quality can be gained.

In counseling the potential estrogen user, the physician must know the fears of his/her clients. In general, these are cancer fears (50%), fear of mental deterioriation (42%), of stroke (37%), of myocardial infarction (33%), of Alzheimer's disease (26%), of breast cancer (26%) and of osteoporosis (18%).[164] All patients fear becoming dependent on others and losing their human dignity and self-determination when old and ill. It is the task of the therapeut to give his/her patient the certainty that he/she will secure for her the best possibilities of a treatment and protect her from harm as far as possible.

If a competent tailored treatment is presumed, then the benefit of long-term ERT/HRT is significantly higher than the possible risk or drawbacks in all possible configurations. The costs are relatively low and, in any case, lower than the treatment of the many diseases, which are partly preventable by estrogens in postmenopausal women. Being free from climacteric complaints, the increase in the quality of life, improvement of psychic stability, of cognitive functions and of psychophysic performance are important items for the individual judgment of benefit and for the preservation of social competence and human dignity in old age.

The mathematical calculation of risk–benefit factors can only be approximate and is by no means exact. They do not stand firm against strict scientific objections, but they are the best available attempt to come as near as possible to conclusive evidence.

In the decision of benefits and possible risks, the woman concerned has the last word, for she alone will bear the risks and earn the benefits of HRT. She should be familiar with all pros and cons (see my formulation for counseling patients). However, the client should know that her physician will do everything to protect her from unnecessary side effects and harm. Each woman experiences her menopause in a unique way. Therefore the risk–benefit equation must be individualized. Lastly the severity of complaints, the ratio of breast cancer risk versus prevention of osteoporosis, cardiovascular protection, maintenance of cognitive function with the addition of more years of a quality of life and the compression of morbidity will be decisive for a yes or no of a long-term preventive treatment. The therapeut should not try to overcome prejudices of his patients by arguments, as he/she will not be successful. It must be remembered that alternative treatments are available. In addition, with respect to dynamic biological changes that occur with aging, and with advancing knowledge, the risk–benefit assessment must be repeated and actualized at yearly intervals.

Correctly performed randomized controlled studies, according to the rules of evidence-based medicine using a practice-conformed design are still awaited. Future controlled trials should be free from the basic mistakes of the HERS and WHI studies. The, by design, disastrous trial of WHI and the unnecessary unwise withdrawal of funding for the WISDOM trial is deplorable, as we now have to wait an indeterminable time for undisputed evidence.

Medical counseling should be based on data that are as firm as possible. It must be improved in practice. However, nothing can replace the trust between a doctor and his/her patient, and a thoughtful experience will always play an important role in the patient's confidence, which determines her adherence to treatment and the success of therapy. The patient's 'Thank you, doctor', will be the best proof of a positive benefit–risk relation of ERT/HRT.

REFERENCES

1. Sarrell L, Sarrel PM. Helping women decide about hormone replacement therapy – approaches to counseling and medical practices. In: (Berg G, Hammar M, eds) *The Modern Management of the Menopause*. (Parthenon: New York, 1994) 499–509.
2. Writing Group for the Women's Health Initiative Investigators. Risks and benefits of estrogen plus progestin in healthy postmenopausal women: principal results from the Women's Health Initiative randomized controlled trial. *JAMA* 2002; **288**: 321–5.
3. Beller FK. Ist die WHI-Studie 'evidenced', d.h. bewiesene Medizin? *Frauenarzt* 2002; **43**: 1299–303.
4. Huber J, Birkhäuser M, Metka M et al. Europäische Gynäkologen analysieren WHI-Hormonstudie amerikanischer Kardiologen, Internat: Menopauseforum Tuohilampi, *J Menopause* 2002; **9**: 7–13.
5. Benson, K, Hartz AI. A comparision of observational studies and randomized clinical trials. *N Engl J Med* 2000; **342**: 1878–86.
6. Guenther C. Nutzen-Risiko-Bilanzierung der Hormonersatztherapie. Bundesinstitut für Arzneimittel und Medizinprodukte, Berlin. *Klinikarzt* 2000; **30**: 2–7.
7. Fioretti et al. Costs of prevention. *Progr Obstet Gynecol* 1987; **30**: 204–7.

8. Barrett-Connor E. Risks and benefits of replacing estrogen. *Ann Rev Med* 1992; **43:** 239–51.

9. Bergner M. Development, use and testing of the sickness impact. In: (Walker S, Rosser M, eds) *Quality of Life Assessment. Key Issues in the 1990s.* (Kluwer Academic Press: Dordrecht, 1993) 201–9.

10. Bosworth, HB, Bastian, LA, Siegler IC. Benefits and drawbacks to hormone replacement therapy among nursing home women. *Women's Health Iss* 1998; **8:** 53–9.

11. Cummings SR. Benefit–risk weighing in HRT. Consensus Conference Copenhagen, 1999. *MMW Extrablatt* 1999; **94:** 12.

12. Daly E. HRT: An analysis of benefits, risks and costs. *Br Med Bull* 1992; **48:** 368–400.

13. Hilard K, Whitcroft S, Ellerington MC, Whitehead MI. Long term risks and benefits of hormone replacement therapy. *J Clin Pharm Ther* 1991; **16:** 231–45.

14. Hunt K, Vessey M. The risks and benefits of hormone replacement therapy: an updated review. *Curr Obstet Gynecol* 1991; **1:** 21–7.

15. Kenemans P. Risk and benefits of long term HRT: a calculated risk? Symposion State of the Art of Practical HRT Report. *Eur Menopause J* 1996; **3:** 7731.

16. Lauritzen C. Das Beratungsgespräch zur Frage Nutzen/Risiko und zu möglichen Nebenwirkungen einer Langzeitsubstitution mit Oestrogenen-Gestagenen in der Postmenopause. Neue Entwicklungen der Substitution mit Hormonen. *Zbl Gynaekol* 2000; **122:** 116–33.

17. Lauritzen C. Hormone in und nach den Wechseljahren: Nutzen und Risiken müssen gegeneinander abgewogen werden. *Inform für die Patientin Gyne,* 2002.

18. Leidenberger F. Nutzen-Risiko Analyse einer Hormonsubstitution. *Gynaekologe* 1997; **30:** 314–25.

19. Lobo RA. Benefit and risk of estrogen replacement therapy. *Am J Obstet Gynecol* 1995; **173:** 982–90.

20. Noji A. Quality of life for changing health: perimenopause among Japanese in Japan and the USA. In: (Aso T, ed) *The Menopause at the Millennium.* (Parthenon: New York, 2000) 127–32.

21. Notelovitz M. Hormone replacement therapy – benefits versus risks. *Eur Menopause J* 1996; **3:** 186–96.

22. Paganini-Hill A. The risk and benefits of estrogen replacement therapy: Leisure World. *Int J Feril Menopause Study* 1995; **40:** 54–62.

23. Palacios S. Current perspectives on the benefits of HRT in postmenopausal women. *Maturitas* 1999; **33:** 1–13.

24. Roche M, Vessey M. Hormone replacement therapy in the menopause. Risks, benefits and costs. In: (Drife JO, Studd JWW, eds) *HRT and Osteoporosis.* (Springer: London, 1990) 363–72.

25. Rozenberg S, Fellemans C, Barudy-Vasquez J et al. Prescription attitudes of gynecologists towards risk and benefit situation. In: (Aso T, ed) *The Menopause at the Milllennium.* (Parthenon: New York, 1999) 415–20.

26. Schneider HPG. Überlegungen zur Nutzen-Kosten-Analyse und Gesundheitseffektivität der Oestrogenbehandlung im Klimakterium. *Med Welt* 1980; **31:** 27–32.

27. Wenderlein M. HRT – eine preiswerte Präventivmedikation. *Frauenarzt* 1999; **40:** 1130–2.

28. Bush JW, Chen MM, Patrick DL. Health status index in cost-effectiveness analysis of PKU program. In: (Berg RL, ed) *Health Status Indices.* (Hospital Research and Educational Trust: Chicago, 1973.)

29. Weinstein MC, Stason WB. Foundations of cost effectiveness analysis for health and medical practice. *N Engl J Med* 1977; **296:** 716–21.

29a. Wiklund I, Karlberg J. Evaluation of quality of life in clinical trials: selecting quality of life measures. *Controlled Clin Trials* 1991; (Suppl;): 204S–16S.

30. Weinstein MC Estrogen use in postmenopausal women, costs, risks and benefits. *N Engl J Med* 1980; **303:** 308–18.

31. Weinstein MC, Schiff I. Cost effectiveness of hormone replacement therapy in the menopause *Obstet Gynecol Surv* 1960; **38:** 445–55.

32. Henderson BE, Paganini-Hill A, Ross RK. Decreased mortality in users of estrogen replacement therapy. *Arch Int Med* 1991; **151:** 75–8.

33. Tosteson ANA, Weinstein MA, Schiff IC. Cost-effectiveness of hormone replacement therapy. In: (Lobo RA, ed) *Treatment of the Postmenopausal Woman.* (Raven Press: 1994) 504–14.

34. Tosteson ANA, Gabriel S, Kneeland T et al. Has the impact of hormone replacement therapy on health-related quality of life been underestimated? *J Women's Health Gender-Based Med* 2000; **9:** 119–30.

35. Daly E, Vessey P, Barlow D et al. Hormone replacement therapy in a risk–benefit perspective. In: (Berg G, Hammar M, eds) *The Modern*

Management of the Menopause. (Parthenon: New York, 1994) 473–90.

36. Cheung D, Wren B. Cost effectiveness of HRT in terms of health care and Qualys. *Med J Aust* 1992; **156:** 312–16.

37. Grady D, Rubin SM, Petitti DB et al. Hormontherapie zur Gesundheitsyorsorge und Lebensverlängerung bei postmenopausalen Frauen. *Menopause J* 1999; **1:** 28–59. [*Ann Intern Med* 1992; **117:** 1016–37.]

38. Sitruk-Ware R, Utian WH. Risk and benefits of hormone replacement therapy. In: (Sitruk-Ware R, Utian WH, eds) *The Menopause and Hormonal Treatment. Therapy. Facts and Controversies.* (Marcel Dekker Inc: New York, 1991) 283–7.

39. Wren BG. Hormone replacement therapy and breast cancer. *Eur Menopause J* 1999; **2:** 11–9.

40. Heinemann K, Assmann A, Möhrer S et al. Reliability of the Menopause Rating Scale. *Zbl Gynaekol* 2002; **124:** 157–9.

41. Schneider HPG. Quality of life assessed by menopause rating scales. In: *Menopause. The State of the Art.* (Parthenon: London, 2003) 314–18.

42. Wenderlein M. Die WHI-Studie – kaum eine Studie zur Primärprävention. *Frauenarzt* 2002; **43:** 1304–10.

43. Michaelsson K, Baron JA, Johnell O, Persson I, Ljunghall S. Variation in the efficacy of hormone replacement therapy in the prevention of hip fracture. Swedish Hip Fracture Study Group. *Osteoporos Int* 1998; **8**(6): 540–6.

44. Ringe JD, Steinhagen-Thiessen. *Osteoporosis Sandorama* 1986; **1:** 10–13.

45. Lip GY, Beevers M, Churchill D, Beevers DG. Hormone replacement therapy and blood pressure in hypertensive women. *J Hum Hypertens* 1994; **8**(7): 491–4.

46. Grodstein F, Newcomb PA, Stampfer MJ. Postmenopausal hormone therapy and the risk of colorectal cancer: a review and meta-analysis. *Am J Med* 1999; **106:** 574–82.

47. Grodstein F, Stampfer MJ, Manson JE et al. Postmenopausal estrogen and progestin use and the risk of cardiovascular disease. *N Engl J Med* 1996; **335:** 453–61.

48. Genazzani AR, Gambacciani M. Cardiovascular disease and hormone replacement therapy. Position paper of an International Menopause Society Expert Workshop, London, 2000. *Cimacteric* 2002; **3:** 233–40.

49. Ginsburg J. *The Circulation in the Female.* (Parthenon: New York, 1989.)

50. Neves e Castro M, Collins P, Clarkson ThB. *Oestrogens and the Cardiovascular System.* (Eska: Paris, 1997.)

51. Grodstein F. Postmenopausal hormone therapy and mortality. *N Engl J Med* 1997; **336:** 1769–75.

52. Bush TI, Cowan L et al. Estrogen use and all causes mortality. *JAMA* 1983; **249:** 903–6.

53. Bush TL, Barrett-Connor E, Cowan LD et al. Cardiovascular mortality and noncontraceptive use of estrogen in women: results from the Lipid Research Clinics Program Follow-up Study. *Circulation* 1987; **75**(6): 1102–9.

54a. Stampfer MJ, Grodstein F. Role of hormone replacement in cardiovascular disease. A quantitative assessment of the epidemiologic evicence. *Press Med* 1991; **230:** 47–63.

54b. Stampfer J. HRT and cardiovascular disease. *Eur Menopause J* 1998; **1:** 7–8.

55. Petitti D, Sidney S, Quesenberg CP, Bernstein A. Ischemic stroke and use of estrogen and estrogen/progestogen as hormone replacement therapy. *Stroke* 1998; **28:** 23–8.

56. Criqui MH, Suarez E, Barret-Connor JB et al. Postmenopausal estrogen use and mortality. Results from a prospective study in a defined homogenous community. *Am J Epidemiol* 1988; **128:** 606–14.

57. Hunt K, Vessey M, McPherson K. Mortality in a cohort of long term users of hormone replacement: an updated analysis. *Br J Obstet Gynaecol* 1990; **97:** 1080–6.

58. Sourander I, Rajala T, Raiha T et al. Cardiovascular and cancer morbidity and mortality and sudden cardiac death in postmenopausal women on oestrogen replacement therapy (ERT). *Lancet* 1998; **152:** 1965–9.

59. Wagner JD, Williams JK, Adams MR et al. Effects of mammalian estrogens and phyto-estrogens on the vascular system. In: (Lippert ThH, Mueck AO, Ginsburg J, eds *Sex Steroids and the Cardiovascular System.* (Parthenon: London, 1996) 21–34.

60. Polder EA. Costs of Alzheimer's disease. *Lancet* 1988; **351:** 359–62.

61. Alzheimer Association. 2000. Press release.

62. Henderson VW. Estrogens and dementia: a clinical and epidemiological update. In: (Wren B, ed). *Progress in the Management of the Menopause.* (Parthenon: New York, 1997): 40–9.

63. Turner JB, Beyreuther K, Theuring F, eds. *Alzheimer's Disease.* (Spinger: Berlin, 1996).

64. Alves SE, McEwen BS. Estrogen and brain function: implications for aging and dementia.

In: (Oettel M, Schillinger E, eds). *Estrogens and Antiestrogens*. (Springer: Berlin, 1999): 315–28.

65. Henderson VW, Watt L, Buckwalter JG. Cognitive skills associated with estrogen replacement in Alzheimer's disease. *Psychoneuroendocrinology* 1886; **21**: 421–30.

66. Nanda K, Bastian LA, Hasselblad V, Simel DL. Hormone replacement therapy and the risk of colorectal cancer: a meta-analysis. *Obstet Gynecol* 1999; **93**: 880–8.

67. Formosa M, Brincat MP, Cardozo LD, Studd JWW. Collagen, the significance in skin, bones and bladder. In: (Lobo R, ed) *Treatment of the Postmenopausal Woman*. (Raven Press: New York, 1993) 143–52.

68. Sawyer Sartori MG, Baracat EC, Girao MJ et al. Menopausal genuine stress incontinence treated with conjugated estrogens plus progestogens. *Int J Gynecol Obstet* 1995; **49**: 165–9.

69. Sherman SS, Goldstein RE, Crawfors SL et al. Menopause and six chronic conditions of aging: the Study of Women's Health Across the Nation (SWAN). In: (Aso T, ed) *The Menopause at the Millennium*. (Parthenon: New York, 2000) 117–26.

70. Alder EM. How to assess quality of life: problems of methodology. In: (Schneider HPG, ed). *Hormone Replacement Therapy and Quality of Life*. (Parthenon: London, 2002) 11–22.

71. Alder EM. How to assess quality of life. In: Schneider HPG, ed) *Menopause. State of the Art*. (Parthenon: London, 2003) 312–3.

72. Dennerstein L. The pursuit of happiness: well being during the menopausal transition: In: (Berg G, Hammar M, eds) *The Modern Management of the Menopause*. (Parthenon; New York, 1994) 151–9.

73. Dennerstein L, Helmes E. The menopausal transition and quality of life: methodological issues. *Qual Life Res* 2000; **9**: 721–31.

74. Derman RJ, Dawood MY, Stone S. Quality of life during sequential hormone replacement therapy – a placebo controlled study. *Int J Fertil* 1990; **40**: 73–8.

75. Eden JA. The risk and benefits of HRT – whom do we select for long term therapy and who will take it? (Birkhäuser MH, Rozenbaum H, eds) *IV European Congress of the Menopause*. (Editions ESKA: Paris, 1998) 385–90.

76. Ernster VL, Bush TL, Huggins GR, et al. Benefits and risks of menopausal estrogen and/or progestine hormone use. *Prev Med* 1988; **17**: 201–23.

77. Gambrell Jr, RD. The menopause. Benefits and risks of estrogen and of estrogen–progestogen replacement therapy. *Fertil Steril* 1982; **37**: 457–62.

78. Gapstur SM, Morrow M, Sellers TA. Hormone replacement therapy and risk of breast cancer with a favorable histology. Results of the Iowa Women's Health Study. *JAMA* 1999; **281**: 2091–7.

79. Gelfand MM. Quality of life issues in the management of the menopause. In: (Popkin DR, Peddle LJ, eds) *Women's Health Today, Procedings of the XIV World Congress of Gynecology and Obstetrics*. (Parthenon: Canforth, 1994) 271–5.

80. Greene JG. Measuring of the symptom dimension of quality of life general and menopause specific scales and their substructures. In: (Schneider HPG, ed). *Hormone Replacement Therapy and Quality of Life*. (Parthenon: London, 2003) 35–43.

81. Kaplan RM, Anderson JP, Ganiats T. The Quality of Well Being Scale: rationale for a single quality of life index. In: (Walker S, Roser M, eds) *Quality of Life Assessment: Key Issues in the 1990s*. (Kluwer Academic Press: Dordrecht, 1993) 65–71.

82. Kingsberg SK. Maintaining and evaluating quality of life after menopause. *Female Patient* 2000; **98** (Suppl May): 19–24.

83. Lauritzen C. Kosten-Nutzen-Risiko-Analyse der Oestrogenbehandlung im Klimakterium. *Gynaekologe* 1986; **19**: 266–75.

84. Löffler H, Saletu B, Gruber L et al. Lebensqualität bei Schlafstörungen im Rahmen eines postmenopausalen Syndroms. *J Menopause* 1997; **4**: 18.

85. Schneider HPG, Schultz-Zehden B, Rosemeier HP, Behre M. Assessing well-being in postmenopausal women. In: (Studd J, ed). *The Management of the Menopause. The Millennium Review*. (Parthenon: New York, 2000) 11–19.

86. Tasaki M, Noji A, Nakane Y. WHGO Quality of Life. *Diagn Treat* 1995; **83**: 133–50.

87. Teichmann AT, Weiland W, Brockerhoff P. Sexual hormone, Arteriosklerose und Fettstoffwechsel der Frau. *Wiss Verlagsanstalt Stuttgart* 1989.

88. Utian WH. Hormonsubstitutionsbehandlung: Allein die Nutzen-Risiko-Bilanz zählt. Gyno Panorama, Geigy, Nr.5 (1990) 5–10. Refer. VI. Internat Congresson the Menopause. Bangkok 1990.

89. Utian WH. Application of cost-effectiveness analysis postmenopausal estrogen therapy. In: (Lauritzen C, van Keep PA, eds). *Estrogen Therapy. The benefits and risks.* (Karger: Basil, 1978): 26–31.

90. Wiklund I, Karlberg J, Mattson L-M. Quality of life of postmenopausal women on a regimen of transdermal estradiol therapy: a double-blind placebo-controlled study. *Am J Obstet Gynecol* 1993; **168**.

91. Williams JK, Adams MR, Klopfenstein HS. Estrogen modulates responses to atherosclerotic coronary arteries. *Circulation* 1990; **81**: 1680–7.

92. Writing Group for the Women's Health Initiative Investigators. Risk and benefits of estrogen plus progestin in healthy post-menopausal women *JAMA* 2002; **17**: 321–33.

93. Zoellner YF. The cost-effectiveness and cost-utility of hormone replacement therapy. In: *Hormone Replacement Therapy and Quality of Life.* (Parthenon: 2002) 123–40.

94. Hunt SM, McKennam SP, McEwen J et al. The Nottingham Health Profile, subjective health and medical consultations. *Soc Sci Med* 1981; **15A**: 221–9.

95. Hunter M. The Women's Health Questionnaire (WHQ): a measure of mid-aged women's perceptions of their emotional and physical health. *Psychol Health* 1972; **7**: 45–52.

96. McHorney CA, Ware JE, Raczek AE. The MOS 36 Items Short form Health Survey (SF 36) II. Psychometric and clinical test validity in measuring physical and mental health constructs. *Med Care* 1993; **31**: 247–63.

97. Utian WH. Application of cost-effectiveness analysis to postmenopausal estrogen therapy. In: (Lauritzen, C, van Keep PA, eds) *Estrogen Therapy: The Benefits and Risks.* Front. Hormone Res. (Karger: Basel, 1978) 26–39.

98. Utian WH. Analysis of hormone replacement therapy. In: (Studd JW, Whitehead MI, eds) *The Menopause* (Blackwell: Oxford, 1988), 262–70.

99. Utian WH. Menopause, hormone therapy, and quality of life. In: (Hammomd ChB, Hasseltine FP, Schiff I, eds) *Menopause, Evaluation and Treatment and Health Concerns.* (Liss: New York, 1989) 193–209.

100. Utian WH, Janata JW, Kingsberg SA, Patrick LD. Determinants of quantification of quality of life after the menopause: The Utian Menopause Quality of Life Score. In: (Aso T, ed) *The Menopause at the Millennium.* (Parthenon: New York, 2000) 141–4.

101. Hauser A, Huber JC, Keller PJ et al. Evaluation of climacteric complaints (Menopause Rating Scale, MRS). *Zbl Gynaekol* 1994; **116**: 16–23.

102. Schneider HPG. Menopause, quality of life, and impact of hormone replacement therapy. *Medicographia* 2001; **69**: 328–33.

103. Schneider HPG, Behre HM. Contemporary evaluation of climacteric complaints, its impacts on quality of life. In: *Hormone Replacement Therapy and Quality of Life.* (Parthenon: London, 2003) 45–61.

104. Schneider HPG, Heinemann L, Rosemeier H-P et al. The Menopause Rating Scale (MRS), reali-bility of scores of menopausal complaints. *Climacteric* 2000; **3**: 59–64. Schneider HPG, Heinemann L, Rosemeir H-P et al. Com-parision with Kuppermann Index and quality of life scale SF 36. *Climacteric* 2000; **3**: 50–8.

105. Hudita D. Impact of urogenital aging on the quality of life. In: (Aso T, ed) *The Menopoause at the Millennium.* (Parthenon: New York, 1999) 504–9.

106. Wiklund I. Methods of assessment of the impact of climacteric complaints on quality of life. *Maturitas* 1998; **29**: 41–50.

107. Tieffenberg JA. Socio-economic and quality analysis in postmenopausal Argentine women. In: (Berg G, Hammar M, eds) *The Modern Management of the Menopause.* (Parthenon: London, 1994), 57–70.

108. Bush TL, Basrret-Connor E, Cowan LD et al. Cardiovascular mortality and noncontraceptive use of estrogens in women: results from the Lipid Research Clinic Program Follow-up Study. *Circulation* 1987; **75**: 1102–9.

109. Paganini-Hill. Morbidity and mortality change with estrogen replacement therapy. In: (Lobo RA, ed): *Treatment of the Postmenopausal Woman.* (Raven Press: New York, 1994) 309–404.

110. Jernström H, Frenander J, Fenö M, Olson H. Hormone replacement before breast cancer diagnosis significantly reduces overall death rate compared with never users. 984 Breast cancer patients. *Br J Cancer* 1999; **80**: 1453–8.

111. Bunker JP, Barnes BA, Mosteller F. Costs, risks and benefits of surgery. (Oxford University Press: New York, 1977.)

111a. Willis DFB, Calle EE, Miracle-McMahill HL, Heath Jr, CW. Estrogen replacement therapy and risk of fatal breast cancer in a prospective cohort of postmenopausal women in the United States. *Cancer Causes Control* 1996; **7**: 449–57.

112. Hoerger TJ, Downs KE. Lakshmanan MC et al. Health care use among US women aged 45 and older: total costs and costs for selected postmenopausal health risks. *J Womens's Health Gender-Based Med* 1999; **8**: 1077–89.

113. Prince RI. The health economics of osteoporosis and estrogen replacement therapy. In: (Wren B, ed). *Progress in the Management of the Menopause.* (Parthenon: New York, 1997) 1780–7.

114. Randell A, Sambrook PN, Nguyen TV et al. Direct clinical and welfare costs of osteoporotic fractures in elderly men and women. *Osteop Int* 1995; **5**: 427–32.

115. Schmidt-Gollwitzer K, Machens, K. Lecture: Socio-economics of HRT. International Menopause Congress, Berlin 2002. In: (Schneider HPG, ed) *Menopause. State of the Art.* (Parthenon: London, 2003) 348–54.

116. Weiss NS. Risk and benefits of estrogen use. *N Engl J Med* 1975; **293**: 1200–5.

117. Zethraeus N, Johannsson M, Henrikson P et al. The impact of hormone replacement therapy on quality of life and willingness to pay. *Br J Obstet Gynaecol* 1997; **104**: 1191–5.

118. Zoellner YF, Brazier JE, Oliver P et al. Development of an algorithm to derive utilities from a validated menopause-specific QoL questionaire (paper discussion). The 59th Health Economist's Study Group (HESG) meeting, London, 2001.

119. Dolan P. Valuing health-related quality of life: issues and controversies. *Pharmacoeconomics* 1998; **15**: 119–27.

120. Hammar M, Christian S, Nathorst-Boos J et al. A double-blind, randomized trial comparing the effects of tibolone and continuous hormone replacement therapy in postmenopausal women with menopausal symptoms. *Br J Obstet Gynaecol* 1998; **105**: 904–11.

121. Armstrong K, Chen TM, Albert D et al. Cost-effectiveness of raloxifen and hormone replacement therapy in postmenopausal women with menopausal symptoms. Impact of breast cancer risk. *Obstet Gynecol* 2001; **6**: 9967–10003.

122. Murphy GK. Undetected cancer. *JAMA* 1977, **237**: 786–8.

123. Lauritzen C, Meier F. Risk of endometrial and mammary cancer morbidity in long term estrogen treatment. In: (Herendael HB, Riphagen FE, Goessens L et al, eds) *The Climacteric. An Update.* (MTP Press: Lancaster, 1984) 207–16.

124. Lauritzen C. Endometrial cancer. In: (Römer Th, Straube, W, eds) *Klimakterium und Hormone.* (Pia: Nürnberg, 1996) 56–62.

125. Persson RI, Yuen J, Bergkvist L, Schairer C. Krebsinzidenz und Mortalität bei Frauen unter Oestrogen und Oestrogen-Gestagentherapie-Langzeit-Beobachtung einer schwedischen Kohorte. *J Menopause* 1999; **1**: 8–27. (Reprint from *Int J Cancer* 1996; **67**: 327–32.

126. Chu J, Schweid AI, Weiss NS. Survival among women with endometrial cancer: a comparison of users and nonusers. *Am J Obstet Gynecol* 1982; **143**: 569–73.

127. McGonigle KF, Karlan BY, Barbuta D et al. Development of endometrial cancer in women on estrogen-progestin replacement therapy. *Gynecol Obstet* 1994; **55**: 126–32.

128. Wuttke W, Weisspflog D. Das Klimakterium und seine Folgeerscheinungen: eine Krankheitsstudie in der Bundesrepublik Deutschland. In: (Schindler A, ed) *Menopause aktuell.* (Aesopus Verlag: Basel, 1996) 77–82.

129. Emmens, Kavanagh. *Hematol Oncol Clin N Am* 1999; **13**: 145.

130. Lacey JV, Mink PJ. Menopausal hormone replacement therapy and risk of ovarian cancer. *JAMA* 2002; **17**: 288–334.

131. Hartge P, Hoover R, McGowan L, Lesher L, Norris HJ. Menopause and ovarian cancer. *Am J Epidemiol* 1988; **127**(5): 990–8.

132. Whittemore AS, Harris R, Itnyre J. Characteristics relating to ovarian cancer risk: collaborative analysis of 12 US case-control studies. IV. The pathogenesis of epithelial ovarian cancer. Collaborative Ovarian Cancer Group. *Am J Epidemiol* 1992; **136**(10): 1212–20.

133. Adami HO, Lund E, Bergstrom R, Meirik O. Cigarette smoking, alcohol consumption and risk of breast cancer in young women. *Br J Cancer* 1988; **58**(6): 832–7.

134. Persson I, Yuen J, Bergkvist L, Adami HO, Hoover R, Schairer C. Combined oestrogen-progestogen replacement and breast cancer risk. *Lancet* 1992; **340**(8826): 1044.

135. Negri E, Tzonou A, Beral V et al. Hormonal therapy for menopause and ovarian cancer in a collaborative re-analysis of European studies. *Int J Cancer* 1999; **80**(6): 848–51.

136. Lando JF, Heck KE, Brett KM. Hormone replacement therapy and breast cancer risk in a national representative cohort. *Am J Prev Med* 1999; **17**: 176–80.

136a. Lafferty FW, Fiske ME. Postmenopausal

estrogen replacement: a long-term cohort study. *Am J Med* 1994; 97(1): 66–77.

136b. Stanford JL, Weiss NS, Voigt LF et al. Combined estrogen and progestin hormone replacement therapy in relation to risk of breast cancer in middle-aged women. *JAMA* 1995; **274**(2): 137–42.

136c. Newcomb PA, Longnecker MP, Storer BE et al. Long-term hormone replacement therapy and risk of breast cancer in postmenopausal women. *Am J Epidemiol* 1995; **142**: 788–95.

137. Colditz GA. Hormones and breast cancer: evidence and implications for consideration of risk and benefits of hormone replacement therapy. *J Women's Health* 1999; **8**: 347–57.

138. Collaborative Group on Hormonal Factors in Breast Cancer. Breast cancer and hormone replacement therapy: collaborative reanalysis of data from 51 epidemiological studies of 52 705 women with breast cancer and 108 411 women without breast cancer. *Lancet* 1997; **350**: 1047–59.

139. Zumoff B. The critical role of alcohol consumption in determining the risk of breast cancer with postmenopausal estrogen administration. *J Clin Endocrinol Metab* 1997; **82**(6): 1656–8.

140. Pike MC, Krailo MD, Henderson BE, Casagrande JT, Hoel DG. 'Hormonal' risk factors, 'breast tissue age' and the age-incidence of breast cancer. *Nature* 1983; **303**: 767–70.

141. Stellungnahme der Kommission Hormontoxikologie der Deutschen Gesellschaft für Endokrinologie. Karzinogene Eigenschaften von Estradiol-17β. *Endokrinologie-Informationen* 2000; **24**: 181–8.

142. Lignieres B de, Vathiare F, Fournier S et al. Combined hormone therapy and risk of breast cancer in a French cohort study of 3175 women. *Climacteric* 2002; **5**: 322–40.

143. Standard of reporting clinical trials. [Editorial]. *Lancet* 22001; **352**: 1–3.

144. Lauritzen C, Frauenarzt: Die präventive Estrogen. *Gestagen-Langzeitprävention*. 2001; **42**: 1214–67.

145. Magnusson C, Baron JA, Correia N et al. Breast cancer risk following long-term estrogen and estrogen–progestin replacement therapy. *Int J Cancer* 1999; **81**: 339–44.

146. Willis DB, Calle EE, Miracle-McMahill HI et al. Estrogen replacement therapy and risk of fatal breast cancer in a prospective cohort of menopausal women in the United States. *Cancer Causes Control* 1996; **7**: 449–57.

147. Hammond CB, Maxson WS. Current status of estrogen therapy in the menopause. *Fertil Steril* 1982; **37**: 407–30.

148. Nachtigall MJ, Smilen RD, Nachtigall RD et al. Incidence of breast cancer in a 22 years' study of women receiving estrogen-progestin replacement therapy. *Obstet Gynecol* 1992; **80**: 827–30.

149. Jick H, Derby LE, Myers MW et al. Risk of hospital admission for idiopathic venous thromboembolism among users of postmenopausal oestrogens. *Lancet* 1996; **348**: 9821–83.

150. Winkler HU, Krämer B, Kwee B, Schindler AE. Östrogensubstitution in der Postmenopause, Blutgerinnung und Fibrinolyse: Vergleich einer neuartigen transdermalen Östradiol-Behandlung mit der oralen Therapie mit konjugierten Östrogenen. *Zbl Gynäkol* 1995; **117**: 540–3.

151. Ettinger B, Golditch IM, Friedman G. Gynecologic consequences of long-term unopposed estrogen replacement therapy. *Maturitas* 1988; **10**: 271–82.

152. Samsioe GN, Mattson LA. Regimens for today and the future. In: (Lobo RA, ed). *Treatment of the Postmenopausal Woman. Basic and Clinical Aspects.* (Raven Press: New York, 1994): 421–6.

153. Raven ML, quoted from *Apothekerzeitung* 1994; **16**: 22–4.

154. German General Insurance. Press release. 1994.

155. German General Health Insurance. Press release. 1991.

156. Fletcher SE, Colditz GA. Failure of estrogen-progestin therapy for the prevention of cardiovascular diseases. *JAMA* 2002; **288**: 366–7.

157. Speroff L. WHI Trial Arm with E/P finds an increase in breast cancer. *Obstet Gynecol Alert* 2002; **19**: 25–30.

158. Writing Group for the Women's Health Initiative Investigators. Risks and benefits of estrogen plus progestin in healthy postmenopausal women: principal results from the Women's Health Initiative, randomized clinical trial. *JAMA* 2002; **288**: 321–3.

159. Lauritzen C. Die prävention der postmenopausen-osteoporose durch östrogen. In: *Prophylaxe und Therapie der Osteoporose mit Östrogenen und Gestagenen.* (Thieme, 1997): 43–85.

159a. Torgerson DJ, Bell-Syer SEM. Hormone replacement therapy and prevention of nonvertebral fractures: a meta-analysis of randomized trials. *JAMA* 2001; **285**(22): 2891–7.

160. Calle EE, Miracle-McMahill HL. Estrogen replacement therapy and risk of colon cancer in

a prospective cohort of postmenopausal women. *J Natl Cancer Inst* 1995; **87**: 517–23.

161. Hebert-Croteau N. A meta-analysis of hormone replacement therapy and colon cancer in women. *Cancer Epidemiol Biomarkers and Prevention* 1995; **18**: 635–9.

162. Gerhardsson de Verdier M, London S. Reproductive factors, exogenous hormones and colorectal cancer by subsite. *Causes Cancer Control* 1992; **3**: 355–60.

163. Furner SE, Davis FG, Nelson RL, Henszel WA. A case-control study of large bowel cancer and hormone exposure in women. *Cancer Res* 1989; **49**: 236–40.

164. Schultz-Zehden B. *Frauengesundheit in und nach den Wechseljahren. Die 1000 Frauen Studie.* (Kempkes: Gladenbach, 1998).

165. Falkeborn M, Persson I, Terent A et al. Hormone replacement therapy and the risk of stroke. *Arch Int Med* 1983; **153**: 1201–9.

166. Burch JC, Byrd BF, Vaughn WK. The effect of long-term estrogen administration to women following hysterectomy. In: (van Keep PA, Lauritzen C, eds). *Estrogen in the Post-Menopause.* (Karger: Basel, 1975): 208–14.

167. Bergkvist L, Adami HO, Persson I et al. Prognosis after breast cancer diagnosis in women exposed to estrogen and estrogen-progestogen replacement therapy. *Am J Epidemiol* 1989; **130**: 221–8.

168. Gambrell RD, jr. Hormone replacement therapy and breast cancer risk. In: (Greenblatt RB, ed). *A Modern Approach to the Perimenopausal Years.* (De Gruyter: Berlin, 1986).

169. Gambrell RD, jr. Hormone replacement therapy and breast cancer risk. *Arch Fam Med* 1996; **5**: 341–8.

170. Hunt K, Vessey M, McPherson K. Mortality in a cohort of long-term users of hormone replacement: an updated analysis. *Br J Obstet Gynaecol* 1990; **79**: 1080–6.

171. Criqui MH, Suarez E, Barrett-Connor JB et al. Postmenopausal estrogen use and mortality. Results from a prospective study in a defined homogenous community. *Am J Epidemiol* 1988; 128: 606–14.

172. Lauritzen C. Ostrogensubstitution vor und nach behandeltem genital- un mammakarzinom. In: (Lauritzen C, ed). Menopause. Hormonsubstitution heute. (PMS Cedip: München, 1994): 89–92.

173. Sellers TA, Mink PJ, Gerham JA et al. The role of hormone replacement therapy in the risk of

breast cancer and total mortality in women with a history of breast cancer. *Ann Inter Med* 1997; **127**: 973–80.

174. Armstrong BK. Oestrogen therapy after menopause – boon or bane. *Med J Austral* 1988; **148**: 213–14.

175. Dupont WD, Page DI. Menopausal estrogen replacement therapy and breast cancer. *Arch Inter Med* 1991; **51**: 61–71.

176. Steinberg KK, Thacker SB, Smith JA et al. A Meta-analysis of the effect of estrogen replacement therapy on the risk of breast cancer. *JAMA* 1991; **265**: 1985–90.

177. Sillero-Arenas M, Delgado-Rodriguez M, Rodigues-Canteras R et al. Menopausal hormone replacement therapy and breast cancer: a meta-analysis. *Obstet Gynecol* 1992; **79**: 286–94.

178. Grady D, Rubin SM, Pettiti H et al. Hormone therapy to prevent diseases and prolong life and postmenopausal women. *Ann Intern Med* 1992; **117**: 1012–37.

179. Bush T, Whitman M, Flaws JA. Hormone replacement therapy and breast cancer: a qualitative review. *Obstet Gynecol* 2001; **98**: 498–503.

180. Campbell S. Double blind psychometric studies on the effects of natural estrogens on post-menopausal women. In: (Campbell S, ed) *The Management of the Menopause and Postmenopausal Years.* (MTP Press: Lancaster, 1976), 149–58.

181. Francis RM, Anderson FCH, Torgerson DJ. A comparison of effectiveness and costs of treatment for vertebral fractures in women *Br J Rheumatol* 1995; **34**: 1167–71.

182. Hammond CB, Jelovsek FR, Lee LK et al. Effects of long-term estrogen therapy. I. Metabolic effects. II. Cancer. *J Obstet Gynecol* 1979; **133**: 525–36.

183. Hulley S, Grady T, Bush et al for the Heart and Estrogen/progestin Replacement Study (HERS). Randomized trial of estrogen plus progestin for secondary prevention of coronary heart disease in postmenopausal women. *JAMA* 1998; **280**: 605–13.

184. Lauritzen C. Möglichkeiten der Prävention des Mammakarzinoms. *Zbl Gynaekol* 2002; **124**: 269–79.

185. Lippert ThH, Mueck AO, Ginsburg J. *Sex Steroids and the Cardiovascular System.* (Parthenon: New York, 1998.)

186. Litschgi M. Nutzen-Risiko-Analyse der Hormonsubstitution. *J Menopause* 1999; **3**: 35–42.

187. Menopausal Hormone Therapy. Scientific Workshop NIH, 23–24 October 2002.

188. Paganini-Hill A. Hormone replacement therapy and stroke: risk, protection or no effects? *Maturitas* 2000; **1:** 811–29.

189. Petitti D, Pertman S, Sidney R. Non-contraceptive estrogen and mortality: long–term follow-up of women in the Walnut Creek Study. *Obstet Gynecol* 1987; **70:** 89–93.

190. Redmond GP. *Lipids and Women's Health*. (Springer: Heidelberg, 1991.)

191. Samsioe G. Statement to evidence based medicine. *Maturitas* 2002; **42:** 38.

192. Schaad MA, Bonjour JP, Rizzoli R. Evaluation of hormone replacement therapy use by sales figures. *Maturitas* 2000; **34:** 185–91.

193. Schairer C, Lubin J, Troisi R et al. Menopausal estrogen and estrogen–progestin replacement therapy and breast cancer risk. *JAMA* 2000; **283:** 485–91.

194. Schneider HPG. HRT and cancer risk. Separating facts from fiction. *Maturitas* 1999; **33** (Suppl 1): 65–72.

195. Stampfer M. Selection bias. *Eur Menopause J* 1994; **1:** 16–17.

196. Sullivan JM, van der Zwag R, Hughes JP et al. Estrogen replacement and coronary disease. Effect on survival in postmenopausal women. *Arch Inern Med* 1982; **150:** 2557–62.

197. Teoh ES, Teoh LKK. Improving the quality of life after 45. In: (Teoh ES, Ratnam S, eds). *The Future of Gynaecology and Obstetrics*. (Parthenon: Carnforth, 1991): 137–50.

198. The Writing Group for the PEPI trial. Effects of estrogens/progestin regimens on heart disease risk factors in postmenopausal women. *JAMA* 1995; **273:** 199–208.

199. Testoson M. *Menopause: Epidemiology*. (Michigan Graduate Course: Ann Arbour, 1998.)

200. Whittington R, Faulds. Hormone replacement therapy II. A pharmacoeconomic appraisal of its role in the prevention of postmenopausal osteoporosis and ischaemic heart disease. *Pharmacoeconomia* 1994; **5:** 513–54.

201. Wilson DH, Taylor AW, MacLennan AH. Estrogen replacement therapy users and non-users as determined by the SF 36 quality of life dimension. *Climacteric* 1998; **1:** 50–4.

202. Wilson L, Brown JS, Shin GP et al. Annual directs cost of urinary incontinence. *Obstet Gynecol* 2002; **98:** 398–406.

203. World Health Organization (WHO). Report of the WHO meeting on the assessment of quality of life in health care: MNH/PSF 91–4, Geneva 1991.

204. Xiao B, Ge QWS. Role or reproductive health in the quality of life in women in the menopause. In: (Aso T, ed) *The Menopause at the Millennium*. (Parthenon: New York, 2000) p 123–8.

205. Zethraeus N, Johannsson M, Jonsson BA. A computer model to analyze the cost-effectiveness of hormone replacement therapy. *Int J Technol Assess Health Care* 2000; **15:** 352–65.

Section 5

Miscellaneous

Chapter 30 Information sheet for climacteric women

Chapter 31 The aging male

Chapter 32 Future developments

Information sheet for climacteric women

C Lauritzen

Complaints? Please let your doctor help you • **Knowledge and understanding are important for reaching the right decision** • **What happens during the change of life (the climacteric)?** • **Estrogen deficiency after the menopause and its consequences** • **Estrogens exert many beneficial effects** • **Elimination of typical climacteric complaints by estrogens** • **Elimination of late consequences of estrogen deficiency by estrogens** • **Quality of life** • **What are the possible side effects and risks of estrogen intake?** • **Thrombosis** • **The cancer problem** • **Other possibilities of treatment for the climacteric** • **Conclusions** • **References**

Dear Visitor to my Practice!
You are at the age of a woman's change of life (climacteric, menopause). According to statistics you still have about 30 years of life before you.

Good years we hope.

They may not begin so well because at about the age of 50 years 80% of women suffer from climacteric complaints caused by the loss of ovarian function. These complaints will probably increase in intensity and last 3–5 years or longer. They have been shown to be severe in about 30% of all cases of the 80% of sufferers.

Therefore, for a woman with postmenopausal ovarian estrogen deficiency symptoms the question arises of whether she will take advantage of the progress of medical science in hormone research. That is, will she consider taking the missing ovarian hormones (an estrogen–progestogen preparation) in order to eliminate climacteric complaints, or would she prefer to bear the symptoms and not take hormones.

This decision will be determined mainly by the severity of the climacteric complaints

experienced, such as hot flushes, sweating, sleeplessness, and depressive moods. Five to 10 years later complaints of the vagina and bladder (urogenital complaints) will appear. All of these symptoms can be very embarrassing, but estrogen replacement therapy (ERT) will quickly and safely eliminate them.

Climacteric and menopause are not a disease. If you have no complaints, then usually you need no ovarian hormones, except in a few special cases which your doctor will indicate for you.

COMPLAINTS? PLEASE LET YOUR DOCTOR HELP YOU

If you suffer from heavy climacteric complaints, which adversely affect your wellbeing and quality of life, then please read the following explanations and recommendations carefully, because your decision will be fundamental for some time to come and will perhaps influence many aspects of your life in future years. It may determine how well you will live in your third phase of life and whether you will be free of troublesome complaints and of diseases that are preventable by estrogen replacement.

Severe climacteric complaints, signaling estrogen deficiency, must not be tolerated passively. They are indeed futile and senseless, and can reduce your daily degrees of freedom and endanger your physical and mental independence. The cause of climacteric symptoms – estrogen deficieny – may even lead to real diseases in later years.

KNOWLEDGE AND UNDERSTANDING ARE IMPORTANT FOR REACHING THE RIGHT DECISION

This information sheet summarizes all necessary facts for your knowledge and understanding of menopausal problems in order to give you a sufficient base for making a well-informed decision, which is thought to be optimal for your wishes and requirements. No one wants to persuade you to make up your mind in any direction. It is completely up to you, after considering all pros and cons, to choose how to deal with the climacteric. Of course, if you want, your doctor will discuss every question you have with you and help you find the best individual solution, tailored to your needs and wishes.

Medical science, which has given females 30 additional years to live after their last menstruation (menopause), accordingly feels responsible for the optimal course of this third phase of female life. The aim of hormone substitution is to prevent unnecessary complaints and diseases, thus securing physical and mental health, social competence and human dignity in old age.

Medicine offers a lot of different hormone preparations, containing an estrogen and usually also a progestogen, which meet all individual reqirements.

WHAT HAPPENS DURING THE CHANGE OF LIFE (THE CLIMACTERIC)?

Normally, every month a follicle is produced in the ovaries which will grow and release an egg for possible fertilization. The estrogen will make the mucous membrane (endometrium) of the womb (uterus) grow. Thereafter, in the ruptured follice a so-called yellow body (corpus luteum) develops, which secretes the yellow-body hormone (luteal hormone = progesterone). This hormone will prepare the endometrium for the implantation of a fertilized egg and protect the pregnancy by relaxing the uterus. If a pregnancy does not occur, the corpus luteum will shrink, its hormone progesterone will decrease and the withdrawal of progesterone will cause the monthly bleed (menstruation), by which the endometrium is shed. A new cycle then begins.

At about the age of 50, follicular growth, ovulation and formation of the corpus luteum and menstrual bleedings will cease, because the ovaries have, during the preceding five decades, lost all their follicles, their eggs and the hormone-producing structures. Accordingly, the follicle hormone (estradiol) will decrease and the luteal hormone (progesterone) will all but vanish. This phase of reproduction is over.

The central regulating organs, diencephalon and anterior pituitary, with their hormones nevertheless try to reactivate the ovaries. But this endeavor is futile because they are 'burnt out'. The estrogen deficiency symptoms begin and will gain increasing intensity over the years that follow.

ESTROGEN DEFICIENCY AFTER THE MENOPAUSE AND ITS CONSEQUENCES

Menopausal estrogen deficiency causes many akward problems These can be prevented or removed by estrogen supply (i.e. substitution by ERT). Progesterone, the luteal hormone, is combined with the estrogen in the second half of the month (hormone replacement therapy = HRT) to secure normal uterine menstrual-like bleedings. These are often irregular during the menopausal transition. They will become regular again with HRT. Thus otherwise necessary surgical interventions to stop the profuse or prolonged bleedings may be prevented. When the uterus has been operatively removed, the addition of progesterone to the estrogen is not necessary.

ESTROGENS EXERT MANY BENEFICIAL EFFECTS

Estrogens are not strictly purpose-restricted hormones, which make possible sexuality and procreation, but they are important general metabolic regulators and stabilizers of the involuntary (autonomous) nervous system. The loss of estrogens causes several, sometimes severe, reactions of the organism, which are expressed as multiple nervous symptoms of functional imbalance – the climacteric complaints – which affect all parts and organs of the body.

ELIMINATION OF TYPICAL CLIMACTERIC COMPLAINTS BY ESTROGENS

Hot flushes, sweating, heart beat irregularities (palpitations, tachycardia), depressive moods and sleeplessness are, in their joint occurrence, typical climacteric complaints. These will, at their most extreme expression, endanger the quality of life. Tiredness, fears, irresolution, despondency and loss of some mental functions, such as drive, zest for life, creativity and loss of short-term memory and creativity, are frequent additional consequences.

It has been shown in innumerable investigations that estrogens can safely remove all these complaint within a few weeks.

ELIMINATION OF LATE CONSEQUENCES OF ESTROGEN DEFICIENCY BY ESTROGENS

Urogenital atrophy

Estrogens guarantee blood supply and optimal nutrition of the sexual organs. Estrogen deficiency will cause shrinking and malnutrition symptoms of these lower abdominal organs. About 10 years after the loss of estrogens, i.e. during postmenopause, atrophic changes of the vagina, urethra and bladder will become symptomatic in more than half of women. Shrinking and descent of the genitalia, dry vagina, itching, discharge and problems in sexual intercourse are frequent complaints. Loss of urine (incontinence), infections and painful frequent voiding will increase with growing old age, and can

gravely restrict social activity and quality of life.

The symptoms of painful urge to urinate are often futilely treated by antibiotics. If atrophic changes are basic, the complaints are, however, safely eliminated by an estrogen treatment, which improves dysfunction and soreness within a few weeks.

Positive influences of estrogens on skin, hair, eyes and connective tissue

Normal thickness of the skin, blood supply and elasticity of the connective tissue will decrease in advancing years. As estrogen deficiency is one of the basic causes, estrogen application can prevent, or at least slow down, the aging changes of the skin, may reduce wrinkling, and increase skin thickness and elasticity to normal. Hair growth is improved. The dry eye (conjuctivitis sicca) and soreness of the eyelid, a frequent complaint in postmenopausal women, is prevented and succesfully treated by estrogens.

Estrogens improve mental functions in states of estrogen deficiency: prevention of Alzheimer's disease

Estrogens can improve brain function in states of estrogen deficiency. Mental functions are dependent on many factors. Estrogens are one of them, consequent to their preventive effect on atherosclerosis, their decreasing effect on cholesterol levels and their dilatating effect on blood vessels, thus improving blood and energy supply of all organs of the body. This includes increase of the brain's blood supply by estrogens. Estrogens also favor the growth of cerebral nerve bundles and protect them from damage. The lessening of vigilance, concentration, memory and word recall, deplored by many older women, can be demonstrably improved by estrogen intake.

There is some evidence that estrogen intake can prevent Alzheimer's disease, which can damage memory and nearly all other mental functions of old people, which will cause them to lose their identity and will leave them totally dependent on external help. The suggested important positive effect of estrogen on Alzheimer's disease must however be further secured by scientific trials.

Positive effects of estrogens on calcium metabolism and bone strength: prevention of bone fractures

In postmenopausal women the calcium content of bones declines. The structure of the bones and their strength is also decreased. Accordingly, the incidence of bone fractures, mainly of the vertebral spine, forearm and hip is greatly increased. Thirty per cent of postmenopausal women will suffer from fractures. Hip fractures occur mostly in women over 70 years of age and, have a mortality of 22%. Chronic illness, pain, dependence and the necessity of permanent care in a nursing home is very often the sad consequence of hip fractures.

Estrogens lead the calcium from food to the bone and optimize vitamin D utilization in the bone by decreasing bone tissue breakdown and by stimulating the build-up of new bone mass. Thus, an intake of estrogen will secure healthy strong bones, prevent bone fractures and secure for this part of organism an unhandicapped life in old age.

Positive effects of estrogens on lipids and atherosclerosis: prevention of myocardial infarction

Estradiol and most other estrogens decrease blood levels of cholesterol by increasing the favorable 'good' fraction [high-density lipoproteins (HDL), anti-atherosclerotic] and by decreasing the 'bad' fraction, detrimental for structure and function of the blood vessels [low-density lipoproteins (LDL), pro-atherosclerotic]. Thus, atherosclerosis is promoted by estrogen deficiency. By this and other beneficial effects on the arteries, estrogens can prevent or postpone atherosclerosis and its consequent complications in aging women, such as coronary infarction.

Animal experiments and studies in postmenopausal females demonstrate that estrogens delay the pathological calcification of the arteries in old age, i.e. the development of atherosclerosis. Moreover, estrogens widen (dilate) blood vessels, including the arteries of the heart (coronaries) and of the brain, thus improving oxygen, nutrient and energy supplies to these important organs. The declining functions of the heart and brain in old age are thus improved by estrogens.

Estrogen replacement, beginning at the age of menopause, will accordingly prevent or slow down atherosclerosis and the resulting diseases. Indeed, 30–50% of myocardial infarctions could be prevented by estrogen replacement. A preventive effect in some forms of stroke is claimed in several studies, but is still controversial.

When atherosclerotic changes are already manifest, an estrogen substitution for prevention is not recommended, because the breakdown effect of estrogens on atherosclerotic lesions (plaques) may cause vascular complications.

The prevention of atherosclerosis, and accordingly of myocardial infarction, will decrease the risk of death from vascular diseases by 20–50% in estrogen takers provided that intake is begun early enough, i.e. at the start of the menopause.

Normally, estrogen–progestogen substitution will be necessary only for as long as the climacteric complaints last, i.e. about 5 years. On the basis of your family history and his findings at check-up, your doctor will advise you of whether or not you are a candidate for long-term estrogen intake (more than 5 years), with the aim of prevention of osteoporosis, atherosclerosis and connected diseases of the heart vessels (coronaries).

Possibly, you will be confronted with the results of recent studies from estrogen medication, e.g. the Women's Health Initiative (WHI) from the US, which found an increase of thromboses, myocardial infarctions, strokes and breast cancers under HRT (not under ERT). However, this investigation was poorly planned, used inappropriate preparations and did not follow the basic rules of 'good clinical practice'. Therefore, the results cannot claim general significance and should not be used in providing advice.

QUALITY OF LIFE

This important criterion of success of a treatment is greatly damaged by severe climacteric complaints such as hot flushes, heavy sweating, sleeping disorders, irregularities of heart function, depressive moods, urinary incontinence, pain during urine voiding, dry vagina, cohabitation problems, discharge, itching and burning, and of decrease of short-term memory and wording. All of these symptoms, if caused by estrogen deficiency, are prevented or removed by early menopausal estrogen intake.

WHAT ARE THE POSSIBLE SIDE EFFECTS AND RISKS OF ESTROGEN INTAKE?

Side effects (such as breast tenderness or water retention) must not occur at all. They are seldom reported (3–5% of cases) and occur mostly only during the first days and weeks of intake, when the optimal dose of hormones has not been found. If such side effects are experienced, the dose of the estrogen is either too high or the mode of application is not optimal. In a few cases the added progestogen may not be well tolerated. Please contact your doctor immediately for a reduction of the dose of the hormones or of the mode of application (e.g. percutaneous by estrogen patch or ointment instead), and all complaints will readily be removed.

Body weight is, contrary to widely held belief, not increased by ERT and HRT. Neither is blood pressure usually increased by estrogens.

Uterine bleedings, if unwanted, can be avoided, by combining estrogen every day of the month with progesterone or a progesterone-like compound continuously. Special preparations are also available which usually do not cause uterine bleedings (e.g. tibolone, estriol). Please ask your therapeut.

To avoid complications, your doctor will ask you questions concerning your family history and your own medical history. This and his/her findings in the medical examination will show whether a hormone treatment should be recommended to you or not. *Indications* are the reasons why you should receive estrogens: *contraindications* are the reasons why you should not receive estrogens. These contraindications, such as hereditary cancer or hereditary cardiovascular diseases, being overweight, varicosis, childlessness and some others factors, are called *risk factors*. These will be considered by your doctor when he/she advises you with regard to possible contraindications to ERT and HRT. Some of the contraindications can be bypassed by the choice of special hormones or modes of application.

Indications

Estrogens should absolutely be prescribed in cases of severe climacteric complaints, early operative loss of the ovaries, in the early stages of osteoporosis and apparent signs of estrogen deficiency of the urogenital organs.

Contraindications

Estrogens should not be prescribed in cases of an accumulation of thrombosis in the family or in the history of the patient (caused by disturbances of coagulation), and also not in cases of an accumulation of cancer in the family and in severe liver diseases. Your doctor will ask you the corresponding questions.

THROMBOSIS

Thrombosis (blood clots in veins) occurs in about 1 per 10 000 cases in untreated women and in 2–3 per 10 000 cases per year under oral estrogen substitution. This is usually the case in inherited disturbances of blood coagulation. A careful ascertainment of accumulation of cases of thromboses in the family history of a patient will ensure that these cases do not receive ERT (i.e. it is a contraindication). Smokers and women with varicosis and who are overweight are especially at risk. The risk can be minimized by use of nonoral estrogens in low doses (e.g. estrogen patches) and by avoidance of triggering events for thrombosis, as well as by weight reduction and treatment of varicosis, and administration of medicaments that strengthen vein function and prevent blood coagulation (e.g. aspirin).

An embolus can result from thrombosis; however, not if thrombosis is prevented or diagnosed early and adequately treated.

THE CANCER PROBLEM

Women fear, most of all, falling ill due to cancer of the breast, uterus, ovaries and/or intestine. Indeed, the incidence of cancer continues to increase steadily in most Western societies. This fear is understandable as these diseases attack the organs of a woman's identity, because the treatment of cancer is stressful and the cure rate is still not satisfactory. However, statistical data show that 42% of women in postmenopausal years and old age die from heart diseases and stroke, and only 20% die of all cancers, from them 2.8% of breast cancer and 0.8% from endometrial cancer. Nevertheless, this is an important psychologic problem.

For the past 70 years there has been a broad discussion in the scientific world about hormones and cancer. However, hormones are not the center of the cancer problem. Women and men must learn that the increase in cancer in the modern world is the price to be paid for the load of heredity, an increased life expectancy, a heavily poisoned environment, damage by ionizing radiation, unhealthy food, smoking and alcohol misuse, overnutrition (especially with animal fats), being overweight, metabolic anomalies (e.g. diabetes), childlessness, late first pregnancy and refraining from breastfeeding. All these are so-called risk factors for the formation of breast and genital cancer.

Hormones like estrogens indeed create a milieu which is optimal for the growth of normal as well of abnormal cells. Estrogens (and other hormones) act like manure or fertilizers: these do, of course, not cause weeds but they do promote the growth of the desired grains and fruits as well as the unwanted weeds. It is the duty and the art of the physician to promote the growth of the grains and fruits (normal cells) and to prevent the growth of the weeds (cancer).

Breast cancer

Ten per cent of the total female population in Western countries will develop a breast cancer during their lifetime. Whether estrogen treatment increases the number of breast cancer cases is, even after 70 years of research, still controversial. This means that the numerical influence of estrogens on the manifestation of breast cancer cases cannot be remarkable.

An evaluation of all reliable epidemiologic studies came to the result that 20% of all publications show a decreased risk of breast cancer in estrogen takers; 44% showed no increase and 30% a small increase.[1] This evaluation could, in summary, not find an increase of breast cancer under ERT or HRT. Another recent evaluation found a small increase under ERT, amounting to a 1.023% increase of breast cancer diagnoses per year of estrogen use after more than 5 years of use.[2] If this is correct, after 10 years of ERT, two additional cases per 1000 women taking ERT would occur. It is believed that these are cancer cases which were already present before but were stimulated to faster growth by the ERT.

Endometrial cancer

Cancer of the lining of the inner womb (endometrium) is not increased when estrogen is combined with an effective progestogen for at least 10 days/month. This combination is ordered according to health authority regulations for women with a uterus. If an endometrial cancer should occur during ERT, the cure rate is increased by 20% as compared to patients not treated by HRT. Only women without a uterus (hysterectomized) must not receive a progestogen.

Cancer of the cervix

Cancer of the neck of the womb is not increased by HRT.

Cancer of the ovaries

Ovarian cancer is not increased by ERT or HRT. A few studies suggested a probable small increase in a small number of cases after long-term treatment, but this is controversial. Besides, the hormonal contraceptive pill prevents ovarian cancer during intake and for many years after withdrawal.

The good news

The cure rate of all cancers is substantially improved in patients who are taking estrogens by about 20–30%. The mortality of breast and genital cancer cases is accordingly decreased by 20–50%. The life expectancy of estrogen takers is prolonged from 0.6 to 2 years. The overall mortality of estrogen takers is decreased by 40–60% as compared to nontakers of the same age, same region and identical social conditions.

OTHER POSSIBILITIES OF TREATMENT FOR THE CLIMACTERIC

Some women want to try so-called natural methods of treatment for climacteric complaints, e.g. plant preparations or homeopathic medicaments. All these are much less effective than ERT and HRT, but they may be sufficient if the complaints are only weak. Most of them exert no preventive effects.

Estrogens from plants (phytoestrogens) have been the focus of interest for some years. They stem mostly from soya or red clover and have only a weak effect on climacteric complaints. However, they do not cause uterine bleeding and do not stimulate the breast as natural estrogens do. Some investigations suggest that breast cancer may even be prevented by phytoestrogens, but this is still not proven. Apparently, phytoestrogens exert positive influences on lipids and osteoporosis, but these claims must be further substantiated.

Preventive effects can be achieved by diet and physical activity. This possibility should consequently be used.

Ask your doctor for more information or consult books on the female climacteric, available in pharmacies or bookstores.

CONCLUSIONS

The benefits of ERT or HRT are considerable and are surely greater than the small possible risks they carry, which can mostly be prevented by well-conducted management. Ask your friends about their experiences. Many thankful women who have had or are having ERT or HRT are witnesses of the noteworthy benefits.

Rely upon your doctor. He/she will ensure that you will gain the benefits, but that unwanted side effects will not occur and that you will be safe from harm. Ask him/her whenever you experience problems or have questions, especially after having read the packaging circular, because this can be difficult to understand and overemphasizes possible risks without duly mentioning the advantages and benefits.

If you regularly see your doctor for prevention or early detection of possible diseases, you will be on the safe side. Please realize, that you can do much for yourself against climacteric complaints and diseases of aging by complying with the advice of your doctor and by following the principles of a healthy lifestyle.

All the best for your menopausal years!

REFERENCES

1. Bush T, Whitmann M, Flaws JA. Hormone replacement therapy and breast cancer: a qualitative review. *Obstet Gynecol* 2001; **98:** 498–508.
2. Beral V, Reeves G, Bull D et al. Breast cancer and hormone replacement therapy: putting the risk into context. In: (Birkhäuser M, Rozenbaum H, eds). *IV European Congress on Menopause*, Eska, Paris, 1998, pp. 2667–77.

31

The aging male

B Lunenfeld

An aging world • Men, aging and health • Partial endocrine deficiency in men (PEDAM) • Body composition and metabolism • Male osteoporosis • Sexual dysfunction and sexuality • Hormone therapy (HT) • Growth hormone (GH) therapy • Improving the health of older men • Strategies to improve and maintain aging men's health • References

AN AGING WORLD

First we were obsessed with the challenge of "population explosion", then we shifted our concern to the problems of global ageing, and only now do we start to grasp the future consequences of a rapid fertility decline

E Diczfalusy 2000

Although the mean life expectancy at birth has been prolonged by more then 25 years within the last century, life expectancy at the age of 65 increased by less then 3 years during the same time (Table 31.1). Moreover, despite the enormous medical progress during the past few decades, 25% of life expectancy after age 65 is spent with some disability, and the last years of life are accompanied by a further increase of incapacity and sickness.

Frailty, disability and dependency will increase immensely the demands on social and health services. The very high cost in relation to these services may strain to the limit the ability of health, social and even political infrastructures not only of developing but also of the most developed and industrialized nations.[1]

The ability to permit men to age gracefully, maintain independent living, free of disability, for as long as possible is a crucial factor in aging with dignity and would furthermore reduce health service costs significantly. To achieve this objective, a holistic approach to the management of aging has to be adopted.[2]

The promotion of healthy aging and the prevention, or drastic reduction, of morbidity and disability of the elderly must now assume a central role in the formulation of the health and social policies of many, if not all, countries. It must emphasize an all-encompassing life-long approach to the aging process, beginning with preconceptual events and focusing on appropriate interventions at all stages of life. Life-history studies of childhood and adolescence demonstrate clearly that social factors probably

Table 31.1 Life expectancy of males at different ages (courtesy of the Registrar General for Scotland, from *Cheating Time* by Roger Gosden)

Year	At birth	At 15 years	At 45 years	At 65 years
1888	43.9	43.9 (58.9)	22.6 (67.6)	10.8 (75.8)
1988	70.5	56.4 (71)	28.2 (73.2)	13.0 (78)

operate in a cumulative fashion. There are significant social class differences in height growth and other aspects of physical development, as well as in incidence of infectious and other diseases, and risk of injury.

The life course perspective leads to important policy and strategy decisions. Firstly, it is clearly possible and desirable to improve the health status of men when they are old, although this approach is still not fully implemented. Secondly, a complementary approach to improving the health of older men would focus on appropriate interventions at all stages of their lives.

The determinants of 'aging' and of 'life expectancy' extend from genetic and molecular determinants to the increasingly powerful forces of environmental, economic, technologic and cultural globalization. Specific measures for the promotion of healthy aging should include:

- the promotion of a safe environment;
- healthy lifestyle including proper nutrition;
- appropriate exercise;
- avoidance of smoking;
- avoidance of drug and alcohol abuses;
- social interactions to maintain good mental health;
- medical health care, including the control of chronic illnesses.

If done effectively, it should result in a significant reduction of the health and social costs, reduce pain and suffering, increase the quality of life of the elderly and enable them to remain productive and contribute to the wellbeing of society. The medical and socioeconomic implication of a demographic reality of a new world will be very different from all preceding epochs in history. Indeed, so new that most people, their governments, national and private pension funds, as well as most health insurers, have not yet had sufficient vision, determination or courage to face up to this immediate challenge. The medical profession, and pharmaceutic and health industries are not yet prepared for these emerging markets.

An increase in the quality of life with a delay, decrease or prevention of disabilities will increase the length of the productive life of aging populations, will decrease dependency, and will decrease health costs related to expensive curative and palliative services.

MEN, AGING AND HEALTH

Before a thing has made its appearance; order should be secured before this order has begun
Lao Tzue

It is impossible to understand aging and health without a gender perspective. Both from a physiologic and psychosocial point of view, the determinants of health as we age are intrinsically related to gender. There is increasing recognition that unless research and programs – on both clinical science and public health – acknowledge these differences, they will not be effective. While women experience greater burdens of morbidity and disability, men die earlier, yet the reasons for such premature mortality are not fully understood. The rapidity with which the worldwide population is aging will require a sharp focus on gender issues if meaningful policies are to be developed. Yet so often gender in the health context is taken as being synonymous only with women's issues.[3]

In contrast to the recent and much needed attention to the social position and health status in women, male health concerns have been relatively neglected. Men continue to have higher morbidity and mortality rates.[3] Life expectancy for men is significantly shorter than that for women in most regions of the world.[1] The course of disease, response to disease and societal response to illness exhibit gender differences, often resulting in different treatments and access to health care. The conventional approach of medical, behavioral and social sciences to the problem of male aging has for a long time been overlooked; there has been an absence of focusing, disconnection and, most of all, lack of interdisciplinary collaboration.

The major causes of morbidity and mortality all take effect over extended periods. DNA is constantly being damaged and repaired; bones are constantly worn away and rebuilt; atheromas are constantly accumulating in side arteries and are constantly being removed. If the rate of decay is faster then the rate of repair, healthy tissue will be lost until the damage produces symptoms of and finally results in disease. Therefore, primary prevention strategies will be most effective when initiated at the earliest opportunity. Prevention of ischemic heart disease, hypertension and stroke, as well as lung cancer, are diseases in which primary prevention needs to be addressed. When problems are more prevalent at older ages, as with prostate and colorectal cancers and osteoporosis, early diagnostic tests, such as appropriate and periodic use of laboratory tests [e.g. prostate specific antigen (PSA)] and screening procedures can play an important role in secondary prevention and self-care strategies.[4]

Significant numbers of male-related health problems such as:

- changes in body constitution;
- fat distribution;
- muscle weakness;
- urinary incontinence;
- loss of cognitive functioning;
- reduction in wellbeing;
- depression;
- sexual dysfunction

could be detected and treated in their early stages if both physicians and public awareness of these problems were more pervasive. This could effectively decrease morbidity, frailty and dependency, increase quality of life and reduce health service costs. Women visit the doctor 150% as often as men, enabling them to detect health problems in their early stages. However, usually men cost the health services more than women since they seek the medical services at a more advanced stage of disease. While women are geared to preventive care, men generally come for 'repair'.

When discussing age-related problems, it is often difficult to separate and to distinguish between:

- the natural aging process, primarily genetically determined and which cannot be changed;

- aging amplifiers determined by environmental and developmental factors, which can be modified;
- an acute or chronic illness or intercurrent disease, which can be prevented, delayed or cured.

It must not be forgotten that aging by itself is associated with reduced productivity, decreased general vigor ('frailty of the aged') as well as with increased incidence of defined diseases, including:

- cardiovascular diseases (CVD);
- malignant neoplasm;
- chronic obstructive pulmonary diseases;
- degenerative and metabolic diseases (arthrosis, diabetes, osteoporosis, etc.);
- visual loss (macular degeneration, cataract);
- hearing loss;
- anxiety, mood, depression and sleep disorders;
- sexual dysfunction;
- various dementias (e.g. Alzheimer's disease).

Five of six men in their sixties have one or more of these diseases. The chronic degenerative diseases have a long latency period before symptoms appear and a diagnosis is finally made. Once the diagnosis is made, drugs may alleviate symptoms but are not very effective in altering the underlying disease, which unfortunately usually continues to worsen.

Heart disease and stroke are the major causes of death and disability in aging men. Approximately 52 million deaths occur worldwide each year, 39 million occurring in developing countries. About one-quarter of all deaths in developing countries and half of all deaths in developed countries are attributed to CVD. Globally, there are more deaths from coronary heart disease (5.2 million) than from stroke (46 million). Age-specific death rates from CVD increase dramatically with age. Within each country, age-specific death rates for all CVD increase at least twofold between the age groups of 65–74 and 75–84 years in both sexes, with consistently at least 50% higher rates for elderly men than for women. Morbidity and disability from these diseases are also high. For example, the Global Burden of Disease project estimates that by 2020, coronary heart disease and stroke will be the first and second leading cause of death, respectively.

For men, prostate cancer is the most prevalent malignancy and the third leading cause of cancer death in men. In 1990, worldwide there were 193,000 deaths from prostate cancer, with 127,000 of those deaths occurring amongst those aged 70 years and over and 51,000 amongst those aged 60–69. Since prostate cancer is primarily a disease affecting men over 50 years of age, the worldwide trend towards an aging population means that the number of prostate cancer deaths is predicted to increase markedly. In the year 2020, a global increase of 393,000 deaths is expected, with 359,000 of those deaths among men over 70 years of age and 103,000 deaths among men aged 60–69.

Worldwide, more than nine million people developed cancer in 1997 and more than six million died of cancer. Cancer deaths increased from 6 to 9% of total deaths from 1985 to 1997 in developing countries, but remained about constant at 21% of total deaths in developed countries. For men, prostate cancer is the most prevalent malignancy. The highest mortality rate was observed for lung cancer with approximately 790,000 deaths in 1997, followed by stomach, liver, colorectal, esophageal and prostate cancers.

Chronic obstructive pulmonary diseases and lung cancer are not only the most frequent problems among men but are also the most easily preventable. In men, 90% of all cases are attributable to cigarette smoking. These data suggest that almost every male lung cancer patient could have prevented his disease. Strategies to promote smoking cessation should be a top public policy priority, especially in those developing countries where aggressive marketing by the tobacco industry is not counterbalanced by adequate public health information advertisements.

The loss of vision, hearing and other senses should be recognized as more than physical problems. Such conditions have profound effects on social and personal interactions, economic viability and the mental health of those affected, and should be treated seriously.

Depression is the most common functional mental disorder affecting aging males, it is both underdiagnosed and undertreated. It has a high rate of recurrence and is associated with significantly increased mortality. Depression is closely linked in this group with physical illness and altered presentation can make diagnosis difficult. Thorough holistic assessment and good communication skills are of utmost importance. Nurses and medical professionals can improve the mental health of these patients with therapeutic attitudes and actions. It must be remembered that about 90% of older men who attempt or complete suicide have depression either not diagnosed or inadequately treated. If men continue to under-report depression, the morbidity of this condition will continue to increase. Proper identification and treatment of depression will have significant public health implications.

Cognitive decline with age is inevitable but the global impairment of the higher cortical functions can be delayed. In women, hormone replacement therapy (HRT) was shown to delay the onset of Alzheimer's disease. There is an urgent need to also obtain such information in men. Dementia is a major public health issue accounting for significant morbidity, loss of independence, loss of dignity and eventual institutionalization. The prevalence of severe dementia increases from 1% at age 65–74, 7% at age 75–84 and 25% after the age of 85. Thirty-seven per cent of patients with Alzheimer's disease live in institutions compared with 1.7% of subjects without dementia.

Many of the chronic disabling genetic and metabolic conditions experienced by aging men are interrelated (comorbidity). The effects of a single minor condition may not be severe but its interaction with other conditions can reduce functional capacity, aggravate pain and cause serious anxiety about the future.

Many men are reluctant to visit their health center or physician due to fear, lack of information and psychologic reasons. Men must be encouraged to *take symptoms more seriously* and seek professional support and advice sooner than they have done in the past. In turn, this will require the availability of services that are suitable for, and sensitive to, the health needs of older men. There may be much to learn from the successes and failures of health services established to meet the specific health needs of women. Educating both the public and health care providers about the importance of early detection of male health problems will result in reducing rates of morbidity and mortality, as well as health costs, for many age-related diseases.

For more than 100 years gynecologists have been specialized physicians for the medical care of women. They have acted as their *homme de confiance* from adolescence to menopause. The modern gynecologist is not only cure oriented but has been trained in preventive strategies and in the maintenance of health and wellbeing. Men's health care is cure and organ specific, and is the responsibility of a variety of medical specialties and subspecialties. No subspecialty has evolved which guarantees high-quality management of men's health care, including curative and preventive strategies, and a holistic approach to the maintenance of health and quality of life. In addition, gender-specific training of primary health care workers who can respond to the unique health concerns of elderly men must be supported. Discussion of medical, psychologic and social problems should be encouraged. To this end, International Society for the Study of the Aging male (ISSAM) and the World Health Organization (WHO) Aging and Health program will work together to develop curricula particular for primary health workers.

PARTIAL ENDOCRINE DEFICIENCY IN MEN (PEDAM)

The law of nature is so unalterable that it cannot be changed by God himself
Hugo Grotius 1625

The most important and drastic gender differences in aging are related to the reproductive organs. In distinction to the course of reproductive aging in women, with the rapid decline in sex hormones expressed by the cessation of menses, men experience a slow and continuous decline of a large number of hormones but do not show an irreversible arrest of reproductive capacity in old age.[5–8]

In the aging male, endocrine changes and decline in endocrine function involve the following.

- Reduced secretory output from peripheral glands due to sclerosis of blood vessels (in the interstitial tissue of Leydig's cells, for example, this process contributes, to a large extent, to the decrease of gonadal androgens).
- Modulation of transcriptional activity: as numbers of CAG repeats in androgen receptors increase the androgenic effect decreases.
- Alterations in the central mechanism controlling the temporal organization of hormonal release. The heterogeneity in basal neuroendocrine function in aging, as reported in the literature, is compounded by the fact that basal hormone levels are far from constant, fluctuating considerably due to the interaction of circadian rhythmicity, sleep and, for some hormones, intermittent pulsatile releases at different intervals. During aging a number of morphologic and neurochemical alterations have been found in the suprachiasmatic nuclei (the central circadian pacemaker) and are likely to be responsible for the dampened circadian hormonal and non-hormonal rhythms.

These are in part responsible for the age-dependent decrease of blood levels of:

- testosterone, with loss of circadian rhythmicity;[9]
- dehydroepiandrosterone (DHEA);
- estradiol;
- growth hormone (GH), e.g. insulin-like growth factor (IGF)-I;
- thyroid hormones;
- night-time prolactin and melatonin concentrations.

Furthermore:

- The circadian rises of cortisol, thyroid-stimulating hormone (TSH), and melatonin continue, to some extent, in aging men, but do however occur 1–1.5 hours earlier;

- the distribution of rapid eye movement (REM) stages during sleep in elderly subjects is similarly advanced;[10]
- sex hormone-binding globulin (SHBG) increases with age, resulting in a further lowering the concentrations of free biologically active androgens;
- luteinizing hormone (LH) and follicle-stimulating hormone (FSH) initially increase with age and later decrease.

The decline with age in the serum concentrations of biologically active forms of testosterone in men is an indisputable fact.[5,11] This decline begins earlier than previously appreciated (approximately at the age of 30) and is progressive and relentless. A 20–30% decline of mean serum testosterone levels is observed between the ages 25 and 75. The fall of the biologically active free testosterone and non-SHBG-bound or bioavailable testosterone in serum is of even greater magnitude, with a reduction of 50% over the same age range as serum levels of SHBG increase.[12,13] Eventually, if men live long enough, serum testosterone levels fall below the threshold for optimal androgen actions (Fig. 31.1).

The decrease in thyroid responsiveness is responsible for the increase of TSH. Moreover, in aging men melatonin secretion also decreases and its circadian periodicity is gradually disrupted. Sleep in these older men is shallow and fragmented.[14] These alterations influence particular GH secretion, which occur with deeper stages of sleep [slow wave (SW) sleep]. In men, approximately 70% of the daily GH output occurs during early (SW) sleep. During aging, SW sleep and GH secretion decrease with the same chronology, raising the possibility that the peripheral effects of the hyposomatotropism of the elderly may partially reflect age-related alterations in sleep–wake homeostasis. While the association between sleep and GH release has been well documented, there is also evidence indicating that components of the somatotropic axes are involved in regulating sleep.[15] It has been shown that in elderly men the decrease in melatonin secretion and its circadian periodicity are correlated with:[16]

- mood disorders;
- decay in cognitive functions;
- increase of sleep disorders;
- regulation of platelet production, probably due to an inhibitory effect of melatonin on macrophage-mediated platelet destruction.

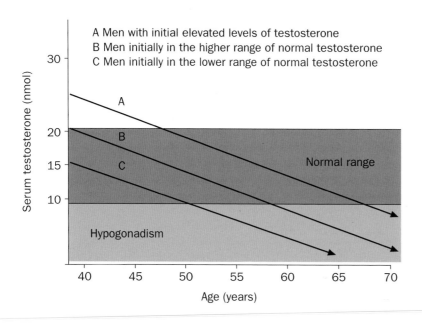

Figure 31.1 Serum testosterone levels (nmol) versus age (years).

Since DHEA, GH and testosterone decrease and only cortisol secretion remains stable during the aging process, the equilibrium between anabolism and catabolism changes towards catabolism.

BODY COMPOSITION AND METABOLISM

Parallel to the decrease of bioavailable testosterone, estrogens and GH, aging men witness a decrease in muscle and bone mass, as well as in muscle strength. Declining bone mass predisposes older men to osteoporosis and hip fracture. Just as with estrogens in women, the decrease in serum testosterone concentrations may be associated with this age-related decline in bone density. Osteoporosis in men occurs about 10 years later than in women. This is due to the fact that the mean peak bone mass in men is higher and estrogen secretion in aging men remains significantly superior compared to postmenopausal women. An increase in body fat, with fat redistribution from peripheral to central stores, also occurs with increasing age.

Aging is associated with a progressive failure of body functions, and particularly with an increasing lack of physical strength and mobility. Many problems of aging are attributable to the progressive loss of lean tissues and to catabolic events. This can be, and often is, associated with a progressive decline in independence and quality of life, leading eventually to a prolonged dependence on others, followed by a distressing process of death. By analogy with the menopause, the fall in GH secretion has been termed the somatopause. In cross-sectional studies on elderly people, the amount of GH secreted spontaneously correlated well with 'good' risk factors such as body composition, mobility, lipid profiles and blood pressure. The question arises whether the fall in GH with aging marks the development of secondary GH deficiency which would benefit from GH supplementation.[17] In 1991, Rudman et al[18] showed beneficial effects in a group of elderly men with low plasma IGF-I values, but no underlying pituitary pathology, which were administered GH. In these adults, low doses of GH increased lean body mass and bone mineral density,

decreased total and abdominal body fat, and lowered low-density liproprotein (LDL) cholesterol and serum leptin levels, resulting in a gain of bone mass after 18–24 months of treatment[19,20] and an improved quality of life.[21] HRT alone is not sufficient to increase muscle strength, decrease fat mass or change the fat contribution and localization in aging men. Proper nutrition and physical exercise targeted at specific muscle groups is mandatory in order to obtain satisfactory results. Moreover, some authors suggest that resistance exercise training improves muscle strength and anabolism in older men, and these improvements were not enhanced when exercise was combined with daily GH administration.[22]

Sleep and exercise are the two major stimuli for secretion of GH in normal people and there is evidence to indicate that the GH response to exercise is essential for developing and maintaining physical fitness. There is also some evidence to suggest that adults who continue to exercise with increasing age better maintain lean body mass and physiologic GH secretion.

Some cognitive functions are known to be sensitive, while others are not, to the process of aging. It is known that general knowledge, vocabulary, basic visual perception and reading ability are not sensitive to aging, while visual–constructive ability and perceptual–motor speed, mental tracking and verbal short- and long-term memory is. Serum IGF-I in elderly men was found to be significantly associated with the performances on the Digit Symbol Substitution test and Concept Shifting Task, which measure perceptual–motor and mental processing speed, both known to decline with age. Subjects with higher IGF-I levels performed better in these tests. This supports the hypothesis that circulating IGF-I may play a role in the age-related reduction of certain cognitive functions, specifically speed of information processing. Exercise could increase the release of GH. In healthy elderly men and women the resistance exercise-induced release of GH is attenuated when compared to younger individuals.[23] Patients can be counseled to start their own antiaging program in becoming more active, starting to exercise and losing weight if obese. This will physiologically lead to tiredness, better sleep and, consequently, higher GH levels. Melatonin secretion will also rise, provided the patient does not sleep in front of the TV or with bright lights on. Eating only small portions or nothing at all before going to bed (dinner canceling) can also increase GH secretion.

A noticeable change during aging is the sleep pattern of the elderly. During the fourth decade (30–40 years of age) the amount of SW sleep decreases dramatically over the same narrow age range, and this change is correlated to a 2–3-fold decrease in the total amount of GH secreted over a 24-hour period. Because the sleep-onset GH pulse is often the major secretory output in adults, age-related decrements in sleep-related GH secretion is likely to play a major role in the hyposomatotropism of senescence.[24] In aging, a decline in sleep continuity, decreased SW sleep, earlier nocturnal cortisol rise and blunted GH secretion occur.

In elderly people, decrements in sleep consolidation and the propensity to awaken from sleep appear to be related to the interaction between a reduction in the homeostatic drive for sleep and a reduced strength of the circadian signal promoting sleep in the early morning.[25]

Low or distorted melatonin rhythms have repeatedly been reported in middle-aged and elderly insomniacs. Melatonin replacement therapy significantly decreased sleep latency and/or increased sleep efficiency, and decreased wake time after sleep onset. In addition, melatonin substitution facilitated benzodiazepine discontinuation in chronic users.[26]

Melatonin is a direct free-radical scavenger and an indirect antioxidant. It has been shown to quench the hydroxyl radical, superoxide anion radical, singlet oxygen, peroxyl radical and peroxynitrite anion. Additionally, melatonin's antioxidant actions probably derive from its stimulatory effect on superoxide dismutase, glutathione peroxidase, glutathione reductase and G6PD, and its inhibitory action on nitric oxide synthase. Melatonin also stabilizes cell membranes, thereby making them more resistant to oxidative attack. Melatonin is devoid of pro-oxidant actions. Thus, in humans, the total antioxidative capacity of serum is related to melatonin levels. Thus, the reduction in melatonin with age may be one of the factors responsible for increased oxidative damage in the elderly.[27]

During childhood (between the sixth and eighth year), DHEA levels increase (adrenarche); peak levels are reached at about 20 years of age. After the age of 35 serum:DHEA levels continuously decrease, reaching very low levels after the age of 70 (adrenopause). Levels of the sulfate of DHEA (DHEAS) in very old people (over 90 years of age), are five times lower than a young control group. Whether this decline represents a harmful hormone deficiency or a beneficial age-related hormonal adaptation is not yet known. As to DHEA and aging, there is no doubt that strong correlations can be established between the declining levels of adrenal androgens and ailments of aging, but whether these statistical associations are causally pathophysiologically interrelated remains to be established.

DHEA plays a role in carbohydrate, fat and bone metabolism, and influences cellular growth, the immune system and brain functions such as sleep, mood, cognition, and memory. Administration of DHEA to elderly men and women has been reported to increase muscle strength, the sense of wellbeing and an increase of serum concentrations of IGF-I.[20–29] In men over 90 years of age, DHEAS levels have positive correlations with body mass index (BMI) and the waist-to-hip ratio, taken as indices of body's energy reserves (fat). In men, the highest functioning levels had the highest levels of DHEAS; hence, a favorable role for DHEAS in successful aging was proposed.[30,31]

DHEA treatment in older individuals was associated with a remarkable increase in perceived physical and psychologic wellbeing for both men and women,[32] with no change in libido. In addition, the augmentation of DHEA and DHEAS in older people to young levels induced an increase in the bioavailability of IGF-I (increase in IGF-I and decrease in IGFBP3), indicating the beneficial effect of

DHEA replacement in age-advanced men and women.[28]

Experimental and clinical investigations suggest the hypothesis that DHEAS can positively influence natural killer (NK) immunity via locally produced IGF-I from NK cells. It was shown that NK-generated IGF-I has a role in the modulation of NK cell cytotoxicity (NKCC) by DHEAS in humans. Although DHEAS may contribute to the interleukin (IL)-2-mediated NKCC, its activity on NK cytolytic function may be dependent on an autocrine mechanism (IGF-I mediated), probably independent of cytokine activation. The higher NKCC response to DHEAS found in old subjects compared to younger ones might counterbalance the age-dependent decline in circulating DHEAS, thus contributing to maintain the pattern of NK immunity during aging.[33] A consequence of the conversion of DHEA to androgens and estrogens is that the effects of DHEA administration are not necessarily harmless. They may influence hormone-sensitive diseases such as breast or prostate cancer. So far there are no reports in the literature of any side effects from self-administration of DHEA, which occurs on a massive scale with DHEA sold as a health product. Well-designed studies investigating the effects of deficiency of adrenal androgens and the results of replacement therapy in humans are required to resolve the long-term effect of levels of adrenal androgens.

Aging in humans is accompanied by a relative increase in adrenal glucocorticoid secretion due to a decline in adrenal androgen synthesis and secretion. The intense interest in adrenal function in aging individuals in recent years is in large measure related to the potential impact of cortisol excess in the development of cognitive impairment and hippocampal neuronal loss, and to the desire to provide hormone replacement and healthy aging. However, an exact relationship remains controversial. DHEAS, but not DHEA, activates peroxisome proliferator-activated receptor alpha (PPAR alpha) in the liver, an intracellular receptor belonging to the steroid receptor superfamily. Thus, DHEAS may serve as a physiologic modulator of liver fatty acid metabolism and peroxi-

somal enzyme expression, and thereby may contribute to the anticarcinogenic and chemoprotective properties of this intriguing class of endogenous steroids. The life-sustaining role of adrenal cortisol secretion and its regulation of metabolism via catabolic actions may be modulated by its partner DHEA and DHEAS. During the anabolic growth period (childhood to early adulthood) the body is exposed to relatively high levels of DHEA/DHEAS; during infancy and aging it is exposed to relatively or absolutely high levels of cortisol. Elevated glucocorticoid levels produce hippocampal dysfunction and correlate with individual deficits in spatial learning in aged rats. It has also been shown that persistent cortisol increases are related to memory impairments in elderly humans, as well as reduced hippocampal volume and deficits in hippocampus-dependent memory tasks. The degree of hippocampal atrophy correlated strongly with both the degree of cortisol elevation over time and current basal cortisol levels. Therefore, basal cortisol elevation may cause hippocampal damage and impair hippocampus-dependent learning and memory in humans.[34]

Estrogen specifically maintains verbal memory in women and may prevent or forestall the deterioration in short- and long-term memory that occurs with normal aging. There is also evidence that estrogen decreases the incidence of Alzheimer's disease or retards its onset, or both.[35] The delayed onset of Alzheimer's disease in men may be due to the fact that estrogen levels are significantly higher in aging men than in postmenopausal women.

Frailty is a wasting syndrome of advanced age that leaves a person vulnerable to falls, functional decline, morbidity and mortality. Men are likely to develop this syndrome later than women, gender difference which is a result of several factors:

- higher baseline levels of muscle mass may protect men from reaching a threshold of weakness and muscle mass loss that may put them into a category of frailty;
- higher GH, testosterone and estrogens, which may provide advantages in muscle mass maintenance;

• cortisol, which is likely less dysregulated in older men as compared to older women.

All the above factors can be considered as neuroendocrine advantages for men over women. There is also evidence of immune system dimorphism that is, in part, responsive to sex steroids, perhaps making men more vulnerable to sepsis and infection and women more vulnerable to chronic inflammatory conditions and muscle mass loss. The net effect of the hormonal dysregulation and immune system dysfunction is an accelerated loss of muscle mass.[36]

In nondiabetic Caucasian subjects of either sex, senescence per se is associated with a progressive decline in both insulin clearance and basal insulin release,[37] the anatomical substrate for emotions. It is now thought that limbic dopamine (DA) represents a precursor of noradrenaline in the biosynthetic pathway of catecholamines.

Dopaminergic innervations are present in the limbic system, which is sensitive to aging. DA levels, biosynthetic and catabolic markers and DA receptors undergo age-related changes. Changes of dopaminergic neurotransmission markers in the limbic system may be associated with cognitive impairment and psychotic symptoms, including dementia and Alzheimer's and Parkinson's diseases.[38]

MALE OSTEOPOROSIS

Youth is the only thing worth having. When I find out that I am growing old, I shall kill myself. To get back my youth I would do anything in the world, except take exercise, get up early, or be respectable
Oscar Wilde (The Picture of Dorian Gray) 1891

Male osteoporosis had a prevalence of around 5% (vertebral fractures) but with the increase in lifespan, osteoporotic fractures are becoming more frequent in men. It has been estimated that 19% of men over the age of 50 in the United States (US) will have one or more fragility fractures in their lifetime; moreover, more than 4 million men in the US have low bone mass and are at risk for fractures.[39] The sequelae of skeletal fractures diminish the quality of life, advance dependency and constitute an important public health problem. Hip fractures in men result in a higher morbidity and mortality than in women. Secondary causes such as gastrointestinal diseases with malabsorption, alcoholism and malignant diseases are common. Hypogonadism and/or decreases of GH are often unfortunately not diagnosed, as clinical signs are subtle.

Criteria for the diagnosis of osteoporosis based on bone density were established by the WHO, using the relationship between risk of fracture and bone mineral density (BMD) in Caucasian women. Such criteria for men have not been defined. Men have larger bones with thicker cortices, although their density and trabecular architecture is similar to that of women.

To date, diagnosis of osteoporosis in men is made by history (risk factors), clinical examination (e.g. reduction of stature, back pain), X-ray, densitometry and laboratory work-up. Cut-off values for WHO classification for male osteoporosis and all densitometry techniques such as dual X-ray absometry (DXA), quantitative ultrasound (QUS) and quantitative computed tomography (QCT) need to be developed. QUS can be measured at the calcaneus and phalanges. Phalangeal ultrasound is especially useful as being easily accessible, fast, radiation free, portable and cheap. Preliminary results show that phalangeal ultrasound might detect structural deterioration, especially in patients on glucocorticoid treatment, earlier than spinal DXA.

The main reason for a gender difference in fracture rates is because men lose less porous (trabecular) bone than women. Many osteoporosis risk factors can be modified without substantially increasing costs for the individual or the health care system. Risk factors for osteoporosis in older men include insufficient calcium intake, cigarette smoking, alcohol abuse and physical inactivity.

The first sign of osteoporosis is often a spontaneous fracture of the lumbar spine, or a fracture of the proximal femur or distal forearm after a fall. Elderly persons are at a higher risk of falling, which can be attributed to use of certain medications, alterations in balance, loss of muscle strength and prolonged reaction times. Preventive measures should target reducing bone loss and factors that contribute to falling. One of the most cost-effective prevention strategies is physical activity,[40] an adequate intake of calcium, adequate vitamin D and an exercise program which maximizes bone and muscle strength. Testosterone administration, together with proper nutrition and targeted physical activity, may postpone the appearance of osteoporosis and delay or prevent bone fractures.

SEXUAL DYSFUNCTION AND SEXUALITY

Dum spiro, spero
'As long as I breath, I hope'

Sexual desire, arousal, performance and activity decrease significantly with age, with a striking increase in the prevalence of impotence in men over 50 years of age. Reasons for decreased sexual activities include loss of libido (partially due to decreased androgen production), lack of partner, chronic illness and/or various social and environmental factors, as well as erectile dysfunction (ED). Studies have shown that aging men with high sexual activity levels have greater plasma testosterone concentrations than men with less sexual activity.[41] Although decreases in serum testosterone may have a correlation with diminished sexual activity in older men, this effect is probably minor compared with the contributions of psychologic, social and health factors.[42] Studies on aging sexuality have been concerned, primarily, with sexual performance, neglecting sexual satisfaction as an independent measure that is theoretically and clinically relevant. Health professionals, educators and elderly men are becoming increasingly aware that libido, interest, capacity and sexual pleasure can remain throughout a lifetime. It was found that sexual information significantly and independently contributed to sexual enjoyment and satisfaction, and that persistent interest in sexual activity results in positive mental and physical healthy benefits.

The frequency, duration and degree of noc-

turnal penile tumescence decreases significantly with age. These events are concomitant with a significant decrease in bioavailable testosterone and a compensatory increase in LH, showing that healthy aging is associated with decreased gonadal activity. Although erectile difficulties were frequently reported, enjoyment of marital sex and men's satisfaction with their own sexuality did not change with aging.

Worldwide, more than a 100 million men are estimated to have some degree of ED. The Massachusetts Male Aging Study reported a combined prevalence of 52% for minimal, moderate and complete impotence in noninstitutionalized 40–70-year-old men in the Boston area.[43] Erection is a neurovascular phenomenon under hormonal control, including arterial dilatation, trabecular smooth muscle relaxation and activation of the corporeal occlusive vein mechanism. Some of the major etiologies of ED are hypertension, diabetes and heart disease. Depression, a disease frequently encountered in aging men, is an important etiology for ED. Furthermore, the antidepressants administered may alleviate the symptoms of depression but may increase ED. Therefore, the antidepressant used should be carefully considered, weighing up the cost and benefit for each product and each individual patient. It should also be remembered that genitourinary and colon surgery very often cause erectile dysfunction. Nerve-sparing surgery, which may reduce the incidence of ED, should be used whenever possible. Patients should be counseled prior to such interventions.

Many drugs, particularly antihypertensive and psychotropic ones, may cause various degrees of ED. When focusing on the maintenance of quality of life among aging men, efforts to maintain, restore or improve sexual function should not be neglected. Recent advances of basic and clinical research has led to the development of new treatment options for ED, including new pharmacologic agents for intracavernosal, intraurethral and oral use. The most important ones are phosphodiesterase inhibitors and apomorphine. The management of ED should only be performed following proper evaluation of the patient and only by physicians with basic knowledge and clinical experience in the diagnosis and treatment of ED.

HORMONE THERAPY (HT)

Old age is the most unexpected of all the things that happen to a man
Leon Trotsky in his diary in exile 1935

The field of hormonal alterations in the aging male is attracting increasing interest in the medical community and in the public at large. Simultaneously, industry has realized the growing importance and enormous potential of the impact of a rapidly mounting population of males over the age of 50 which will be positioned for special health needs in the first quarter of this century and probably beyond. Among these needs HT may find its proper place, as it has for postmenopausal women over the last 25 years. The track record of medical care for the aging male has not been meritorious. Up to the present day there is a considerable misuse of hormonal preparations in the medical care of aging men.

In cases of endocrine deficiencies, traditional endocrinology aims to replace the missing amounts of hormone or hormones with substitutes. It has been demonstrated that interventions such as hormone therapies and use of antioxidant drugs may favorably influence some of the pathologic conditions in aging men, by avoiding the preventable and delaying the inevitable.

Comprehensive medical, psychosocial and lifestyle histories, physical examination and laboratory testing are essential for the diagnosis and management of PEDAM. Acute, chronic or intercurrent diseases must be taken into consideration prior to initiating any hormonal substitution therapy. Hormone substitution should only be performed by physicians with basic knowledge and clinical experience in diagnosis, treatment and monitoring of endocrine deficiencies.

Testosterone (T) therapy

The understanding of androgen deficiency in aging men among large sections of the medical profession dealing with mature men (i.e. primary care, internists, urologists, etc.) has not kept pace with developments in the field. A great deal of confusion and misunderstanding surrounds the four main issues – definition, diagnosis, treatment and monitoring – of acquired hypogonadism of the aging male. For a full discussion of this subject and guidelines for T therapy see Morales and Lunenfeld.[44]

In the era of evidence-based medicine, we have however to acknowledge that data on HRT in the aging male are mostly circumstantial, based on experience of treatment of transitional hypogonadism in young men or of chronic hypogonadism due to disease or experiments of nature. However, over the past several years there has been an increasing interest in evaluating whether T therapy (male HRT) might be beneficial for certain older men in preventing or delaying some aspects of aging. In this regard, a number of prospective studies on HRT in the aging male have been performed.

Peter Marin[45] performed a randomized, placebo-controlled study of 8-months duration with testosterone undecanoate (TU) 160 mg/day in healthy, obese (BMI > 25 kg/m²), middle-aged (> 45 years of age) men. Their mean plasma testosterone was 16 nmol/l (range 9–21 nmol/l); their body composition was measured by a computerized tomography (CT) scan. Within 8 months the sagittal abdominal diameter decreased from 27.0 to 24.6 cm ($P < 0.01$), whereas with placebo no change was observed. Marin[45] also reported improved general wellbeing ($P < 0.05$), feelings of improved energy ($P < 0.1$), improvement of cardiovascular safety aspects such as increased insulin sensitivity after glucose load ($P < 0.01$) and reduced fasting glucose ($P < 0.05$).

Morley[46] reported that males who received testosterone showed a significant increase in both testosterone and bioavailable testosterone concentrations, hematocrit, right-hand muscle strength and osteocalcin concentration. However, they showed a decrease in cholesterol [without a change in high-density lipoprotein (HDL) cholesterol] levels and decreased blood urea nitrogen (BUN):creatinine ratios. These results were confirmed by Snyder et al,[47] who concluded that increasing the serum testosterone concentrations of normal men over 65 years of age to the mid–normal range for young men decreased fat mass, principally in the arms and legs, and increased lean mass, principally in the trunk. Snyder et al[47] also showed that increasing the serum testosterone concentrations of normal men over 65 years of age to the mid–normal range for young men did not increase lumbar spine bone density overall, but did increase it in those men with low pretreatment serum testosterone concentrations (< 7 nmol/l). The prospective studies of Arver et al,[48] Tenover,[49,50] Bebb,[51] and Wang et al,[52] performed on elderly men with verified testosterone deficiency, confirmed earlier work and indicated that androgen replacement increases bone density, the joy of life and aggression in business, improvement of physical and psychic wellbeing, libido, a decrease of fat mass, a change in fat contribution and localization, as well as a decrease in cardiovascular accidents.

The decision to start HRT in men should only be taken after obtaining objective evidence of hormone deficiencies, after exclusion of secondary causes of endocrine dysfunction and after making the balance of risks and expected benefits of the replacement therapy. Prior to initiation of T therapy all patients should have a digital rectal examination (DRE) or an ultrasonographic assessment of the prostate and their PSA level measured; this should be < 3 ng/ml and should be repeated within 3 months of initiation of therapy. Transrectal ultrasonography guided biopsies of the prostate are indicated only if the DRE or the PSA are abnormal. Liver function studies are advisable prior to onset of therapy during the first year and on a yearly basis thereafter during treatment. A fasting lipid profile prior to initiation of treatment and at regular intervals (no longer than 1 year) during treatment is recommended.

If there is no history of adverse effects with regard to urinary obstructive symptoms, sleep apnea, polycythemia (hematocrit < 42% and platelets < 600,000), and if no significant increase in PSA is found, patients should continue with T therapy and have a DRE and a PSA determination, lipid profile, hemoglobin and serum calcium at yearly intervals. T administration should be stopped if PSA increases by 2.0 ng/ml at any time or if an increase of 0.75 ng/ml occurs over a 2-year period

It is common clinical wisdom that a firm diagnosis is desirable prior to embarking in any therapeutic plan. This also applies to the treatment of the hypogonadal man. The goals of treatment most commonly include the restoration of sexual functioning as well as libido and sense of wellbeing. Equally important, T therapy can prevent or improve already established osteoporosis and optimize bone density, restore muscle strength and improve mental acuity and normalize GH levels, especially in elderly males. T therapy should maintain not only physiologic levels of serum testosterone but also the metabolites of testosterone, including estradiol (E2), to optimize maintenance of bone and muscle mass, libido, virility, and sexual function. Because some of the manifestations of late-onset hypogonadism are shared with other conditions independent of a man's androgenic status, appropriate biochemical confirmation of hypogonadism should be sought prior to initiation of treatment. In the absence of defined contraindications, age is not a limiting factor in initiating T therapy in aged men with hypogonadism. The purpose of T therapy is to bring and maintain serum testosterone levels within the physiologic range (supraphysiologic levels are to be avoided). For the diagnosis of acquired hypogonadism, the following algorithm has been suggested (Fig. 31.2). If the patient's history, signs, symptoms, questionnaire and physical examination make the diagnosis of hypogonadism likely, biochemical tests should be used to confirm the diagnosis prior to initiation of treatment.

Total testosterone levels < 250 ng/dl (7 nmol/l) clearly indicate hypogonadism and, in most instances, indicate that benefits may be derived from T therapy. Men with a total testosterone

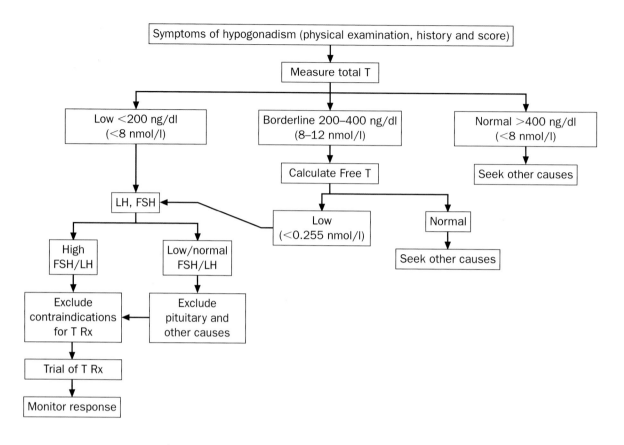

Figure 31.2 Algorithm for the diagnosis of acquired hypogonadism.

level < 150 ng/dl (4.5 nmol/l), a subnormal or inappropriately normal serum LH, level or elevated prolactin levels should be further evaluated with a magnetic resonance imaging (MRI) of the sella turcica area (with and without contrast) to visualize both the hypothalamus and pituitary gland. To exclude hypothalamic or pituitary disease, total testosterone levels of between 250 and 400 ng/dl (7–12 nmol/l) should be repeated and followed up by calculation of free testosterone from total testosterone and SHBG concentrations, or by measurement of free testosterone levels by the dialysis method, or bioavailable testosterone by the ammonium sulfate precipitation method. Calculated free testosterone < 0.255 nmol/l or bioavailable testosterone < 3.8 nmol/l confirms hypogonadism. A number of systemic disorders may suppress testosterone levels, includ-

ing hepatic cirrhosis, chronic renal failure, sickle cell anemia, thalassemia, hemochromatosis, human immunodeficiency virus, amyloidosis, chronic obstructive pulmonary disease (COPD), rheumatism, chronic infections and inflammatory or debilitating conditions. The confirmation of hypogonadism, whether it is late onset (e.g. age dependant) or acquired due to systemic disorders, iatrogenic causes or environmental conditions, merit a trial with T therapy.

If a healthy man has a serum testosterone level > 400 ng/dl (> 12 nmol/l) it is unlikely that he is testosterone deficient and, therefore, clinical judgment should guide the next steps, even if he has symptoms suggestive of testosterone deficiency. Age-related aquired Leydig's cell insufficiency in the aging man can often be reversed by stimulation with human chorionic gonadotropin (hCG).[53] But this kind of therapy is only recommended if the testosterone level doubles within 72 hours following the injection of 5000 IU of hCG.[54,55] If testosterone levels do not double within 72 hours following injection of hCG then T therapy should be considered if clinical history and physical examination show improvement (body composition, muscle mass and strength, sense of wellbeing and energy level, as well as an improvement of sexual function and libido); there is no history of adverse effects, particularly with regard to urinary obstructive symptoms, polycythemia (Hct > 42% and platelets <600,000), sleep apnea; and if no significant increase in PSA is found. Patients should continue with T therapy and have a DRE and a PSA determination, lipid profile, hemoglobin and serum calcium at yearly intervals. Testosterone administration should be stopped if PSA increases by 2.0 ng/ml at any time or if an increase of 0.75 ng/ml occurs over a 2-year period.[4]

Mild benign prostate hypertrophy is a relative, not absolute, contraindication to T therapy. Patients with PEDAM with few or no urinary tract obstructive symptoms may be suitable for T therapy, but patients with advanced obstructive symptoms are not. The addition of 5α-reductase inhibitors to T therapy or the use of a testosterone preparation not reducible by dehydrotestosterone (DHT) may be indicated for hypogonadal patients with benign prostate hypertrophy.

Absolute contraindications for T therapy are known to be prostate cancer and known existence of sleep apnea. Testosterone treatment may result in increased estrogen levels and is therefore contraindicated in men with breast cancer. These patients could be treated with an aromatizable testosterone preparation, but for the time being no hard data with such drugs are available.

Current, generally available, treatment options include buccal and oral tablets and capsules, intramuscular preparations, both long and short acting, implantable long-acting slow-release pellets, transdermal scrotal and non-scrotal patches, and gels. Neither injectable preparations nor slow-release pellets reproduce

the circadian pattern of testosterone production of the testes. This is best accomplished by the transdermal preparations, although oral testosterone may also approximate a circadian rhythm by dose adjustment. The relevance of reproducing a circadian rythmicity during T therapy remains unknown. Common testosterone preparations and their recommended doses are shown in Table 31.2.

DHEA therapy

Arlt et al[55] have examined the pharmacokinetics and peripheral biotransformation of different dosages of *oral DHEA* demonstrating the feasibility of an oral replacement strategy in men and women.[56,57] Despite the fact that the specific biosynthetic enzyme complex 17α-hydroxylase-17-20-desmolase has not been localized in the brain,[58] DHEA and DHEAS can be produced in the central nervous system (CNS), where they reach concentrations higher than those present in plasma,[59,60] and affect the gamma-amihobrtyric acid (GABA)ergic and glutamergic neuro-transmission directly by binding to neural membrane receptors.[61–63] Moreover, it has recently been suggested a specific plasma membrane receptor coupled to $G\alpha i_{2,3}$[64] leading to mitogen-activated protein kinase (MAPK) signaling cascade and to rapid nitric oxide synthesis in endothelial cells.[65]

As to DHEA and aging, there is no doubt that strong correlations can be established between the declining levels of adrenal androgens and ailments of aging, but whether these statistical associations are causally pathophysiologically interrelated remains to be established. The beneficial effects of DHEA in laboratory animals are impressive (for a review see Nippoldt and Nair)[66] and effects on processes such as atherosclerosis, type 2 diabetes, obesity, immune function/cancer prevention and brain function have been reported. However, it has to be remembered that laboratory animals, such as rats and rabbits, do not physiologically produce adrenal androgens, and, if some species do, not in the quantities that the human species does. So far, studies in humans are limited. While some studies have

Table 31.2 Common testosterone preparations and their recommended doses. (From Morales and Lunenfeld)[44]

	Generic name	Trade name	Dose
Injectable	Testosterone cypionate	Depotestosterone cypionate	200–400 mg every 3–4 weeks intramuscular
	Testosterone enanthate	Delatestryl	200–400 mg every 4 weeks intramuscular
	Mixed testosterone esters	Sustanon 250	250 mg every 3 weeks intramuscular
Oral	Fluoxymesterone*	Halotestin	5–20 mg daily
	Methyltestosterone*	Metandren	10–30 mg daily
	Testosterone undecanoate	Andriol Testocap	120–200 mg daily
	Mesterolone	Proviron	25–75 mg daily
Subcutaneous	Testosterone implants	–	1200 mg every 6 months
Transdermal	Testosterone patches	Androderm	6 mg daily
		Testoderm	10–15 mg/day
	Testosterone gel	Androgel Testim TostrexTM	Starting dose of 1% testosterone in gel in 5 g applied once daily. Depending on clinical response, dose may be increased to 7.5 g and then to 10 g

* 17α-alkylated testosterone preparations fluoxymesterone and methyltestosterone are both associated with serious liver toxicity.

found correlations between circulating levels of adrenal androgens and age-related ailments, others have not. Intervention studies present an equally sober picture. One study has found a positive effect on wellbeing.[28] The positive effect on self-esteem and maybe also on wellbeing found in men argues more in favor of an independent effect of DHEA on the brain, since the men were not testosterone deficient. A 100 mg daily dose of DHEA for 6 months restored serum DHEA levels to those of young adults and serum DHEAS to levels at or slightly above the young adult range.[29] Serum cortisol levels were unaltered, consequently the DHEAS:cortisol ratio was increased to pubertal (10:1) levels. Relative to baseline, DHEA administration

resulted in an elevation of serum IGF-I levels in men ($16\pm6\%$; $P = 0.04$). Serum levels of IGFBP-1 and IGFBP-3 were unaltered, fat body mass decreased 1.0 ± 0.4 kg ($6.1\pm2.6\%$; $P = 0.02$), and knee muscle strength ($15.0\pm3.3\%$; $P = 0.02$) and lumbar back strength ($13.9\pm5.4\%$; $P = 0.01$) increased. However, well-designed studies are necessary before final conclusions on patient selection and the usefulness of treatment in aging males can be recommended.

GROWTH HORMONE (GH) THERAPY

In 1991, Rudman et al[67] showed beneficial effects in a group of elderly men with low plasma IGF-I values, but no underlying pituitary pathology, which were administered GH. In these adults low doses of GH increased lean body mass and bone mineral density, decreased body fat and lowered LDL cholesterol. The similarities with the phenotype of adult GH deficiency and the success of GH treatment in reversing many structural and functional abnormalities in that condition have led to speculation that the age-related decline in GH is also a hormone-deficiency syndrome, and that reversing the decline by administering GH or stimulating its secretion would confer clinical benefits.

The starting dose of GH administration is not well established but a dose of 0.05–0.1 U/kg subcutaneously seems reasonable. Once placed on GH administration, individual dose titration must be done on the basis of the IGF-I levels resulting from GH administration and the occurrence of side effects. The aim to produce IGF-I levels in the normal range or only slightly above normal (0–1 standard deviations above mean levels of IGF-I). Secondly, if side effects occur (flu-like symptoms, myalgia, arthralgia, carpal tunnel syndrome, edema, impairment of glucose homeostasis), GH dosage is reduced in steps of 25%. Contraindications against GH use include type I diabetes, active (or a history of) cancer, intracranial hypertension, diabetic retinopathy or carpal tunnel syndrome and severe cardiac insufficiency.

Large long-term, placebo-controlled, prospective well-designed studies are still missing. They are necessary before final conclusion on patient selection and the usefulness of treatment in aging males can be recommended.

HRT alone is not sufficient to increase muscle strength, decrease fat mass and change in fat contribution and localization in aging men. Proper nutrition and physical exercise targeted at specific muscle groups is Administration of GH induces increases in both bone and lean mass and a decrease in fatty tissue in elderly men with GH deficiency.[67,68] The dose of GH required to maintain serum IGF-I levels in the normal range while minimizing side effects in this group of patients, however, has not been fully assessed. Toogood and Shalet[69] demonstrated that the GH replacement dose in

elderly subjects is considerably lower than that required by younger adults with GH deficiency. According to Janssen et al,[70] GH therapy at doses of 0.6 and 1.2 IU/day in male and female patients, respectively, is, in general, able to increase serum IGF-I into the normal range after 12 weeks of treatment, without reaching supranormal levels of serum IGF-I. This dose could, therefore, be a starting dose in GH-deficient elderly patients. None of the low-dose GH-treated patients exhibited supernormal IGF-I levels.[69]

HRT alone is not sufficient to increase muscle strength, decrease fat mass and change the fat contribution and localization in aging men. Proper nutrition and physical exercise targeted at specific muscle groups is mandatory in order to obtain satisfactory results.

The decision to start HRT in men should only be taken after obtaining objective evidence of hormone deficiencies, after exclusion of secondary causes of endocrine dysfunction and after making the balance of risks and expected benefits of the replacement therapy. When data of long-term well-controlled studies have become available, long-term substitution therapy with one or more hormonal preparations will most probably, if used correctly, improve the quality of life of aging men, delay symptoms of aging and maybe even delay the aging process.

Although it is probably not unrealistic that in future HT in men will become as common as HRT in women today, it goes without saying that even today there is strong evidence that a healthy lifestyle with regular physical activity has significant physiologic, psychologic and social benefits for older persons.

IMPROVING THE HEALTH OF OLDER MEN

The prolongation of a good life, happy and healthy, is fully in keeping with the spirit of medicine and is in a sense the very consummation of all that medical research has worked towards
Nobel Laureate Sir Peter Medawar while coping with the after effects of a stroke

Although it is now well established that significant physiologic, psychologic, social and societal benefits accrue from participation in physical activity,[71] the proportion of older individuals who participate regularly in physical activity is generally low. For example, the US Surgeon General's Report on Physical Activity and Health[72] estimates that only about 17% of older persons exercise at or above recommended levels of physical activity. A significant problem is motivating individuals of all ages to begin and to continue to participate in regular exercise.

Appropriate nutrition and a healthy and safe environment are critically important in preventing or reducing morbidity and disability. It is not just the quantity of food which is required to provide an energy balance, but also the quality and timing of the dietary intake. Adequate hydration is also essential. An aging male counseling session will not be complete before detailed information is obtained on nutritional habits and daily food and liquid consumption. Individualized supplementation of antioxidants, phytonutrients (including fibers) and vitamins will often be required in men over 50 years of age.

The impact of diet and specific food groups on aging and age-associated degenerative diseases has been widely recognized in recent years. The modern concept of the free-radical theory of aging takes as its basis a shift in the antioxidant/pro-oxidant balance that leads to increased oxidative stress, impaired regulation of cellular function and aging. In the context of this theory, antioxidants can influence the primary 'intrinsic' aging process as well as several secondary age-associated pathologic processes. For the latter, several epidemiologic and clinical studies have revealed potential roles for dietary antioxidants in the age-associated decline of immune function, and the reduction of risk of morbidity and mortality from cancer and heart disease. It is often assumed that antioxidant nutrients contribute to the protection afforded by fruit, vegetables and red wine against diseases of aging. However, the effect of fruit, vegetables and red wine consumption on the overall antioxidant status in humans is unclear. The total antioxidant capacity of serum determined as oxygen radical absorbance capacity

(ORAC) assay, trolox equivalent antioxidant capacity (TEAC) and ferric-reducing ability (FRAP) assay, using the area under the curve, increased significantly by 7–25% during the 4 hours following consumption of red wine, strawberries, vitamin C or spinach. The consumption of strawberries, spinach or red wine, which are rich in antioxidant phenolic compounds, can increase the serum antioxidant capacity in humans. Meydani[73] reported that long-term supplementation with vitamin E enhances immune function in aged animals and elderly subjects. The addition of the trace element selenium (60–200 µg/day) to vitamin E is recommended, since this will significantly increase the antioxidant properties. Larry Clark from the University of Arizona claimed a significant reduction of prostate, colon/rectal and lung cancers.[81] These and other observations indicate that, at present, the effects of dietary antioxidants are mainly demonstrated in connection with age-associated diseases in which oxidative stress appears to be intimately involved.

Many potential cardioprotective phytonutrients have been incorporated into functional foods. A meta-analysis of 38 clinical studies showed that an average of 47 g of soy protein significantly reduced total cholesterol LDL and triglycerides.[74]

Dietary fiber (from oats, beans, barley, rye, fruit and vegetables,) besides lowering cholesterol influences on both small and large intestine function. In addition to the effects on fermentation, dietary fiber fragments which have not been degraded by bacteria swell and hold water, thus having a stool bulking effect. This in turn stimulates colon motility, shortens the transit time through the colon and increases the amount of stool passes each day. This in turn seems to decrease the risk of colon and colon/rectal cancer. Usually, one daily portion of a very-high-fiber breakfast cereal (containing 9.8 g fiber/standard portion of 40 g) plus some fruit or vegetables is sufficient. Dietary guidance should however always be given on an individual basis, based on the patient's existing diet and lifestyle. It appears that nutritional modulation and manipulation represents one possible approach to successful aging and a healthy longevity.

Patients can be counseled to start their own antiaging program in becoming more active, starting to exercise and losing weight if obese. This will physiologically lead to tiredness, better sleep and, consequently, higher GH levels. Melatonin secretion will also rise, provided the patient does not sleep in front of the TV or with full lights on. Eating only small portions or nothing at all before going to bed (dinner canceling) can also increase GH secretion.

STRATEGIES TO IMPROVE AND MAINTAIN AGING MEN'S HEALTH

Aging no physician can stop. But he can if he is good, do a lot to reduce the symptoms
Johann Wolfgang von Goethe

Men who are educated about the value that preventative health care can play in prolonging their lifespan, quality of life and their role as a productive family member will be more likely to participate in health screening. To obtain this goal it will be necessary to:

- make available a group of trained medical professionals who can understand, guide, educate and manage the problems of the aging men;
- provide more information about the normal male aging process, and to advertise and promote aging in a positive and active way. Men should receive education and be prompted to take on teaching roles themselves, leading self-help groups and advocating on behalf of their aging communities;
- establish programs empowering men to become well-informed, active managers of their own health and the health of their surrounding social environments;
- obtain essential epidemiologic data and to intensify basic and clinical research on aging men;
- assess age-related nutritional needs;
- develop strategies for physical exercise (aerobic for maintaining cardiac function, and anerobic targeted to specific muscle groups and stretching);

- develop and assess new and improved drugs for the prevention and treatment of pathologic changes related to aging.

To this end, the efforts of all governmental and nongovernmental organizations to promote aging men's health on local, national and international levels must be strongly encouraged.

A holistic approach to this new challenge of the twenty-first century will necessitate a quantum leap in multidisciplinary and internationally coordinated research efforts, supported by new partnerships between industry and governments, and philanthropic and international organizations.

It is my sincerest hope that the next few years will enrich us with facts and clarify the state of our present knowledge, permitting us to recognize some of the missing links and give us the tools and methodology to design and plan ways to understand the aging of men. This would permit us to help improve the quality of life, avoid the preventable, and postpone and decrease the pain and suffering of the inevitable for aging men.

REFERENCES

1. Lunenfeld B. Aging male. *Aging Male* 1998; **1:** 1–7.
2. Lunenfeld B. Hormone replacement therapy in the aging male. *Aging Male* 1999; **2:** 1–6.
3. Kalache A, Lunenfeld B. Health and the ageing male. *Aging Male* 2000; **3:** 1–36.
4. Tremblay RR, Morales AJ. Canadian practice recommendations for screening monitoring and treating men affected by andropause or partial androgen deficiency. *Aging Male* 1998; **1:** 213–18.
5. Gray A, Feldman A, Mckinlay JB, Longcope C. Age, disease, and changing sex hormone levels in middle-aged men: results of the Massachusetts Male Aging Study. *J Clin Endocr Metab* 1991; **73:** 1016–25.
6. Vermeulen A. Clinical review 24. Androgens in the aging male. *J Clin Endocr Metab* 1991; **73:** 221–4.
7. Kaufman JM, Vermeulen A. Declining gonadal function in elderly men. *Baillière's Clin Endocr Metab* 1997; **11:** 289–300.
8. Gooren LJL. Endocrine aspects of aging in the male. *Molec Cell Endocr* 1998; **145:** 153–9.
9. Bremner WJ, Vitiello MV, Prinz PN. Loss of

circadian rhythmicity in blood testosterone levels with aging in normal men. *J Clin Endocr Metab* 1983; **56**: 1278–81.

10. Van Coevorden A, Mockel J, Laurent E et al. Neuroendocrine rhythms and sleep in aging men. *Am J Physiol* 1991; **260**: E651–E661

11. Swerdloff RS, Wang C. Androgen deficiency and aging in men. *West J Med* 1993; **159**: 579–85.

12. Vermeulen A, Kaufman JM, Giagulli VA. Influence of some biological indices on sex hormone binding globulin on androgen levels in aging and obese males. *J Clin Endocr Metab* 1996; **81**: 1821–27.

13. Ferrini R, Barrett-Connor E. Sex hormones and age: a cross-sectional study of testosterone and estradiol and their bioavailable fractions in community-dwelling. *Am J Epidemiol* 1998; **147**: 750–4.

14. Copinschi G, Van Cauter E. Effects of ageing on modulation of hormonal secretion by sleep and circadian rhythmicity. *Horm Res* 1995; **43**: 20–24.

15. Van Cauter E, Plat L, Copinschi G. Interrelations between sleep and the somatotropic axis. *Sleep*, 1998; **21**: 553–66.

16. Waldhauser F, Kovacs J, Reiter E. Age-related changes in melatonin levels in humans and its potential consequences for sleep disorders. *Exp Gerontol* 1998; **33**: 759–72.

17. Savine R, Sonksen PH. Is the somatopause an indication for growth hormone replacement? *J Endocr Invest* 1999; **22**: 142–9.

18. Rudman D, Feller AG, Cohn L et al. Effects of human growth hormone on body composition in elderly men. *Horm Res* 1991; **36**: 73–81.

19. Johannsson G, Rosen T, Bosaeus I et al. Two years of growth hormone (GH) treatment increases bone mineral content and density in hypopituitary patients with adult-onset GH deficiency. *J Clin Endocr Metab* 1996; **81**: 2865–73.

20. Johannsson G, Grimby G, Sunnerhagen KS, Bengtsson B-A. Two years of growth hormone (GH) treatment increase isometric and isokinetic muscle strength in GH-deficient adults. *J Clin Endocr Metab* 1997; **82**: 2877–84.

21. Burman P, Broman JE, Hettat J et al. Quality of life in adults with growth hormone (GH) deficiency: response to treatment with recombinant human GH in a placebo-controlled 21-month trial. *J Clin Endocr Metab* 1995; **80**: 3585–90.

22. Yarashesky KE, Zachwieja JJ, Campbell JA, Bier DM. Effect of growth hormone and resistance exercise on muscle growth and strength in older men. *Am J Physiol* 1995; **268**: E268–E276.

23. Pyka G, Wiswell RA, Marcus R. Age-dependent effect of resistance exercise on growth hormone secretion in people. *J Clin Endocr Metab* 1992; **75**: 404–7.

24. Van Cauter E, Plat L. Physiology of growth hormone secretion during sleep. *J Pediatr* 1996; **128**: S32–S37.

25. Guldner J, Schier T, Friess E et al. Reduced efficacy of growth hormone-releasing hormone in modulating sleep endocrine activity in the elderly. *Neurobiol Aging* 1997; **18**: 491–5.

27. Reiter RJ, Guerrero JM, Garcia JJ, Acuna-Castroviejo D. Reactive oxygen intermediates, molecular damage, and aging. *Ann NY Acad Sci* 1998; **854**: 410–24.

28. Morales AJ, Nolan JJ, Nelson JC, Yen SS. Effects of replacement dose of dehydroepiandrosterone in men and women of advancing age. *J Clin Endocr Metab* 1994; **78**: 1360–7.

29. Morales AJ, Haubrich RH, Hwang JY et al. Dehydroepiandrosterone (DHEA) on circulating sex steroids, body composition and muscle strength in age-advanced men and women. *Clin Endocr (Oxf)* 1998; **49**: 421–32.

30. Ravaglia G, Forti P, Maioli F et al. The relationship of dehydroepiandrosterone sulfate (DHEAS) to endocrine-metabolic parameters and functional status in the oldest-old. Results from an Italian study on healthy free-living over-ninety-year-olds. *J Clin Endocr Metab* 1996; **81**: 1173–8.

31. Yen SS, Laughlin GA. Aging and the adrenal cortex. *Exp Gerontol* 1998; **33**: 897–910.

32. Stomati M, Rubino S, Spinetti A et al. Endocrine, neuroendocrine and behavioral effects of oral dehydroepiandrosterone sulfate supplementation in postmenopausal women. *Gynecol Endocr* 1999; **13**: 15–25.

33. Solerte SB, Fioravanti M, Vignati G et al. Dehydroepiandrosterone sulfate enhances natural killer cell cytotoxicity in humans via locally generated immunoreactive insulin-like growth factor I. *J Clin Endocr Metab* 1999; **84**: 3260–7.

34. Lupien SJ, de Leon M, de Santi S et al. Cortisol levels during human aging predict hippocampal atrophy and memory deficits. *Nat Neurosci* 1998; **1**: 69–73.

35. Sherwin BB. Can estrogen keep you smart? Evidence from clinical studies. *J Psychiatry Neurosci* 1999; **24**(4): 15–21.

36. Walston J, Fried LP. Frailty and the older man. *Med Clin N Am* 1999; **83**: 1173–94.

37. Iozzo P, Beck-Neilsen H, Laakso M et al.

Independent influence of age on basal insulin secretion in nondiabetic humans. European Group for the Study of Insulin Resistance. *J Clin Endocr Metab* 1999; **84:** 863–8.

38. Barili P, De Carolis G, Zaccheo D, Amenta F. Sensitivity to ageing of the limbic dopaminergic system: a review. *Mech Ageing Dev* 1998; **106:** 57–92.

39. Melton 3rd LJ. Evidence-based assessment of pharmaceutical interventions. *Osteoporosis Int* 1998; **8:** 17–21.

40. Nordin C. *Scope for the Prevention and Treatment of Osteoporosis in Improving the Health of Older People: A World View.* (Oxford University Press: Oxford, 1990) 160.

41a. Schiavi RC, Schreiner-Engel P, Mandeli J et al. Healthy aging and male sexual function. *Am J Psychiatry* 1995; **147:** 766–71.

41b. Sih R, Morley JE, Kaiser FE et al. Testosterone replacement in older hypogonadal men: a 12 monthy randomized controlled trial. *J Clin Endocr Metab* 1997; **82:** 1661–4.

42. Harman SM, Blackman MR. Is there an andropause, the analogue to menopause, and if so what tissues are affected and how? In: Rabaire B, Pryor JL, Trasler JM, eds. *Handbook of Andrology.* (American Society of Andrology: Lawrence, 1995) pp 72–5.

43. Feldman HA, Goldstein I, Hatzichristou DG et al. Impotence and its medical psychological correlates; results of the Massachusetts Male Aging Study. *J Urol* 1994; **151:** 54–61.

44. Morales A, Lunenfeld B. Androgen replacement therapy in aging men with secondary hypogonadism. *Aging Male* 2001; **4:** 151–62.

45. Marin P, Holmang S, Jonsson L et al. The effects of testosterone treatment on body composition and metabolism in middle-aged obese men. *Int J Obes Metab Disord* 1992; **16**(12)**:** 991–7.

46. Morley JE, Perry HM, Kaiser FE et al. Effect of testosterone replacement therapy in old hypogonadal males: a preliminary study. *J Am Geriatr Soc* 1993; **41:** 149–52.

47. Snyder PJ, Peachey H, Hannoush P et al. Effect of testosterone treatment on body composition and muscle strength in men over 65 years of age. *J Clin Endocr Metab* 1999; **84:** 2647–53.

48. Arver S, Lönn L, Ekström U et al. The effects of physiological androgen replacement in aging diabetic men. A placebo controlled study. *Aging Male* 2000; **3:** 4.

49. Tenover JL. Testosterone and the aging male. *J Androl* 1997; **18:** 103–6.

50. Tenover JL. Male HRT in the new millennium: an update. *Aging Male* 2000; **3:** 7.

51. Bebb RA, Wade J, Frohlich J et al. A randomized, double blind, placebo controlled trial of testosterone undecanoate administration in aging hypogonadal men: effects on bone density and body composition. *Aging Male* 2000; **3:** 2.

52. Wang C, Eyre DR, Clark R et al. Sublingual testosterone replacement improves muscle mass and strength, decreases bone resorption, and increases bone formation markers in hypogonadal men. *J Clin Endocr Metab* 1996; **81:** 3654–62.

53. Lunenfeld B, Eshkol A, Glezerman M. Male climacteric? In: (Bandhauer E, Frick J, eds) *Handbook of Urology, Volume XVI. Disturbances in Male Fertility.* (Springer Verlag: Berlin, 1982) 421–7.

54. Lunenfeld B, Berezin M. L'insuffisance leydigienne liée au vieillissement. *Androcrinologie* 1989; **8:** 691–702.

55a. Arlt W, Callies F, Allolio B. DHEA replacement in women with adrenal insufficiency – pharmacokinetics, bioconversion and clinical effects on well-being, sexuality and cognition. *Endocr Res* 2000; **26:** 505–11.

55b. Arlt W, Callies F, van Vlijmen JC et al. Dehydroepiandrosterone replacement in women with adrenal insufficiency. *N Engl J Med* 1999; **341:** 1013–20.

56. Tomer Y, Lunenfeld B, Berezin M. Andropause: myth or reality? *Harefuah* 1995; **128:** 785–8.

57. Arlt W, Callies F, Koehler I et al. Dehydroepiandrosterone supplementation in healthy men with an age-related decline of dehydroepiandrosterone secretion. *J Clin Endocr Metab* 2001; **86:** 4686–92.

58. Baulieu EE, Robel P. Neurosteroids: a new brain function? *J Steroid Biochem Mol Biol* 1990; **37**(3)**:** 395–403.

59. Corpechot C, Robel P, Axelson M et al. Characterization and measurement of dehydroepiandrosterone sulfate in rat brain. *Proc Natl Acad Sci USA* 1981; **78:** 4704–7.

60. Majewska MD. Neurostereoids: endogenous bimodal modulators of the $GABA_A$ receptor. Mechanism of action and physiological significance. *Prog Neurobiol* 1992; **38:** 379–95.

61. Majewska MD, Demigoren S, Spivak CE, London ED. The neurosteroid dehydroepiandrosterone sulfate is an allosteric antagonist of the $GABA_A$ receptor. *Brain Res* 1990; **526:** 143–6.

62. Demigoren S, Majewska MD, Spivak CE,

London ED. Receptor binding and electrophysiological effects of dehydroepiandrosterone sulfate, an antagonist of the GABA$_A$ receptor. *Neuroscience* 1991; **45**: 127–35.

63. Debonnel G, Bergeron R, de Montigny C. Potentiation by dehydroepiandrosterone of the neural response to N-methyl-D-aspartate in the CA$_3$ region of the rat dorsal hippocampus: an effect mediated via sigma receptors. *J Endocr* 1996; **150**: S33–S42.

64. Liu D, Dillon JS. Dehydroepiandrosterone activates endothelial cell nitric-oxide synthase by a specific plasma membrane receptor coupled to Galpha(i2,3). *J Biol Chem* 2002; **277**(24): 21379–88. (Epub 2002, April 2004).

65. Simoncini T, Mannella P, Fornari L et al. Dehydroepiandrosterone (DHEA) modulates endothelial nitric oxide synthesis via direct genomic and non-genomic mechanisms. *Endocrinology* 2003 (in press).

66. Nippoldt TB, Nair KS. Is there a case for DHEA replacement? *Baillière's Clin Endocr Metab* 1998; **12**: 507–20.

67. Rudman D, Feller AG, Nagraj HS et al. Effect of human growth hormone in men over 60 years old. *N Engl J Med* 1990; **323**: 1–6.

68. Goh VHH, Mu SC, Gao F, Lim KS. Changes in body composition, and endocrine and metabolic functions in healthy elderly Chinese men following growth hormone therapy. *Aging Male* 1998; **1**: 264–9.

69. Toogood AA, Shalet SM. Growth hormone replacement therapy in the elderly with hypothalamic–pituitary disease: a dose-finding study. *J Clin Endocr Metab* 1999; **84**: 131–6.

70. Janssen YJ, Frolich M, Roelfsema F. A low starting dose of genotropin in growth hormone-deficient adults. *J Clin Endocrinol Metab* 1997; **82**(1): 129–35.

71. World Health Organization (WHO). *Jakarta Declaration on Leading Health Promotion into the 21st Century*. (WHO: Geneva, 1997.)

World Health Organization (WHO). *International Classification of Impairments, Disabilities and Handicaps*. (WHO: Geneva, 1980.)

72. United States Surgeon General Report on Physical Activity and Health. 1996.

73. Meydani M, Lipman RD, Han SN et al. The effect of long-term dietary supplementation with antioxidants. *Ann NY Acad Sci* 1998; **854**: 352–60.

74. Anderson JW Meta-analysis of the effects of soy protein intake on serum lipids. *N Engl J Med* 1995; **333**: 276–82.

75. Rudman D. Growth hormone, body composition and aging. *J Am Geriatr Soc* 1985; **33**: 800–7.

76a. Tenover JS. Effects of testosterone supplementation in the aging male. *J Clin Endocr Metab* 1992; **75**: 1092–8.

76b. Zisapel N. The use of melatonin for the treatment of insomnia. *Biol Signal Recep* 1999; **8**: 84–9.

77. United Nations. *World Population Prospects. The 1998 Revision*. (United Nations: New York, 1999.)

78. Vermeulen A. Androgen replacement therapy in the aging male – a critical evaluation. *J Clin Endocr Metab* 2001; **86**: 2380–90.

79. Wang C, Swerdloff RS, Iranmanesh A et al and the Testosterone Gel Study Group. Transdermal testosterone gel improves sexual function, mood, muscle strength, body composition parameters in hypogonadal men. *J Clin Endocr Metab* 2000; **85**: 2839–53.

80. Wilkins R, Adams OB. Health expectancy in Canada, demographic, regional and social dimensions. *Am J Public Health* 1983; **73**: 1073–80.

81. Duffield-Lillico AJ, Dalkin BL, Reid ME et al. Nutritional Prevention of Cancer Study Group. Selenium supplementation baseline plasma selenium status and incidence of prostate cancer: an analysis of the complete treatment period of the Nutritional Prevention of Cancer Trial. *BJU Int* 2003; **91**: 608–12.

32

Future developments

C Lauritzen

General remarks • Woman-specific medicine • Prevention of diseases • Costs of prevention • Prediction of risk, risk factors, special markers • Women's perception of risks • Coronary heart diseases • Selective estrogen receptor modulators (SERM) • Stroke • Obesity • Cancer • Future scientific cooperation • Future controlled trials on estrogens • Information of the patient • Mental disorders • Cognitive functions • Osteoporosis • Urogenital conditions • Esthetic medicine and antiaging • Thromboembolism • Gallbladder diseases • Patient information • The menopause as an occasion for health promotion • Improving compliance • Importance of political health measures • Markers for the question of who will profit from hormonal substitution • Old and new preparations • Influence of genetic variants on effects of hormones • Summary • References • Further reading

GENERAL REMARKS

Science continues to progress. In the last few decades scientists have learned that sex and gender are important determinants not only of personal psychology and social positions in life, but also in understanding diseases, their course and outcome, and their prevention and treatment. Many scientists, e.g. gynecologists, gynecologic endocrinologists and their societies, have the privilege of assisting women in the existential problems of their lives, and are endeavoring to deal more competently with the special conditions of women in health and disease, helping them to solve their health problems by basic research and by converting the results into successful practical management.

Menopause societies, dealing with the successive phases of menopause, postmenopause and senium, have their particular justification by the normal early cessation of ovarian function in women and the resulting sequelae of fate-determining, but partially preventable, diseases.

For the average 30 postmenopausal years, without the beneficial effects of estrogens, medicine has taken the responsibility to prevent unnecessary diseases, suffering and harm, thus trying to secure social competence and human dignity for the aging woman.

The following exposition of the thus-defined subject will formulate probable future developments and the wishes of the hormone therapeut for scientific research.

WOMAN-SPECIFIC MEDICINE

There exist more than 100 known differences between females and males of anatomical, physical, genetic, biochemical, hormonal, metabolic, behavioral, mental and psychic character. Therefore, woman-specific medicine must be created. Women live (not least thanks to ovarian hormonal function up to the age of 50), on average, longer than men and make up the majority of the population over 65 years of age.

They suffer from diseases, disorders and conditions different to those of men. Even when women have the same diseases as males, women often experience different symptoms and responses to treatment to their male counterparts. Women have often not been included in scientific studies due to the commonly held belief that what was true for men was also true for women. Because this assumption is not true, woman-specific medicine must be developed urgently, to provide older women with the best possible care.

Research has shown that, apart from sex-specific diseases, cancers and climacteric symptomatology, women more often suffer from certain particular diseases, and for twice as many years as men.

The concerns of the menopause must be extended to the senium, and should be combined and with geriatric gynecology, including geriatric oncology. The discussion of the gynecologist as the family doctor of the woman must be maintained and made concrete without violating the competence of internists and osteologists. More cooperation with these specialties is very necessary for optimal management, welfare and wellbeing of our postmenopausal patients.

PREVENTION OF DISEASES

The aim of gynecomedical care for postmenopausal women is to avoid preventable dieases. This endeavor is intended to postpone diseases leading to disability and death, the so-called compression of morbidity. Management of the menopause tries to secure the possibility of living in as good health as possible up to the age of 80 plus, and for minimizing suffering from disease or lessening vigor for life, leading ultimately to death.

The medicine to come is a medicine of prevention of diseases rather than of treatment. Anyway, repair is not always possible. Of course, treatment of diseases will always be necessary, but prophylaxis and avoidance of disease will, in the future, prevail before repair of established diseases. Prevention should start early but it is never too late to begin.

The methods and relative effectiveness, as well as the cost–benefit relations, of prevention must be assessed according to the rules of evidence-based medicine and improved according to the progress of science. Lifestyle counseling, mainly diet and age-adapted physical activity, will be the most important and effective measures, as about only 30% of diseases in aged women are genetically determined but as many as 70% are caused by a poor lifestyle.

Treatment with medicaments, including estrogens, must be performed on the basis of well-established and carefully documented methods and evidence-based results. However, the controlled trials of intervention must be designed as near as is practical to realistic conditions. This was not always the case in some recent trials.

COSTS OF PREVENTION

The general introduction of prevention to the health service will, in the beginning, perhaps increase costs. However, in the long term, although women will become older, if prevention works they will have more healthy years free of handicaps, resulting in a compression of morbidity. Older women will therefore more often live independently, having a good quality of life, in their own homes. An enormous amount of money could thus be saved.

The costs of treatment for women over 50 years of age in Germany are, for the time being, twice that of women during maturity, doubling thereafter every 10 years, increasing to six times at the age of 80.

Changing to preventive medicine would, as said, substantially decrease the costs. At present, the amount of money spent by the German health insurance for treatment is 3000 Euro/person/year and only 2.56 Euro for prevention. The allowance for the money used for prevention is limited by statutory requirements.[1] The medical profession, health insurances and government authorities must consequently be convinced to change the trend from treatment of diseases to their prevention for the sake both of reduction of costs and of human suffering.

PREDICTION OF RISK, RISK FACTORS, SPECIAL MARKERS

Medicine to come will, as explained above, be predominantly preventative. Prevention is based on the assumption that *risk factors* determine the incidence of manifestation of diseases and that the recognition and influencing of these factors will decrease the probability of manifestation of the relevant disease.

The concept of taking risk factors into account, as derived from clinical experience and epidemiologic studies, for prediction of future disease is, however, still unsatisfactory. It is a statistical parameter derived from large populations. In practice, a woman with risk factors may not become ill, while a woman without risk factors may develop the disease. The meaning, importance or significance of risk factors for the individual case must therefore be further elucidated. Genetics will become more important in this regard. New, better predictive risk factors and risk markers must be found.

Ideally, each patient should have a risk profile done by her doctor for her most important risks, and be counseled as appropriate, considering lifestyle as well as prevention by effective medicaments. On this basis, one could manage an individual behavior pattern and concentrate on specific measures of prevention and early diagnostics. This is an important area for more research.

WOMEN'S PERCEPTION OF RISKS

It is astonishing that women's awareness of their perceived and real risks differ so much, and are so far from reality and much more psychological than factual in character. More than half of all climacteric women fear breast or other gynecologic cancers. In our experience, only 4% fear cardiovascular diseases or premature death from such a disease. However, the real causes of death in late postmenopausal women are exactly the reverse: about 34% will die of heart diseases, 8% of stroke, 4% of breast cancer and 21% of all other cancers.

Thus, information correcting this common misjudgment is one of the most important tasks of physicians counseling menopausal clients, to improve their motivation for hormone replacement therapy (HRT) and their adherence to the proposed therapy.

CORONARY HEART DISEASES

These constitute the number one illness and the most frequent cause of death for women. Women account for 52% of all deaths due to heart diseases and 61% of all deaths due to stroke. As applying to many other diseases, this cardiovascular syndrome has a particular profile in women because, among the female patients who die suddenly from coronary heart attacks, 64% have had no previous symptoms.

When symptoms occur they may be different from those in males: women are treated and hospitalized later than males; women may respond differently to treatment; women experience their cardiovascular diseases later than males, especially during late postmenopause when protection from ovarian estrogens has ceased. Thirty-four per cent of all unnecessary premature deaths of women are due to cardiovascular diseases. Heart attacks are more deadly for women (44%) than for men (27%). Nevertheless, women are less frequently treated for their cardiovascular diseases prior to death.

It will therefore be the task of the medical profession to instruct all menopausal patients on the high actual risks of myocardial infarction and stroke, to transfer the knowledge of risk factors, and to develop and apply biochemical markers for early recognition and preventative treatment cardiovascular risks, e.g. high-density lipoprotein (HDL), low-density lipoprotein (LDL), lipoprotein (a) Lp(a), hyperhomocysteinaemia and C-reactive protein.

In basic research, the early changes playing a crucial role in atherogenesis must be further analyzed. The influence of estrogens and progestogens on the early and late stages of atherosclerosis and thrombotic changes, such as on thrombin receptor, cell adhesion molecules such as A-selectin and intracellular adhesion molecules (ICAM), must be tested further. Better understanding will mean better prevention and more effective treatment.

Primary prevention

The beneficial effect of primary prevention by long-term estrogen substitution, beginning in early menopause, was doubted on the grounds of controversial and disputed controlled trials, but is probably true providing it is started in early menopause and if appropriate estrogens and progestogens are used. The problem must be further investigated in controlled trials, which should be properly designed and closer to practice than those published so far.

The relative indications, benefits and drawbacks of the different estrogens, progestogens and their individual modes of application must be clarified concerning their special therapeutic effects and side effects in long-term preventive treatment. The role of estrogens and their metabolites, designer hormones and progestogens in primary and secondary prevention of cardiovascular diseases, and optimal management, must be clarified. The role of statins, also in combination with estrogens, in primary and secondary prevention of cardiovascular diseases should also be investigated further.

In any case, it is remarkable that when cardiovascular events occur, the post-infarction and the post-stroke mortality is generally lower in women who experience the event under ERT or HRT. All trials agree in this respect. A reduction of mortality is also seen in estrogen takers suffering from cancerous diseases of the breast, genitalia and colon. This is what the doctor is entitled to tell his/her patients when counseling them on long-term ERT or HRT.

A primary or secondary prevention with the only indication of prevention of cardiovascular events has never been practiced by gynecologists in Europe. The positive effects on the incidence of myocardial infarction, and perhaps also on stroke, suggested by American epidemiologic studies was taken by estrogen therapeuts in Europe as a very welcome additional beneficial effect of long-term HRT, and was used in some special cases as an argument for initiation of long-term treatment and to improve adherence to long-term therapy.

Secondary prevention

Secondary prevention following myocardial infarction is not and never has been a sole indication for estrogen therapy, but rather for statins or a combination of statins and estrogen, and for dietary measures such as addition of unsaturated fatty acids. These cases should be treated by the internist. The suggested combination of statins and estrogens in secondary prevention of cardiovascular diseases should be subject to controlled trials.

SELECTIVE ESTROGEN RECEPTOR MODULATORS (SERM)

Today we have estrogen-active compounds called SERM that are free of unwanted effects on the endometrium and breast. The SERM raloxifene seems to reduce the incidence of coronary events. This compound and some other SERM do not stimulate the endometrium and breast, but do reduce the risk for osteoporosis

New SERM or designer hormones, which also abolish climacteric complaints without influencing the endometrium and breast, must be found, thus overcoming some of the objections against classic ERT and HRT.

The influence of estrogens and the different progestogens on early and late atherosclerosis and their consequences must be further analyzed, including the role of statins or of a combination of statins and estrogen.

Phytoestrogens seem to act similarly to SERM. They inhibit aromatase, 5α-reductase and tyrosinase, which all play a role in the development of mammary cancer. The effect of these substances on climacteric complaints, and the assumed preventative effect on cardiovascular diseases and breast cancer, must be subjected to further biochemical, and controlled clinical and epidemiologic trials.

STROKE

The influence of estrogens on stroke is controversial. Some studies have found prevention by estrogens, some no change and others an increase of risk. Apparently, the incidence of subarachnoidal bleeding is slightly increased under estrogen intake (especially in combination with hypertension), while intracerebral bleeding and thromboembolic stroke seem to be decreased under estrogens. Modern biochemical tools and cerebral imaging will probably promote our basic and clinical knowledge of stroke. In any case, the indication for estrogens with respect to stroke must be clarified.

The effects of estrogens, SERM designer hormones and phytoestrogens, as well as of the progestogens, on cerebral perfusion, metabolism and the incidence of the different forms of stroke must therefore be the subject of further investigations.

The climacteric woman must know the risk factors and be informed about the postmenopausal risks of stroke so that these factors will be better appreciated by the women concerned.

OBESITY

Being overweight is becoming more and more prevalent, particularly in postmenopausal women. It is an important risk factor for cardiovascular diseases, the metabolic syndrome, diabetes types 1 and 2, thrombosis, and for breast, ovarian and endometrial cancers. Further research on the causal effects of insulin, insulin-like growth factor (IGF)-2 and leptin in atherosclerosis, the metabolic diseases and in carcinogenesis are warranted. The knowledge concerning the role of obesity and of lifestyle factors in the genesis of atherosclerosis and cancer, and on their fatal course, is not sufficiently known to most women. Therefore, relevant information must be conveyed to climacteric women in order to improve the motivation for initiation of preventative measures and to improve compliance.

CANCER

Cancer is the leading cause of death in postmenopausal women. It is only after the age of 75 that death from heart diseases becomes the number one killer. Breast cancer is the most common form of cancer in women; lung cancer is the leading cause of cancer deaths in women, followed by breast cancer and colorectal cancer.

Cancer is mostly seen by lay people as a predetermined fate that cannot be influenced. Prevention is however apparently possible by changing lifestyle in order to eliminate risk and triggering factors. Age-adapted physical motion and gymnastics will add to the success of prevention.

Much research has been devoted to the question of estrogens and carcinogenesis of breast and genital cancers. However, it is now largely clear that estrogens are rather creating an internal milieu of general growth and stimulation of the mitoses, so that faulty copies of genetic material increase in statistic probability. However, estrogens act mainly as a promotional factor for pre-existing cancer clones originating from the receptor-positive cells of the reproductive system.

The population must be made aware that cancer is in essence the duty that humankind has to pay for the load of heredity, an increased life expectancy, a poisoned environment and food, and for ionizing radiation. Overnutrition, especially with animal fats, being overweight, tallness, metabolic anomalies, smoking and alcohol abuse, influence of free radicals, childlessness or late first pregnancy, avoiding breastfeeding, and mitogenic hormones can promote the risk for and the manifestation of cancerous disease, but only if the body's normal multiple defense mechanisms have been damaged.

Cancer can be prevented, at least in part. Many of the risk factors affecting cancer incidence are known, as cited before. Our patients should know that most cancer risks can be influenced by compliance of a healthy lifestyle.

Research has to analyze the role of the different exogenous carcinogens, radicals, endogenous metabolism and the conversion of precancerous cells in the body to active cancer, and their influence on the different cancers.

The role of hormones and their metabolites in concert with carcinogens and promotors, and finally the real possibilities of prevention by hormones, antihormones, SERM and designer hormones, must be completely elucidated.

Early diagnostics, for instance by determination of relevant markers [such as prostate-specific antigen (PSA) for prostatic cancer] must be developed.

The experience with contraceptive hormones in the prevention of ovarian, endometrial and colon polyposis and cancer, and the effects of SERM, aromatase inhibitors and phytoestrogens in the prevention of breast cancer, as well as the prevention of ovarian and colon cancer with nonsteroidal antirheumatics, and some anthypertensive drugs, must be systematically extended.

There are hopeful starting points for genetic engineering of cancer and for preventing the metastatic spread of cancer cells. Immunopotentiation, tumor vaccination, molecular chemotherapy, genetic response of tumor cells against tumoricides, introduction of apoptotic medicaments and genes, as well as inactivation of oncogenic products, will probably bring progress in prevention and treatment of cancers. This must be the direction of future research.

Breast cancer

The generally held opinion is, as stated above, that estrogens are not carcinogenic themselves but rather promotors of benign as well as pre-existent malign cell growth. Some authors suppose that oxidative estrogen metabolites may be potentially directly carcinogenic, as for instance 4OH-, 2OH- and 16OH-estradiol, which may be metabolized to electrophilic catechol estrogen-3,4-chinones. The results were primarily produced with hamster kidneys and human MCF 104 breast epithelial cells. The hypothesis of induction of mutations by these metabolites neglects the fact that some rodents – irrelevant to the human condition – are prone to spontaneous or induced mutations of genes and that during in vitro experiments using cells, the normal mechanisms of apoptosis, DNA repair, effects of radical scavengers, and of tumor suppressor genes and of controls in the cell cycle cannot exert their in vivo normal inhibitory effect on a carcinogenic development. In addition, some endocrine anomalies of the thyroid

and several medicaments influence 16- and 4-hydroxylation and methylation. The correlation of this questionable hypothesis to reality and its possible quantitative importance deserves clarification.

The female breast is a potent endocrine gland exhibiting aromatization, 17β-hydroxysteroid dehydrogenase activity, sulfoconjugation and sulfatase activity, and produces several growth factors. The role of these local metabolic events in promoting carcinogenesis or growth factors, and on mitosis and proliferation of existing cancer cell clones, as well as the influence of sytemic estrogen–progestogen levels on this complex – the endocrine-metabolic system of the breast – must be intricately explored, as this may be important for understanding breast cancer development, prevention and treatment.

The influence of aromatase inhibitors on the aromatization in breast tissue and the resulting decrease of breast cancer risk has already been shown. The role of the different aromatase inhibitors versus SERM in the prevention and treatment of patients at high risk for breast cancer must be further clarified, and the appropriate patients for such a treatment must be selected by relevant criteria which must still be determined.

Endometrial cancer

The addition of a potent progestogen for at least 10 days normalizes or even decreases the risk of endometrial cancer development. The optimal progestogen and the optimal duration of progestogen medication (14 days or continuously) to prevent hyperplasia and endometrial cancer must still be found. Local application of progesterone to the endometrium by progestogen-secreting intrauterine devices (IUD) and vaginally applied progesterone must be tested futher by appropriate trials.

The height and structure of the endometrium should ideally be assessed during each regular check-up every year, at least in high-risk cases. Our patient biopsy of the endometrium should be technically further improved.

Cancer of the ovaries

An early diagnosis must be promoted especially for ovarian cancer, as diagnosis is mostly late and more than 50% of patients die from this disease within 5 years. Every patient should at the regular check-up receive an ultrasound scan of the ovaries (and of the endometrium). Early diagnosis by determination of labelled autoantibodies, e.g. of p53 or others, seems to be not far off.

The questionable small increase in ovarian cancer under long-term ERT/HRT is still controversial, but must be taken in account and discussed in counseling the patient.

However, it should also be made known to the public that oral hormonal contraception reduces the risk of endometrial, mammary and colon cancers, and that all cancers under estrogens are mostly localized and less aggressive, and that the cure rate of endometrial, breast and colon cancers is improved in patients under postmenopausal estrogen substitution. Could this indication of the contraceptive pill perhaps be used as a measure of prevention and protection for patients with an increased risk of these cancers?

General remarks on gynecologic cancers

Most important in basic research will be the identification of those risk groups who will develop breast and genital cancers. Genetic factors interact with exogenous factors in the etiology of gynecologic carcinoma. *BRCA* genes are responsible for only 5% of all breast cancers. Low penetrance genes influence the risk for sporadic and familial breast cancer. Low penetrance genes for breast cancer susceptibility modify the effects of estrogens and progestogens and of exogenous carcinogens on the breast. The inclusion of genetic analyses in epidemiologic studies may in future identify those subgroups of women who exhibit an elevated breast or genital cancer risk. Candidate genes would be genes affecting the estrogen biosynthesis within the breast, influencing androgen aromatization, estrogen–progesterone catabolism in the direction of 16-, 2- and 4-hydroxy-lation, methylation and sulfoconjugation or deconjugation.

Investigations on receptors, co-repressors and co-activators of estrogen and progesterone, and target genes for these receptors and their specific proteins, are necessary. Thus, methods of preventing or modifying cancer risk could be developed.

DNA chips will become important in breast and gynecologic cancer clinics for the development of new therapies. With the help of the individual, activation responses may help predict the risk and probability of possible metastasis. DNA chips may also give hints for the response of certain tumors to specific hormonal or chemotherapy.

Colon cancer

Normal colon epithelial cells and cancer cells express estrogen receptors. Prevention, early diagnosis and treatment of this cancer must be intensified by forcing the age group concerned to perform regular hemoccult tests and to undergo sigmoidoscopies. Intestinal polyps should be removed. The influence of estrogens and nonsteroidal antirheumatics in the prevention of colon cancer should be investigated further, as this might promote our understanding of carcinogenesis. It would certainly be elucidating to know why estrogens and nonsteroidal antirheumatics reduce the incidence of colon polyps and cancers.

FUTURE SCIENTIFIC COOPERATION

Gynecologists, internists and orthopedists should cooperate more closely than they have done so far in clinical and epidemiologic research. Each specialty can learn much from the others. The scientific questions posed today can only be solved by the combined research of many jointly planned and cooperating clinics and research institutes of different specializations. Gynecologic clinics should integrate departments of clinical or experimental gynecologic endocrinology and biochemical sections headed by competent scientists in well-established positions.

Epidemiologic studies should be planned by statisticians, practitioners, and clinicians of the specialties concerned, to prevent trials which are irrelevant to practice and contrary to well-established facts. Thus, wrong paths of considerable disadvantage for patients and their doctors will be avoided.

Scientific results should not be given to the lay public before being published and, if problematic, should be simultaneously accompanied by an expert commentary in the same issue of the journal concerned.

FUTURE CONTROLLED TRIALS ON ESTROGENS

We learnt from the WHI study that certain hormone combinations are not optimal and that postmenopausal women should not be treated with estrogens without a clear indication. Climacteric complaints and low levels of estradiol must be present. Starting treatment with oral estrogens in older women with the usual hormonal preparations is not recommended and may cause, if not strongly indicated and controlled, an increase in side effects and risk. Low-dose parenteral or local treatment would be optimal for women in the senium needing estrogens. This recognition and knowledge is however not new to the experienced and competent hormone therapeut.

Future randomized controlled trials are necessary to secure the primary preventative effects of estrogens on cardiovascular diseases, Alzheimer's disease and to determine the real effect of estrogens on breast and ovarian cancer incidence. Such investigations should however – in contrast to the WHI study – be performed on so-far healthy menopausal patients between the ages of 50 and 55, who have climacteric complaints (low estrogen levels) and should use natural estradiol and progesterone, including parenteral medication (e.g. patches). Such studies should be planned under consideration of adequacy of the experimental design to clinical practice. It is to be hoped that the Cochrane Institute will contribute to the collection of unfalsified useful knowledge.

INFORMATION OF THE PATIENT

The role of estrogen for the development of gynecologic cancers is certainly basic in the sense of creating a *milieu interne* for optimal conditions of mitosis and growth of normal and cancerous cells possessing estrogen receptors. However, this is only one factor in the multifactorial and multistep event of cancer development. Other factors are causally more important, e.g. genetics, family history, metabolic diseases, lifestyle, radiation, alcohol and reproductive factors.

Questionable theories of a direct carcinogenic action of certain estrogen metabolites are not to be included in the information given to patients. The advocates of such a theory have no data on the frequency of the occurrence of such anomalies, do not take into account the many anticancer regulations of the intact organism and are not in agreement with the epidemiologic data, as the cancer incidence in the statistics decreases after withdrawal of the estrogen.

The female population has consequently, as explained above, to learn that cancer is lastly the duty that humankind has to pay for the load of heredity, old age, poisoning of the environment, ionizing radiation and that the realization of cancer is promoted by metabolic diseases, being overweight, overnutrituion, consumption of too much animal fat, childlessness, late first pregnacy and not breastfeeding. Only on this basis will comprehensive prevention be necessary.

The future counseling of patients should, as far as possible, be free of any doubts and uncertainties of personal judgment and scientifically unsolved problems, which will hopefully be ascertained by increased acquisition of evidence-based knowledge.

MENTAL DISORDERS

Endogenous depression is becoming a global epidemic. It is second to heart disease as the reason for losing healthy years in old age. This fact is important to know for the gynecologist as the primary carer of women. There is however no special increase in incidence during the climacteric, but there is a spreading in old age.

The role of estrogens in the prevention of Alzheimer's disease and schizophrenia is still controversial, as controlled studies with greater numbers of women are lacking. Much circumstantial evidence argues for the reality of the preventive effect of estrogens on morbus Alzheimer. The confirmation of a preventative effect of estrogens would have an enormous impact on the summary of benefits of estrogen substitution, and on the incidence and costs of this disease. Therefore, there is great interest in clarification of this question. Menopausal depressive mood (melancholia) can be improved by estrogen medication.

COGNITIVE FUNCTIONS

Concentration, drive, vigilance, word recall and short-term memory, which normally all deteriorate during postmenopausal estrogen deficiency, are improved by estrogen medication. Hormones have an impact on brain development, promotion of growth and regeneration of neurons and dendrites, and offer protection against toxic influences. The production and metabolism of cerebral neurohormones is an extremely interesting subject. A more in-depth knowledge of this intricate matter would probably lead to inconceivable therapeutic consequences.

The need for basic and clinical research in this field seems especially urgent and promising, and may open new possibilities to influence multiple cerebral regulations. The improvement of cognitive functions is one of the most important aims of estrogen substitution, securing social competence and human dignity in old age. Basic and epidemiologic research on the effect of estrogen on cerebral functions therefore is of high priority.

OSTEOPOROSIS

Osteoporosis occurs more often in postmenopausal women than in men, as females build up less bone mass in early life and lose gonadal hormonal function earlier than males. The supply of calcium and vitamin D is deficient in older women. Therefore, dietary or medical supplementation is important during the postmenopause and senium. Estrogens are effective in primary prevention of osteoporosis only for as long as they are given. If estrogens are withdrawn in patients who exhibit side effects or are at risk, alternatives such as calcium, vitamin D, age-adapted gymnastics and bisphosphonates should be considered as a continuation of the prevention. Hip protectors are apparently very effective in the prevention of hip fractures.

Although estrogens are effective in the therapy of osteoporosis, a primary oral therapy with estrogens for a treatment of osteoporosis is not indicated in older women, as the impact of unwanted side effects may increase in old age. We recommend calcium, vitamin D and bisphosphonates after the age of 60, but treatment should be performed by, or in cooperation with, an osteologist.

Raloxifene reduces the risk of osteoporosis and fractures without stimulating the endometrium and breasts. Other SERM will probably be found that will also abolish climacteric complaints.

Osteoarthritis (excluding rheumatoid forms) affects twice as many women as men. In all its forms, arthritis is the third leading cause of disability, preventing work and the performance of normal daily activities. Estrogens seem to have a beneficial influence on the resulting complaints in the small joints. This effect should be used much more than at present. The mechanism of action awaits elucidation.

UROGENITAL CONDITIONS

Urogenital conditions afflict many women at all ages. These include urinary incontinence, pollakiuria/strangury and urinary tract infections. These complaints have a profound influence on quality of life, and social and sexual relations. They are often taboo and in addition are misdiagnosed and inadequately treated by antibiotics without realizing the basic cause of atrophia. An estrogen treatment, which can remove the basic atrophic changes, is often not considered. Of approximately 30% of women suffering urologic problems during the postmenopause only 10% seek medical care. This percentage must be increased by improving information for doctors and patients concerning the effects of estrogens, progesterone and testosterone on blood supply, epithelial proliferation and function of the bladder.

ESTHETIC MEDICINE AND ANTIAGING

The beneficial cosmetic effect of estrogens and progesterone on the aging of the skin and connective tissue should be used to improve the motivation of women to take estrogens long term. Locally, estriol has been shown in randomized double-blind studies to smooth wrinkles and to improve the quality of the skin (epidermis and subcutis) of the face. Estrogens and progesterone (via an effect on metalloproteinases) will certainly play a part in the new antiaging branch of medicine, which has yet to become more scientific and serious than it is now. Many questions in this area await a solution.

THROMBOEMBOLISM

This is a rare complication of estrogen–progestogen medication, which occurs mostly during the first year of treatment, adding to the possible risks of HRT. Its occurrence can be partly prevented by inquiry of the family and patient history, by which 60–80% of risk cases could be recognized and prevented. Being overweight and varicosis as risk factors can be treated. Patients at risk must be made aware of triggering events of thrombosis and how to avoid them. The effects of the different estrogens and progestogens, and their application forms, on the coagulation mechanisms and the respective receptors in the vessel walls must be further clarified by using modern diagnostic methods. The diagnosis of thrombosis must be improved. Progestogens exerting a prothrombotic effect should not be used. Measures of prevention of thrombosis under ERT/HRT and use of hormones without unwanted effects on the incidence of thrombosis must be found.

GALLBLADDER DISEASES

Clinical measures (e.g. cholagogue, diet) to prevent an unwanted increase in the incidence of gallbladder diseases should be tested, especially the effect of bypass of the first liver passage by parenteral application of low-dose hormones and application of additional preventive treatment.

PATIENT INFORMATION

The role of estrogens in the development of gynecologic cancers is certainly basic in the sense of creating a *milieu interne* for optimal conditions of mitosis of growth of normal and cancerous cells possessing estrogen receptors. However, this is only one factor of a multifactorial occurrence. Other factors are causally more important, e.g. genetic damage, metabolic diseases and poor lifestyle.

Again, the female population has to made aware of the fact that cancer is the duty that humankind has to pay for a load of familial heredity, old age, poisoning of the environment and ionizing radiation, and that the realization of cancer is promoted by metabolic diseases, being overweight, overnutrition, consumption of too much animal fat and by childlessness, late first pregnancy and not breastfeeding. Official guidelines of competent gremia and guides for disease management need to be prepared to optimize the treatment and care of postmenopausal women.

Up-to-date, identically worded information sheets for menopausal patients who consider hormonal substitution, discussing all aspects of ERT and HRT, should be available in all practices.

THE MENOPAUSE AS AN OCCASION FOR HEALTH PROMOTION

The menopause is an extraordinary occasion for health promotion and prevention of diseases of old age. The North American Menopause

Society (NAMS) has published a survey that indicated that the majority of women (75%) made lifestyle changes around the time of the menopause. Changes in diet and nutrition were the most frequent alterations (51%). The next most frequent alteration was to increase the amount of exercise (34%) and finally a reduction of stress by taking more vacations, getting massages or spending more time on themselves. Nearly 9% said they reduced their alcohol intake and a similar portion said they reduced smoking. About 10% tried alternative holistic remedies and treatments to fight climacteric complaints. Women who had discussed using HRT with their doctors were more likely to modify their lifestyle.

In addition, patients, who had seen a health provider, in most cases, took the opportunity to participate in regular screenings for early detection of gynecologic diseases and other postmenopausal disturbances which could possibly limit their lifespan. They were also more likely to have regular mammograms and bone density measurements. The data from NAMS revealed that both education and income level were related to whether a woman received counseling about hormone therapy.

Investigations from Japan show that health promotion measures like lifestyle changes and medical treatment like hormone substitution reduce the number of lost working days due to disease.[2]

The physician should support menopausal patients by giving useful hints and tips and detailed instructions, more so than is presently usual.

IMPROVING COMPLIANCE

The dropout of patients from treatment is a significant problem of HRT and one that must be solved. In Germany, more than 70% of patients leave ERT/HRT within 5 years.

Compliance is dependent primarily on motivation. Motivation is determined and created by the severity of the climacteric complaints, the quality of medical counseling, effectively of treatment and possible side effects.

Consequently, we have to increase and optimize the counseling of climacteric women, and to create HRT without significant side effects and which will not damage motivation.

IMPORTANCE OF POLITICAL HEALTH MEASURES

The medical profession alone cannot introduce and substantially improve prevention. The support of government, and the laws and regulations of the health system, are also necessary. The medical profession must, by their leading gremia, influence the health insurers and governmental authorities to introduce prevention plans. Financial resources must be provided by the health system and by personal provision to pay for expensive new methods of treatment in order to avoid a two-tier medical system.

MARKERS FOR THE QUESTION OF WHO WILL PROFIT FROM HORMONAL SUBSTITUTION

Low HDL, and high LDL, Lp(a), homocysteine, hyperuricemia and C-reactive proteins are known to be markers for atherosclerosis, myocardial infarction and stroke, and may, if increased, predict a possible risk of cardiovascular diseases.

Further development of ultrasonography and enzyme diagnostics would secure prevention and early treatment of osteoporosis. Cancer markers (such as p53) would ideally show who is at risk for cancer and should perhaps not receive conventional estrogen substitution but eventually SERM or phytoestrogens. Better markers for the risk of thrombosis as are available now would be desirable.

OLD AND NEW PREPARATIONS

Concerning the old preparations, it seems necessary to improve the pharmacodynamics of estradiol in order to bring it as near as possible to the dynamics of physiologic ovarian secretion. This also applies to progesterone. As concerns progestogens, if used at all the great number of different compounds should be reduced to a few, allowing a targeted influence, e.g. an antiandrogenic effect.

Clinical epidemiologic studies must test further whether parenteral (transdermal) application has the same preventive effect on cardiovascular diseases as oral medication.

Knowledge of α- and β-receptors of estrogens, and the different receptors of progesterone and receptor adaptor proteins, has led to progress in understanding cellular hormonal mechanisms and has opened new possibilities of treatment. This progress will continue and create new modes of management.

New preparations and new forms of administration will broaden the possibilities of bypass of the first liver passage and of individualization of hormone substitution. Nasal application and vaginal rings secreting estrogens and progesterone, producing therapeutic blood levels, are interesting new possibilities of parenteral application in ERT.

Progesterone

The problem with oral progesterone is its rapid metabolism and inactivation by the first liver passage. The development of a compound which after oral intake is resorbed by the lymphatic system (such as testosterone undecanoate) is promising. Such a progesterone derivate would not be subject to the first liver passage and would consequently not be inactivated early but metabolized in a similar way to normal ovarian secretion.

A progesterone preparation that is applied vaginally is available. An effective nasal application could perhaps also be developed.

Progesterone is resorbed to optimal therapeutic concentrations in breast tissue when applied locally to the skin over the breast. This mode of application results in a significant reduction of mitosis in the breast tissue. It should therefore be used in cases of breast complaints, with estrogen monotherapy, in simple epithelial hyperplasia and in increased density in the mammogram. Could the application method perhaps be preventive for breast cancer?

Designer hormones

Hormones that do not cause bleeding, do not influence the endometrium or breast and do not promote cancer of the breast and genital organs will be found. Tamoxifen, raloxifene, 17α-estradiol and phytoestrogens are the first of such hormones, and must be further investigated. In particular, the effects of isoflavones on lipids, atherosclerosis, osteoporosis, and breast and genital cancers should be better known. Their possible side effects must be tested. The prevention of breast cancer with a combination of SERM and phytoestrogens, or with therapeutic human estrogens and SERM should be tried.

INFLUENCE OF GENETIC VARIANTS ON EFFECTS OF HORMONES

Protein PGP, which in the cell membrane is responsible for multidrug resistance, and gene MDR1 influence resorption, blood levels and metabolism of hormones, and apparently influence on hormonal cellular effects and responses of the organism. A better insight into these mechanisms might be helpful for the individual dosage of hormones and the control of their effects.

Investigations on genetic polymorphism may pave the way towards hormone-dependent cancer promotion. High-risk genotypes for cancer development will be found and improve the understanding of cancer development and its prevention.

SUMMARY

It can be predicted that ERT/HRT, possibly in substantially modified form, will increase in importance for the management of the postmenopausal woman. New hormones, hormone-like substances and new methods of prediction of risks will be found. Improvement of quality of life and compression of morbidity will however remain the preferential aims of menopausal management. In view of the overwhelming abundance of scientific data, the transformation of basic scientific findings into clinical practice will be the most difficult task.

REFERENCES

1. Lee LY, Ku SY. Health aging in the new millennium. In: (Schneider HPG, ed). *Menopause. The state of the art.* (Parthenon: Carnworth, 2003), 344–7.
2. Asdo T. The significance of the menopause in human life in the present and next centuries. In: (Asdo T, Yanaihara T, Fijimoh S, eds). *The Menopause in the Millennium.* (Partzjhenon, 2000), 88–94.

FURTHER READING

National Institutes of Health (NIH). *Agenda for Research on Women's Health for the 21st Century. Volume 7. New Frontiers of Women's Health.* (NIH Publications: Bethesda) No. 01–4319.

Speroff L. *The menopause. A signal for the future.* In: (Lobo RA, ed) *Treatment of the Postmenopausal Woman: Basic and Clinical Aspects.* (Raven Press: New York, 1994) 1–8.

Teoh E-S, Ratnam Sh. *The Future of Gynaecology and Obstetrics.* (Parthenon: 1991.)

Index

Page numbers in italics refer to *tables* and *figures*.

abdominal obesity 119, 236, 237–8, 332
Aβ42 (β-amyloid 1–42) 174–5, 177
acetylcholine *20*
acne 134, 234–5, 248
activated protein C (APC) resistance 287, 288
AD *see* Alzheimer's disease
adenomatous hyperplasia 303–4
adenomatous polyposis 339
adhesion molecules 164
adipose tissue, endocrine functions 119
adrenomedullin 311
aging, molecular basis 229–30
aging in males 399–420
  body composition and metabolism 405–8
  common diseases 401–2
  endocrine changes 403–5
  health improvement
    diet 416–17
    physical activity 415–16
    strategies 417
    see also nutrition in the elderly
  hormone therapy 410
    DHEA 413–14
    growth hormone 414–15
    testosterone 410–13, *414*
  life course perspective 399–400
  life expectancies 9–11, *399*
  need for disease prevention strategies 401
  osteoporosis 405, 408–9
  promotion of healthy aging 400, 417
  sexual dysfunction and sexuality 190–1, 409–10
alcohol
  breast cancer risk 265–6, 329–30

  cardiovascular risk 264–5
  colon cancer risk 340
  endometrial cancer risk 335
  ovarian cancer risk 338
  and women's health 15
alendronate *143*, 144
allopregnanolone 24, 25
alopecia, hormone treatment 233–4
alpha-lipoic acid 260
alpha-tocopherol (vitamin E) 259, 333, 416
Alzheimer's disease (AD)
  24S-hydroxycholesterol levels 178–9
  costs 365
  delayed onset in men 407
  disease progression 173–4
  endogenous estrogen levels
    CSF 177–8
    serum 175–7
  ERT 22, 174, 365, 393–4, 429
  estrogen and hippocampal glucose metabolism
    179–80
  future studies 181
  incidence in women 13
  molecular biology 174–5
β-amyloid 1–42 (Aβ42) 174–5, 177
amyloid plaques 174, 175
anastrozole 312
androgen receptors (AR)
  characteristics 102
  pontine micturition center 208
  urogenital tract 207
androgen replacement therapy (ART) 6, 192
  effects on liver 133–4

androgen replacement therapy (ART) *continued*
  men 410–13, *414*
  subjective side-effects 134
  topical
    abdominal obesity 237–8
    cellulite 237
    clitoral arousal improvement 195, 196–7
  women xxiv, 64, 89, 192
  see also dehydroepiandrosterone (DHEA);
      testosterone: therapy
androgens
  effects on hair 233
  effects on subcutaneous tissue 236–7
  physiologic activities 102
androstanolone 237
angina pectoris 61
angiogenesis 160
angiotensin II receptor type 1 (AT1) 166
angiotensinogen 294
anti-aging diets 230, 255–6
anti-androgens 102
antidepressants, sexual dysfunction due to 192, 197
antiestrogens 100, *101*
antioxidant(s)
  dietary 416
  enzymes 258
  melatonin 23, 406
  vitamins 258–60, 332–3, 339–40, 416
antithrombin deficiency 288, 290
apomorphine 195, 200
apoptosis 304
aromatase gene 307
aromatase inhibitors 311–12, 426
articular climacteric symptoms 64–5, 66, 72
artificial estrogens 7
ascorbic acid *see* vitamin C
aspirin 340
AT1 (angiotensin II receptor type 1) 166
atherogenesis
  delay by estrogens 159, 165, 394
  inflammatory markers 164
  smooth muscle cell proliferation 165
atherosclerotic vascular disease 151–8
  genetic factors in HRT response 156–7
  HRT clinical trials
    patient recruitment issues 155
    results 152–5
  risk factors 151–2
  risk prediction 156
autoimmune hepatitis 299

Battey's operation 220
benefit–risk considerations 351–88
  basics 354–5
  benefit:risk ratios 351–2
  ERT 357–9, 360, 361, 362
  estrogen–progestogen sequential HRT *358*, 359–62
  healthy user bias 355–6
  individualized 380

lifetime risks of menopausal diseases 354
  new preparations 368–9
  objective measures 357
  patients' opinions 356–7
  risks of HRT outlined 353–4
  summary of results of assessments 377–8, 379
  see also specific studies
benign prostate hypertrophy 413
biochanin A 272, 276
bisphonates 144
bladder function 208, 209
Blatt Menopause Index 66
bleeding with HRT 46, 109, 132, 373
bone
  effects of exercise 264
  effects of phytoestrogens 277
  loss 139
    see also osteoporosis
bone mass measurement 48, 140–1, 408
brain
  actions of sex hormones
    mechanisms 19–20
    neuropeptide modulation 22–4, *25*
    neurosteroid modulation 24–5
    neurotransmitter modulation 20–2, *25*
  effects of phytoestrogens 277
  estrogen and hippocampal glucose metabolism
      179–80
  locations of sex hormone receptors 19
  menopause and function 20
  neuropeptide/neurotransmitter levels and HRT *20*
BRCa genes 319
breast
  estrogen formation 306
  local progesterone application 85, 88, 432
  tenderness 132–3
  tissue sensitivity to estrogen 307
breast cancer
  biological and molecular basis 306–7
  carcinogen levels in tissue 331
  contraceptive pill and 323
  electromagnetic fields and 331
  ERT/HRT 305, 325–7
    effect on mortality 368, *369*, 372
    influence on risk 370–3
    information for patients 396
    Million Women Study (MWS) xxii–xxiv
    WHI study *xvi*, xvii, *xviii*, xx, 304
  estrogen and carcinogenesis 305
    biological demonstration 308–11, 426
    estrogen metabolites 307–8, *309*, 426
    glandular breast 306–7
    individual patient differences 307
  estrogen formation in tissues 306
  future research 426, 427
  hormone therapy 311–12, *313*, 323–4, 426
  incidence and mortality 14, 317
  phytoestrogen effects 278–9, 324
  prevention

breastfeeding 322
breast reduction 322
diet 257, 327–9
early pregnancy 321
exercise 263–4, 332
oophorectomy 324–5
raloxifene 311, 323
recommendations 333
tamoxifen 311, 323
vitamins 332–3
progestogen selection 326–7
as reason for stopping HRT 46
risk calculation using Gail model *321*
risk factors
alcohol misuse 265–6, 329–30
benign breast changes 322
body weight factors 331–2
breast size 322
childlessness 321–2
early menarche 321
genetic factors 318–19, 427
ionizing radiation exposure 331
late menopause 325
mammographic density 322–3
smoking 330
sterility treatment 322
summarized *319*
tallness 322
xenoestrogen exposure 330–1
risk profiles 318
as basis for HRT *320*
undetected 372
Breast Cancer Prevention Trial (BCPT) 311
breastfeeding 322
Budd–Chiari syndrome 299

caffeine 266–7
calcium 144–5, 165–6, 260–1
caloric restriction 255–6
cancer
basis of prevention 318
diet and risk 256–8, 262, 327–9
future research 425–7
and HRT (patient information sheet) 396–7
incidence and mortality rates 14
initiation 328–9
occult 369–70, 372
overweight and 16
prevention 317, 425, 426
progression 329
promotion 329
smoking and 266
see also carcinogenesis; *specific cancers*
carbohydrate metabolism
effects of combined HRT 123–5
effects of estrogen deficiency 120–1
effects of estrogen replacement 121–3
see also diabetes mellitus; metabolic syndrome
carcinogenesis 318, 328–9

apoptosis 304
endometrial cancer 303–4
estrogen and breast cancer 305–11
role of catechol estradiol metabolites 304–5, 307–8, *309*, 426
cardiovascular diseases (CVD)
alcohol and risk 264–5
diet and prevention 256
in elderly men 401–2
metabolic syndrome and 119–20
protective effects of exercise 263
vitamin E effects 259
in women 13–14, 423
primary prevention with estrogen 83, 364–5, 378–9, 394, 424
risk factors 15, 151–2
secondary prevention 81, 424
see also atherosclerotic vascular disease
cardiovascular system, effects of phytoestrogens 278
carers, women's roles as 13
β-carotene 332
carotenoids 262
catecholamine *20*
catecholaminergic system, sex hormone effects 20–1
catechol estrogen metabolites 168, 304–5, 307–8, *309*, 426
catechol-O-methyltransferase (COMT) 307, 308, *309*
cellulite 236–7
chloasma 230
cholelithiasis 297–8
cholestasis 296–7
cholesterol
in bile 297
brain turnover 178, 179
synthesis 294
cholesterol ester transfer protein (CETP) 119
choline acetyltransferase (ChAT) 21, 22
cholinergic system, effects of estrogen 21–2
cirrhosis 298–9
climacteric
defined 5
explained for patients 392
historical theories 37–9
introduction of term 37
climacteric depression 224–5
climacteric syndrome
assessment rating scales 66–75, *68, 69*
cause 57
defined 5
domino effect 58–9
placebo effect 59
sociocultural factors 43–4, 58
symptoms 57, 59–66
frequency 57–8, *74*
MRS I 71–2
speed of responses to HRT 66, 85, *86*
clitoral cavernosal tissue, age-related changes 196
clonidine 23
clover leaves 272

cobalamin (vitamin B12) 260
coenzyme Q_{10} (ubiquinone) 232, 260
cognitive function 22, 63, 393, 402, 405, 429
  see also Alzheimer's disease
collagen 243, 244
  changes in urogenital atrophy 208
  hormonal influences 231
  HRT effects 231, 246, 247
    topical estrogen 231, 232
  menopausal changes 245, 246
colon cancer
  future research 427
  incidence and mortality 317, 339
  prevention 340
  protective effects of hormones
    ERT/HRT 340, 365–6
    oral contraception 340
  risk factors 258, 339–40
compliance with HRT 47–9, 85–6, 131, 431
congestive heart failure 14
conjugated estrogens 6–7
connective tissue 243–4
  see also collagen
continence, roles of estrogen 207, 208
continuous combined therapy (CCT) 111–13
contraception
  patients with premenopausal cycle anomalies 32–3
  see also oral contraception
coronary heart disease (CHD)
  alcohol and risk 264–5
  diet and 257
  in elderly men 401, 402
  metabolic syndrome and 119–20
  in women 423–4
  see also cardiovascular diseases (CVD)
corpus luteum 392
corticosteroid-binding globulin (CBG) 294
corticosteroids
  chemical structures *94*
  therapy and skin 246
cortisol *94*, 236, 237, 405, 407
cost-effectiveness analysis
  ERT 357–9
  HRT 360, 362–3, 374–6
  weighting schemes 357
costs
  consequences of longevity 354
  disease treatment *360*, 365
  ERT and HRT 368, 374
  postmenopausal estrogen deficiency 375–6
  preventive medicine 422
  screening 376
coumestrol 272, 277
C-reactive protein (CRP) 164
CREB binding protein/p300 (CBP/p300) *96*, 97
cultural views of menopause 43–4, 58
curettage 373
cyproterone acetate 234–5
cystitis, postcoital 199

cytochrome CYP-1A1 308, *309*
cytochrome CYP-17 306, 308, *309*
cytochrome CYP-19 306
cytochrome P-450 hepatic enzymes 293

daidzein *101*, 272, 276, 277
danazol 221
deep vein thrombosis 373
definitions of terms 4–8
dehydroepiandrosterone (DHEA)
  chemical structure *94*
  effects on sexual function 200
  hepatic dysfunction 134
  production 24, 406
  replacement therapy 24–5, 89, 406–7, 413–14
delta (8, 9)-dehydroestrone sulfate (DHES) 7
dementia 402
  see also Alzheimer's disease
demographic challenge 9
depression
  climacteric 224–5
  elderly men 402
  excess in women 219
  first use of estrogen 220
  links with hormonal fluctuations 219–20
  postnatal 223–4
  progestogen intolerance and 133, 222, 224, 225–6
  see also premenstrual syndrome (PMS)
depressive mood (melancholia) 63, 66, 71, 429
dermis
  composition 243
  HRT effects 246
  menopausal changes 245
designer hormones 432
detrusor function 208, 209
DHEA *see* dehydroepiandrosterone
diabetes mellitus
  and cardiovascular disease 15, 119–20
  effects of HRT 125–6
  endometrial cancer risk factor 335
  incidence and prevalence rates 14–15
  type 1 117, 125
  type 2 117, 119–20, 122, 125–6, 335
  see also metabolic syndrome
Dickens, Charles 219
diet
  anti-aging 230, 255–6
  and breast cancer 257, 327–9
  and colon cancer 339
  in disease prevention 256–8
  for health in the elderly 254–5, 416–17
  and ovarian cancer 338
dietary fiber 257, 327–8, 339, 416
dihydroxytestosterone (5α-DHT) 102
disability adjusted life expectancy (DALE) 11
DNA-binding domain (DBD), sex steroid 95, *96*
DNA chips 427
doctor–patient relationship 46–7, 79
doctors, as lifestyle counselors 267

dopamine 20–1
drug-dependent female sexual dysfunction 193
dry mouth 195
dual energy X-ray absorptiometry (DEXA) 140–1
ductulogenesis *in vitro* 310
dydrogesterone 125
dyspareunia 197–200

eating difficulties in the elderly 252
  see also nutrition in the elderly
eicosanoids 261
elastin 243
electromagnetic fields and breast cancer risk 331
employment and health 12
endometrial cancer
  adenomatous hyperplasia 303–4
  endogenous estrogen production 334
  ERT/HRT 334–5
    information for patients 396
    long-term sequential estrogen–progestogen 107
    role of progestogen 106
    unopposed estrogen 106, 370
  future research 426
  Health Status Index risk quantification *370*
  incidence and mortality 14, 317, 333
  oral contraception 334
  prevention 336
  risk factors 333–4, 335–6
  tamoxifen-related 311, 323, 335
endometrial hyperplasia
  continuous combined therapy 12, 111
  malignant potential 109
  sequential estrogen–progestogen HRT 107, *108*
    long-cycle 110, 111
  unopposed estrogen 105–6
endometrium, effects of HRT
  continuous combined therapy 111–13
  intrauterine progestogen delivery 33, 85, 113–14,
    222
  sequential estrogen–progestogen 107–8
    bleed timing and histology 109, *110*
    long-cycle 109–11
  unopposed estrogen 105–6
β-endorphin (β-EP) *20*, 22–3
endothelial cell migration and proliferation 160
endothelin 163
epidermis 243, 246
equilenin 36
equilin 36, 294
equol 272, 276, 277
erectile dysfunction (ED) 409–10
Eros clitoral therapy device (EROS-CTD) 200
E-selectin 164
esterified estrogens 7
esthetic endocrinology 229
estradiol
  17α-estradiol 89, *90*
    scalp preparation 234
  chemical structure *94*

metabolism after oral administration 295
  preparations 7, 83–5
  see also estrogen replacement therapy (ERT);
    estrogens
estradiol-releasing vaginal rings (Estrings) 212–13
estradiol sulfate 295
estriol 36, 211, 212, 294
estrogen receptors
  breast tissue 307
  diversity 323
  epidermis 230
  ERα and ERβ expression 99
  rat brain 19
  urogenital tract 207
  see also steroid hormone nuclear receptors
estrogen replacement therapy (ERT)
  Alzheimer's disease 22, 174, 365, 429
  benefit–risk considerations 357–9, 360, 361, 362
  cancer risks
    breast *see* breast cancer: ERT/HRT
    colon 340, 365–6
    endometrium 106, 370
    ovary 337–8, 370, 396–7
  cardiovascular disease prevention 83, 364–5, 378–9,
    394, 424
  contraindications 80–1, *82*, 395
  cost–effectiveness analysis 357–9
  current advice xxiv
  defined 6
  depressive mood treatment 63, 66, 429
  duration 85
  effects on carbohydrate metabolism 121–3
  established principles 352
  eye disorders 238
  female pattern hair loss prevention 234
  goals 352
  and hypertension 364
  indications 81, 83, 395
  and life expectancy 368
  ocular reactions to patches 134
  osteoporosis prevention 83, 142–4, 363–4
  patient information sheet 391–7
  perimenopausal depression 225
  PMS 222–3
  postnatal depression 223–4
  preparation selection 83, *84*, 85, 87–8
  pulsed therapy 7
  risks outlined 353–4
  skin anti-aging therapy 231–2, 245, 247, 248, 393,
    430
  skin reactions to patches 134
  urinary incontinence management 209–11
  urinary tract infection management 211–12
  urogenital atrophy management 212–13, 366, 378,
    393, 429–30
  see also hormone replacement therapy (HRT)
estrogen response elements 307
estrogens
  alcohol and metabolism of 329

estrogens *continued*
  artificial 7
  and bladder function 208
  breast, formation in tissues 306
  breast cancer involvement *see* breast cancer:
    estrogen and carcinogenesis
  breast tissue sensitivity to 307
  catechol 168, 304–5, 307–8, *309*, 426
  CNS effects 175
  conjugated 6–7
  deficiency and carbohydrate metabolism 120–1
  deficiency and liver function 295–6
  designer *90*
  effects on Aβ42 metabolism 175
  effects on insulin secretion 122, *123*
  endogenous
    CSF levels in AD 177–8
    and endometrial cancer 334
    serum levels in AD 175–7
  endometrial proliferation mechanism 106
  esterified 7
  extraction and synthesis 36
  hepatic metabolism 293–5
  and hippocampal glucose metabolism in AD
    179–80
  isolation and identification 35–6
  in lower urinary tract cell proliferation 207–8
  natural 6
  in neurologic control of micturition 208
  neuropeptide modulation 22–4, *25*
  neurosteroid modulation 24
  neurotransmitter modulation 20–2, *25*
  and pancreatic function 299–300
  physiologic activities 99–100
  production in postmenopausal women 306–7
  roles in continence 207
  synthetic 7
  urethral effects 208
  vascular actions *see* vascular actions of estrogens
    and progestins
  see also estrogen replacement therapy (ERT); sex
    steroid hormones
estrone 35–6, 83, 295
estrone sulfate 294, 295
ethinylestradiol 36, 294
ethisterone 36
etidronate 144
exemestane 312
exercise
  breast cancer prevention 263–4, 332
  cardiovascular disease reduction 263
  colon cancer prevention 339
  elderly people 16, 415–16
  growth hormone secretion and 405
  osteoporosis reduction 264, 409
extracellular matrix 230
eye
  hormone therapy of aging diseases 238
  reactions to estradiol patches 134

Factor V Leiden 288, 290, 373
fat consumption
  breast cancer risk 257, 328
  colon cancer risk 339
  daily limit 255
fat deposition, hormonal influences 236–7
female pattern hair loss 233, 234
female sexual dysfunction (FSD) 185–203
  classification 186
  as climacteric syndrome symptom 63–4, 66
  diagnostic work-up 201
  orgasmic disorders 195–7
  sexual arousal disorders 193–5
  sexual desire disorders 186–93
  sexual pain disorders 197–200
  studies 200
female sexual response models *187, 189*
Feminine Forever (Wilson) 39
fertility decline, European Union 9
fiber *see* dietary fiber
fibroblasts, dermal 230–1
finasteride 235
'five-a-day' campaign 257
flavonoids 262
flaxseed 306
fluid intake, recommendations for the elderly 255
fluoride treatment 145, *147*
flutamide *101*, 102, 235
folic acid 254, 257–8, 260, 329, 332
follicle stimulating hormone (FSH) 31
  effects of phytoestrogens *273–5*
folliculin 35, 36
formication 67
formononetin 272, 276
fracture prevention
  bisphonates 144
  calcium and vitamin D 144–5
  costs 363–4, 368
  estrogen 142–3, *144, 361*, 363
  parathyroid hormone 145
  raloxifene 144
fractures, risk factors 140
Framingham algorithm 156
free radicals 258–9, 332, 416

galanin *20*, 23
gallbladder disease 133, 297–8, 373, 430
gender differences
  aging and health 400
  cardiovascular diseases 13–14
  employment rates 12
  frailty onset 407–8
  incomes of elderly 12–13
  life expectancy and healthy life expectancy 9–11
  marital status in elderly 13
  medical 421–2
  self-perceived health 11–12
  socioeconomic inequalities in mortality 16

see also aging in males
gene silencing 229–30
genistein *101*, 272
glaucoma 238
glucagon, estrogen-induced resistance to 122–3
glucose homeostasis, effects of insulin resistance 118
glucose tolerance, effects of combined HRT 123–4
glucosinolates 262
glycitein 272
glycosaminoglycans (GAG) 245
gonadotrophin-releasing hormone (GnRH), effects of
    sex hormones 22
gonadotrophin-releasing hormone (GnRH)
    analogues 221
Green's Menopause Index 69
green tea extracts 232
growth hormone (GH)
    response to exercise 405
    secretion during sleep 404, 406
    therapy in elderly men 405, 414–15
gynecologic cancers, future research 427

hair loss, hormone therapy 233–4
health
    employment and 12
    lifestyle factors 15–16, 251–69
    political support 431
    promotion 430–1
    self-perceived 11–12
health status indices 357
healthy life expectancy *10*, 11
healthy user bias 355–6
hearing loss, effect of tibolone 238–9
heart, functional disorders 61, 66, 71
Heart and Estrogen/progestin replacement Study
    (HERS) xviii–xix, 152–4, 155, 210, 285–6
    NAMS response xx–xxi
hepatic tumors 298
hepatitis 299
hip fractures 13, 363
hippocampus, estrogen and glucose metabolism
    179–80
hirsutism 235–6
hormone replacement therapy (HRT) 79–91
    acne 234–5, 248
    adverse publicity xv–xvi
    androgens *see* androgen replacement therapy
        (ART)
    and atherosclerosis 151–8, 165, 394
    basic considerations 79
    benefits/risks *see* benefit–risk considerations
    breast tenderness 132–3
    cancer promotion effect 369
    cancer risks
        breast *see* breast cancer: ERT/HRT
        colon 340, 365–6
        endometrium *see* endometrial cancer: ERT/HRT
        ovary 338, 370, 396–7
    cardiovascular disease prevention 83, 364–5, 378–9,

        394, *424*
    clinical trials
        future 428
        HERS *see* Heart and Estrogen/progestin
            Replacement Study (HERS)
        Million Women Study (MWS) xv–xvi, xxii–xxiv
        NAMS report on HERS and WHI xx–xxi
        WHI *see* Women's Health Initiative (WHI) study
    combined treatment 6
    compliance 47–9, 85–6, 131, 431
    consultations 134–5
    continuous combined therapy 111–13
    contraindications 80–1, *82*, 395
    cost 368, 374
    cost-effectiveness analysis *see* cost–effectiveness
        analysis: HRT
    current advice xxiv
    defined 6
    depressive mood treatment 63, 66, 429
    diabetic patients 125–6
    duration 85, 352
    effects on carbohydrate metabolism 123–5
    endometrial effects *see* endometrial cancer:
        ERT/HRT; endometrium, effects of HRT
    β-endorphin levels *20*, 22–3
    established principles 352
    fracture prevention 142–3, *144*, *361*, 363
    galanin levels *20*, 23
    genetic factors 156–7
    goals 352
    history 35–40
    and hypertension 364
    indications *80*, 81, 83, 395
        long-term therapy 85, *87*
    intraocular pressure reduction 238
    justification for 3–4
    and life expectancy 368, 374
    liver function and 296
        see also liver: HRT and disease
    long-cycle regimens 109–11
    long-term 85, *87*, 352–3, 378
    males *see* aging in males: hormone therapy
    markers predicting benefit from 431
    neuropeptide and neurotransmitter levels *20*
    neurosteroid modulation 24
    one woman's experience 51–3
    organ-specific *90*
    osteoporosis prevention 83, 142–4, 363–4
    pancreatitis 300
    patient information 45–6, 391–7, 428
    patients' opinions 356–7
    PMS 222–3
    preparation selection 83–5, 87–8, 326–7
    psychologic effects 133
    risks
        management of 86
        outlined 353–4
        see also benefit–risk considerations
    sequential treatment 6

hormone replacement therapy (HRT) *continued*
   side-effects 83, 88–9, 131–6, 395
   skin anti-aging 231–3, 245, 247, 248, 393, 430
   speed of symptom response 66, 85, *86*
   success rates 85, *86*
   vaginal bleeding 46, 109, 132, 373
   water retention 132
   weight gain 131–2
   see also specific climacteric symptoms; vascular
      actions of estrogens and progestins
hormones 93
   changes in aging males 403–5
   designer 432
   influences on skin 230–1
   influences on subcutaneous tissues 236–7
   ovarian 3, 4
   roles in carcinogenesis 303–15
   see also sex steroid hormones, *specific hormones*
hospital admissions 368
hot flashes 59
hot flushes
   biochemical causes 61
   clinical features 59–61
   differential diagnosis 61
   effects of phytoestrogens 272, *273–5*, 277
   HRT efficacy *62*, 66
   incidence variation between countries 271
   MRS I definition 71
   secondary consequences 58
human breast epithelium (HBEC MCF-10F) cell line 310
human chorionic gonadotrophin (hCG) 412–13
24S-hydroxycholesterol levels in AD 178–9
hyperandrogenism 32, 134, 234–6
hyperchylomicronemia 300
hyperhomocysteinemia 288
hyperinsulinemia 119, 257
hypertension
   effects of insulin resistance 119
   and HRT 364
hyperthyroidism 32
hypertriglyceridemia 119, 300
hyperuricemia 119
hypoactive sexual desire disorder
   defined 186
   see also sexual desire disorders
hypogonadism (male)
   acquired
      diagnosis 411–12
      testosterone therapy 410–11
   subcutaneous tissue 236–7
hypothermia, anti-aging effects 230
hypothyroidism 32
hysterectomy
   and ovarian cancer risk 337
   and PMS 221, 223, 226
   risks, costs and benefits 373
   urogenital atrophy prevalence 206

ibandronate 144

idiopathic recurrent jaundice of pregnancy 296
idoxifene 213
immunosenescence 253
indoles 262
induced menopause, defined 6
inflammation 287–8
inflammatory markers 164
information sheet for climacteric women 391–7
insulin
   estrogen therapy and sensitivity 121
   progestogen therapy and sensitivity 123, *124*
   resistance 117–19, 120
insulin-like growth factor-I (IGF-I) 405, 406–7, 414–15
intercellular adhesion molecule-1 (ICAM-1) 164
intrauterine progestogen delivery 33, 85, 113–14, 222
ionizing radiation and breast cancer risk 331
ipriflavone 277
irritability 63
isoflavones
   compounds 272
   see also phytoestrogens
isotretinoin 234

jaundice 296, 297
joint symptoms, climacteric 64–5, 66, 72

keratinocytes 230, 243
keratoconjunctivitis sicca 238, 393
kidneys, changes in the elderly 253
Klinefelter's syndrome 237
Kupperman Index 66–8

Langerhans cells 230
late menopause 5
Lawson Tait's operation 220
letrozole 311–12
levonorgestrel
   induction of insulin resistance 123, *124*
   see also intrauterine progestogen delivery
levormeloxifene 213
Leydig's cell insufficiency, age-related 412–13
libido, loss 63, 64
   see also sexual desire disorders
lichen sclerosus, vulvular 192, 196
life expectancy 9–11
   caloric restriction and 255–6
   estrogen–progestogen therapy 374
   estrogen therapy 368
   males at different ages *399*
lifestyle counseling 251–69
ligand-binding domain (LBD), sex steroid 94, *95*
lignans 262, 271–2, 278–9
lipids, effects of phytoestrogens 278
lipoprotein(a)(Lp(a)) and estrogens 157
lipoprotein lipase 118
liver
   effects of oral androgens 133–4
   estrogen metabolism 293–5
   estrogens and function 133, 295–6

HRT and disease 296
    cholelithiasis 297–8
    cholestasis 296–7
    cirrhosis 298–9
    hepatitis 299
    porphyria 297
    sarcoidosis 299
    tumors 298
    venous thrombosis 298
HRT post-transplantation 299
longevity, costs of 354
low-density lipoproteins (LDL)
    effects of estrogens/progestins on oxidation 166, *167*
    effects of phytoestrogens 278
lower urinary tract symptoms 209
lung cancer 14, 15, 402
lutein 262
lycopene 262

magnesium 261
male pattern baldness in women 233–4
male sexual dysfunction 190–1, 409–10
mammary cancer *see* breast cancer
mammographic density and breast cancer risk 322–3
mammography 14, 305
mastectomy, preventive 319
matrix metalloproteinases (MMP) 165, 231
MCF-10F cell line 310
MCP-1 (monocyte chemoattracting protein-1) 164–5
MDR1 gene 432
medroxyprogesterone acetate (MPA) xvii, xviii, 83, 123, *124*
megestrol acetate 312
melancholia 63, 66, 71
melanocytes 230, 243
melatonin 20, 23–4, 404, 406
memory 63, 71, 407
men
    history of HRT 39
    life expectancies 9–11, *399*
    provision of health needs 403
    self-perceived health 11–12
    sexual dysfunction 190–1, 409–10
    socioeconomic inequalities in mortality 16
    see also aging in males; gender differences
menopausal transition, defined 5
menopause
    carbohydrate metabolism 120–1
    CNS effects 20
    cultural views of 43–4, 58
    defined 4
    historical theories 37–9
    history of the term 37
    induced 6
    late
        breast cancer risk 325
        defined 5
        endometrial cancer risk 335
        ovarian cancer risk 337

one woman's experience 51–3
    as opportunity for health promotion 430–1
    patient information 44–5, 391–7
    premature 5, 44
    rating scales 66–75, *68, 69*
    socioeconomic effects 366
    women's concerns 45, *81*
    see also climacteric syndrome
Menopause Rating Scale I (MRS I) *68, 69,* 70–2
Menopause Rating Scale II (MRS II) 72–5
menstrual cycle anomalies, premenopausal 31–3
metabolic syndrome
    cardiovascular disease risk 119–20
    concept 117
    effects of estrogen replacement 121–3
    hyperinsulinemia 119
    hypertriglyceridemia 119
    insulin resistance 117–19, 120
    menopausal 120–1, *122*
methylene tetrahydrofolate reductase, thermolabile variant 288
mifepristone (RU486) 101
migraine 132
migration studies 251, 256, 324
Million Women Study (MWS) xv–xvi, xxii–xxiv
minerals 260–1
minimax concept 369
minoxidil lotion 233
MONICA study 14
monocyte chemoattracting protein-1 (MCP-1) 164–5
mood
    effects of HRT 133
    see also depression; depressive mood (melancholia)
MRS I *see* Menopause Rating Scale I
Multiple Outcomes of Raloxifene Evaluation (MORE) study 134, 311
muscular climacteric symptoms 64–5, 66, 72
MWS (Million Women Study) xv–xvi, xxii–xxiv
myocardial infarction 154, 394

naloxone 23
natural estrogens 6
nervousness 63, 66, 71
neurofibrillary tangles 174
neuropeptides
    levels before and after HRT *20*
    modulation by sex hormones 22–4, *25*
neuropeptide Y (NPY) *20*, 23
neurosteroids
    actions 98, *99*
    levels before and after HRT *20*
    modulation by sex hormones 24–5
neurotransmitters
    levels before and after HRT *20*
    modulation by sex hormones 20–2, *25*
niacin (vitamin B3) 260
nitric oxide (NO) 160–1, 238
noncoital sexual pain disorders 197, 198
No Reason for Panic (Zelinsky) 53

norepinephrine (NE) 20–1
norethisterone 36, 37, 123–5, 142, 222
norethynodrel 37
North American Menopause Society (NAMS)
    response to HERS and WHI xx–xxi
nuclear localization sequence (NLS) 95
Nurses' Health Study xx, 15, 153, 285
nutrition in the elderly
    anti-aging diets 230, 255–6
    causes of poor nutrition 253
    digestive organ changes 252–3
    fluid intake 255
    food supplements 255
    handicaps of aging 252
    healthy diet composition 254–5, 416–17
    minerals and trace elements 260–1
    problems 252
    vitamins 259–60, 416

obesity 425
    abdominal 119, 236, 237–8, 332
    cancer risks 16
        breast 331–2
        colon 339
        endometrium 335
        ovary 338
    prevalence 15–16
ocular reactions to estradiol patches 134
oestrogens see estrogens
oestrus 5
omega-3 fatty acids 255, 261, 328
omega-6 fatty acids 261
oophorectomy and breast cancer 324–5
opioids, endogenous 22–3
opotherapy 39
oral contraception
    cancer risks
        breast 323
        colon 340
        endometrium 334
        ovary 337
    and carbohydrate metabolism 121, 125
    patients with premenopausal cycle anomalies 32
orgasmic disorders
    definition 195
    diagnostic work-up 196–7
    physiological setting 196
    prevalence 195–6
osteoarthritis 429
osteopenia *141*
osteoporosis 139–50, 429
    antiresorptive therapies
        bisphonates 144
        calcium and vitamin D 144–5, 261
        HRT and alternatives 83, 142–4, 363–4
    benefits of exercise 264, 409
    diagnostic criteria *141*, 408
    formation stimulating therapies 145, *147*
    hip fracture rates 13, 363

individualization of therapy 146
    ipriflavone treatment 277
    male 405, 408–9
    MWI study *xvi, xvii, xviii*
    pathogenesis 139
    prevention benefits, risks and costs 363–4, 368
    prevention and treatment 141–2, 409
    risk markers 139, *140*
    skin thickness screening tests 247
    treatment monitoring 145–6, *147*
ovarian cancer
    early diagnosis 427
    effects of ERT and HRT 337–8, 370, 396–7
    etiologic hypotheses 336–7
    incidence and mortality 317, 336
    national differences 14
    oral contraceptives and 337
    prevention 318, 337, 338
    risk factors 337, 338
ovarian cycle syndrome 221
ovaries
    consequences of loss of function 3–4
    discovery of relationship with menstruation 35
    functions 3

P-450 aromatase gene 307
PAI-1 (plasminogen-activator inhibitor type 1) 119,
    163–4
palpitations 61
pancreas 299–300
pancreatic cancer 300
pancreatitis 300
parathyroid hormone 145
paresthesia 67
paroxonase 157
partial endocrine deficiency in men (PEDAM) 403–5
patient–doctor relationship 46–7, 79
patient information
    HRT side-effects 45–6, 428
    information sheet 391–7
    menopause 44–5
patients' opinions of HRT 356–7
peak bone mass 139, *140*
PEPI trial 112, 132
perimenopausal endogenous ovarian
    hyperstimulative syndrome 31
perimenopause, defined 5
PGP 432
phenylpropanolamine 211
physical activity see exercise
phytoestrogens 89, 100, 271–83
    chemical structures *101*
    clinical effects 262–3
        bone 277
        brain 277
        breast 278–9, 306, 324
        cardiovascular system and lipids 278
        menopausal symptoms 272–7
    compounds 271–2

mode of action 262
    patient information 397
placebo effect 59
plasminogen activator inhibitor type 1 (PAI-1) 119,
        163–4
PMS *see* premenstrual syndrome (PMS)
polycystic ovary syndrome 334
polyunsaturated fatty acids (PUFA) 254–5, 261
porphyria 297
postcoital cystitis 199
Postmenopausal Estrogen/Progestin Interventions
        (PEPI) trial 112, 132
postmenopause, defined 5
postnatal depression 223–4
pregnenolone 93, *94*, 98, *99*
premature menopause 5, 44
premenopausal cycle anomalies
    clinical examination 32
    contraception 32–3
    symptoms 31
    treatment 33
premenopause, defined 5
premenstrual syndrome (PMS)
    cause 221
    historical aspects 220
    progestogen intolerance 222, 226
    symptoms 221
    treatment 221–3
primary biliary cirrhosis 298
primary prevention, defined 8
PROCAM algorithm 156
progesterone
    chemical structure *94*
    defined 8
    and detrusor activity 209
    effect on carbohydrate metabolism 123
    effects on neurotransmission 21
    endothelin suppression 163
    history 36
    physiologic activities 101–2
    roles in skin 231
    therapy
        breast application 85, 88, 432
        preparations 83–5, 88, 326–7, 432
        skin anti-aging 232–3
        see also hormone replacement therapy (HRT)
    see also progestogens
progesterone-medicated IUDs 33, 85, 113–14, 222
progestins
    defined 8
    see also progestogens
progestogen receptors (PR) 101
    urogenital tract 207
    see also steroid hormone nuclear receptors
progestogens
    defined 8
    effects on neuropeptides 22–3
    effects on neurotransmission 21
    physiologic activities 101–2

synthesis 36–7
therapeutic use
    adverse psychologic effects 133
    agent selection 83, 326–7
    breast cancer 312
    current advice xxiv
    effects on carbohydrate metabolism 123–5
    endometrial cancer protection 106, 107, 334–5
    intolerance and depression 133, 222, 224, 225–6
    see also hormone replacement therapy (HRT)
    see also progesterone; vascular actions of estrogens
        and progestins
prolactin 192, 193
Propionibacterium acnes 234
prostacyclin 161–3
prostate cancer 369, 402
protein-C deficiency 288, 290
protein-S deficiency 288
prothrombin 20210A 288, 290
pudendal nerve entrapment syndrome 199
pulsed estrogen therapy 7
pyridoxine (vitamin B6) 260

quality of life
    adjustments 367
    defined 47, 69, 366, *367*
    impact of estrogen therapy 367, 368
    measurement 357
    questionnaires 68–9, 366–7
quantitative computed tomography (QCT), bone
        mass measurement 141
quercetin 262
quinoids 307–8

raloxifene
    allopregnanolone release 25
    chemical structure *101*
    clinical effects 323
        bone 144, 145, *146*
        breast 311
        endometrium 113, 311
        summarized *90*
        urogenital prolapse 213
    mode of action 100
    side-effects 134
rating scales, climacteric assessment 66–75, *68*, *69*
5α-reductase 233, 234, 235
relaxin 168
resveratrol 262
retinoids 332
risedronate 144
risk factors, significance of 423
risks
    women's perceptions of 423
    see also benefit–risk determinations
RU486 (mifepristone) 101

salicylic acid 234
sarcoidosis 299

Scandinavian Long Cycle Study Group 110–11
scar treatment 248
scavestrogens *90*
secondary prevention, defined 8
selective androgen receptor modulators (SARM) 8,
    102
selective estrogen receptor modulators (SERM) 8,
    100, *101*, 323–4, 424
    see also raloxifene; tamoxifen
selective progestogen receptor modulators (SPRM) 8
selective serotonin reuptake inhibitors (SSRIs)
    sexual dysfunction due to 192, 197
    vasomotor symptom alleviation 33
selenium 416
self-assessment Menopause Rating Scale (MRS II)
    72–5
self-perceived health 11–12
senium 5
SERM *see* selective estrogen receptor modulators
serotonergic system
    HRT and serotonin levels *20*
    sex hormone effects 21, 167–8
sex hormone-binding globulin (SHBG) 294, 404
sex steroid hormone antagonists 100, *101*
sex steroid hormones
    mechanisms of action in the CNS
        genomic 19
        non-genomic 19–20
        see also steroid hormone nuclear receptors
    neuropeptide modulation 22–4, *25*
    neurosteroid modulation 24–5
    neurotransmitter modulation 20–2, *25*
    physiologic effects 102–3
    see also specific hormones; steroid hormones
sexual activity outcomes, factor analysis *188*
sexual arousal disorders
    definition 193
    diagnostic work-up 194–5
    physiological setting 193–4
    prevalence 193
    role of HRT 195
sexual aversion disorder
    definition 186, 187
    see also sexual desire disorders
sexual desire disorders
    definitions 186–7
    diagnostic work-up 189–93
    physiological setting 188
    prevalence 187–8
    role of HRT 189
sexual dysfunction
    definitions 186
    see also female sexual dysfunction; male sexual
        dysfunction
sexual history-taking 190–3, 194–5, 196–7, 198–200
sexual pain disorders
    definition 197–8
    diagnostic work-up 198–200
    physiological setting 198

    prevalence 198
sexual response models, female *187, 189*
sildenafil treatment, female arousal disorders 195, 200
silent information regulator (SIR) system 230
Sjögren's syndrome 200
skin
    composition 243
    effects of corticosteroids 246
    hormonal influences 230–1
    hormone therapy for aging symptoms 231–3, 245,
        247, 248, 393, 430
    menopausal changes 245–6, 247–8
    reactions to estradiol patches 134
    thickness measurement 245–6
        in osteoporosis screening 247
    vascular changes during menopause 244–5
sleep
    disorders 62, 66, 71
    in the elderly 404, 406
    improvement with estrogen therapy 367
smoking
    cancer risks 266
        breast 330
        colon 340
        endometrium 335–6
        lung 15, 402
    cardiovascular risks 151, 266
    cessation strategies 266
    effect on estrogen metabolism 293
    and women's health 15, 266
sociobehavioral changes 13
socioeconomic inequalities in mortality 16
somatopause 405
soy 271
    see also phytoestrogens
spironolactone 235
SSRIs *see* selective serotonin reuptake inhibitors
statins xx, 81, 154, 155, 164
steroid hormone nuclear receptors
    activation 96–7
    characteristics 94
    modular structure 94–6
    transcriptional activity 97–8
steroid hormones
    chemical structures *94*
    mechanisms of action
        genomic *see* steroid hormone nuclear receptors
        nongenomic 98–9
        see also sex steroid hormones: mechanisms of
            action in the CNS
    synthesis 93
steroid receptor coactivator 1 (SRC-1) *96, 97*
stomach cancer 257
stroke
    gender difference 14
    influence of estrogens *361, 365,* 424–5
        WHI study xvi, xvii, *xviii*
    influence of estrogen and sequential progestogen
        361

subcutaneous tissues
    hormonal influences 236–7
    hormone therapy
        abdominal obesity 237–8
        cellulite 237
suicide, elderly men 402
synthetic estrogens 7

Tait, Lawson (operation) 220
tamoxifen
    breast cancer prevention and treatment 311, 312, 323
    chemical structure *101*
    clinical effects summarized *90*
    endometrial cancer risk 311, 323, 335
    ovarian cancer treatment 370
tau protein 174
testosterone
    changes in aging men 404, 409
    chemical structure *94*
    physiologic activities 102
    systemic disorders which suppress levels 412
    see also androgen replacement therapy (ART)
thirst, reduction in the elderly 252
thromboembolism *see* venous thromboembolism
thrombophilias 288–9, 290
thrombosis 395–6
    see also venous thromboembolism
thromboxane 162, 163
thyroxine-binding globulin (TBG) 294
tibolone 89, *90*
    auditory brainstem response modification 238–9
    bone mass conservation 144, *145*
    breast cancer risk xxii, xxiv
    effects on female sexual function 192
    endometrial effects 113, 144
tiredness 63, 66, 71
tissue inhibitors of metalloproteinases (TIMP) 231
tocopherol (vitamin E) 259, 333, 416
toremifene *90*, 323
transactivation domains (TAF) 95
transcription factors 97–8
tretinoin 231, 234
triglycerides 118, 119, 121, 126, 300
tubal ligation 336, 337
Turner's syndrome 295
type 1 diabetes 117, 125
type 2 diabetes 117, 119–20, 122, 125–6, 335

ubiquinone (coenzyme Q_{10}) 232, 260
ultrasound measurements
    bone mass 141
    skin thickness 246
ultra-violet (UV) irradiation, skin aging 231
urethra, effects of estrogen 208
urinary incontinence
    economic costs 206–7
    epidemiology 206, 209

estrogen therapy
    meta-analyses 209–10, 211
    stress incontinence 210–11
    urge incontinence 211
    leakage at orgasm 196
urinary tract infections 209
    estrogen therapy 211–12
urodilatin 168
urogenital atrophy
    economic costs 206–7
    epidemiology 205–6
    estrogen therapy 212–13, 366, 378, 393, 429–30
    symptoms 64, 71–2, 205, 208–9
Utian Menopause Quality of Life Score 68–9

vaginal bleeding with HRT 46, 109, 132, 373
vaginal dryness 64, 66, 67, 72, 194
vaginal receptiveness 198
vaginal rings 432
vaginismus 197
vascular actions of estrogens and progestins 159–72
    effects on LDL oxidation 166, *167*
    endothelium dependent
        effects on inflammatory markers 164
        endothelin suppression 163
        MCP-1 production 164–5
        migration and proliferation of endothelial cells 160
        MMP-1 production 165
        nitric oxide synthesis 160–1
        PAI-1 production 163–4
        prostacyclin synthesis 161–3
    estradiol metabolite effects 168
    smooth muscle cells
        AT1 regulation 166
        calcium influx inhibition 165
        cell migration and proliferation 165
    other vasoactive markers 166–8
vascular cell adhesion molecule-1 (VCAM-1) 164
vascular effects of hyperinsulinemia 119
vasoactive intestinal peptide (VIP) 194
venous thromboembolism (VTE)
    increased risk with HRT 157, 285–9, 373, 430
        risk management 289–90
    information for patients 395–6
    liver 298
    risk factors 289
very low density lipoproteins (VLDL), effects of insulin 118, 119
vestibulitis 199
viral hepatitis 299
vitamin A 332
vitamin B3 260
vitamin B6 260
vitamin B12 260
vitamin C 254, 259–60, 332
vitamin D 144–5, 261, 332–3
vitamin E 259, 333, 416

vitamins
    antioxidant 258–60, 332–3, 339–40, 416
    breast cancer prevention 332–3
    dietary sources 254, 255
    increased demand in the elderly 252, 253
    supplementation 259–60
VTE *see* venous thromboembolism (VTE)

water retention 132
weight
    effects on health 15–16
    effects of HRT 131–2
    and longevity 256
    and menstrual cycle irregularities 32
    and phytoestrogen effects 276
    see also obesity
Western lifestyle, impact on health 251–2
WHI *see* Women's Health Initiative (WHI) study
woman-specific medicine 421–2
women
    carers 13
    employment and health 12

income among elderly 12–13
life expectancies 9–11
mortality and morbidity 13
one woman's experience of HRT 51–3
perceptions of health risks 423
self-perceived health 11–12
socioeconomic inequalities in mortality 16
Women's Health Initiative (WHI) study xv–xviii,
        xix–xx, 113, 153–5, 355
    information gained from 378–9
    informing patients about 45
    NAMS response xx–xxi
wound healing 248

xanthophylls 262
xeaxanthin 262
xenoestrogens and cancer 330–1

yoga 89

zinc 252, 261
Zoladex 221